T0191958

Mathematical and Statistical Applications in Life Sciences and Engineering

Avishek Adhikari · Mahima Ranjan Adhikari
Yogendra Prasad Chaubey
Editors

Mathematical and Statistical Applications in Life Sciences and Engineering

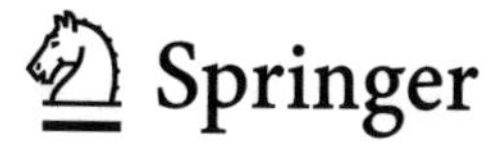

Editors
Avishek Adhikari
Department of Pure Mathematics
University of Calcutta
Kolkata, West Bengal
India

Yogendra Prasad Chaubey
Department of Mathematics and Statistics
Concordia University
Montreal, QC
Canada

Mahima Ranjan Adhikari
IMBIC
Kolkata, West Bengal
India

ISBN 978-981-13-3854-0 ISBN 978-981-10-5370-2 (eBook)
https://doi.org/10.1007/978-981-10-5370-2

Printed on acid-free paper

This Springer imprint is published by Springer Nature
The registered company is Springer Nature Singapore Pte Ltd.
The registered company address is: 152 Beach Road, #21-01/04 Gateway East, Singapore 189721, Singapore

Preface

This is the commemoration volume celebrating the 10th foundation anniversary of the Institute for Mathematics, Bioinformatics, Information Technology and Computer Science (IMBIC), a research institute that was founded in India in 2006 with branches in Sweden and Japan, and is dedicated to the scientific and technical activities at the forefront of various areas across interdisciplinary Mathematics, Statistics, and Computer Science.

To achieve its objectives, IMBIC organizes international interdisciplinary conferences in every December in Kolkata on "Mathematical Sciences for Advancement of Science and Technology (MSAST)." The conference MSAST 2016 was the 10th of the series of these conferences. Prominent mathematicians and statisticians were invited to contribute articles to the celebration of this milestone. The response was overwhelming. The present volume was conceived in order to exhibit the beauty of mathematics and statistics and emphasize applications in allied sciences. In order to achieve this goal, eminent scientists featuring such contributions were invited to contribute to the volume. As a culmination of this effort, the present volume contains articles covering a wide range of topics of current importance.

The articles on mathematical applications cover the topics of coloring problem, control of stochastic structures, and information dynamics, whereas the articles on statistical applications cover the areas on image denoising, life testing and reliability, survival and frailty models, analysis of drought periods, prediction of genomic profiles, competing risks, environmental applications, and chronic disease control. The articles contained in this volume present state-of-the-art material along with a detailed and lucid review of the relevant topics and issues concerned. This volume reports on the newest developments in some of the interesting and promising areas of mathematical and statistical research today, and is expected to provide an important resource for researchers and practitioners in the relevant areas mentioned above. The key features of this volume such as

- Focus on mathematical and statistical applications in a single volume,
- Accessible and lucid presentation,
- Detailed review of the cutting edge technologies,
- Articles from the worldwide experts in the field, and
- Wide range of topics on applications of modern relevance,

are expanded in 16 book chapters.

Mathematical applications span the first three chapters. Chapter 1 deals with the problem of allocating radio frequencies to the base stations of the cellular network such that interference between stations at a different distance can be avoided while keeping the range of distinct frequencies to a minimum. Chapter 2 discusses the use of vibration control techniques in order to control or suppress wild vibrations in structures caused by resonance or flutter due to external sources along with a numerical example with a recorded dataset from a California earthquake. Chapter 3 discusses the solutions of Hamilton ODE's and Hamilton–Jacobi PDE's involving single-time and multi-time higher-order Lagrangians, and is expected to be of interest to engineers and applied mathematicians.

Statistical applications span the next 13 chapters. Chapter 4 presents a comprehensive overview of the *denoising* problem and subsequent development in the context of cDNA microarray images, in the context of genomic research, where wavelet-based methods have been quite useful. Chapter 5 introduces a transformation-based distribution family appropriate for hazard modeling where the well-known Weibull model may fail, and Chap. 6 introduces yet another family based on the so-called *mode-centric Gaussian* distribution as a fraternal twin of the Gaussian distribution appropriate for life-data models.

Chapter 7 considers the use of *stochastic volatility* models for analyzing drought periods with discussions of real examples. Chapter 8 gives a new estimator of the *mean residual life function* and compares its performance with other nonparametric estimators available in the literature while illustrating the relevance of the results on a real dataset. Chapter 9 gives a detailed overview of techniques for predicting outcomes such as colon cancer survival from diverse genomic profiles whereas Chap. 10 discusses a bivariate frailty model with an application to competing risk theory. Chapter 11 considers the estimation of the stress strength parameter under the Bayesian paradigm with illustrations on a real dataset.

Chapter 12 reports on the spatiotemporal analysis of air pollution effects on clinic visits using the data from Taiwan that is based on several Bayesian techniques, and Chap. 13 gives a comprehensive review of statistical inference procedures in the context of competing risks when the cause of failure may be missing or masked for some units. Chapter 14 discusses and illustrates several environmental applications based on the Birnbaum–Saunders model, and Chap. 15 considers multistate modeling in the context of data on chronic conditions from individuals in disease registries. The final chapter, Chap. 16, presents estimation for lifetime characteristics in connection with a time-constrained life-testing experiment.

We had invited more than 50 potential contributors, and 19 articles were submitted. After a careful review, 16 articles were selected that make the 16 chapters of the present volume. We are thankful to all the contributors to this volume and especially to the corresponding authors for their cooperation and timely submission of the articles and revisions. We have derived substantial help in reviewing these articles from the following reviewers to whom we owe our immense gratitude:

Jorge A. Achcar (Brazil), Koby Asubonteng (USA), Saria Awadalla (USA), M. L. Lakhal-Chaieb (Canada), Ashish K. Chattopadhyay (India), Propser Donovon (Canada), Sujit K. Ghosh (USA), David Hanagal (India), Tamanna Howlader (Bangladesh), Abdulkadir Hussein (Canada), Nachimuthu Manickam (USA), Manoel Santos-Neto (Brazil), Partha Sarathi Roy (Japan), Satyajit Roy (India), Helton Saulo (Brazil), and Jingjing Wu (Canada).

We apologize for any omissions. We are also grateful to Springer for publishing this volume and to all individuals who have extended their support and cooperation in order to bring the project of IMBIC for publishing this commemorative volume to fruition.

Kolkata, India
Kolkata, India
Montreal, Canada
August, 2017

Avishek Adhikari
Mahima Ranjan Adhikari
Yogendra Prasad Chaubey

Contents

Editors and Contributors

About the Editors

Avishek Adhikari, Ph.D. is Assistant Professor of Pure Mathematics at the University of Calcutta. He is a recipient of the President of India Medal and Young Scientist Award. He was a post-doctorate fellow at the Research Institute INRIA, Rocquencourt, France. He was a visiting scientist at Indian Statistical Institute, Kolkata, and Linkoping University, Sweden. He visited many institutions in India, Japan, Sweden, France, England, Switzerland, and South Korea on invitation. His main interest lies in algebra, cryptology, discrete mathematics, theoretical computer science, and their applications. He has published four textbooks on mathematics including one book *Basic Modern Algebra with Applications* (Springer) and edited one research monograph. He has published several papers in foreign journals of international repute, conference proceedings, and book chapters. Four students have already been awarded Ph.D. degree under his guidance. He successfully completed several projects funded by the Government of India and is a member of the research teams from India for collaborative Indo-Japan (DST-JST and DST-JSPS) research projects. He is a member on editorial board of several journals and Founder Secretary (honorary) of the Research Institute IMBIC and Treasurer (honorary) of the Cryptology Research Society of India (CRSI).

Mahima Ranjan Adhikari, Ph.D. is the Founder President of the Institute for Mathematics, Bioinformatics, Information Technology and Computer Science (IMBIC), Kolkata, and former Professor of Pure Mathematics at the University of Calcutta. He has published a number of papers in several Indian and foreign journals including *Proceedings of American Mathematical Society* and eight textbooks including *Basic Modern Algebra with Applications* (Springer) and *Basic Algebraic Topology and its Applications* (Springer). Twelve students have already been awarded Ph.D. degree under his guidance on various topics such as algebra, algebraic topology, category theory, geometry, analysis, graph theory, knot theory, and history of mathematics. He is a member of American Mathematical Society and on the editorial board of several Indian and foreign journals and research monographs. He was elected as the president of the Mathematical Science Section (including Statistics) of the 95th Indian Science Congress, 2008. He visited several institutions in India, USA, UK, China, Japan, France, Greece, Sweden, Switzerland, Italy, and many other countries on invitation.

Yogendra Prasad Chaubey, Ph.D. is Professor of Statistics in Department of Mathematics and Statistics at Concordia University, Montreal, Canada. His research interests include Sampling, Linear Models, Distribution Theory, and Nonparametric Smoothing. His current research is focused on nonparametric functional estimation that has been funded by discovery grant program from Natural Sciences and Engineering Research Council of Canada. He has been active in promoting Statistics through membership in various capacities of several statistical associations and organization of scholarly conferences such as Statistics 2001 Canada, Statistics 2011 Canada, and the workshop on Nonparametric Curve Smoothing during July 2001, July 2011, and December 2013, respectively, that were held at Concordia University. He served and is currently serving on the editorial board of several statistical journals and has trained approximately 40 masters and 6 doctoral students. He was elected as a member of the prestigious International Statistical Institute in 2005 and was later inducted as a member of the Provost Circle at Concordia University. He was awarded P. Stat. designation by the Statistical Society of Canada in 2014 for his professional statistical qualifications and was given Life Achievement Award for his leadership and contributions to Statistics by Forum for Interdisciplinary Studies in 2016. He has edited three research monographs and published over 130 research articles in scholarly statistical journals of international repute, conference proceedings, and book chapters.

Contributors

Jorge Alberto Achcar Medical School, University of São Paulo, Ribeirão Preto, SP, Brazil; Department of Social Medicine, FMRP University of São Paulo, Monte Alegre Ribeirão Preto, SP, Brazil

Jean-Francois Angers University of Montreal, Montreal, QC, Canada

Kobby Asubonteng AstraZeneca Pharmaceuticals, Gaithersburg, MD, USA

Saria Salah Awadalla Division of Epidemiology and Biostatistics, UIC School of Public Health (SPH-PI), Chicago, IL, USA

N. Balakrishnan Department of Mathematics and Statistics, McMaster University Hamilton, Hamilton, ON, Canada

Atanu Biswas Applied Statistics Unit, Indian Statistical Institute, Kolkata, India

Emílio Augusto Coelho-Barros Federal Technological University of Paraná, Cornélio Procópio, PR, Brazil

Richard J. Cook Department of Statistics and Actuarial Science, University of Waterloo, Waterloo, ON, Canada

Sonjoy Das Department of Mechanical and Aerospace Engineering, University at Buffalo, Buffalo, NY, USA

Biswa Nath Datta Department of Mathematical Sciences, Northern Illinois University, De Kalb, IL, USA

Isha Dewan Theoretical Statistics and Mathematics Unit, Indian Statistical Institute, New Delhi, India

Jie Fan Division of Biostatistics, Department of Public Health Sciences, Miller School of Medicine, University of Miami, Miami, FL, USA

Sujit K. Ghosh Department of Statistics, NC State University, Raleigh, NC, USA

Kundan Goswami Department of Mechanical and Aerospace Engineering, University at Buffalo, Buffalo, NY, USA

Ramesh C. Gupta University of Maine, Orono, ME, USA

Tamanna Howlader Institute of Statistical Research and Training, University of Dhaka, Dhaka, Bangladesh

Alan Hutson Department of Biostatistics, University at Buffalo, Buffalo, NY, USA

Erin Kobetz Division of Biostatistics, Department of Public Health Sciences, Miller School of Medicine, University of Miami, Miami, FL, USA

Debasis Kundu Department of Mathematics and Statistics, Indian Institute of Technology Kanpur, Kanpur, India

Jerald F. Lawless Department of Statistics and Actuarial Science, University of Waterloo, Waterloo, ON, Canada

Víctor Leiva School of Industrial Engineering, Pontificia Universidad católica de Valparaíso, Valparaíso, Chile

Shufang Liu Department of Statistics, NC State University, Raleigh, NC, USA

Roberto Molina de Souza Federal Technological University of Paraná, Cornélio Procópio, PR, Brazil

Govind S. Mudholkar Department of Statistics and Biostatistics, University of Rochester, Rochester, NY, USA

Uttara Naik-Nimbalkar Department of Mathematics, Indian Institute of Science Education and Research (IISER), Pune, India

S. M. Mahbubur Rahman Department of Electrical and Electronic Engineering, University of Liberal Arts Bangladesh, Dhaka, Bangladesh

Ushnish Sarkar Department of Pure Mathematics, University of Calcutta, Kolkata, India

Helton Saulo Department of Statistics, University of Brasília, Brasília, Brazil

J. Sunil Rao Division of Biostatistics, Department of Public Health Sciences, Miller School of Medicine, University of Miami, Miami, FL, USA

Daniel Sussman Division of Biostatistics, Department of Public Health Sciences, Miller School of Medicine, University of Miami, Miami, FL, USA

Savin Treanţă Faculty of Applied Sciences, Department of Applied Mathematics, University “Politehnica” of Bucharest, Bucharest, Romania

Constantin Udrişte Faculty of Applied Sciences, Department of Mathematics-Informatics, University "Politehnica" of Bucharest, Bucharest, Romania

Ziji Yu Biostatistics Department, Jazz Pharmaceuticals, Palo Alto, CA, USA

Xiaojun Zhu Department of Mathematics and Statistics, McMaster University Hamilton, Hamilton, ON, Canada

Part I
Mathematics

Chapter 1
Hole: An Emerging Character in the Story of Radio k-Coloring Problem

Ushnish Sarkar and Avishek Adhikari

Abstract Frequency assignment problem (FAP) of radio networks is a very active area of research. In this chapter, radio networks have been studied in a graph-theoretic approach where the base stations of a cellular network are vertices and two vertices are adjacent if the corresponding stations transmit or receive broadcast of each other. Here, we deal with the problem of allocating frequencies to the base stations of the cellular network such that interference between stations at different distances can be avoided and at the same time, and the range of distinct frequencies used can be kept minimum. A certain variant of FAP on such network is radio k-coloring problem ($k \geq 2$ being a positive integer) where stations (vertices) are assigned frequencies (colors) in such a way that the frequency difference increases (using k as a parameter) with the growing proximity of the stations. The focus has been laid on unused frequencies in the spectrum. These unused frequencies are referred as holes, and they are found to heavily influence the structure of the network (graph). In this chapter, we highlight many combinatorial aspects of holes in the context of radio k-coloring problem and its applicability as well as importance in real life.

1.1 Introduction

1.1.1 Motivation

Channel assignment problem or frequency assignment problem is one of the most important problems in the design of cellular radio networks. A geographical area covered under a cellular network is divided into smaller service areas referred as cells. Every cell has a base station and communications among all the wireless terminals or

U. Sarkar · A. Adhikari (✉)
Department of Pure Mathematics, University of Calcutta, 35 Ballygunge Circular Road, Kolkata 700019, India
e-mail: avishek.adh@gmail.com

U. Sarkar
e-mail: usn.prl@gmail.com

A. Adhikari et al. (eds.), *Mathematical and Statistical Applications in Life Sciences and Engineering*, https://doi.org/10.1007/978-981-10-5370-2_1

the users in these cells are made through their corresponding cell area base stations. Now the base stations transmit or receive any communication in specified frequencies which are obtained by dividing the radio spectrum uniformly into disjoint frequency bands. Suppose a radio receiver is tuned to a signal on channel c_0, broadcast by its local transmitter (i.e., the closest one). The quality of reception will be degraded if there is excessive interference from other nearby transmitters. Also, due to the reuse of the same channel c_0 in the vicinity, there will be "co-channel" interference. Moreover, since in reality, as the signal energy from one channel spills over into its nearby channel, neither transmitters nor receivers operate exclusively within the frequencies of their assigned channel. Hence, stations using channels close to c_0 are also potential source of interference. Imposing constraints to channel separations between pair of transmitters, potentially capable of interference, is a way to maintain signal quality of the broadcast. Let $d(x, y)$ be the distance between transmitter sites x and y in some suitable metric and $\delta_c(x, y)$ be the minimum allowed spectral separation of the channels assigned to sites x and y. Then for any two pairs of transmitter sites (x_1, y_1) and (x_2, y_2), if $d(x_1, y_1) \geq d(x_2, y_2)$, then $\delta_c(x_1, y_1) \leq \delta_c(x_2, y_2)$. Thus there is a monotonic trade-off between distance and spectral separation. Moreover, the physical assumptions made above imply that the spectral constraints are determined only by distances, in the sense that if $d(x_1, y_1) = d(x_2, y_2)$, then $\delta_c(x_1, y_1) = \delta_c(x_2, y_2)$. In other words, if the distance between two stations is small, the difference in their assigned channels must be relatively large, whereas two stations at a larger distance may be assigned channels with a smaller difference. Thus, if the channels assigned to the stations x and y are $f(x)$ and $f(y)$, respectively, then

$$|f(x) - f(y)| \geq l_{xy}, \tag{1.1}$$

where l_{xy} depends inversely on the distance between x and y. Also, the range of frequencies, from which the assignment is to done, should be kept as narrow (and hence economic) as possible keeping in mind the scarcity and dearness of the radio spectrum.

Now the problem of channel assignment was first interpreted in a graph-theoretic approach by Hale [19]. Here, we consider the base stations, i.e., the transceivers in the network as vertices. Two vertices are adjacent if the corresponding stations can broadcast or receive the transmission of each other, i.e., if their transmission ranges intersect. Also, as the channels are uniformly spaced in the radio spectrum, we can consider the channel assignment of networks as an integer coloring or integer labeling problem of graphs.

Chartrand et al. [8, 9] have introduced the radio k-coloring problem of a simple finite graph by taking $l_{xy} = k + 1 - d(x, y)$ in Eq. 1.1. Formally, for any positive integer $k \geq 2$, a radio k-coloring L of a finite simple graph G is a mapping $L : V \rightarrow \mathbb{N} \cup \{0\}$ such that for any two vertices u, v in G,

$$|L(u) - L(v)| \geq k + 1 - d(u, v) \tag{1.2}$$

While assigning colors (i.e., frequencies) to the vertices (i.e., transceivers) of a graph (i.e., radio network) in an economic manner keeping in mind the distance constraints of the radio k-coloring problem, some integers are found to be left unassigned to any vertex. Such integers represent unused frequencies in the radio spectrum allotted for the network and they will be termed as holes in our subsequent discussion. These holes are found to exhibit splendid properties. Studying them enables us to understand various important structural properties of the graph representing the radio network. Exploiting these properties, we may even construct a larger network whose frequency assignment (radio k-coloring) can be done without changing frequencies of the older stations and using the unassigned frequencies of the previous network for the new stations. Thus, our new network shall not need to procure any additional frequency. Besides, these holes possess some beautiful combinatorial features which make them worth studying on their own.

1.1.2 Important Definitions, Notations, and a Brief Survey

First, we have to be acquainted with some important notions. Throughout this chapter, graphs have been taken as simple and finite. The number of vertices of a graph is its order. Let G be any graph. Then $V(G)$ and $E(G)$ denote the vertex set and the edge set of G, respectively. Also, let L be any radio k-coloring of G. Then $(max_{v \in V} L(v) - min_{v \in V} L(v))$ is referred as the span of L, denoted by $span(L)$, and $min_L\{span(L) : L\ is\ a\ radio\ k - coloring\ of\ G\}$ is referred as the *radio k-chromatic number* of G, denoted by $rc_k(G)$. Interestingly, if L be a radio k-coloring of G, then $L + a$ is the same. Therefore, without loss of generality, we shall assume $min_{v \in V} L(v) = 0$, for any radio k-coloring L on G. Any radio k-coloring L on G with span $rc_k(G)$ is referred as $rc_k(G)$-coloring or simply rc_k-coloring (when the underlying graph is fixed).

So far, the radio k-coloring problem has been mostly studied for $k = 2$, $k = 3$, $k = diam(G) - 2$, $k = diam(G) - 1$, $k = diam(G)$. The radio k-coloring is referred as *radio coloring*, *antipodal coloring*, and *near-antipodal coloring*, and the corresponding radio k-chromatic numbers are known as *radio number*, *antipodal number*, and *near-antipodal number* of G for $k = diam(G)$, $k = diam(G) - 1$ and $k = diam(G) - 2$, respectively, where $diam(G)$ denotes the diameter of G, i.e., the maximum distance between any two vertices of G. For $k = 2$, the problem becomes the $L(2, 1)$-coloring problem introduced by Griggs and Yeh [18] and for $k = 3$, the problem is often referred as $L(3, 2, 1)$-coloring. Note that the radio 2-chromatic number $rc_2(G)$ is also often denoted as $\lambda_{2,1}(G)$ and termed as $\lambda_{2,1}(G)$-*number* or simply $\lambda_{2,1}$-*number*. Also, rc_2-coloring of G is referred as $\lambda_{2,1}$-*coloring of* G. In fact, in our subsequent discussion, we will mostly use $\lambda_{2,1}(G)$ instead of $rc_2(G)$.

For an rc_k-coloring L on a graph $G = (V, E)$, let $L_i^k(G) = \{v \in V | L(v) = i\}$ and $l_i^k(G) = |L_i^k(G)|$. We replace $L_i^k(G)$ by L_i and $l_i^k(G)$ by l_i if there is no confusion regarding G and k. The vertices of L_i are represented by v_j^i, $1 \leq j \leq l_i$, and if $l_i = 1$, we replace v_j^i by v^i. In a rc_k-coloring L on G, a color i is referred as a *multiple color* if $l_i \geq 2$. Sometimes colors are referred as labels too. If two vertices u and v of G are adjacent, then we write $u \sim v$; otherwise, we write $u \nsim v$. Let G be a graph and $e = uv$ be an edge of G. If the edge e is deleted, then the resulting graph, which has same vertex set as that of G, is denoted by $G - e$. If $S \subset V(G)$, then $G - S$ is the graph obtained by deleting the vertices in S and the edges incident to the vertices in S.

Compared to other radio k-coloring problems, the $L(2, 1)$-coloring, the radio coloring, and the antipodal coloring of graphs have received extensive attention. A thorough survey of $L(2, 1)$-coloring may be found in [5]. For $k \neq 2$, the radio k-coloring problem has been studied for comparatively fewer families of graphs including paths, trees and cycles [7, 22, 25, 28], powers of paths and cycles [26, 29, 36], toroidal grids [37], etc. Saha et al. studied lower bound for radio k-chromatic number in [38]. Readers may go through [35] for a detailed survey in radio k-coloring problem.

1.1.3 Introduction to Holes

An interesting difference between general graph coloring and radio k-coloring is that an optimal general graph coloring uses every color between maximum color and minimum color, whereas an rc_k-coloring may not do the same (see Figs. 1.2 and 1.3). If i is an integer, $0 < i < rc_k(G)$, such that it is not assigned to any vertex of G as a color by an rc_k-coloring L of G, then i is called a *hole* of L. Any rc_k-coloring has at most $(k - 1)$ consecutive holes [39]. The minimum number of occurrences of $(k - 1)$ consecutive holes in any rc_k-coloring on G is said to be the *$(k - 1)$-hole index of G* and denote by $\rho_k(G)$ or simply ρ_k if there is no confusion regarding the graph [40]. Also, exploiting the maximum number of consecutive holes in any rc_k-coloring on G, the notion of $(k-1)$-hole has been defined in [40]. A *$(k-1)$-hole* in a rc_k-coloring L on a graph G is a sequence of $(k - 1)$ consecutive holes in L. If L has $(k - 1)$ consecutive holes $i + 1, i + 2, \dots, i + k - 1$, then the corresponding $(k - 1)$-hole is denoted by $\{i + 1, i + 2, \dots, i + k - 1\}$. Clearly then, the minimum number of $(k-1)$-holes in any rc_k-coloring on G is the $(k-1)$-hole index of G. We refer the collection of all rc_k-colorings on G with $\rho_k(G)$ number of $(k - 1)$-holes as $\Lambda_{\rho_k}(G)$. Moreover, the minimum span of a radio k-coloring on G with at most $(k - 2)$ consecutive holes is defined as max-$(k - 2)$-hole span of G and denoted by $\mu_k(G)$. Note that the 1-hole index and 2-hole index of the graph in Fig. 1.1 is 2. Again, the 1-hole index and 2-hole index of the same graph are zero as shown in Figs. 1.2 and 1.3.

Now, an rc_2-coloring, i.e., a $\lambda_{2,1}$-coloring does not have two consecutive holes. Clearly then, $\rho_2(G)$ is the minimum number of holes in any $\lambda_{2,1}$-coloring on G which is often referred as *hole index of* G, denoted by $\rho(G)$. Thus, the 1-hole index and hole index of G are same. Also, $\Lambda_{\rho_2}(G)$ is referred as $\Lambda_\rho(G)$. Moreover, the max-0-hole span of G is referred as *no-hole span of* G, and $\mu_2(G)$ is alternatively written

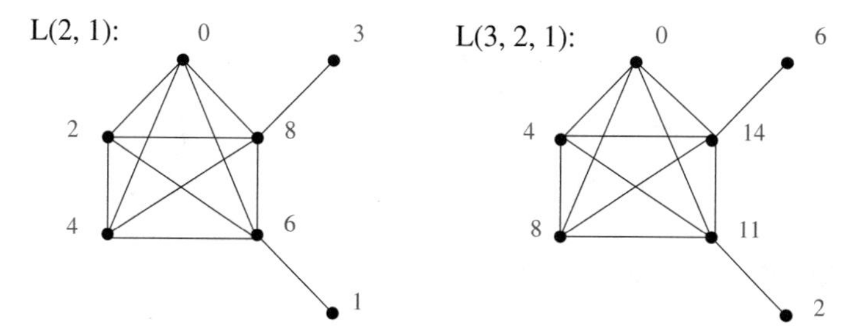

Fig. 1.1 Example of graph with positive 1-hole index and 2-hole index

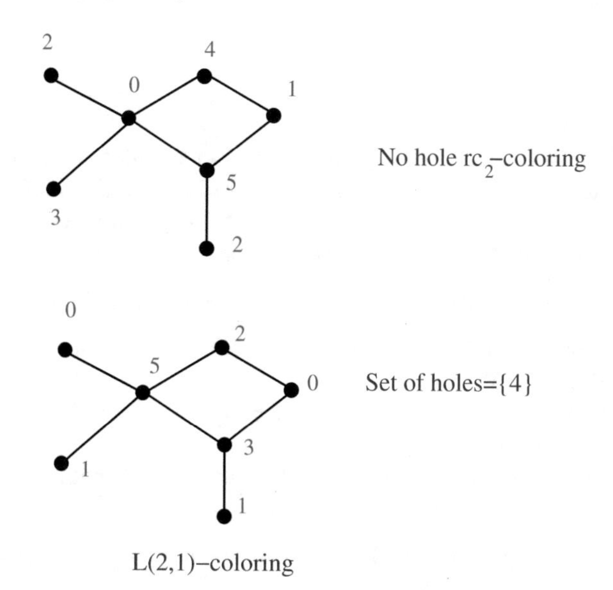

Fig. 1.2 Examples of rc_2-colorings with and without holes

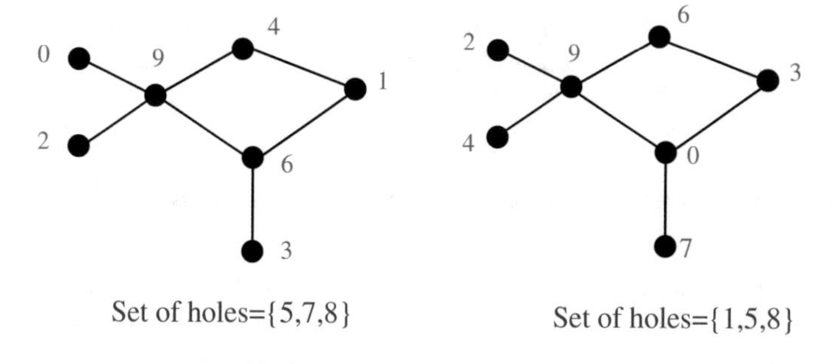

Fig. 1.3 Examples of rc_3-colorings/radio colorings with holes

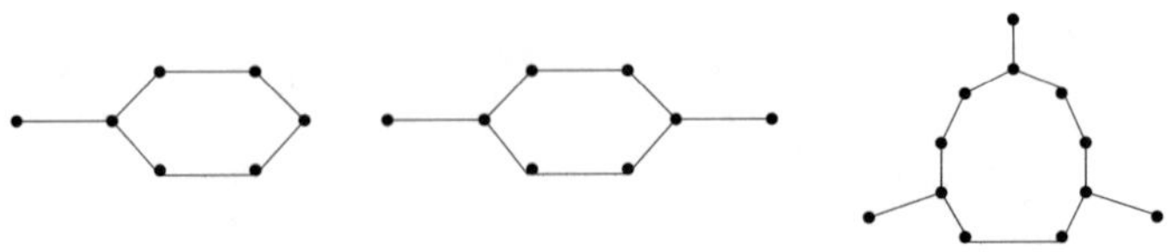

G_1 G_2 G_3

Fig. 1.4 Examples of non-full colorable graphs

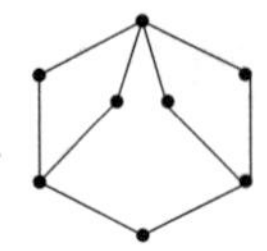

Fig. 1.5 One more example of non-full colorable graphs

as simply $\mu(G)$. Note that $rc_k(G) \leq \mu_k(G)$ and in particular, $\lambda_{2,1}(G) \leq \mu(G)$. If $\lambda_{2,1}(G) = \mu(G)$, then the graph G admits a $\lambda_{2,1}$-coloring with no hole. Such $\lambda_{2,1}$-coloring of G is said to be no hole $\lambda_{2,1}$-coloring or *consecutive* $\lambda_{2,1}$-*coloring* of G and the graph G is said to be a *full colorable* graph.

It has been shown in [13] that the following graphs are full colorable:

(i) any connected graph G with $\Delta(G) = 2$ except P_3, C_3, C_4 and C_6;
(ii) any tree T with $\Delta(T) \geq 3$ except stars;
(iii) any connected non-tree graph G of order at least six with $\Delta(G) = 3$ and $\lambda_{2,1}(G) = 4$ except the graphs in the Fig. 1.4;
(iv) any connected non-tree graph G of order either 7 or 8 with $\Delta(G) = 4$ and $\lambda_{2,1}(G) = 5$ except the graph in the Fig. 1.5.

Several interesting combinatorial properties of holes in a $\lambda_{2,1}$-coloring as well as existence of full colorable graphs have been studied in [1, 13, 16, 30, 31]. Recently, holes in a rc_k-coloring has been studied in [40], and several interesting properties have been explored. In fact, the study of holes in an rc_k-coloring on a graph is an emerging topic in literature. However, this problem is comparatively more explored for rc_2-coloring, i.e., a $\lambda_{2,1}$-coloring of a graph than for general k.

1.2 k-Islands and an Equivalence Relation on $\Lambda_{\rho_k}(G)$

We now define k-islands and using this notion, we will define an equivalence relation on $\Lambda_{\rho_k}(G)$. These notions will be very helpful in our subsequent discussion. Based on the fact that an rc_k-coloring of a graph G may have at most $(k-1)$ consecutive holes [39], an Ω-set and a k-island have been defined in [40]. Let $L \in \Lambda_{\rho_k}(G)$. An *$\Omega$-set of* L is a non-empty set A of non-negative integers, assigned by L as colors, such that $s \in A$ only if $0 \leq |s - s'| < k$, for some $s' \in A$. A maximal Ω-set of $L \in \Lambda_{\rho_k}(G)$ is a *k-island* or simply an *island of* L, if there is no confusion regarding

k. The minimum and maximum element of an island I are said to be the left and right coast of I, respectively, denoted by $lc(I)$ and $rc(I)$ accordingly. The left and right coasts of I are together called the coastal colors or coastal labels of I. If the set of coastal colors of some island is a singleton set, then the island is said to be an *atoll*.

An Equivalence Relation on $\Lambda_{\rho_k}(G)$:

First, we discuss a recoloring of an rc_k-coloring in $\Lambda_{\rho_k}(G)$, referred as an α-recoloring (see [40]), which eventually will induce an equivalence relation on $\Lambda_{\rho_k}(G)$. Let $L \in \Lambda_{\rho_k}(G)$ and $I_0, I_1, \ldots, I_{\rho_k}$ be the islands of L such that $lc(I_{j+1}) = rc(I_j) + k, 0 \leq j \leq \rho_k - 1$. For any $i, 0 \leq i \leq \rho_k$, and $m, 0 \leq m \leq (\rho_k - i)$, let us define a new radio k-coloring $\hat{L}$ on G as follows:

$$\hat{L}(u) = \begin{cases} L(u), \text{ if } L(u) \notin \bigcup_{s=i}^{i+m} I_s, \\ rc(I_{i+m}) - t, \text{ if } L(u) \in \bigcup_{s=i}^{i+m} I_s \text{ and } L(u) = lc(I_i) + t, t \geq 0. \end{cases}$$

It is easy to verify that $\hat{L} \in \Lambda_{\rho_k}(G)$ and the islands $I'_0, I'_1, \ldots, I'_{\rho_k}$ of $\hat{L}$ are such that $I'_j = I_j$, for $j \notin \{i, i+1, \ldots, i+m\}$ and $rc(I'_{i+m-t}) = rc(I_{i+m}) - (lc(I_{i+t}) - lc(I_i))$, $lc(I'_{i+m-t}) = rc(I_{i+m}) - (rc(I_{i+t}) - lc(I_i))$, for $0 \leq t \leq m$. This recoloring $\hat{L}$ is an α-recoloring of L.

Let η be a relation on $\Lambda_{\rho_k}(G)$ defined by $L_1 \eta L_2$ if and only if L_2 is obtained from L_1 using of finite α-recolorings. It is easy to verify that η is reflexive, symmetric, and transitive. Thus, η is an equivalence relation on $\Lambda_{\rho_k}(G)$. Therefore, any rc_k-coloring in $\Lambda_{\rho_k}(G)$ is η-related to some $L \in \Lambda_{\rho_k}(G)$ with islands $I_0, I_1, \ldots, I_{\rho_k}$ such that $lc(I_{j+1}) = rc(I_j) + k, 0 \leq j \leq \rho_k - 1$ and $|I_0| \leq |I_1| \leq \cdots \leq |I_{\rho_k}|$. Thus, we may assume, without loss of generality, that for any $L \in \Lambda_{\rho_k}(G)$, if the islands of L are $I_0, I_1, \ldots, I_{\rho_k}$ with $lc(I_{j+1}) = rc(I_j) + k, 0 \leq j \leq \rho_k - 1$, then $|I_0| \leq |I_1| \leq \cdots \leq |I_{\rho_k}|$. We refer this finite sequence $(|I_0|, |I_1|, \ldots, |I_{\rho_k}|)$ as the *k-island sequence of L* or simply the *island sequence of L*, if there is no confusion regarding k. For the graph G in Fig. 1.1, the $\lambda_{2,1}$-coloring in $\Lambda_{\rho_2}(G)$, i.e., $\Lambda_\rho(G)$, has 2-islands $I_0 = \{0, 1, 2, 3, 4\}$, $I_1 = \{6\}$, $I_2 = \{8\}$, and the rc_3-coloring in $\Lambda_{\rho_3}(G)$ has 3-islands $I_0 = \{0, 2, 4, 6, 8\}$, $I_1 = \{11\}$, $I_2 = \{14\}$. Hence, $(1, 1, 5)$ is a 2-island sequence as well as a 3-island sequence of G.

1.3 An Upper Bound of $\rho_k(G)$nd Related Issues

In this section, an upper bound of $\rho_k(G)$ has been given. Moreover, various interesting features regarding order, regularity (i.e., each vertex having the same degree), radio k-chromatic number, domination number as well as perfect domination number of G (defined later) can be found when $\rho_{k(G)}$ attains its upper bound. We will start with the following results which will give a structural insight of a graph G in presence of a $(k-1)$-hole of an rc_k-coloring in $\Lambda_{\rho_k}(G)$. But first, we need this definition. Let G

and H are two graphs. Then $G + H$ is the *disjoint union* of G and H having vertex set $V(G) \cup V(H)$ and edge set $E(G) \cup E(H)$. Thus, mG is the disjoint union of m pairwise disjoint copies of G.

Lemma 1.1 [40] *Let G be a graph with $\rho_k(G) \geq 1$ and $L \in \Lambda_{\rho_k}(G)$. If $\{i+1, i+2, \ldots, i+k-1\}$ is a $(k-1)$-hole in L, then $l_i = l_{i+k}$ and the subgraph of G induced by $L_i \cup L_{i+k}$ is $l_i K_2$.*

Proof **Case I**: Let $l_{i+k} \geq 2$. If possible, let $x \in L_{i+k}$ be such that $x \nsim v$, where v is an arbitrary vertex in L_i. We define $\hat{L}$ by

$$\hat{L}(u) = \begin{cases} L(u), \text{ if } u \neq x, \\ i + k - 1, \text{ if } u = x. \end{cases}$$

Clearly, $\hat{L}$ is an rc_k-coloring with fewer $(k-1)$-holes, leading to a contradiction.

Case II: Let $l_{i+k} = 1$ and $L_{i+k} = \{x\}$. If possible, let $x \nsim v$, where v is an arbitrary vertex in L_i. We define $\hat{L}$ by

$$\hat{L}(u) = \begin{cases} L(u), \text{ if } L(u) \leq i, \\ L(u) - 1, \text{ if } L(u) \geq i + k. \end{cases}$$

Then $\hat{L}$ is a radio k-coloring with span $rc_k(G) - 1$, a contradiction.

Hence, every vertex of L_{i+k} is adjacent to a unique vertex in L_i. Similarly, any vertex L_i is adjacent to a unique vertex in L_{i+k}. From this, the proof follows.

The following result is going to play a key role in our subsequent discussion.

Corollary 1.1 [40] *Let G be a graph with $\rho_k(G) \geq 1$ and I, J are two distinct islands of $L \in \Lambda_{\rho_k}(G)$ with x and y as two coastal colors of I and J, respectively. Then $l_x = l_y$ and the subgraph of G induced by $L_x \cup L_y$ is $l_x K_2$.*

Proof Applying finite number of suitable α-recolorings, we assume, without loss of generality, that $x = rc(I)$, $y = lc(J)$ and $y = x + k$. The proof follows from Lemma 1.1.

We are now in a position to obtain an upper bound of $\rho_k(G)$.

Theorem 1.1 [40] *Let G be a graph with $\rho_k(G) \geq 1$. Then $\rho_k(G) \leq \Delta(G)$, where $\Delta(G)$ is the maximum degree of any vertex in G.*

Proof Let $I_0, I_1, \ldots, I_{\rho_k}$ be the islands of any $L \in \Lambda_{\rho_k}(G)$. Let x be any coastal color of I_0 and $u \in L_x$. Then by Corollary 1.1, $u \sim v_y$, where $v_y \in L_y$ in G, for each coastal color y of I_j, $1 \leq j \leq \rho_k(G)$. Hence, $d(u) \geq \rho_k(G)$. Therefore, $\rho_k(G) \leq \Delta(G)$.

When $\rho_k(G)$ attains its upper bound, G shows some interesting structural properties. Before we discuss the situation, let us take a look at few definitions. In a graph

G, a set $S \subseteq V(G)$ is a *dominating set* if for every vertex $u \in V(G) \setminus S$, there is a $v \in S$ such that $u \sim v$ (see [42]). The minimum order of a dominating set is the *dominating number* of G, denoted by $\gamma(G)$. A set $S \subset V(G)$ is said to be a *perfect dominating set* if every vertex in $V(G) \setminus S$ is adjacent to exactly one vertex in S (see [20]). The minimum cardinality of a perfect dominating set of G is the *perfect domination number* of G, denoted by $\gamma_p(G)$. Clearly $\gamma(G) \leq \gamma_p(G)$.

Now, we state the following lower bound for domination number. It will help us to prove Theorem 1.3.

Theorem 1.2 [20, 41] *For any graph G of order n, $\gamma(G) \geq \lceil \frac{n}{\Delta(G)+1} \rceil$.*

Now, we explore the structure of G, including its regularity, order, domination number, etc., when $\rho_k(G) = \Delta(G)$.

Theorem 1.3 [40] *Let G be a graph of order n with $\rho_k(G) \geq 1$ and $\rho_k(G) = \Delta(G) = \Delta$. Then*

(i) G is a Δ-regular graph;
(ii) $rc_k(G) = k\Delta$;
(iii) $n \equiv 0 \ (mod\ \Delta + 1)$;
(iv) $\gamma(G) = \gamma_p(G) = \frac{n}{\Delta+1}$;
(v) If $n \neq \Delta + 1$, then $\mu_k(G) = rc_k(G) + 1$.

Proof Let $I_0, I_1, \ldots, I_{\rho_k}$ be the islands of any $L \in \Lambda_{\rho_k}(G)$ with $lc(I_{j+1}) = rc(I_j) + k, 0 \leq j \leq \rho_k - 1$ such that $|I_0| \leq |I_1| \leq \cdots \leq |I_{\rho_k}|$. Then the number of islands of L is $\rho_k + 1$.

We claim that every island of L is an atoll. If not, then there exists an island I of L such that $lc(I) \neq rc(I)$. Then by Corollary 1.1, for any vertex v with $L(v)$ as a coastal color of any other island J of L, $d(v) \geq \rho_k + 1 = \Delta + 1$, which is a contradiction. Hence, every island is a singleton set, i.e., an atoll. Thus, for every vertex v of G, $L(v)$ is a coastal color of some island of L and therefore every vertex has same degree, by Corollary 1.1. Hence, G is Δ-regular.

Since each island of L is atoll, $I_j = \{kj\}, 0 \leq j \leq \Delta$. Hence, $rc_k(G) = k\Delta$.

Moreover, by Corollary 1.1, $l_{ki} = l_{kj} = l$ (say), $0 \leq i < j \leq \Delta$. Therefore, $n = l(\Delta + 1)$, i.e., $n \equiv 0$ (mod $\Delta + 1$).

Again, by Corollary 1.1, the subgraph induced by $L_{ki} \cup L_{kj}$ is lK_2, for any i, j with $0 \leq i < j \leq \Delta$. Also, $I_i = \{ki\}, 0 \leq i \leq \Delta$. Therefore, L_{ki} is a dominating set as well as a perfect dominating set of G, for every $i, 0 \leq i \leq \Delta$. Hence, $\gamma(G) \leq \frac{n}{\Delta+1}$. Using Theorem 1.2, we get $\gamma(G) = \frac{n}{\Delta+1}$. Hence, $\gamma_p(G) = \frac{n}{\Delta+1}$.

Let $n \neq \Delta + 1$. Then $l \geq 2$. Since $lc(I_j) = rc(I_j)$, for every $0 \leq j \leq \Delta$, using Corollary 1.1, we get a path $P : v_0, v_1, \ldots, v_\Delta$ in G such that $L(v_j) \in I_j = \{kj\}$, $0 \leq j \leq \Delta$. Now, the new coloring $\hat{L}$ on G defined by

$$\hat{L}(u) = \begin{cases} L(u), \text{ if } u \neq v_j, 0 \leq j \leq \Delta, \\ L(u) + 1, \text{ if } u = v_j, 0 \leq j \leq \Delta. \end{cases}$$

is a radio k-coloring of G with no $(k-1)$-hole. Hence, $\mu_k(G) \leq span(\hat{L}) = rc_k(G)+1$. But since $\rho_k(G) > 0$, $\mu_k(G) > rc_k(G)$. Therefore, $\mu_k(G) = rc_k(G)+1$.

1.4 A New Family of Graphs: $\mathscr{G}_{\Delta,t}$

Things become very interesting when $\rho_2(G) = \Delta(G)$, i.e., $\rho(G) = \Delta(G)$. By Theorem 1.3, the order of G is $t(\Delta+1)$, for some integer $t \geq 1$. Let $\mathscr{G}_{\Delta,t}$ be the family of connected graphs G with $\rho(G) = \Delta(G) = \Delta$ and order $t(\Delta+1)$, for some integer $t \geq 1$. Then using Theorem 1.3, $l_i = t$, for $i = 0, 2, 4, \ldots, \lambda_{2,1}(G) = 2\Delta$. Note that $\mathscr{G}_{\Delta,1} = \{K_{\Delta+1}\}$.

1.4.1 A Characterization of $\mathscr{G}_{\Delta,2}$

We now focus on $t = 2$. For any $\Delta \geq 2$, let G be the bipartite graph obtained by deleting a perfect matching from $K_{\Delta+1,\Delta+1}$, where a perfect matching is a set M of edges such that no two edges in M share a vertex, and each vertex of the graph is incident to exactly one edge in M. Then G is connected Δ-regular graph with order $2(\Delta+1)$. It can be easily verified that $G \in \mathscr{G}_{\Delta,2}$. Now, the question is **whether every connected Δ-regular graph with order $2(\Delta+1)$ belongs to $\mathscr{G}_{\Delta,2}$**.

Before we answer this question, we will state the following result which will be helpful in the subsequent discussion. Note that a cycle through all the vertices of a graph is a *Hamiltonian cycle* and any graph having a Hamiltonian cycle is a *Hamiltonian graph*. Also, any path through all the vertices of a graph is a *Hamiltonian path* in the graph. Clearly, a Hamiltonian graph contains a Hamiltonian path.

Theorem 1.4 [42] *Let G be a graph on $n \geq 3$ vertices having minimum degree $\delta(G) \geq \frac{n}{2}$. Then G is a Hamiltonian graph.*

Now we are in a position to prove the following result.

Lemma 1.2 [16] *If G is a connected Δ-regular graph of order $2(\Delta+1)$, then $G \in \mathscr{G}_{\Delta,2}$ or $\lambda_{2,1}(G) = 2\Delta+1$.*

Sketch of proof. Clearly, G^c is a $(\Delta+1)$ regular graph of order $2(\Delta+1)$. As $\delta(G^c) = \frac{1}{2}|V(G^c)|$, by Theorem 1.4, G^c has a Hamiltonian path, say, $P : v_0, v_1, \ldots, v_{2\Delta+1}$. Hence by assigning color i to v_i, $0 \leq i \leq 2\Delta+1$, we get $\lambda_{2,1}(G) \leq 2\Delta+1$.

We shall now show that if $\lambda_{2,1}(G) \leq 2\Delta$, then $G \in \mathscr{G}_{\Delta,2}$. For this, using the distance condition of $L(2,1)$-coloring and regularity as well as order of G, we would show that if α is a multiple color of any $\lambda_{2,1}$-coloring L, then $l_\alpha = 2$ and $\alpha-1$, $\alpha+1$ are two holes in L which in turn will help us to show $|V(G)| = \Sigma_{i=0}^{\lambda_{2,1}(G)} m_i \leq 2\lfloor \frac{\lambda_{2,1}(G)+2}{2} \rfloor$, implying $\lambda_{2,1}(G) \geq 2\Delta$. Hence, $\lambda_{2,1}(G) = 2\Delta$ and using this we can show $\rho(G) = \Delta$. □

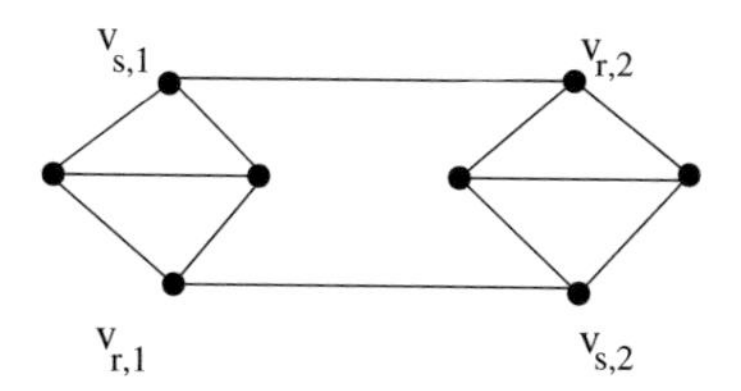

Fig. 1.6 Illustrating an example of e-exchange

Remark 1.1 The above result says about the radio 2-chromatic number of G if G is a connected Δ-regular graph of order $2(\Delta + 1)$ and $G \notin \mathcal{G}_{\Delta,2}$.

We now discuss a graph construction (introduced in [16]) which will be helpful in characterizing $\mathcal{G}_{\Delta,2}$.

The S-Exchange of Sum of Two Graphs:

Let G_1, G_2 be two graphs both isomorphic to G with $V(G) = \{v_1, v_2, \ldots, v_n\}$ and ϕ_i $(i = 1, 2)$ be graph isomorphisms from G to G_i, where $\phi_i(v_j) = v_{j,i}$. Also let $e = v_r v_s$ be an edge of G. Let $T(e) = \{v_{r,1}v_{s,2}, v_{r,2}v_{s,1}\}$. Then the *e-exchange of graph* $G_1 + G_2$, denoted by $X_e(G_1 + G_2)$, is the graph with the vertex set $V(G_1 + G_2)$ and edge set $(E(G_1 + G_2) - \{\phi_1(e), \phi_2(e)\}) \cup T(e)$.

Let $S \subseteq E(G)$. Then the S-exchange of $G_1 + G_2$, denoted by $X_S(G_1 + G_2)$, is the graph with vertex set $V(G_1 + G_2)$ and the edge set $(E(G_1 + G_2) - \cup_{e \in S}\{\phi_1(e), \phi_2(e)\}) \cup (\cup_{e \in S} T(e))$, where for each e, $T(e)$ is defined earlier.

For example, if G is isomorphic to the complete graph K_3 and $S = E(G)$, then $X_S(G_1 + G_2)$ is isomorphic to the cycle C_6. Also if G is isomorphic to the complete graph K_4 and $e = v_r v_s$ is any edge of G, then $X_e(G_1 + G_2)$ is isomorphic to the graph shown in Fig. 1.6.

We now state the following theorem which gives a characterization of $\mathcal{G}_{\Delta,2}$ in terms of S-exchange.

Theorem 1.5 [16] *Let G be a connected Δ-regular graph of order $2(\Delta + 1)$. Then $G \in \mathcal{G}_{\Delta,2}$ if and only if there is a set $S \subseteq E(K_{\Delta+1})$ such that G is isomorphic to $X_S(K_{\Delta+1} + K_{\Delta+1})$.*

1.4.2 $\mathcal{G}_{\Delta,t}$ *and the t-Neighborhood Property*

We shall now address the more general issue of connected Δ-regular graphs having order $t(\Delta + 1)$, for any $t \geq 2$. Král' et al. [24] identified a special property of connected Δ-regular graph with order $t(\Delta + 1)$. A connected Δ-regular graph with order $t(\Delta + 1)$ is said to have *the t-neighborhood property* if for any two disjoint sets U and W of vertices of G, the following holds: If no vertex of U is adjacent to any vertex of W and any pair of vertices in U or W are at least three distance apart, then $|U| + |W| \leq t$.

We now have the following result.

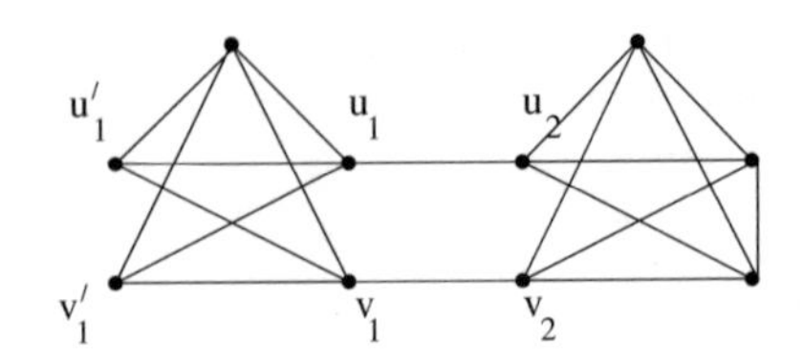

Fig. 1.7 Illustrating H_4

Theorem 1.6 [24] *Let G be a connected Δ-regular graph of order* $t(\Delta + 1)$ *with* $\lambda_{2,1}(G) \leq 2\Delta$ *such that G satisfies the t-neighborhood property. Then* $\lambda_{2,1}(G) = 2\Delta$ *and* $\rho(G) = \Delta$ *and hence* $G \in \mathcal{G}_{\Delta,t}$.

Sketch of proof. Clearly, there is an $L(2, 1)$-coloring of G with span at most 2Δ. Using the t-neighborhood property of G, $m_i + m_{i+1} \leq t$. For any odd integer i_0, $1 \leq i_0 \leq 2\Delta, t(\Delta+1) = \Sigma_{i=0}^{2\Delta} m_i = (\Sigma_{i=0}^{\frac{i_0-1}{2}} m_{2i} + m_{2i+1}) + (\Sigma_{i=\frac{i_0+1}{2}}^{\Delta} m_{2i-1} + m_{2i}) - m_{i_0} \leq t(\Delta + 1) - m_{i_0}$. Therefore, $m_{i_0} = 0$, for every odd integer i_0, $1 \leq i_0 \leq 2\Delta$. So $m_{2i} = t, 0 \leq i \leq \Delta$. From this, the proof follows. □

Thus, Theorem 1.6 says that if G is a connected Δ-regular graph of order $t(\Delta+1)$ with $\lambda_{2,1}(G) \leq 2\Delta$, then satisfying the t-neighborhood property is a sufficient condition for obtaining $\lambda_{2,1}(G) = 2\Delta$ and $\rho(G) = \Delta$. We now show that the condition is not necessary. In fact, we will prove that there is a connected Δ-regular graph of order $3(\Delta + 1)$ which does not satisfy the 3-neighborhood property and for which $\lambda_{2,1}(G) = 2\Delta$ and $\rho(G) = \Delta$.

Before we prove this, we shall state the following lemmas whose proofs follow easily.

Lemma 1.3 [31] *Let G be a graph isomorphic to* $K_{m+1} - e$, *where the edge* $e = uv$. *Then* $\lambda_{2,1}(G) = 2m - 1$ *and for any* $\lambda_{2,1}$*-coloring L of G,* $\{L(u), L(v)\} = \{2i, 2i+1\}$ *for some* $i \in \{0, 1, \ldots, m - 1\}$.

Lemma 1.4 [18] *Let H be a subgraph of G. Then* $\lambda_{2,1}(H) \leq \lambda_{2,1}(G)$.

Now, we construct a graph H_m ($m \geq 3$) consisting of two components. First one is $K_{m+1} - \{e_1, e_2\}$, where $e_1 = u_1v_1$ and $e_2 = u_1'v_1'$ are two non-incident edges (called the left component of H_m); the other component of $K_{m+1} - e$, where $e = u_2v_2$ (called the right component of H_m). Now, we add two edges u_1u_2 and v_1v_2 (See Fig. 1.7). We prove the following result.

Lemma 1.5 [31] $\lambda_{2,1}(H_m) = 2m$, *for* $m \geq 3$.

Proof Label $u_1, v_1, u_2, v_2, u_1', v_1'$ by $0, 2, 2, 0, 2m - 2, 2m$, respectively, and the remaining $(m - 3)$ vertices in the left component by $4, 6, \ldots, 2m - 4$ and the remaining $(m-1)$ vertices in the right component by $4, 6, \ldots, 2m$. This is an $L(2, 1)$-coloring of H_m of span $2m$ and so $\lambda_{2,1}(H_m) \leq 2m$.

If possible, let $\lambda_{2,1}(H_m) < 2m$. Since H_m has $K_{m+1} - u_2v_2$ as its subgraph (the right component), so by Lemma 1.4, $\lambda_{2,1}(H_m) = 2m - 1$. Let L be a $\lambda_{2,1}$-coloring of H_m. Without loss of generality, we can assume that $L(u_2) = 2i$ and

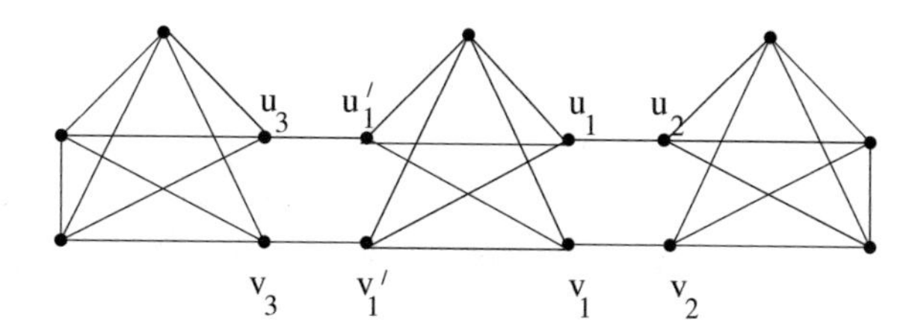

Fig. 1.8 Illustrating G_4

$L(v_2) = 2i + 1$, by Lemma 1.3. Then the vertices in the right component of H_m are colored with $0, 2, 4, \ldots, 2i, 2i+1, 2i+3, \ldots, 2m-1$. Therefore, $\{L(u_1), L(v_1)\} \subseteq \{1, 3, 5, \ldots, 2i-1, 2i+2, 2i+4, \ldots, 2m-2\}$ as L satisfies the distance two condition. Hence, $|L(u_1) - L(v_1)| \geq 2$. Therefore, $\{L(u_1'), L(v_1')\} = \{2j, 2j+1\}$, for some $j \in \{0, 1, \ldots, m-1\}$ and so the vertices in the left component are colored by $0, 2, 4, \ldots, 2j, 2j+1, 2j+3, \ldots, 2m-1$. But as $i \neq j$ and $L(u_2) = 2i$, $L(v_2) = 2i + 1$, so this leads to a contradiction. Hence, $\lambda_{2,1}(H_m) = 2m$.

We now construct a graph G_m which consists of three components: one is $K_{m+1} - \{e_1, e_2\}$, where $e_1 = u_1v_1$ and $e_2 = u_1'v_1'$ are two non-incident edges (called middle component); the other two components are $K_{m+1} - e_i'$, where $e_i' = u_iv_i$, $i = 2, 3$ (called left and right components, respectively). Now, add edges $u_1u_2, v_1v_2, u_1'u_3$ and $v_1'v_3$ (See Fig. 1.8).

Lemma 1.6 [31] *$\lambda_{2,1}(G_m) = 2m$, for $m \geq 3$.*

Proof Since H_m is a subgraph of G_m, $\lambda_{2,1}(G_m) \geq 2m$, by Lemmas 1.4 and 1.5. Again, label the vertices $u_1, v_1, u_1', v_1', u_2, v_2, u_3, v_3$ with $0, 2, 2m-2, 2m, 2, 0, 2m, 2m-2$, respectively; the remaining $(m-1)$ vertices of the left (right, respectively) component by distinct colors from the set $\{0, 2, \ldots, 2m-4\}$ ($\{4, 6, \ldots, 2m\}$, respectively). Lastly, label the remaining $(m-3)$ vertices in the middle component by the distinct colors from $\{4, 6, \ldots, 2m-4\}$. This is an $L(2, 1)$-coloring of G_m and hence $\lambda_{2,1}(G_m) = 2m$.

Now we are in a position to discuss the following result.

Theorem 1.7 [31] *For each integer $m \geq 3$, there exists a connected m-regular graph G of order $3(m+1)$ without 3-neighborhood property such that $\lambda_{2,1}(G) = 2m$ and $\rho(G) = m$.*

Sketch of proof. Clearly G_m is a connected m-regular graph of order $3(\Delta + 1)$. By Lemma 1.6, $\lambda_{2,1}(G_m) = 2m$. Consider the set of vertices $U = \{u_2, u_3\}$ and $W = \{v_2, v_3\}$ in G_m. Clearly, each pair of vertices of U or W is three distance apart, and no vertex of U is adjacent to any vertex of W. Moreover, $|U| + |W| = 4 > 3$. Hence, G_m does not satisfy the 3-neighborhood property.

Now, it can be shown (see [31]) that for any $\lambda_{2,1}$-coloring L of G_m, if u, v are any two vertices in the same component, i.e., in the middle or left or right component, of G_m, then $L(u), L(v)$ cannot be consecutive integers. Hence, $1, 3, 5, \ldots, 2m-1$ are holes in L. So, $\rho(G_m) = m$. □

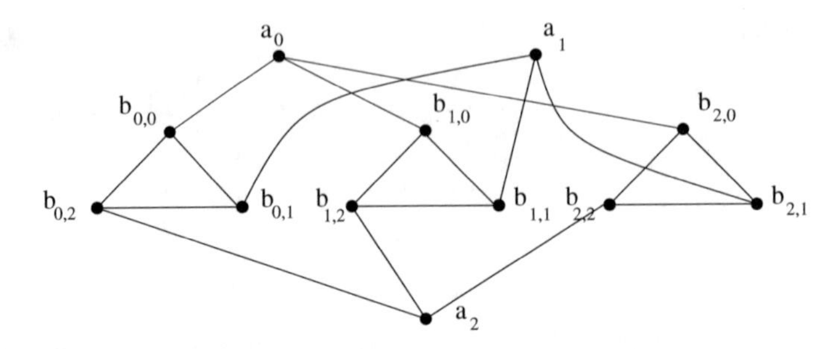

Fig. 1.9 Illustrating Ω_3

1.4.3 A Conjecture on $\mathcal{G}_{r,t}$

In this subsection, we study a conjecture regarding $\mathcal{G}_{r,t}$ and its disproof. But first we need to understand the backdrop in which the conjecture shall find its relevance. For this, we will study the following two families of connected r-regular graphs.

We begin with a class Ω_r of connected r-regular graphs, for any $r \geq 1$, introduced in [16]. Let $X = rK_r$ and $Y = rK_1$. Let $V(\Omega_r) = V(X) \cup V(Y)$, where

(i) $V(X) = \cup_{i=0}^{r-1} B_i$, $B_i = \{b_{i,j} | \ 0 \leq j \leq r-1\}$ and (ii) $V(Y) = \{a_0, a_1, \ldots, a_{r-1}\}$.

Let $E(\Omega_r) = R \cup S$ where (i) $R = \cup_{i=0}^{r-1} R_i$, $R_i = \{b_{i,j}b_{i,k} : 0 \leq j < k \leq r-1\}$ and (ii) $S = \cup_{i=0}^{r-1} S_i$, $S_i = \{a_i b_{m,i} : 0 \leq m \leq r-1\}$. Clearly, Ω_r is a connected r-regular graph with order $r(r+1)$ (See Fig. 1.9).

It can be easily verified that Ω_1 and Ω_2 are isomorphic to K_2 and C_6, respectively.

We now observe the following facts regarding distances in Ω_r.

For $0 \leq i < j \leq r-1$, $d(a_i, a_j) = 3$.

For $0 \leq i, j, k, l \leq r-1$,

$$d(b_{i,j}, b_{k,l}) = \begin{cases} 1, & \text{if} \quad i = k \text{ and } j \neq l, \\ 2, & \text{if} \quad i \neq k \text{ and } j = l, \\ 3, & \text{otherwise;} \end{cases}$$

Also for $0 \leq i, j, k \leq r-1$,

$$d(a_i, b_{j,k}) = \begin{cases} 1, & \text{if} \quad i = k, \\ 2, & \text{otherwise;} \end{cases}$$

Using these facts, we can say that Ω_r satisfies the r-neighborhood property.

Now let $B_k = \{b_{i,j} | \ (j - i) \equiv k \ (mod \ r)\}$, $0 \leq k \leq r-1$. Clearly, $|B_k| = r$ and each pair of vertices of B_k and Y are at distance three. Hence, we can assign an $L(2, 1)$-coloring on Ω_r as follows:

Fig. 1.10 Illustrating $\Omega_{4,2}$

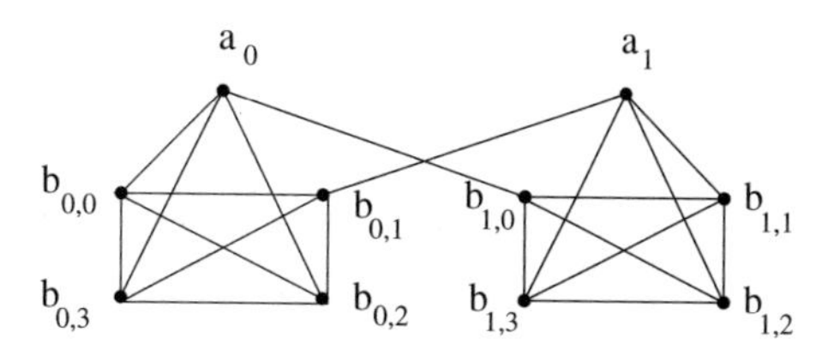

$$L(v) = \begin{cases} 2k, \text{ if } v \in B_k, \\ 2r, \text{ if } v = a_i, \text{ where } i = 0, 1, \ldots, r-1. \end{cases}$$

Hence, $\lambda_{2,1}(\Omega_r) \leq 2r$. Therefore by Theorem 1.6, $\Omega_r \in \mathscr{G}_{r,r}$, for every $r \geq 1$. Thus, for every $r \geq 1$, $\mathscr{G}_{r,r}$ is non-empty.

Given any $r \geq 2$, to show that $\mathscr{G}_{r,t}$ is non-empty for every $t < r$, Georges et al. constructed another graph $\Omega_{r,t}$ in [16]. Let $X = tK_r$ and $Y = tK_1$. Then $V(\Omega_{r,t}) = V(X) \cup V(Y)$, where

(i) $V(X) = \cup_{i=0}^{t-1} B_i$, $B_i = \{b_{i,j} | 0 \leq j \leq r-1\}$ and (ii) $V(Y) = \{a_0, a_1, \ldots, a_{t-1}\}$. Also $E(\Omega_{r,t}) = R \cup S \cup T$, where (i) $R = \cup_{i=0}^{t-1} R_i$, $R_i = \{b_{i,j}b_{i,k} : 0 \leq j < k \leq r-1\}$, (ii) $S = \cup_{i=0}^{t-1} S_i$, $S_i = \{a_i b_{m,i} : 0 \leq m \leq t-1\}$ and (iii) $T = \cup_{i=0}^{t-1} T_i$, $T_i = \{a_i b_{i,j} : t \leq j \leq r-1\}$ (See Fig. 1.10). Clearly $\Omega_{r,t}$ is a connected r-regular graph with order $t(r+1)$. It can be easily verified that $\Omega_{2,1}$ is isomorphic to K_3 and in general $\Omega_{r,1}$ is isomorphic to K_{r+1}. Argument similar to the analysis of Ω_r can show that $\Omega_{r,t} \in \mathscr{G}_{r,t}$.

Georges et al. were unable to prove that $\mathscr{G}_{r,t}$ is non-empty for $t > r$ and at this point they conjectured in [16] that $\mathscr{G}_{r,t} = \emptyset$, for every $t > r$. This conjecture was proven to be wrong by Král' et al. in [24]. For this, they constructed an $(\alpha + \beta - 1)$-regular connected graph $\Gamma_{\alpha,\beta}$ of order $\alpha\beta(\alpha + \beta)$ with $\rho(\Gamma_{\alpha,\beta}) = \Delta(\Gamma_{\alpha,\beta}) = \alpha + \beta - 1$. Now, $V(\Gamma_{\alpha,\beta})$ consists of two sets $V_g = \{[a, b, \bar{a}] : 1 \leq a \leq \alpha, 1 \leq b \leq \beta \text{ and } 1 \leq \bar{a} \leq \alpha\}$ and $V_r = \{[a, b, \bar{b}] : 1 \leq a \leq \alpha, 1 \leq b \leq \beta \text{ and } 1 \leq \bar{b} \leq \beta\}$. The vertices of V_g and V_r are called green and red vertices, respectively. Two distinct green vertices $[a, b, \bar{a}]$ and $[a', b', \bar{a}']$ are adjacent if and only if $b = b'$ and $\bar{a} = \bar{a}'$. Similarly, two distinct red vertices $[a, b, \bar{b}]$ and $[a', b', \bar{b}']$ are adjacent if and only if $a = a'$ and $\bar{b} = \bar{b}'$. A green vertex $[a, b, \bar{a}]$ is adjacent to a red vertex $[a', b', \bar{b}']$ if and only if $a = a'$ and $b = b'$ (Fig. 1.11).

We now prove the following theorem.

Theorem 1.8 [24] *For every $\alpha, \beta \geq 1$, $\lambda_{2,1}(\Gamma_{\alpha,\beta}) \leq 2(\alpha + \beta - 1)$.*

Proof For $i = 0, 1, \ldots, \alpha - 1$, define $A_i = \{u = [a, b, \bar{a}] \in V_g : i \equiv a + \bar{a} \ (mod\ \alpha)\}$. Also, for $j = 0, 1, \ldots, \beta - 1$, define $B_j = \{v = [a, b, \bar{b}] \in V_r : j \equiv b + \bar{b} \ (mod\ \beta)\}$. Then A_i and B_j are independent sets for all i and j. Also, $V_g = \cup_{i=0}^{\alpha-1} A_i$ and $V_r = \cup_{j=0}^{\beta-1} B_j$. Moreover, we claim that any two vertices in an A_i or B_j are at least three distances apart. If not, then without loss of generality, we may assume that two green vertices $u = [a, b, \bar{a}]$ and $v = [a', b', \bar{a}']$ in A_i are two distance apart. Let the common neighbor of u and v be a green vertex. Then $b = b'$

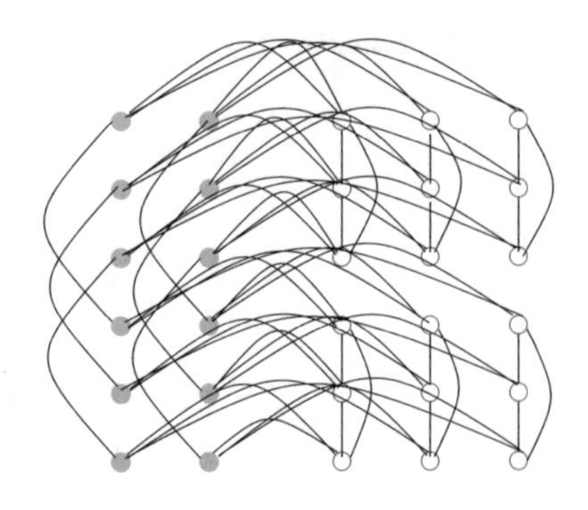

Fig. 1.11 Illustrating $\Gamma_{2,3}$, where the solid circles are green vertices and empty circles are red vertices

and $\bar{a} = \bar{a}'$. Therefore, $a \equiv a' \ (mod\ i)$ implying $a = a'$, i.e., $u = v$. Similarly, if the common neighbor of u and v is a red vertex, then u and v become identical.

Now, we color each vertex of A_i by $2i$, for $i = 0, 1, \ldots, \alpha - 1$, and each vertex of B_j by $2j + 2\alpha$, for $j = 0, 1, \ldots, \beta - 1$. Hence, $\lambda_{2,1}(\Gamma_{\alpha,\beta}) \leq 2(\alpha + \beta - 1)$.

We now state the following result without proof.

Theorem 1.9 [24] *For every $\alpha, \beta \geq 1$, $\Gamma_{\alpha,\beta}$ has the $\alpha\beta$-neighborhood property.*

Therefore by Theorems 1.6, 1.8 and 1.9, we have $\lambda_{2,1}(\Gamma_{\alpha,\beta}) = 2(\alpha+\beta-1)$ and $\rho(\Gamma_{\alpha,\beta}) = \alpha+\beta-1$, i.e., $\Gamma_{\alpha,\beta} \in \mathcal{G}_{\alpha+\beta-1,\alpha\beta}$. Putting $\alpha = \lfloor \frac{r}{2} \rfloor + 1$ and $\beta = \lceil \frac{r}{2} \rceil$, we get $\alpha\beta(\alpha+\beta) = (r+1)\lfloor \frac{(r+1)^2}{4} \rfloor$. Hence, for the graph $\Gamma_{\alpha,\beta}$, we get the following result.

Corollary 1.2 [24] *For every $r \geq 1$, there exists a r-regular connected graph G of order $(r+1)\lfloor \frac{(r+1)^2}{4} \rfloor \approx \frac{r^3}{4}$ with $\rho(G) = r$.*

This disproves the conjecture that $\mathcal{G}_{r,t} = \emptyset$, for every $t > r$.

1.5 Relation Between the Hole Index of G and the Path Covering Number of G^c and Its Generalization for the Radio k-Coloring Problem for Any $k \geq 2$

1.5.1 *Relation Between Hole Index of G and Path Covering Number of G^c*

In [15], Georges et al. investigated the $L(2, 1)$-coloring problem from a completely different viewpoint. In this paper, the $L(2, 1)$-coloring problem of a graph has been studied in the light of another graph parameter known as path covering number of the complement graph, where the path covering problem is actually an extension of Hamiltonian path problem. The minimum number of vertex-disjoint paths required to exhaust all the vertices of a graph G is the path covering number of G, denoted by $c(G)$ and a set of minimum number of vertex-disjoint paths exhausting all the vertices of G is a minimum path covering of G. Note that $c(G) = 1$ if G has a Hamiltonian path. Finding a minimum path covering has applications in establishing ring protocols, codes optimization, and mapping parallel programs to parallel architectures [3, 4, 33, 34].

In [15], it is shown that if $c(G) = r$, $\lambda_{2,1}(G) \leq n + r - 2$, and the upper bound is attained if and only if $r \geq 2$. Exploiting this, an elegant relation between the hole index of G and the path covering number of G^c has been obtained in [16].

Let $c(G^c) = r$ and $\{P^1, P^2, \ldots, P^r\}$ be a collection of paths in G^c exhausting all the vertices. For $1 \leq i \leq r$, let v^i_j be the jth vertex along P^i and p_i be the number of vertices in P^i. If V is the vertex set of G and $\mathbb{N}$ be the set of natural numbers, then defining the mapping $f : V \to \mathbb{N} \cup \{0\}$ by

$$f(v^i_j) = i + j - 2 + \Sigma_{t=1}^{i-1} p_t, \tag{1.3}$$

we obtain the upper bound described above.

In [15], Georges et al. identified a certain kind of hole and referred it as gap. A hole i of a $\lambda_{2,1}$-coloring L is said to be a *gap* if $l_{i-1} = l_{i+1}$ and if $v^{i-1} \sim v^{i+1}$ in G. Let us now have a look into the following results regarding existence of gaps without proof.

Lemma 1.7 [15] *Let $L \in \Lambda_\rho(G)$. Then $G(L)$ is empty or $M(L)$ is empty, where $G(L)$ and $M(L)$ are the sets of gaps and multiple colors of L, respectively.*

Lemma 1.8 [15] *Let $L \in \Lambda_\rho(G)$ be such that $G(L)$ is empty. Then G^c has a Hamiltonian path.*

Now if G^c has a Hamiltonian path, i.e., $c(G^c) = 1$, then by the above upper bound of $\lambda_{2,1}(G)$, $\lambda_{2,1}(G) \leq n - 1$, where n is the number of the vertices.

Conversely, let $\lambda_{2,1}(G) \leq n - 1$. Let $L \in \Lambda_\rho(G)$. If L has no hole, then $G(L)$ is empty and so G^c has a Hamiltonian path, by Lemma 1.8. If L has hole, then by pigeon-hole principle, L has multiple colors and so by Lemma 1.7, again $G(L)$ is empty and so G^c has a Hamiltonian path, by Lemma 1.8.

The above argument and suitable induction principle on $r \geq 2$ prove the following result which gives a very elegant characterization of the radio 2-coloring problem, i.e., the $L(2, 1)$-coloring problem in terms of path covering problem.

Theorem 1.10 [15] *Let G be a graph on n vertices and $r = c(G^c)$. Then*

(i) $\lambda_{2,1}(G) \leq n - 1$ *if and only if* $r = 1$;
(ii) $\lambda_{2,1}(G) = n + r - 2$ *if and only if* $r \geq 2$.

Remark 1.2 Let G be a graph on n vertices and $\lambda_{2,1}(G) = n - 1$. Then using Theorem 1.10, we can say that G admits a $\lambda_{2,1}$-coloring which has no hole. Hence, $\mu(G) = \lambda_{2,1}(G)$.

Now, we are in a position to establish the relation between $\rho(G)$ and $c(G^c)$.

Theorem 1.11 [16] *Let G be a graph on n vertices and* $\lambda_{2,1}(G) \geq n - 1$. *The* $\rho(G) = c(G^c) - 1$.

Proof Let $\mathscr{P}$ be a minimum path covering of G^c with $\mathscr{P} = \{P^1, P^2, \ldots, P^r\}$. For $1 \leq i \leq r$, Let v^i_j be the jth vertex along P^i and p_i be the number of vertices in P^i. Define $f : V \to \mathbb{N} \cup \{0\}$ by $f(v^i_j) = i + j - 2 + \Sigma_{t=1}^{i-1} p_t$, as discussed earlier. Then f is a $\lambda_{2,1}$-coloring with $c(G^c) - 1$ holes. Therefore, $\rho(G) \leq c(G^c) - 1$.

Let $L \in \Lambda_\rho(G)$ and l be the number of distinct colors in L. Then $\lambda_{2,1}(G) = l + \rho(G) - 1 \leq n + \rho(G) - 1$ implying $\rho(G) \geq \lambda_{2,1}(G) - (n - 1) = c(G^c) - 1$, using Theorem 1.10. This completes the proof.

Now a conjecture was proposed in [16] **that for any** r**-regular graph** G **with** $\rho(G) \geq 1$, $\rho(G)$ **divides** r. This was disproved by Adams et al. in [1]. They constructed an r-regular graph G such that $\rho(G)$ and r are relatively prime integers.

Theorem 1.12 [1] *For each* $s \geq 2$, *there exists an* r*-regular graph G with* $\rho(G) = s$ *such that* $\rho(G)$ *and r are relatively prime integers.*

Proof For any $s \geq 2$, construct a graph G such that $G^c = H_1 + H_2 + \ldots + H_{s+1}$, where H_{s+1} is cycle with four vertices and each H_i is isomorphic to K_3, for $i = 1, 2, \ldots, s$. Therefore, G has $3s + 4$ vertices and is $3s + 1$-regular. Now, $c(G^c) = s + 1$ and so, by Theorem 1.11, $\rho(G) = s$. Clearly, $\rho(G)$ and $3s + 1$ are relatively prime.

1.5.2 Relating the (k − 1)-Hole Index of G and the Path Covering Number of G^c

In [39], the entire thing as described in the previous subsection has been re-explored for a general $k \geq 2$, i.e., for the radio k-coloring problem. In fact, the Theorem 1.10 has been extended for any rc_k-coloring problem of G, $k \geq 2$, where $G \in \mathscr{G}_1 \cup \mathscr{G}_2$, $\mathscr{G}_1$ **being the family of triangle-free graphs** and $\mathscr{G}_2$ **being the family of graphs** G **such that each connected component in** G^c **has a Hamiltonian path**. Based on it, for the family $\mathscr{G}_1 \cup \mathscr{G}_2$, Theorem 1.11, which says about relation between the hole index of G and the path covering number of G^c, has been extended for a radio k-coloring problem, where $k \geq 2$ is an arbitrary integer.

Before we dig further, first we state the following two results.

Lemma 1.9 [42] *A graph G has a Hamiltonian path if and only if the graph* $G \vee K_1$ *has a Hamiltonian cycle, where* $G \vee K_1$ *is the graph obtained by adding edges between all the vertices of G and* K_1.

Before we state the following theorem, we need two definitions. Let G be a graph. Then the *connectivity* of G, denoted by $\kappa(G)$, is the minimum size of a vertex set S such that $G - S$ has more connected components than G or has only one vertex.

Also, the independence number, denoted by $\alpha(G)$, is the maximum size of a pairwise nonadjacent vertex set.

Theorem 1.13 [11] *If $\kappa(G) \geq \alpha(G)$, then G has a Hamiltonian cycle (unless $G = K_2$).*

Now we prove the following important lemma which will be used frequently in our subsequent discussion.

Lemma 1.10 [39] *Let L be a rc_k-coloring of a graph G, for $k \geq 2$. Let u, v be two distinct vertices of G such that $u \in L_i$ and $v \in L_j$. If $0 \leq |i - j| \leq k - 1$, then u and v are adjacent in G^c and if $0 \leq |i - j| \leq k - 2$, then for any vertex $w \in V \setminus \{u, v\}$, w is adjacent to either of u, v in G^c.*

Proof If $0 \leq |i - j| \leq k - 1$, then $d(u, v) \geq 2$ in G and therefore $u \sim v$ in G^c.

If $0 \leq |i - j| \leq k - 2$, then $d(u, v) \geq 3$ in G. Therefore, for any vertex $w \in V \setminus \{u, v\}$, we must have either $w \sim u$ or $w \sim v$ in G^c, because otherwise $d(u, v) = 2$ in G, a contradiction.

The following two theorems give the number of connected components of G^c in terms of $rc_k(G)$.

Theorem 1.14 [39] *Let G be a graph of order n and with $rc_k(G) \leq (n - 1)(k - 1)$, $k \geq 2$. Then G^c is connected.*

Proof If L have a multiple color i, there are two distinct vertices u, v in L_i. Hence by Lemma 1.10, G^c is connected.

If not, then L has no multiple colors. Let L have ρ_L number of holes. Then $rc_k = n + \rho_L - 1$ and so $n + \rho_L - 1 \leq (n - 1)(k - 1)$, i.e. $\rho_L \leq (n - 1)(k - 2)$.

If any two successive colors i, j have exactly $(k - 2)$ successive holes between them, then $|i - j| = k - 1$. Therefore, $v^i \sim v^j$ in G^c, by Lemma 1.10. Thus, we get a path P in G^c given by $P : v^0, v^{k-1}, v^{2k-2}, \ldots, v^{(n-1)(k-1)}$. Hence, G^c is connected.

Otherwise, there are successive colors i, j having at most $(k - 3)$ holes between them i.e. $0 \leq |i - j| \leq k - 2$. Then by Lemma 1.10, we have G^c is connected.

Now, we state the following result regarding the number of connected components of G^c when $rc_k(G) > (n - 1)(k - 1)$ without proof.

Theorem 1.15 [39] *Let G be a graph of order n and with $rc_k(G) = (n-1)(k-1)+t$, $t \geq 1$, $k \geq 2$. Then G^c has at most $t + 1$ components.*

The above discussion enables us to obtain an upper bound of $rc_k(G)$ in terms of $c(G^c)$.

Theorem 1.16 [39] *Let G be a graph with $c(G^c) = r$. Then for any $k \geq 2$, $rc_k(G) \leq n(k - 1) + r - k$.*

Proof Let $\{P_1, P_2, \ldots, P_r\}$ be a minimum path covering of G^c, where p_i is the number of vertices of P_i. We denote the jth vertex $(1 \leq j \leq p_i)$ of the ith path $(1 \leq i \leq r)$ as x^i_j.

Now, we define a radio k-coloring f of G as $L(x^i_j) = (\Sigma_{t=1}^{i-1} p_t - i + j)(k-1) + (i-1)k$.
Since $span(f) = (n-r)(k-1) + (r-1)k = n(k-1) + r - k$, therefore for $k \geq 2$, $rc_k(G) \leq n(k-1) + r - k$.

The next theorem shows that for a triangle-free graph G, the upper bound for $rc_k(G)$ obtained in Theorem 1.16 is a necessary and sufficient condition for having a Hamiltonian path in G^c.

Theorem 1.17 [39] *Let G be a triangle-free graph with n vertices. Then for any $k \geq 2$, $rc_k(G) \leq (n-1)(k-1)$ if and only if G^c has a Hamiltonian path.*

Proof Suppose $rc_k(G) \leq (n-1)(k-1)$. Using Theorem 1.14, G^c is connected and hence $\kappa(G^c \vee K_1) \geq 2$. Since G is triangle-free, therefore $\alpha(G^c) \leq 2$ and so $\alpha(G^c \vee K_1) \leq 2$. Thus, $\kappa(G^c \vee K_1) \geq \alpha(G^c \vee K_1)$. So $G^c \vee K_1$ has a Hamiltonian cycle, by Theorem 1.13 and hence by Lemma 1.9, G^c has a Hamiltonian path.

Conversely, if G^c has a Hamiltonian path, then by Theorem 1.16, $rc_k(G) \leq (n-1)(k-1)$.

This completes the proof.

Using Theorems 1.16, 1.17 and an induction on $r = c(G^c)$, we can prove next theorem that provides a closed formula for $rc_k(G)$ when G^c has no Hamiltonian path and G is triangle-free.

Theorem 1.18 [39] *Let G be a triangle-free graph with n vertices. Then for any $k \geq 2$, $rc_k(G) = n(k-1) + r - k$ if and only if $c(G^c) = r$, when $r \geq 2$.*

The next results similar to the above ones deal with graphs in $\mathcal{G}_2$.

Theorem 1.19 [39] *Let $G \in \mathcal{G}_2$ be a graph with n vertices. Then for any $k \geq 2$, $rc_k(G) \leq (n-1)(k-1)$ if and only if G^c has a Hamiltonian path.*

Proof If G^c has a Hamiltonian path, by Theorem 1.16, we have $rc_k(G) \leq (n-1)(k-1)$.
Conversely, let $rc_k(G) \leq (n-1)(k-1)$. Then by Theorem 1.14, G^c is connected and hence has a Hamiltonian path as $G \in \mathcal{G}_2$.

By using Theorems 1.15, 1.16, and 1.19 and an induction on $r = c(G^c)$, the next theorem is obtained to give a closed formula for $rc_k(G)$ when $G \in \mathcal{G}_2$.

Theorem 1.20 [39] *Let $G \in \mathcal{G}_2$ be a graph with n vertices. Then for any $k \geq 2$, $rc_k(G) = n(k-1) + r - k$ if and only if $c(G^c) = r$, when $r \geq 2$.*

Now, we are in a position to extend Theorem 1.11, for any $k \geq 2$ and for any graph $G \in \mathcal{G}_1 \cup \mathcal{G}_2$, to obtain a relation between the $(k-1)$-hole index of G and the path covering number of G^c.

Theorem 1.21 [40] *For any graph $G \in \mathscr{G}_1 \cup \mathscr{G}_2$, $\rho_k(G) = c(G^c) - 1$, if $rc_k(G) \geq (n-1)(k-1)$.*

Proof Let $r = c(G^c)$.

Case I: Suppose $rc_k(G) = (n-1)(k-1)$. Then by Theorems 1.17 and 1.19, G^c has a Hamiltonian path. Let a Hamiltonian path in G^c be $P : x_0, x_1, \ldots, x_{(n-1)}$. We now define a radio k-coloring L on G by $L(x_i) = i(k-1), 0 \leq i \leq n-1$. Clearly, $span(L) = (n-1)(k-1)$ and so L is an rc_k-coloring on G and $\rho_k(G) = 0 = c(G^c) - 1$.

Case II: Let $rc_k(G) > (n-1)(k-1)$. Then by Theorems 1.18 and 1.20, $r \geq 2$ and $rc_k(G) = n(k-1) + r - k$. Let G^c has a minimum path covering $\mathscr{P} = \{P^{(1)}, P^{(2)}, \ldots, P^{(r)}\}$. Also let the j-th vertex, $1 \leq j \leq p_i$, of the $P^{(i)}$, $1 \leq i \leq r$, be x^i_j, where p_i is the number of vertices of $P^{(i)}$. Let us define a radio k-coloring L of G as $L(x^i_j) = (\Sigma_{t=1}^{i-1} p_t - i + j)(k-1) + (i-1)k$. Then $span(L) = n(k-1) + r - k$, i.e., L is a rc_k-coloring on G and L has $(r-1)$ number of $(k-1)$-holes. Hence, $\rho_k(G) \leq r - 1 = c(G^c) - 1$.

Suppose $\hat{L} \in \Lambda_{\rho_k}(G)$ and $I_0, I_1, \ldots, I_{\rho_k(G)}$ be the islands of $\hat{L}$. Now, using Lemma 1.10, the vertices in the set $A_i = \{u : \hat{L}(u) \in I_i\}$ form a path $Q^{(i)}$ (say) in G^c, for $0 \leq i \leq \rho_k(G)$. Thus, $\{Q^{(0)}, Q^{(1)}, \ldots, Q^{(\rho_k(G))}\}$ is a path covering of G^c. Hence, $c(G^c) \leq \rho_k(G) + 1$.
Therefore $\rho_k(G) = c(G^c) - 1$. This completes the proof.

The next result shows that the value of $\rho_k(G)$ remains unchanged for any $k \geq 2$.

Corollary 1.3 [40] *For any graph $G \in \mathscr{G}_1 \cup \mathscr{G}_2$, let $c(G^c) \geq 2$. Then $\rho_{k_1}(G) = \rho_{k_2}(G)$, for any integers $k_1, k_2 \geq 2$ and hence $\rho_k(G) = \rho(G)$, for every integer $k > 2$.*

Proof Proof follows directly from Theorems 1.18, 1.20 and 1.21.

We now study the $(k-1)$-hole index of some families of graphs. The following discussion is the consequences of Theorem 1.20 in [39] and Theorem 1.21 in [40].

Corollary 1.4 *Let $G = K_{m_1, m_2, \ldots, m_r}$ $(r \geq 2)$ be a complete multipartite graph of order n. Then $\rho_k(G) = r - 1$, for $k \geq 2$.*

Proof Clearly, $G^c = K_{m_1} + K_{m_2} + \cdots + K_{m_r}$ and thus $G \in \mathscr{G}_2$. Hence by Theorem 1.20, $rc_k(G) = n(k-1) + r - k$. Therefore, the proof follows by Theorem 1.21.

Let F be a group and $S \subset F$ be such that S does not contain the identity element and $g \in S$ if and only if $g^{-1} \in S$. Then the Cayley graph $G = Cay(F, S)$ is the graph with the vertex set F and the edge set $\{gh : hg^{-1} \in S\}$.

Corollary 1.5 *Let $G = Cay(\mathbb{Z}_n, S)$ where $S = \mathbb{Z}_n \setminus \{\overline{0}, \overline{m}, -\overline{m}\}$ such that $gcd(m, n) > 1$. Then for any $k \geq 2$, $\rho_k(G) = gcd(m, n) - 1$, when $k \geq 2$.*

Proof Now $G^c = Cay(\mathbb{Z}_n, \{\pm\overline{m}\})$. Since the element $\overline{m}$ in the group $(\mathbb{Z}_n, +)$ is of order $\frac{n}{gcd(m,n)}$, therefore $\mathbb{Z}_n \neq <\overline{m}>$ and $<\overline{m}>$ has $gcd(m,n)$ number of cosets in $\mathbb{Z}_n$. Now, the subgraphs induced by the elements of cosets of $<\overline{m}>$ in $\mathbb{Z}_n$ are the connected components of G^c. Let $a+<\overline{m}>$ be a coset of $<\overline{m}>$ in $\mathbb{Z}_n$. Then $P: a, a+\overline{m}, a+2\overline{m}, \ldots, a+(\frac{n}{gcd(m,n)}-1)\overline{m}$ is a path through the vertices of the connected component of G^c induced by the elements of $a+<\overline{m}>$ and therefore $G \in \mathscr{G}_2$. Hence, the number of cosets is the path covering number of G^c, i.e., $c(G^c) = gcd(m,n)$. Using Theorem 1.20, $rc_k(G) = n(k-1) + gcd(m,n) - k$ and so the proof follows by Theorem 1.21.

1.6 Some Interesting Properties of Island Sequence

First, we recall that the nondecreasing sequence of cardinalities of islands of an rc_k-coloring in $\Lambda_{\rho_k}(G)$ is the island sequence of the coloring. The island sequences of rc_k-colorings in $\Lambda_{\rho_k}(G)$ exhibit several interesting properties. Some of them hold for any $k \geq 2$ and the others hold for the particular case $k = 2$. The first subsection deals with an issue for general k, and the last two subsections are about $k = 2$.

1.6.1 Can a Finite Sequence Be a k-Island Sequence for the Same Graph and for Every $k \geq 2$?

In [40], a question was raised and solved regarding whether there may be a finite sequence such that it would be a k-island sequence of some rc_k-coloring in $\Lambda_{\rho_k}(G)$ for every $k \geq 2$. The following result deals with this issue.

Theorem 1.22 [40] *For any graph $G \in \mathscr{G}_1 \cup \mathscr{G}_2$, if $c(G^c) \geq 2$, then there exists a finite sequence of positive integers which is admitted as a k-island sequence by some $L \in \Lambda_{\rho_k}(G)$, for every $k \geq 2$.*

Proof Suppose $r = c(G^c) \geq 2$ and $\mathscr{P} = \{P^{(1)}, P^{(2)}, \ldots, P^{(r)}\}$ be a minimum path covering of G^c. Also, let p_i be the number of vertices of $P^{(i)}$. Now, for any $k \geq 2$, $rc_k(G) = n(k-1)+r-k$, using Theorems 1.18 and 1.20. Without loss of generality, let $p_1 \leq p_2 \leq \cdots \leq p_r$. Let the jth vertex, $1 \leq j \leq p_i$, of $P^{(i)}$, $1 \leq i \leq r$, be x^i_j. We now define a radio k-coloring L of G by $L(x^i_j) = (\Sigma_{t=1}^{i-1} p_t - i + j)(k-1) + (i-1)k$. Clearly, L is a rc_k-coloring on G and L has $(r-1) = \rho_k(G)$ number of $(k-1)$-holes, by Theorem 1.21. Hence, $L \in \Lambda_{\rho_k}(G)$. Since the colors of vertices in each path $P^{(i)}$ together form a k-island of L and each vertex receives distinct color, therefore the k-island sequence of L is $(p_1, p_2, \ldots, p_r)$. As $k \geq 2$ is an arbitrary integer, the proof is complete.

In the rest of this section, by islands we will mean only 2-islands.

1.6.2 On Graphs Admitting Different 2-Island Sequences

In [16], a very interesting question regarding island sequence has been raised in the perspective of radio 2-coloring i.e., $L(2,1)$-coloring problem. To understand the question, we need to take a look into Figs. 1.12 and 1.13. Figure 1.12 illustrates existence of two $\lambda_{2,1}$-labelings on the connected graph $K_{2,3}$ admitting two distinct sets of islands with the same island sequence (2, 3), whereas Fig. 1.13 is an example of the existence of a disconnected graph $K_5 + K_2$ which admits two distinct island sequences (1, 1, 5) and (1, 3, 3).

Keeping this in mind, Georges et al. [16] raised the question that **whether there exists a connected graph admitting distinct island sequences**. In [2], this problem was handled. But before we dig further, we need to be acquainted with the following terms proposed in [2].

A vertex in a graph is said to be *heavy vertex* if its degree is at least three; otherwise, the vertex is a *light vertex*. An edge incident to two heavy vertices is a *heavy edge*. A graph is a *2-sparse graph* if no two heavy vertices in it are adjacent.

Now, we prove the following results.

Lemma 1.11 [2] *Let v be a heavy vertex in a 2-sparse graph G. Then v is an internal vertex in every minimum path covering of G.*

Proof If possible, let v be an end vertex of a path P in a minimum path covering $\mathscr{P}$ of G. As v is a heavy vertex and G is a 2-sparse graph, v has a light neighbor, say, u which is an end vertex of a path, say, Q, another member of $\mathscr{P}$. Therefore, $(P + Q) + e$, where the edge $e = uv$, is a path and so G has a path covering with fewer cardinality, a contradiction.

Lemma 1.12 [2] *Let e be an edge incident to two light vertices of a tree T. Then e is contained in every minimum path covering of T.*

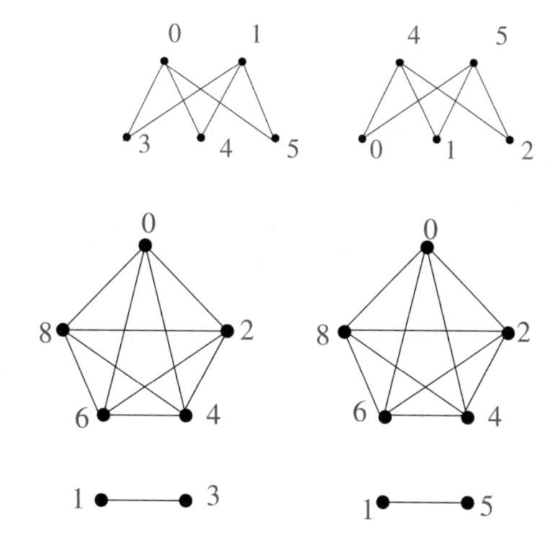

Fig. 1.12 Examples of distinct $\lambda_{2,1}$-labeling on same graph admitting same island sequence

Fig. 1.13 Examples of two $\lambda_{2,1}$-labelings on same graph admitting distinct island sequences

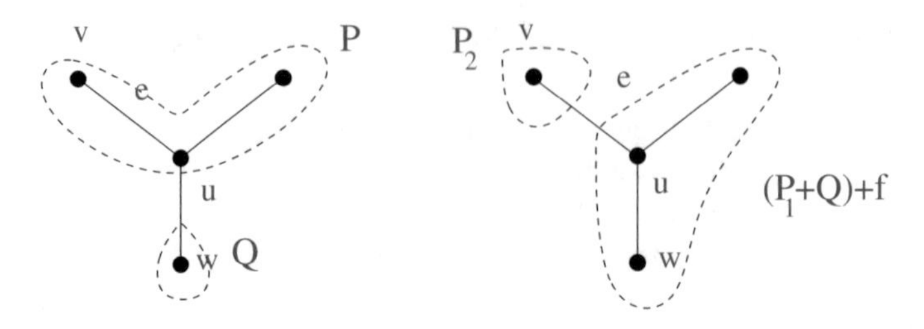

Fig. 1.14 Illustrating swapping

Proof If not, then the two light vertices incident to e are end vertices of two distinct paths, say, P and Q in a minimum path covering of T, and hence, the path $(P+Q)+e$ is a member of a new path covering of T with fewer cardinality, a contradiction.

Let T be a tree. Then a maximal path S, with a leaf as one end, in T is *a vine* in T if each vertex in S is a light vertex of T. If T is not a path, then there is a heavy vertex adjacent to one end of the vine other than the leaf. This unique heavy vertex is called *the center* of the vine S.

With the above result, the following lemma is an easy observation.

Lemma 1.13 [2] *Every vine in a 2-sparse tree T is a subgraph of every minimum path covering of T.*

We now develop a tool that constructs two different vertex-disjoint paths from two given vertex-disjoint paths P and Q where P contains an edge $e = uv$, u being an internal vertex of P, and u is adjacent to one end vertex w of Q. Deleting e gives two paths P_1 and P_2 such that one of them, say, P_1 has u as an end vertex. Then $(P_1 + Q) + f$, where the edge $f = uw$, and P_2 are two vertex-disjoint paths containing the same vertices exhausted by P and Q. This construction is referred in [2] as *swapping e with f* (illustrated in Fig. 1.14).

Let S be a vine in a 2-sparse tree T with p leaves. Now, by Lemma 1.13, S is a subgraph of a path P in an arbitrary minimum path covering $\mathscr{P}$ of T. If the center v of S is included in P, then v must be an internal vertex of P, by Lemma 1.11, and v is adjacent to an end vertex of another path Q of $\mathscr{P}$ through an edge f. Let the edge be $e = uv$, where u is an end vertex of S. Then swapping e with f gives a new minimum path covering of T.

Using this argument and induction principle on p along with the fact that $T - S$ is a 2-sparse tree with $(p - 1)$ leaves, we obtain the following result.

Theorem 1.23 [2] *If T is a 2-sparse tree with p leaves and T is not a single vertex, then $c(T) = p - 1$.*

Now using Theorems 1.10, 1.11, and 1.23, the next result follows.

Theorem 1.24 [2] *Let T be a 2-sparse tree with p leaves and n vertices. If T is not a path, then $\lambda_{2,1}(T^c) = n + p - 3$ and $\rho(T^c) = p - 2$.*

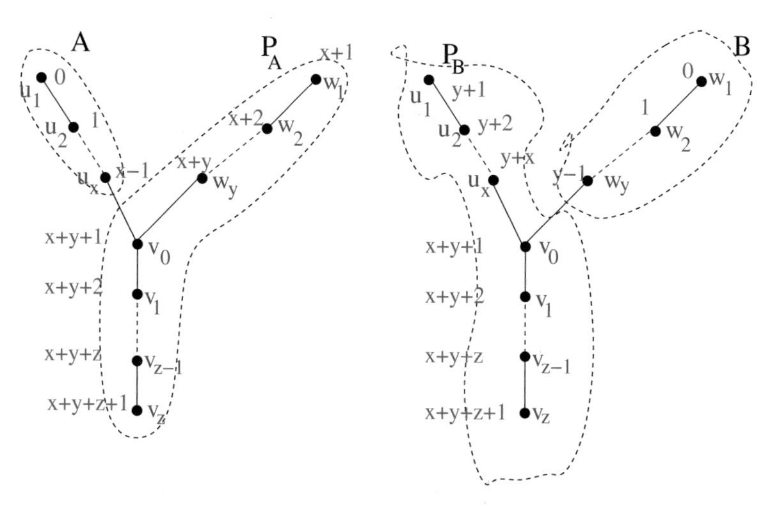

Fig. 1.15 Two minimum path coverings of T with colors written in red

Before we proceed further, let us extend the classical notion of star. A tree with exactly one heavy vertex and same number of vertices in all its vines is a *generalized star*. Now, we are in a position to discuss the following theorem.

Theorem 1.25 [2] *Let T be a 2-sparse tree. If T is neither a path nor a generalized star, then T^c admits two different island sequences.*

Sketch of proof. Let p be the number of leaves in T. Then $p \geq 3$.

First we assume that T has exactly three leaves. Then T has exactly three vines, say, $A = u_1u_2 \ldots u_x$, $B = w_1w_2 \ldots w_y$ and $C = v_1v_2 \ldots v_z$ with same center, say, v_0 adjacent to u_x, w_y and v_1. Since T is not a generalized star, without loss of generality, we can assume $x < y$. By Theorem 1.23, $c(T) = 2$ and by Theorem 1.24, $\lambda_{2,1}(T^c) = x + y + z + 1$ and $\rho(T^c) = 1$.

Now, the vine A, together with the path P_A induced by vertices of the vines B and C, along with the center v_0, forms a minimum path covering of T. Again, the vine B, together with the path induced by vertices of the vines A and C, along with the center v_0, forms a minimum path covering of T. From Fig. 1.15, it is evident that T^c admits two distinct island sequences $(x, y + z + 1)$ and $(x + y + z, y)$, ignoring the nondecreasing order.

Applying induction on p, the proof follows. □

Now we prove the following result.

Lemma 1.14 [2] *Let T be a 2-sparse tree. If T is neither a path nor a generalized star, then T^c is connected.*

Proof **Case I** Let u, v be two leaves of T such that u and v are not adjacent to the same vertex in T. Then every vertex is adjacent to either of u, v in T^c. Also, u and v are adjacent in T^c. Hence, T^c is connected.

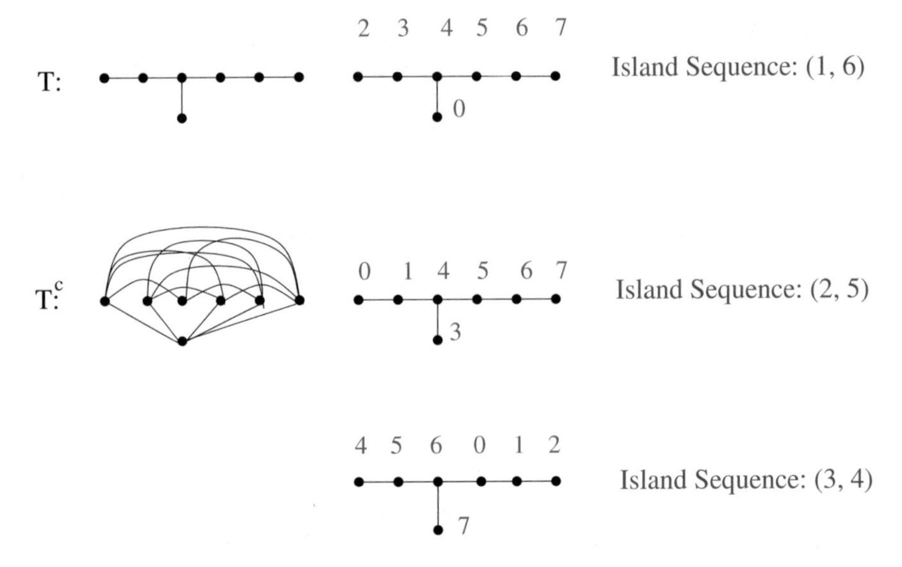

Fig. 1.16 Different $\lambda_{2,1}$-colorings and island sequences of T^c

Case II Let u, v be two leaves of T such that u and v are adjacent to the same vertex, say, w in T. As T is not a star, so T has at least one vine of length at least two with w as its center. Therefore, using Case I, it can be shown that T^c is connected.

Theorem 1.25 and Lemma 1.14 together prove the main result of this subsection.

Theorem 1.26 [2] *There exists an infinite family of connected graphs that admit at least two different island sequences.*

Figure 1.16 gives an example of a 2-sparse tree T such that $\lambda_{2,1}(T^c) = 7, \rho(T^c) = 1$ and T^c admits three different island sequences.

1.6.3 On Graphs Admitting Unique 2-Island Sequence

In light of the previous discussion, a natural question arises: **whether there is graph admitting a unique island sequence in the perspective of radio 2-coloring i.e., $L(2,1)$-coloring problem**. The answer is affirmative (see [32]). But before we explore the solution, we need the following terms.

First, we define the path sequence which is a complementary notion of island sequence. Let $\mathscr{P}$ be a minimum path covering of G. The *path sequence of* $\mathscr{P}$ is the ordered sequence of the numbers of vertices of each path in $\mathscr{P}$ listed in nondecreasing order.

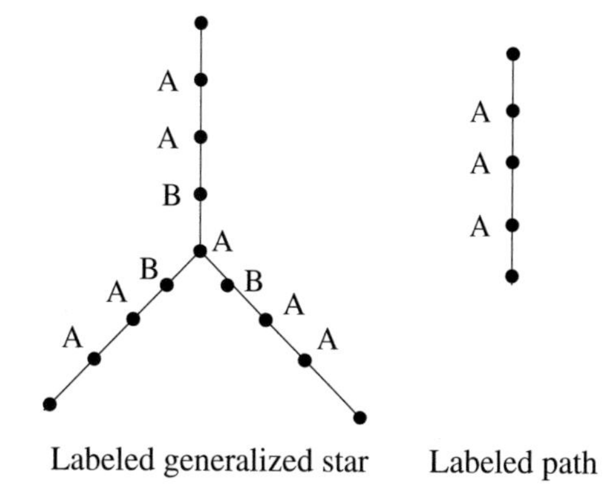

Fig. 1.17 Illustrating labeled generalized star and labeled path

Remark 1.3 By the $L(2, 1)$-coloring in Eq. 1.3 in Sect. 1.5 for obtaining the upper bound of $\lambda_{2,1}(G)$ and the subsequent discussion in subsection 1.5.1, we can say that if $c(G^c) \geq 2$, then a minimum path covering of G^c can induce a $\lambda_{2,1}$-labeling f of G with $\rho(G) = c(G^c) - 1$ holes [see Theorem 1.11]. Now, the island sequence of f is same as the path sequence of G^c. Thus, G admits a unique island sequence if and only if G^c admits a unique path sequence and $c(G^c) \geq 2$.

We now define a labeled generalized star and labeled path. A *labeled generalized star* is a generalized star in which every non-leaf neighbor of its center is labeled B and every other non-leaf vertex is labeled A. A *labeled path* is a path with at least three vertices in which every non-leaf vertex is labeled A (see Fig. 1.17).

Before we proceed further, we state the following lemmas without proof.

Lemma 1.15 [32] *Let S be a vine of a graph G. Then S is a subgraph of every minimum path covering of G.*

Lemma 1.16 [32] *Let v be a vertex of a tree T. If v has at least two light neighbors, then v is an internal vertex in any minimum path covering of T.*

Lemma 1.17 [32] *Let v be a heavy vertex of a tree T and e be an edge incident to v. Then e is not used in some minimum path covering of T and hence $c(T) = c(T - e)$ if one of the following conditions holds.*
(a) v has at least three light neighbors;
(b) v has exactly two light neighbors, and e is not incident to any light vertex.

We now define a family of labeled trees introduced in [32]. Let $\mathscr{F}$ be a family of labeled trees. A labeled tree T is an element of $\mathscr{F}$ if and only if T is a labeled generalized star with at least three vines or a labeled path or T can be constructed by using at least one operations among Type-1, Type-2, and Type-3 to some element T' of $\mathscr{F}$, where all the non-leaf vertices of T' are labeled A or B. The operations are described below.

Type-1 operation: Attach a labeled generalized star S with at least three vines to T' by adding an edge uv, u being an A-labeled vertex in T' and v being an A-labeled

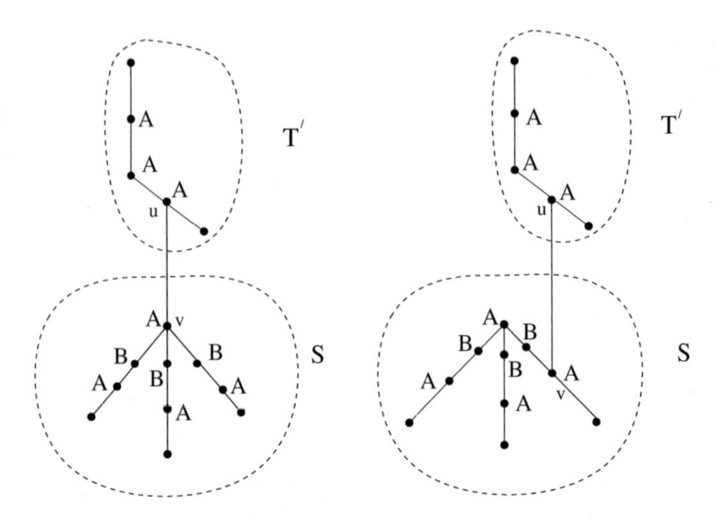

Fig. 1.18 Illustrating Type-1 operation

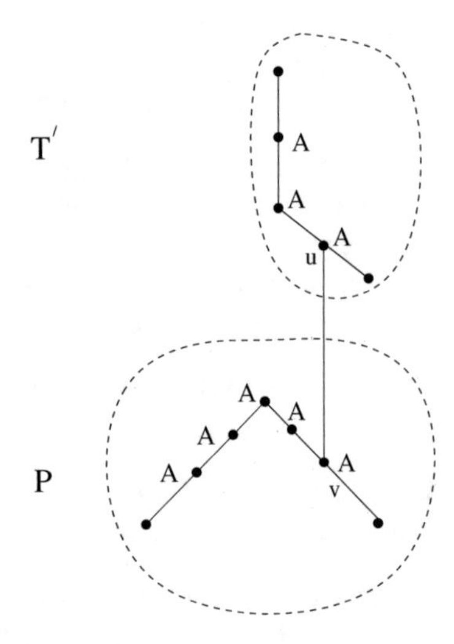

Fig. 1.19 Illustrating Type-2 operation

vertex in S. Clearly, v can be chosen in two ways: (i) v is the center of S, or (ii) v is a vertex labeled A in a vine of S (see Fig. 1.18).

Type-2 operation: Attach a labeled path P to T' by adding an edge uv, u being an A-labeled vertex in T' and v being any non-leaf vertex in P (see Fig. 1.19).

Type-3 operation: Attach a labeled generalized star S to T' by adding an edge uv, u being an B-labeled vertex in T' and v being the center of S such that the length of each vine in S is the same as that of the labeled generalized star S', which is the original/previously attached labeled generalized star containing u (see Fig. 1.20).

Now we focus on the main result of this subsection.

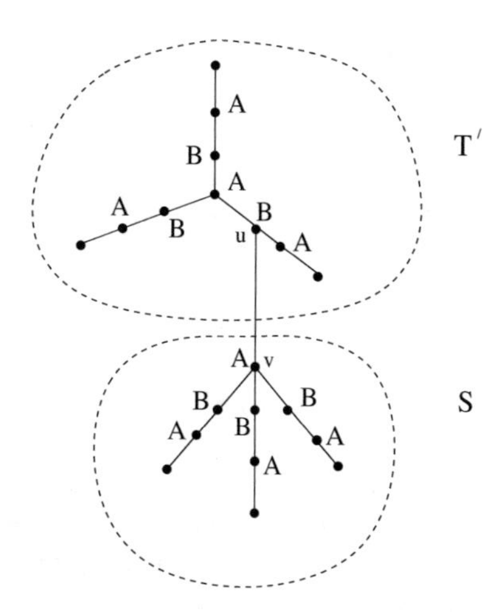

Fig. 1.20 Illustrating Type-3 operation

Theorem 1.27 [32] *Every labeled tree in $\mathscr{F}$ admits a unique path sequence.*

Sketch of proof. Let T be a labeled tree in $\mathscr{F}$ and $s(T)$ be the number of operations required to construct T. To prove that T admits a unique path sequence, we use induction on $s(T)$.

If $s(T) = 0$, T is either a labeled path or a labeled generalized star with at least three vines. In either case, T admits a unique path sequences.

Let all trees T' in $\mathscr{F}$ with $s(T') < k$, $k \geq 1$ being an integer, admit a unique path sequence.

Let $T \in \mathscr{F}$ with $s(T) = k$. Then T must be obtained from a $T' \in \mathscr{F}$ with $s(T') < k$ by using any one of Type-1, Type-2, and Type-3 operations. By induction hypothesis, T' admits a unique path sequence.

Case I: Let T be obtained from T' by using a Type-1 operation. Since v (labeled A) has at least three light neighbors distinct from u or exactly two light neighbors distinct from u, therefore by Lemma 1.17 and Theorem 1.23, $c(T) = c(T') + l - 1$, where $l \geq 3$ is the number of leaves of S.

If possible, let the edge uv be included in some path, say, P of a minimum path covering of T. Now, by Lemma 1.16, v is an internal vertex of P. Let w be a neighbor of v in S such that w is not in P. Swapping uv with vw gives a new minimum path covering of T avoiding uv. This induces a minimum path covering of T' with u (labeled A) as an end vertex of path in it. But it can be shown that every vertex, which is labeled A, is an internal vertex in any minimum path covering of a tree in $\mathscr{F}$. Hence, we arrive at a contradiction.

Thus every minimum path covering of T avoids the edge uv. Also, by induction hypothesis, T' and S admit unique path sequences. Therefore, T admits a unique path sequences.

Case II: Similar argument follows if T is obtained by Type-2 operation, and it can be shown that the edge uv does not belong to any path in any minimum path covering of T. This concludes the case.

Case III: Let T be obtained from T' by a Type-3 operation. As v has at least three light neighbors in S, by Lemma 1.17(a) and by Theorem 1.23, $c(T) = c(T') + l - 1$, where $l \geq 3$ is the number of leaves of S. By induction hypothesis, T' and S admit unique path sequences, say, $(x_1, x_2, \ldots, x_{c(T')})$ and $(s_1, s_1, \ldots, 2s_1 + 1)$, respectively, where the length of the path sequence of S is $l - 1$, and s_1 is the number of vertices in a vine in S. Therefore, ignoring the nondecreasing order, we can say $(x_1, x_2, \ldots, x_{c(T')}, s_1, s_1, \ldots, 2s_1 + 1)$ is a path sequence of T, as the edge uv is not included in a minimum path covering of T, by Lemma 1.17.

We now consider the situation when uv is in a path, say, P with p vertices in a minimum path covering $\mathscr{P}$ (say) of T. By Lemma 1.16, v is an internal vertex of P which must contain a vine of S. Since S has at least three vines, therefore using Lemma 1.15, there exists a vine of S as a path in $\mathscr{P}$. Let w be an end of this vine of S such that w is adjacent to v. Swapping uv by vw gives a new minimum path covering $\mathscr{P}'$, say, of T avoiding uv. Clearly, u is at the end of a path, say, P' in $\mathscr{P}'$ with $p - (s_1 + 1)$ vertices.

It can be shown that the vine in T' containing u is a path in the minimum path covering of T' induced by $\mathscr{P}'$. Since T is obtained by Type-3 operation, this vine is in the original/previously attached labeled generalized star S' while obtaining T'. Moreover, length of vines of S and S' are the same. Thus, P' also has s_1 vertices. Hence, $p - (s_1 + 1) = s_1$, i.e., $p = 2s_1 + 1$. Using induction hypothesis on T' and S, we can again have a path sequence of T induced by $\mathscr{P}'$ is $(x_1, x_2, \ldots, x_{c(T')}, s_1, s_1, \ldots, 2s_1 + 1)$. Clearly, the sequence does not get changed if we swap vw with uv to obtain $\mathscr{P}$ from $\mathscr{P}'$. This concludes the case. □

The above theorem implies the following result which establishes the existence of connected graph with a unique island sequence.

Corollary 1.6 [32] *Let $T \in \mathscr{F}$. Then T^c admits a unique island sequence.*

1.7 Some Extremal Problems Related to 1-Hole Index of Graphs

In this section, we study some extremal situations regarding $\rho_2(G)$, i.e., $\rho(G)$ and $\mu_2(G)$, i.e., $\mu(G)$.

1.7.1 An Extremal Situation Regarding $\mu(G)$

Here, we discuss an extremal situation regarding $\mu(G)$. But to appreciate its importance, first, we need the following result which gives an upper bound of $\mu(G)$ in terms of $\lambda_{2,1}(G)$ and $\rho(G)$. After proving this upper bound, we will see that for every positive integer m, there is a graph G with $\rho(G) = m$ such that $\mu(G)$ attains the upper bound.

Theorem 1.28 [12] *Let G be a graph with order $n \geq \lambda_{2,1}(G) + 2$ and $\rho(G) \geq 1$. Then $\mu(G) \leq \lambda_{2,1}(G) + \rho(G)$.*

Proof Let $L \in \Lambda_\rho(G)$ and $h_1, h_2, \ldots, h_{\rho(G)}$ be the holes in L where $0 < h_1 < h_2 < \ldots < h_{\rho(G)} < \lambda_{2,1}(G)$. Since $n \geq \lambda_{2,1}(G) + 2$, therefore L must have multiple colors, and hence, L has no gap, by Lemma 1.7. Then by Corollary 1.1, $l_{h_i-1} = l_{h_i+1} = l_{h_j-1} = l_{h_j+1} > 1$, for all i, j with $1 \leq i < j \leq \rho(G)$.

Let $u \in L_{h_i-1}$. Then there is a vertex $v \in L_{h_i+1}$ such that $u \sim v$ and $w \in L_{h_{i+1}+1}$ such that $v \nsim w$.

Case I: Let $I_i(L)$ be not an atoll. Then let $p \in L_{h_{i+1}-1}$ such that $p \sim w$. We define a new $L(2, 1)$-coloring f on G as follows:

$$\begin{aligned}
&u \mapsto h_i;\\
&v \mapsto \text{first unused integer} > \lambda_{2,1}(G);\\
&p \mapsto h_{i+1};\\
&w \mapsto f(v) + 1;\\
&f(x) = L(x), \text{if} x \neq u, v, p, w.
\end{aligned}$$

Case II: Let $I_i(L)$ be an atoll. Then we define a new $L(2, 1)$-coloring f on G as follows:

$$\begin{aligned}
&u \mapsto h_i;\\
&v \mapsto h_i + 2;\\
&w \mapsto \text{first unused integer} > \lambda_{2,1}(G), \text{ if } I_{i+1}(L) \text{ is not an atoll;}\\
&\text{or } w \mapsto h_{i+2}, \text{ if } I_{i+1}(L) \text{ is an atoll.}
\end{aligned}$$

Repeating the same argument for each $i = 1, 2, \ldots, \rho(G)$, the proof follows.

We now study the possibility of equality of the relation in Theorem 1.28, which is an extremal situation of the said theorem.

Theorem 1.29 [12] *For every $m \geq 1$, there is a graph G with $\rho(G) = m$ and $\mu(G) = \lambda_{2,1}(G) + m$.*

Proof First we construct a graph G_m with $5(m + 1)$ vertices, for every $m \geq 2$, by taking two disjoint copies of $K_{2(m+1)}$, say, A and B, and a copy C (say) of K_{m+1}, disjoint from $A + B$. Let the vertices of A are $a_0, a_2, a_4, \ldots, a_{4m+2}$; the vertices of B are $b_0, b_2, b_4, \ldots, b_{4m+2}$ and the vertices of C are $c_1, c_5. c_9, \ldots, c_{4m+1}$.

Apart from the edges in between the vertices of A, B and C, there are additional edges in G_m described as follows.

(i) edges between c_1 and each of $a_4, a_6, \ldots, a_{4m+2}$;
(ii) edges between c_5 and each of a_0, a_2;
(iii) edges between c_5 and each of $b_8, b_{10}, \ldots, b_{4m+2}$;
(iv) edges between c_i and b_k if $|j - k| \geq 2$, for every $j \geq 9$.

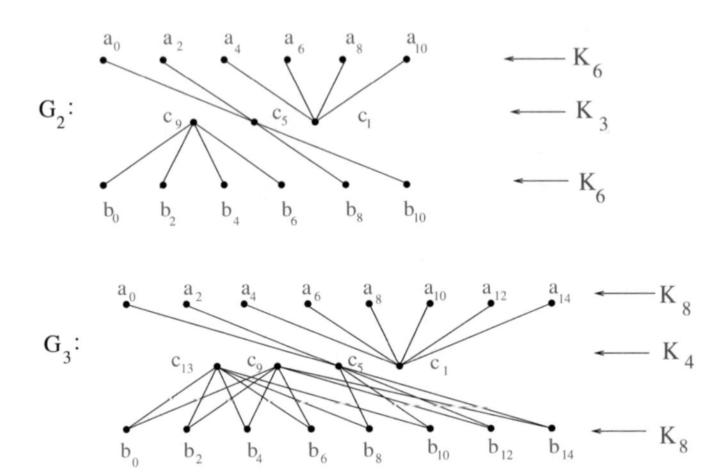

Fig. 1.21 Examples of G_2 and G_3

We illustrate G_2 and G_3 in the Fig. 1.21.

Note that $d(a_i, b_i) = 3$, for each $i = 0, 2, 4, \ldots, 4m + 2$. Also, in view of the additional adjacency conditions described above, we assign color f on G_m given by $f(a_i) = i$ and $f(b_j) = j$, for $i, j = 0, 2, 4, \ldots, 4m + 2$. Moreover, $f(c_t) = t$ for $t = 1, 5, 9, \ldots, 4m + 1$. Clearly f is an $L(2, 1)$-coloring of G_m with span $4m + 2$. But $\lambda_{2,1}(K_{2m+2}) = 4m + 2$. Therefore, $\lambda_{2,1}(G_m) = 4m + 2$. Also $\rho(G_m) \leq m$.

Again, since G_m contains K_{2m+2}, every $\lambda_{2,1}$-coloring on G_m assigns the colors in $\{0, 2, 4, \ldots, 4m + 2\}$ to precisely one vertex in each of A and B. Also, the $(m + 1)$ vertices of C can engage at most $(m + 1)$ vertices distinct from colors of A and B. Hence in any $\lambda_{2,1}$-coloring on G_m has at least $(4m + 3) - (2m + 2) - (m + 1) = m$ holes. Therefore, $\rho(G_m) = m$.

Let L be an $L(2, 1)$-coloring of G_m so that L assigns every color in $\{0, 1, 2, \ldots, span(L)\}$ to some vertex in G_m. Let k be a multiple color in L. Since any vertex in C is at a distance at most 2 from any other vertex, k cannot be assigned to c_i, for $i = 1, 5, 9, \ldots, 4m + 1$. Then k is assigned to one vertex in each of A and B such that these two vertices are not adjacent to the same vertex in C. Also, note that these two vertices of A and B are together adjacent to m vertices in C. So none of these m vertices of C and no vertex in A as well as B can be assigned colors from $\{k - 1, k + 1\}$. Hence, only one vertex in C is left to be colored from $\{k - 1, k + 1\}$. This contradicts the prerequisite of L, unless $k = 0$ or $span(L)$. Hence, no color other than 0 and $span(L)$ can be a multiple color. Also $l_k = 2$.

Thus at most four vertices can receive multiple colors (i.e., 0 and $span(L)$ can be assigned to two vertices each). Hence, each of the remaining $(5m + 1)$ uncolored vertices will be assigned a distinct color in $\{1, 2, \ldots, span(L) - 1\}$. Hence, $\mu(G) \geq span(L) = 5m + 2$, i.e., $\mu(G) \geq \lambda_{2,1}(G_m) + m$.

Using Theorem 1.28, we have $\mu(G) = \lambda_{2,1}(G_m) + m$.

1.7.2 An Extremal Situation Regarding $\rho(G)$

For any graph G with $\lambda_{2,1}(G) = 2m$, for some integer $m \geq 2$, any $\lambda_{2,1}$-coloring of G uses at most $(2m + 1)$ colors and since it does not have two consecutive holes, therefore $\rho(G) \leq m$. In this scenario, the natural question arises: **Given an integer $m \geq 2$, is there any graph G with $\lambda_{2,1}(G) = 2m$ such that $\rho(G) = m$?**

We now assume that G_1 and G_2 are two isomorphic copies of K_{m+1} under the isomorphisms ϕ_1 and ϕ_2, respectively, where $V(K_{m+1}) = \{x_1, x_2, \ldots, x_{m+1}\}$. Also let $V(G_1) = \{u_1, u_2, \ldots, u_{m+1}\}$ and $V(G_2) = \{v_1, v_2, \ldots, v_{m+1}\}$ such that $\phi_1(x_i) \mapsto u_i$ and $\phi_2(x_i) \mapsto v_i$. Let $e = x_1 x_{m+1}$. Then the e-exchange G of the graph $G_1 + G_2$ (defined in Sect. 1.4) is a connected m-regular graph of order $2(m + 1)$. Therefore by Theorem 1.5, $\lambda_{2,1}(G) = 2m$ and $\rho(G) = m$ (See Fig. 1.6 for an example when $m = 3$).

From the above discussion, the following theorem follows.

Theorem 1.30 [12] *For every integer $m \geq 2$, there exists a connected graph G with $n = 2(m + 1)$ vertices such that $\lambda_{2,1}(G) = 2m$ and $\rho(G) = m$.*

1.7.3 A New Family and a Characterization of Graphs G with $\lambda_{2,1}(G) = 2m$ and $\rho(G) = m$

We now focus on the graphs G with $\lambda_{2,1}(G) = 2m$ and $\rho(G) = m$. We define a new family of graphs. For positive integers s, m, let $G(s, m)$ denotes the family of $(m + 1)$-partite graphs G with partite sets $V_0, V_1, \ldots, V_m$ such that $|V_0| = |V_1| = \cdots = |V_m| = s$ and for any i, j $(0 \leq i < j \leq m)$, the subgraph induced by $V_i \cup V_j$ is a perfect matching (defined in Sect. 1.4). Now, we prove the following theorem.

Theorem 1.31 [31] *For every integer $m \geq 1$, if a graph G has $\lambda_{2,1}(G) = 2m$ and $\rho(G) = m$, then $G \in G(s, m)$, for some integer $s \geq 1$.*

Proof Let $\lambda_{2,1}(G) = 2m$ and $\rho(G) = m$. Then any $L \in \Lambda_\rho(G)$ has $(m + 1)$ islands and every island is an atoll. Therefore, the proof follows using Corollary 1.1.

Thus, if $\lambda_{2,1}(G) = 2m$ and $\rho(G) = m$, then G has $s(m + 1)$ vertices. It is easy to see that $G \in G(1, m)$ if and only if G is isomorphic to K_{m+1}. Thus, G has $(m + 1)$ vertices, $\lambda_{2,1}(G) = 2m$ and $\rho(G) = m$, for some integer $m \geq 1$, if and only if $G \in G(1, m)$. This raises a natural question that **whether $G \in G(2, m)$ is a necessary and sufficient condition for $|V(G)| = 2(m + 1)$, $\lambda_{2,1}(G) = 2m$ and $\rho(G) = m$**. The following theorem gives an affirmative answer to this issue.

Theorem 1.32 [31] *For every integer $m \geq 1$ and any graph G, $|V(G)| = 2(m+1)$, $\lambda_{2,1}(G) = 2m$ and $\rho(G) = m$ if and only if $G \in G(2, m)$.*

Sketch of proof. Using Theorem 1.31 and the fact that $|V(G)| = 2(m+1)$, it can be easily proved that $G \in G(2, m)$ is a necessary condition.

To prove that it is a sufficient condition, let $G \in G(2, m)$. Then $V(G) = \cup_{i=0}^{m} V_i$, where $V_i = \{x_i, y_i\}$ is an independent set for each i, $0 \leq i \leq m$, and the subgraph induced by $V_i \cup V_j$ is a perfect matching, for all i, j with $0 \leq i < j \leq m$. Then $d(x_i, y_i) \geq 3$ for all $i, 0 \leq i \leq m$. We define an $L(2, 1)$-coloring L on G by assigning color $2i$ to each vertex in V_i, for all i, $0 \leq i \leq m$. Then $\lambda_{2,1}(G) \leq 2m$.

Now, since $\lambda_{2,1}(G) \leq 2m$ and $|V(G)| = 2(m+1)$, therefore any $\lambda_{2,1}$-coloring of G has a multiple color. Let f be any coloring in $\Lambda_\rho(G)$ and i be a multiple color of f. We can show that for any pair of vertices x, y with $d(x, y) \geq 3$ and a vertex $z \in V(G) \setminus \{x, y\}$, either $x \sim z$ or $y \sim z$. Hence, it can be proved that $l_i = 2$.

Also, we can show that every color in f is a multiple color. Hence, $l_j = 2$ for $j = 0, 2, 4, \ldots, 2m$ and consequently, $1, 3, \ldots, 2m-1$ are holes in f. Hence, the proof follows. □

Until now, we have discussed different theoretical aspects of hole related issues. Now, we turn our attention towards a practical scenario.

1.8 Construction of Larger Graph Without Increasing Radio k-Chromatic Number When $(k-1)$-Hole Index Is Positive

The scarcity and the high cost of radio spectrum bandwidth are pushing the need for an extension of a network without procuring additional frequencies such that the allocated frequencies assigned to the old stations remain unchanged. This problem may be interpreted as a construction of a new graph G^* such that G is an induced subgraph of a graph G^* in the same class such that $rc_k(G^*) = rc_k(G)$ where the $rc_k(G)$-coloring and the $rc_k(G^*)$-coloring use same color to the vertices of G. If we allow the new stations of the extended network to be assigned with the frequencies left unused for the old network, then the colors of the newly introduced vertices of G^* should be the holes in the preexisting rc_k-coloring of G since the unused frequencies are represented by holes of a rc_k-coloring (optimum frequency assignment) on a graph G (network of transmitters). To address this issue, we exploit a structural property of graph with positive $(k-1)$-hole index as can be found in the following result.

Lemma 1.18 [40] *For $k \geq 2$, let L be an rc_k-coloring of a graph G with a $(k-1)$-hole $\{i+1, i+2, \ldots, i+k-1\}$, where $i \geq 0$. Then there are two vertices $u \in L_i$ and $v \in L_{i+k}$ such that u and v are adjacent in G.*

Proof If possible, let no vertex of L_i be adjacent to any vertex in L_{i+k} in G. By defining a new coloring $\hat{L}$ as follows:

$$\hat{L}(u) = \begin{cases} L(u), \text{ if } L(u) \leq i, \\ L(u) - 1, \text{ if } L(u) \geq i + k. \end{cases}$$

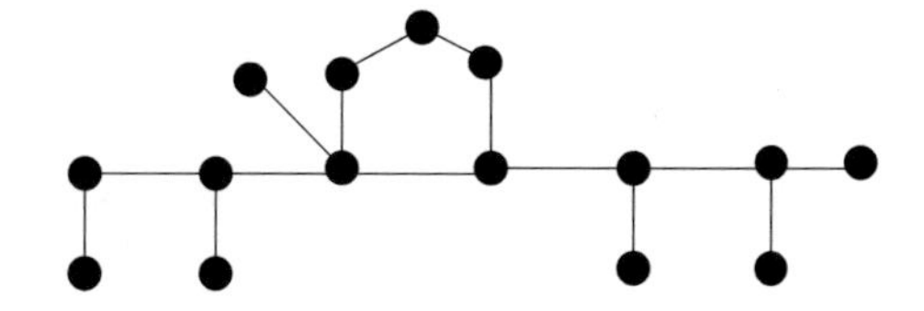

Fig. 1.22 Illustrating an example of $\mathscr{H}_k$, for $2 \leq k \leq 7$

we obtain a proper radio k-coloring of G with span $rc_k(G) - 1$, a contradiction. This completes the proof.

In [40], a new family $\mathscr{H}_k, k \geq 2$, of graphs has been introduced. It is the family of graphs G such that for every edge e in G, there exists a vertex $\omega_e \in V(G)$ which is at a distance $\lfloor \frac{k}{2} \rfloor$ from one vertex incident to e and at a distance $\lceil \frac{k}{2} \rceil + 1 - k(mod\ 2)$ from another vertex incident to e.

Before we give examples of this family, we need some definitions. The *cartesian product* of G and H, denoted by $G \Box H$, is the graph with vertex set $V(G) \times V(H)$ and a vertex (u, v) is adjacent to another vertex (u', v') if and only if (i) $u = u'$ and $v \sim v'$ in H, or (ii) $v = v'$ and $u \sim u'$ in G. Also note that the *eccentricity* of a vertex u of G, denoted by $\varepsilon(u)$, is $max_{v \in V(G)} d(u, v)$. The *radius* of a graph, denoted by $rad\ G$, is $min_{u \in V(G)} \varepsilon(u)$. The *center* of G is the subgraph induced by the vertices of minimum eccentricity.

Now, some examples of $\mathscr{H}_k$ are given below (see [40]):

(i) $C_n \in \mathscr{H}_k$, where $n \geq 4$ and $2 \leq k \leq n - 1 - n\ (mod\ 2)$.
(ii) $C_n \Box P_m \in \mathscr{H}_k$, where $n \geq 4$, $m \geq 2$ and $2 \leq k \leq n - 1 - n\ (mod\ 2) + m - m\ (mod\ 2)$.
(iii) Let T be a tree. Then $T \in \mathscr{H}_k$, where $2 \leq k \leq 2.rad\ T + (-1)^{|C(T)|-1}$ and $|C(T)|$ is the number of vertices in the center of T.
(iv) The graph in Fig. 1.22 (see [40]) is an example of $\mathscr{H}_k$, for $2 \leq k \leq 7$.

Now, we are in a position to prove the following theorem.

Theorem 1.33 [40] *Let $G \in \mathscr{H}_k$ with $\rho_k(G) \geq 1$. Then there is a graph $G^* \in \mathscr{H}_k$ such that*

(i) G is an induced subgraph of G^*;
(ii) $rc_k(G^*) = rc_k(G)$;
(iii) $\rho_k(G^*) = \rho_k(G) - 1$.

Sketch of proof. Let L be any rc_k-coloring on G. Since $\rho_k(G) \geq 1$, let $\{i+1, i+2, \ldots, i+k-1\}$ be a $(k-1)$-hole in L with $i \geq 0$. By Lemma 1.18, we have $x \in L_i$ and $y \in L_{i+k}$ such that $x \sim y$.

Case I: Let ω_e be the vertex in G such that $d(x, \omega_e) = \lfloor \frac{k}{2} \rfloor$ and $d(y, \omega_e) = \lceil \frac{k}{2} \rceil + 1 - k(mod\ 2)$. Let us construct a new graph G^* by introducing a new vertex ω^* and a new edge $\omega^* \omega_e$ to G. Clearly $G^* \in \mathscr{H}_k$ and G is an induced subgraph of G^*. We define a new coloring L^* on G^* given by

$$L^*(u) = \begin{cases} L(u), \text{ if } u \in V(G) \\ i + \lceil \frac{k}{2} \rceil, \text{ if } u = \omega^* \end{cases}$$

Since $i+1, i+2, \ldots, i+k-1$ are consecutive holes in L, either

$$L^*(\omega_e) \geq L^*(y) + k + 1 - d(\omega_e, y) = i + k + \lfloor \frac{k}{2} \rfloor + k(mod\ 2) \quad (1.4)$$

or

$$L^*(\omega_e) \leq L^*(x) - (k + 1 - d(\omega_e, x)) = i - \lceil \frac{k}{2} \rceil - 1 \quad (1.5)$$

From Eqs. (1.4) and (1.5), we get $|L^*(\omega^*) - L^*(\omega_e)| \geq k$

Also, $|L^*(\omega^*) - L^*(x)| = k + 1 - d(\omega^*, x)$ and $|L^*(\omega^*) - L^*(y)| \geq k + 1 - d(\omega^*, y)$.

Let $u \in V(G^*) \setminus \{x, y, \omega_e, \omega^*\}$ such that there exists a path from u to ω^* in G^*.

Case I.(a) Let $d(x, u) = k - r_1$ and $d(y, u) = k - r_2$, where $0 \leq r_1, r_2 \leq k - 1$. Using the fact that $i+1, i+2, \ldots, i+k-1$ are holes in L and the distance constrains of the radio k-coloring L^*, we can say either $L^*(u) \leq i - r_1 - 1$ or $L^*(u) \geq i + k + r_2 + 1$. Using the inequalities $d(\omega_e, u) \geq d(x, u) - d(\omega_e, x)$ and $d(\omega_e, u) \geq d(y, u) - d(\omega_e, y)$, we have

$|L^*(\omega^*) - L^*(u)| \geq k + 1 - d(\omega^*, u)$.

Case I.(b) Let $d(x, u) = k$ and $d(y, u) = k + 1$. Then $L^*(u) \leq i - 1$ or $L^*(u) \geq i + k$. Now, using the inequality $d(\omega_e, u) \geq d(x, u) - d(\omega_e, x)$, we can show $k + 1 - d(\omega^*, u) \leq |L^*(\omega^*) - L^*(u)|$.

But $x \sim y$ in G implies $|d(x, u) - d(y, u)| \leq 1$. Therefore, Case I.(b), together with Case I.(a), implies $|L^*(\omega^*) - L^*(u)| \geq k + 1 - d(\omega^*, u)$, whenever $u \in V(G^*) \setminus \{x, y, \omega_e, \omega^*\}$ with $d(x, u) = k - r, 0 \leq r \leq k - 1$.

Case I.(c) Let $d(x, u) = k + r, r \geq 1$. Then $d(y, u) \geq k + r - 1 \geq k$. Using similar argument as before, L^* can be shown to be a radio k-coloring of G^*.

The discussion suggest that L^* is a proper radio k-coloring of G^*.

Case II Let ω_e be a vertex in G such that $d(y, \omega_e) = \lfloor \frac{k}{2} \rfloor$ and $d(x, \omega_e) = \lceil \frac{k}{2} \rceil + 1 - k(mod\ 2)$. Similar to *Case I*, we construct a new graph G^* by introducing a new vertex ω^* and a new edge $\omega^*\omega_e$ to G. Clearly, $G^* \in \mathscr{H}_k$, since $G \in \mathscr{H}_k$ and $y = \omega_{e'}$, where $e' = \omega_e\omega^*$. We define a new coloring $\hat{L}$ on G^* by

$$\hat{L}(u) = \begin{cases} L(u), \text{ if } u \in V(G) \\ i + \lfloor \frac{k}{2} \rfloor, \text{ if } u = \omega^* \end{cases}$$

Similar argument, as in Case I, proves $\hat{L}$ is a radio k-coloring of G^*.

The rest of the proof follows easily. □

The following results are easy consequences of the above result.

Theorem 1.34 [40] *Let $G \in \mathscr{H}_k$ be a graph with $\rho_k(G) \geq 1$. Then there exists a graph $G^* \in \mathscr{H}_k$, such that*

(i) G is an induced subgraph of G^*;
(ii) $rc_k(G^*) = rc_k(G)$;
(iii) $\rho_k(G^*) = 0$.

Remark 1.4 The above two theorems are all about extending a graph in $\mathscr{H}_k$ with a positive $(k-1)$-hole index without changing the radio k-chromatic number as well as colors of the existing vertices until the $(k-1)$-hole index becomes zero.

Theorem 1.34 can also be presented in the following way for general k as well as for the particular case $k = 2$.

Theorem 1.35 [40] *Let n be a positive integer such that* $n = rc_k(G)$, *for some* $G \in \mathscr{H}_k$. *Then there exists a graph* $G^* \in \mathscr{H}_k$, *containing G as its induced subgraph, such that* $rc_k(G^*) = n$ *and* $\mu_k(G^*) = rc_k(G^*)$.

Corollary 1.7 [40] *Let n be a positive integer such that* $n = \lambda_{2,1}(G)$, *for some* $G \in \mathscr{H}_2$. *Then there exists a graph* $G^* \in \mathscr{H}_2$, *such that*
(i) G is an induced subgraph of G^*;
(ii) $\lambda_{2,1}(G^*) = n$;
(iii) G^* *is full colorable.*

Acknowledgements The research is supported in part by National Board for Higher Mathematics, Department of Atomic Energy, Government of India (No 2/48(10)/2013/NBHM(R.P.)/R&D II/695).

References

1. Adams, S.S., M. Tesch, D.S. Troxell, B. Westgate, and C. Wheeland. 2007. On the hole index of L(2,1)-labelings of r-regular graphs. *Discrete Applied Mathematics* 155: 2391–2393.
2. Adams, S.S., A. Trazkovich, D.S. Troxell, and B. Westgate. 2010. On island sequences of labelings with a condition at distance two. *Discrete Applied Mathematics* 158: 1–7.
3. Arikati, S.R., and C.P. Rangan. 1990. Linear algorithm for optimal path cover problem on interval graphs. *Information Processing Letters* 35: 149–153.
4. Boesch, F.T., and J.F. Gimpel. 1977. Covering the points of a digraph with point-disjoint paths and its application to code optimization. *Journal of Association for Computing Machinery* 24: 192–198.
5. Calamoneri, T. 2011. The L(h, k)-labelling problem: An updated survey and annotated bibliography. *Computer Journal* 54: 1344–1371.
6. Chang, G.J., and D. Kuo. 1996. The L(2,1) coloring problem on graphs. *SIAM Journal on Discrete Mathematics* 9: 309–316.
7. Chartrand, G., D. Erwin, and P. Zhang. 2000. Radio antipodal coloring of cycles. *Congressus Numerantium* 144: 129–141.
8. Chartrand, G., D. Erwin, F. Harrary, and P. Zhang. 2001. Radio labeling of graphs. *Bulletin of the Institute of Combinatorics and its Applications* 33: 77–85.
9. Chartrand, G., D. Erwin, and P. Zhang. 2005. A graph labeling problem suggested by FM channel restrictions. *Bulletin of the Institute of Combinatorics and its Applications* 43: 43–57.
10. Cockayne, E.J., B.L. Hartnell, S.T. Hedetneimi, and R. Laskar. 1993. Perfect domination in graphs. *Journal of Combinatorics, Information & System Sciences* 18: 136–148.

11. Chavátal, V., and P. Erdős. 1972. A note on Hamiltonian circuits. *Discrete Mathematics* 2: 111–113.
12. Fishburn, P.C., and F.S. Roberts. 2003. No-hole L(2,1)-colorings. *Discrete Applied Mathematics* 130: 513–519.
13. Fishburn, P.C., and F.S. Roberts. 2006. Full color theorems for $L(2, 1)$-labelings. *SIAM Journal on Discrete Mathematics* 20: 428–443.
14. Fotakis, D., G. Pantziou, G. Pentaris, and P. Spirakis. 1999. Frequency assignment in mobile and radio networks. Networks in distributed computing. *DIMACS Series in Discrete Mathematics and Theoretical Computer Science* 45: 73–90.
15. Georges, J.P., D.W. Mauro, and M.A. Whittlesey. 1994. Relating path coverings to vertex colorings with a condition at distance two. *Discrete Mathematics* 135: 103–111.
16. Georges, J.P., and D.W. Mauro. 2005. On the structure of graphs with non-surjective $L(2, 1)$-labelings. *SIAM Journal on Discrete Mathematics* 19 (1): 208–223.
17. Godsil, C., and G. Royle. 2001. *Algebraic graph theory*. Graduate text in mathematics. Springer.
18. Griggs, J.R., and R.K. Yeh. 1992. Labeling graphs with a condition at distance two. *SIAM Journal on Discrete Mathematics* 5: 586–595.
19. Hale, W.K. 1980. Frequency assignment: Theory and applications. *Proceedings of the IEEE* 68: 1497–1514.
20. Haynes, T.W., and S.T. Hedetniemi, P.J. Slater. 1998. *Fundamentals of domination in graphs*. Marcel Dekker Inc.
21. Kchikech, M., R. Khennoufa, and O. Togni. 2008. Radio k-labelings for Cartesian products of graphs. *Discussiones Mathematicae Graph Theory* 28 (1): 165–178.
22. Khennoufa, R., and O. Togni. 2005. A note on radio antipodal colorings of paths. *Mathematica Bohemica* 130 (1): 277–282.
23. Khennoufa, R., and O. Togni. 2011. The radio antipodal and radio numbers of the hypercube. *Ars Combinatoria* 102: 447–461.
24. Král', D., R. Škrekovski, and M. Tancer. 2006. Construction of large graphs with no optimal surjective $L(2, 1)$-labelings. *SIAM Journal on Discrete Mathematics* 20 (2): 536–543.
25. Li, X., V. Mak, and S. Zhou. 2010. Optimal radio colorings of complete m-ary trees. *Discrete Applied Mathematics* 158: 507–515.
26. Liu, D.D.-F., and M. Xie. 2004. Radio number for square of cycles. *Congressus Numerantium* 169: 105–125.
27. Liu, D.D.-F., and X. Zhu. 2005. Multi-level distance labelings for paths and cycles. *SIAM Journal on Discrete Mathematics* 19 (3): 610–621.
28. Liu, D.D.-F. 2008. Radio number for trees. *Discrete Mathematics* 308: 1153–1164.
29. Liu, D.D.-F., and M. Xie. 2009. Radio number for square paths. *Ars Combinatoria* 90: 307–319.
30. Lu, C., L. Chen, and M. Zhai. 2007. Extremal problems on consecutive $L(2, 1)$-labelling. *Discrete Applied Mathematics* 155: 1302–1313.
31. Lu, C., and M. Zhai. 2007. An extremal problem on non-full colorable graphs. *Discrete Applied Mathematics* 155: 2165–2173.
32. Lu, C., and Q. Zhou. 2013. Path covering number and $L(2, 1)$-labeling number of graphs. *Discrete Applied Mathematics* 161: 2062–2074.
33. Moran, S., and Y. Wolfstahl. 1991. Optimal covering of cacti by vertex disjoint paths. *Theoretical Computer Science* 84: 179–197.
34. Ntafos, S.C., and S.L. Hakim. 1979. On path cover problems in digraphs and applications to program testing. *IEEE Transactions on Software Engineering* 5: 520–529.
35. Panigrahi, P. 2009. A survey on radio k-colorings of graphs AKCE. *Journal of Graphs and Combinatorics* 6 (1): 161–169.
36. Saha, L., and P. Panigrahi. 2012. Antipodal number of some powers of cycles. *Discrete Mathematics* 312: 1550–1557.
37. Saha, L., and P. Panigrahi. 2013. On the radio number of toroidal grids. *Australasian Journal of Combinatorics (Center for Discrete Mathematics and Computing, Australia)* 55: 273–288.
38. Saha, L., and P. Panigrahi. 2015. A lower bound for radio k-chromatic number. *Discrete Applied Mathematics* 192: 87–100.

39. Sarkar, U., and A. Adhikari. 2015. On characterizing radio k-coloring problem by path covering problem. *Discrete Mathematics* 338: 615–620.
40. Sarkar, U., and A. Adhikari. A new graph parameter and a construction of larger graph without increasing radio k-chromatic number. *Journal of Combinatorial Optimization*. https://doi.org/10.1007/s10878-016-0041-9.
41. Walikar, H.B., B.D. Acharya, and E. Sampathkumar. 1979. *Recent developments in the theory of domination in graphs*. MRI Lecture Notes in Mathematics, vol 1. Allahabad: Mahta Research Institute.
42. West, D.B. 2001. *Introduction to graph theory*. Prentice Hall.
43. Yeh, R.K. 2006. A survey on labeling graphs with a condition at distance two. *Discrete Mathematics* 306: 1217–1231.

Chapter 2
Robust Control of Stochastic Structures Using Minimum Norm Quadratic Partial Eigenvalue Assignment Technique

Kundan Goswami, Sonjoy Das and Biswa Nath Datta

Abstract The use of active vibration control technique, though typically more expensive and difficult to implement compared to the traditionally used passive control approaches, is an effective way to control or suppress dangerous vibrations in structures caused by resonance or flutter due to the external disturbances, such as winds, waves, moving weights of human bodies, and earthquakes. From control perspective, it is not only sufficient to suppress the resonant modes of vibration but also to guarantee the overall stability of the structural system. In addition, the no-spillover property of the remaining large number of frequencies and the corresponding mode shapes must be maintained. To this end, the state-space based linear quadratic regulator (LQR) and H_∞ control techniques and physical-space based robust and minimum norm quadratic partial eigenvalue assignment (RQPEVA and MNQPEVA) techniques have been developed in the recent years. In contrast with the LQR and H_∞ control techniques, the RQPEVA and MNQPEVA techniques work exclusively on the second-order model obtained by applying the finite element method on the vibrating structure, and therefore can computationally exploit the nice properties, such as symmetry, sparsity, bandness, positive definiteness, etc., inherited by the system matrices associated with the second-order model. Furthermore, the RQPEVA and MNQPEVA techniques guarantee the no-spillover property using a solid mathematical theory. The MNQPEVA technique was originally developed for the deterministic models only, but since then, further extension to this technique has been made to rigorously account for parametric uncertainty. The stochastic MNQPEVA technique is capable of efficiently estimating the probability of failure with high accuracy to ensure the desired resilience level of the designed system. In this work, first a brief

K. Goswami · S. Das (✉)
Department of Mechanical and Aerospace Engineering, University at Buffalo,
318 Jarvis Hall, Buffalo, NY 14260, USA
e-mail: sonjoy@buffalo.edu

K. Goswami
e-mail: kundango@buffalo.edu

B. N. Datta
Department of Mathematical Sciences, Northern Illinois University,
361 Watson Hall, De Kalb, IL 60115, USA
e-mail: profbiswa@yahoo.com

A. Adhikari et al. (eds.), *Mathematical and Statistical Applications in Life Sciences and Engineering*, https://doi.org/10.1007/978-981-10-5370-2_2

review of the LQR, H_∞, and MNQPEVA techniques is presented emphasizing on their relative computational advantages and drawbacks, followed by a comparative study with respect to computational efficiency, effectiveness, and applicability of the three control techniques on practical structures. Finally, the methodology of the stochastic MNQPEVA technique is presented and illustrated in this work using a numerical example with a representative real-life structure and recorded data from a California earthquake.

2.1 Introduction

Structural systems (e.g., high-rise buildings, bridges, wind turbines, aircraft, etc.) may undergo high amplitude vibration due to resonance or flutter when subjected to various dynamic loads (e.g., earthquake, wind, wave, moving weights of human bodies, etc.). If not suppressed, such high amplitude vibration may lead to collapse (e.g., failure of the Tacoma Narrows Bridge, Washington in 1940 [1]) or loss of functionality (e.g., wobbling of the Millennium Bridge, London in 2000 [2]) of the structures. Currently, there exist various strategies for vibration suppression, among which the most popular is the active vibration control (AVC). Large number of AVC techniques, for example, linear quadratic regulator (LQR) [3–5] and H_∞ [4–9] have been developed in the last three decades. The LQR and H_∞ techniques are based on the state-space representation of the dynamics of structural systems. In recent years, minimum norm quadratic partial eigenvalue assignment (MNQPEVA) and robust quadratic partial eigenvalue assignment (RQPEVA) techniques have been developed for AVC, which are based on the physical-space based representation of the dynamics of structural systems [10–12]. The MNQPEVA and RQPEVA techniques are computationally more efficient than the LQR and H_∞ techniques as (i) the system matrices in the state-space approach have twice the dimension of the system matrices in the physical-space based approach, (ii) the system matrices in the state-space approach lose the computationally exploitable properties, for example, symmetry, definiteness, sparsity, bandness, etc., inherited by the system matrices in the physical-space based approach, (iii) unlike the LQR and H_∞ techniques, the MNQPEVA and RQPEVA techniques require only partial information of the eigenpairs (i.e., eigenvalues and associated eigenvectors) to be shifted for the design of controlled/closed-loop systems, and (iv) the MNQPEVA and RQPEVA techniques ensure the *no-spillover property* in terms of sophisticated mathematical theory [13].

In practice, structural systems are plagued with uncertainties from several primitive sources including, but not limited to, variability in input parameters (e.g., material, geometric, loading) often modeled as *parametric uncertainty* [14] and system-level structural complexities typically modeled as *model form uncertainty* or *model uncertainty* [15]. If the available AVC techniques fail to account for the effects of these uncertainties, the designed control systems might not be able to reduce the vibration level of the structures. In the recent past, state-space approach-based H_∞ control technique has been extended to incorporate several sources of uncertainties mentioned above [9, 16–22]. Recently, physical-space based stochastic MNQPEVA technique has been developed that is computationally more effective than the H_∞ technique for large-scale systems due to the reasons mentioned earlier in this section [23].

In this work, a brief review of three AVC strategies, viz., the LQR, the H_∞, and the MNQPEVA techniques is presented first highlighting their relative computational advantages and drawbacks (see Sects. 2.2.1–2.2.3). Using a representative real-life structure, a comparison of the three techniques is presented next that (i) emphasizes on the computational efficiency and effectiveness of the MNQPEVA technique over the LQR and H_∞ techniques and (ii) provides motivation for extending the MNQPEVA technique to account for various uncertainties in structural systems (see Sect. 2.2.4). The comparative study is followed by a discussion on the stochastic MNQPEVA technique developed earlier in the literature [23] (see Sects. 2.3.1–2.3.2). Finally, the stochastic MNQPEVA technique is illustrated in this work through a numerical example with a representative real-life structure and recorded data from a California earthquake (see Sect. 2.3.3).

2.2 Brief Review and Comparison of LQR, H_∞, and MNQPEVA Techniques

In this section, brief description of the LQR, H_∞, and MNQPEVA control techniques are presented first followed by comparison of these three techniques illustrated using a numerical example. To understand the working principle of the three techniques, let us first consider the governing equation representing the dynamics of structural systems given by

$$\mathbf{M}\ddot{\boldsymbol{\eta}}(t) + \mathbf{C}\dot{\boldsymbol{\eta}}(t) + \mathbf{K}\boldsymbol{\eta}(t) = \mathbf{f}(t) \tag{2.1}$$

Equation (2.1) is obtained via the finite element (FE) discretization of the governing partial differential equations (PDEs) approximating the dynamic response of the physical structural system. In Eq. (2.1), the matrices **M**, **C**, and **K** denote the mass, damping, and stiffness matrices of the system, respectively, vector $\boldsymbol{\eta}(t)$ denotes the displacement response of the system at any instant t, $\mathbf{f}(t)$ denotes the dynamic load acting on the system at instant t, and the dot $(\dot{\ })$ denotes time derivative. Note that **M**, **C**, and **K** are real symmetric positive-definite matrices of size $n \times n$, where n is the degrees of freedom (dof) associated with the FE model of the system. Since **M**, **C**, and **K** are generated by FE technique, they are very large and often inherit nice structural properties, such as definiteness, bandness, sparsity, etc., which are useful for large-scale computing. The system is, in general, known as open-loop system. The dynamics of the open-loop system can also be represented in the linear state-space format as follows:

$$\begin{aligned}\dot{\mathbf{x}}(t) &= \mathbf{A}\mathbf{x}(t) + \mathbf{E}\mathbf{d}(t)\\ \mathbf{z}(t) &= \mathbf{W}\mathbf{x}(t)\end{aligned} \tag{2.2}$$

where $\mathbf{A}$, $\mathbf{E}$, $\mathbf{W}$, $\mathbf{x}(t)$, $\mathbf{d}(t)$, and $\mathbf{z}(t)$ denote the system matrix, external disturbance matrix, output matrix, state vector, external disturbance vector, and output vector, respectively. The quantities $\mathbf{A}$, $\mathbf{E}$, $\mathbf{x}(t)$, and $\mathbf{d}(t)$ appearing in Eq. (2.2) are related to the quantities $\mathbf{M}$, $\mathbf{C}$, $\mathbf{K}$, $\boldsymbol{\eta}(t)$, and $\mathbf{f}(t)$ present in Eq. (2.1) via the relations given by

$$\begin{aligned}\mathbf{A} &= \begin{bmatrix} \mathbf{0} & \mathbf{I} \\ -\mathbf{M}^{-1}\mathbf{K} & -\mathbf{M}^{-1}\mathbf{C} \end{bmatrix} \\ \mathbf{E} &= \begin{bmatrix} \mathbf{I} & \mathbf{0} \\ \mathbf{0} & -\mathbf{M}^{-1} \end{bmatrix} \\ \mathbf{x}(t) &= [\boldsymbol{\eta}(t), \dot{\boldsymbol{\eta}}(t)]^T \\ \mathbf{d}(t) &= [\mathbf{0}, \mathbf{f}(t)]^T \end{aligned} \tag{2.3}$$

where $\mathbf{I}$ is the identity matrix and $\mathbf{0}$ denotes both the null matrix and the null vector. It will be clear from the context whether $\mathbf{0}$ refers to a null matrix or a null vector. The real matrices $\mathbf{A}$ and $\mathbf{E}$ that appear in Eqs. (2.2) and (2.3) are typically highly populated and have dimensions twice as that of the original system matrices $\mathbf{M}$, $\mathbf{C}$, and $\mathbf{K}$. Therefore, more computation memory and time will be required, if the state-space approach (see Eq. (2.2)) is adopted instead of the physical-space based approach (see Eq. (2.1)), to estimate the displacement response $\boldsymbol{\eta}(t)$ (and/or velocity and acceleration responses) of a large-scale open-loop system (i.e., system matrices with large n).

2.2.1 Brief Review of LQR Technique

The objective of the traditional LQR technique is to design a control input $\mathbf{u}(t)$ for the nominal open-loop system given by

$$\begin{aligned}\dot{\mathbf{x}}(t) &= \mathbf{A}\mathbf{x}(t) \\ \mathbf{z}(t) &= \mathbf{W}\mathbf{x}(t)\end{aligned} \tag{2.4}$$

such that the nominal closed-loop system given by

$$\begin{aligned}\dot{\mathbf{x}}(t) &= \mathbf{A}\mathbf{x}(t) + \mathbf{B}_L\mathbf{u}(t) \\ \mathbf{z}(t) &= \mathbf{W}\mathbf{x}(t) + \mathbf{D}\mathbf{u}(t)\end{aligned} \tag{2.5}$$

is asymptotically stable, i.e., $\mathbf{x}(t) \to 0$ as $t \to \infty$ [3–5]. In Eq. (2.5), the matrices $\mathbf{B}_L$ and $\mathbf{D}$ denote the control matrix and the direct transmission matrix, respectively, and they are real valued. It is important to note that the control input $\mathbf{u}(t)$ designed via the traditional LQR technique does not account for the dynamic load $\mathbf{f}(t)$ as the nominal open-loop, and the nominal closed-loop systems are independent of the external disturbance $\mathbf{d}(t)$ (see Eqs. (2.4) and (2.5)). Details pertaining to the design of $\mathbf{u}(t)$ following the traditional LQR technique are presented in Sect. 2.2.1.1.

2.2.1.1 Traditional LQR Technique

In traditional LQR technique, the control input $\mathbf{u}(t)$ is typically obtained by minimizing the quadratic cost function given as follows:

$$J = \int_{t=0}^{\infty} \left[\mathbf{x}^T(t)\,\mathbf{Q}\mathbf{x}(t) + \mathbf{u}^T(t)\,\mathbf{R}\mathbf{u}(t)\right] dt \tag{2.6}$$

where $\mathbf{Q} = \mathbf{Q}^T \geq \mathbf{0}$ and $\mathbf{R} = \mathbf{R}^T > \mathbf{0}$ are the weight matrices associated with the norms $\|\mathbf{x}(t)\|_2$ and $\|\mathbf{u}(t)\|_2$, respectively. In practice, $\mathbf{Q} = \mathbf{W}^T\mathbf{W}$, $\mathbf{R} = \rho\mathbf{D}^T\mathbf{D} = \rho\mathbf{I}$, and $\mathbf{D}^T\mathbf{W} = \mathbf{0}$ are typically assumed. With these assumptions and $\rho = 1$, the cost function can be expressed as $J = \int_{t=0}^{\infty} \|\mathbf{z}(t)\|_2 dt$, where $\mathbf{z}(t) = \mathbf{W}\mathbf{x}(t) + \mathbf{D}\mathbf{u}(t)$. Note that, by minimizing J, two conflicting quantities $\|\mathbf{x}(t)\|_2$ (i.e., the response of the system) and $\|\mathbf{u}(t)\|_2$ (i.e., the input required for vibration control) are simultaneously minimized in the traditional LQR technique.

The form $\mathbf{u}(t) = -\mathbf{G}_L\mathbf{x}(t)$, where $\mathbf{G}_L$ denotes the feedback gain matrix, is typically chosen in the traditional LQR technique with the assumption that all the states $\{x_i(t)\}_{i=1}^{2n}$ are observable at any instant t. Note that the matrix $\mathbf{G}_L$ is a real valued matrix of dimension $m_L \times 2n$ with $m_L \leq 2n$. With $\mathbf{u}(t) = -\mathbf{G}_L\mathbf{x}(t)$, the dynamics of the nominal closed-loop system can be written as follows:

$$\begin{aligned} \dot{\mathbf{x}}(t) &= (\mathbf{A} - \mathbf{B}_L\mathbf{G}_L)\,\mathbf{x}(t) \\ \mathbf{z}(t) &= (\mathbf{W} - \mathbf{D}\mathbf{G}_L)\,\mathbf{x}(t) \end{aligned} \tag{2.7}$$

Assuming (i) the pair $(\mathbf{A}, \mathbf{B}_L)$ be stabilizable and (ii) the pair $(\mathbf{A}, \mathbf{Q})$ be detectable, there exists a unique optimal control input $\mathbf{u}^*(t) = -\mathbf{G}_L^*\mathbf{x}(t)$. The unique optimal feedback gain matrix $\mathbf{G}_L^*$ is given by

$$\mathbf{G}_L^* = \mathbf{R}^{-1}\mathbf{B}_L^T\mathbf{X} = \frac{1}{\rho}\mathbf{B}_L^T\mathbf{X} \tag{2.8}$$

where $\mathbf{X} = \mathbf{X}^T \geq \mathbf{0}$ is the unique solution of the algebraic Riccati equation (ARE) given as follows:

$$\begin{aligned} &\mathbf{A}^T\mathbf{X} + \mathbf{X}\mathbf{A} - \mathbf{X}\mathbf{B}_L\mathbf{R}^{-1}\mathbf{B}_L^T\mathbf{X} + \mathbf{Q} = \mathbf{0} \\ \Rightarrow\ &\mathbf{A}^T\mathbf{X} + \mathbf{X}\mathbf{A} - \frac{1}{\rho}\mathbf{X}\mathbf{B}_L\mathbf{B}_L^T\mathbf{X} + \mathbf{W}^T\mathbf{W} = \mathbf{0} \end{aligned} \tag{2.9}$$

Existence of $\mathbf{u}^*(t)$ indicates that (i) the closed-loop system given by Eq. (2.5) or (2.7) is asymptotically stable irrespective of the stability of the open-loop system given by Eq. (2.4), and (ii) the decay in response of the closed-loop system is faster than the decay in response of the corresponding open-loop system. It should be noted here that the optimal control input $\mathbf{u}^*(t)$ and the associated optimal feedback gain matrix $\mathbf{G}_L^*$ can also be obtained by solving an alternate optimization problem involving linear matrix inequalities (LMIs) [24, 25], which is not presented here to save space.

2.2.1.2 Modified LQR Technique

The feedback gain matrix $\mathbf{G}_L$ obtained via the traditional LQR technique depends on the weight coefficient ρ (see Eq. (2.9)). Therefore, the required maximum control force, which is associated with the maximum value of control input $\mathbf{u}(t)$, is influenced by the choice of ρ. It can be observed from Eq. (2.6) that, by choosing large ρ, the cost function J can be heavily penalized for small increase in control input $\mathbf{u}(t)$ [3, 5, 26]. Hence, the maximum value of control input $\mathbf{u}(t)$ can be reduced by increasing the weight coefficient ρ, however, at the cost of increase in system response (i.e., increase in $\mathbf{x}(t)$).

The dynamics of a nominal closed-loop system, which is designed following the traditional LQR technique, subjected to some external disturbance $\mathbf{d}(t)$ can be written as follows:

$$\begin{aligned} \dot{\mathbf{x}}(t) &= (\mathbf{A} - \mathbf{B}_L\mathbf{G}_L)\,\mathbf{x}(t) + \mathbf{E}\mathbf{d}(t) \\ \mathbf{z}(t) &= (\mathbf{W} - \mathbf{D}\mathbf{G}_L)\,\mathbf{x}(t) \end{aligned} \tag{2.10}$$

As mentioned earlier in Sect. 2.2.1, the effect of external disturbance $\mathbf{d}(t)$ (or dynamic load $\mathbf{f}(t)$) is not accounted for in the design of control input $\mathbf{u}(t)$ (and feedback gain matrix $\mathbf{G}_L$) by the traditional LQR technique. Therefore, the response (e.g., displacement, inter-story drift, velocity, acceleration, stress, etc.) of the closed-loop system given by Eq. (2.10) be within certain user-prescribed limit is not always guaranteed. In this regard, a new optimization problem, which can reduce the required control input and simultaneously constrain the closed-loop system response within certain user-prescribed limit, can be formulated as follows:

$$\begin{aligned} &\max_{\rho}\ \rho \\ &\text{s.t.}\ \ y_i\left(\mathbf{x}(t;\,\rho), \dot{\mathbf{x}}(t;\,\rho)\right) \le y_{i_{cr}};\ \ i = 1, \ldots, n_y \end{aligned} \tag{2.11}$$

In Eq. (2.11), $y_i\left(\mathbf{x}(t;\,\rho), \dot{\mathbf{x}}(t;\,\rho)\right)$ represents the ith response quantity of interest with the associated critical value given by $y_{i_{cr}}$ and n_y denotes the number of response quantities. The term $\mathbf{x}(t;\,\rho)$, which is parameterized with respect to ρ, represents the state of the closed-loop system given by Eq. (2.10). To evaluate the term $y_i\left(\mathbf{x}(t;\,\rho), \dot{\mathbf{x}}(t;\,\rho)\right)$, one needs to solve for $\mathbf{x}(t;\,\rho)$ and $\dot{\mathbf{x}}(t;\,\rho)$ using

$$\dot{\mathbf{x}}(t;\rho) = \left(\mathbf{A} - \frac{1}{\rho}\mathbf{B}_L\mathbf{B}_L^T\mathbf{X}(\rho)\right)\mathbf{x}(t;\rho) + \mathbf{E}\mathbf{d}(t) \tag{2.12}$$

where $\mathbf{X}(\rho)$ can be obtained by solving Eq. (2.9).

2.2.2 Brief Review of H_∞ Technique

The objective of the H_∞ technique is to design a control input $\mathbf{u}(t)$ for the open-loop system given by Eq. (2.2) such that the influence of external disturbance $\mathbf{d}(t)$ on the output $\mathbf{z}(t)$ of the closed-loop system is minimized. Assuming all the states $\{x_i(t)\}_{i=1}^{2n}$ are observable at any instant t, the form $\mathbf{u}(t) = \mathbf{G}_H\mathbf{x}(t)$ is typically chosen in state-feedback H_∞ technique. Note that the matrix $\mathbf{G}_H$ is the feedback gain matrix of dimension $m_H \times 2n$ with $m_H \leq 2n$. With the control input $\mathbf{u}(t) = \mathbf{G}_H\mathbf{x}(t)$, the dynamics of the closed-loop system can be written as follows:

$$\begin{aligned} \dot{\mathbf{x}}(t) &= (\mathbf{A} + \mathbf{B}_H\mathbf{G}_H)\,\mathbf{x}\,(t) + \mathbf{E}\mathbf{d}(t) \\ \mathbf{z}(t) &= (\mathbf{W} + \mathbf{D}\mathbf{G}_H)\,\mathbf{x}(t) \end{aligned} \tag{2.13}$$

where $\mathbf{B}_H$ denotes the control matrix and the definitions of $\mathbf{A}$, $\mathbf{E}$, $\mathbf{W}$, $\mathbf{D}$, $\mathbf{x}(t)$, and $\mathbf{z}(t)$ are same as defined earlier in Sect. 2.2.

In the Laplace domain, the influence of the external disturbance $\mathbf{d}(s)$ on the output $\mathbf{z}(s)$ of the closed-loop system can be characterized by the transfer function matrix which is given as follows:

$$\mathbf{T}_{zd}(s) = (\mathbf{W} + \mathbf{D}\mathbf{G}_H)\,(s\mathbf{I} - \mathbf{A} - \mathbf{B}_H\mathbf{G}_H)^{-1}\,\mathbf{E} \tag{2.14}$$

In this regard, the design objective of H_∞ technique is to obtain a feedback gain matrix $\mathbf{G}_H$ which minimizes the H_∞-norm of the transfer function matrix denoted by $\|\mathbf{T}_{zd}(s)\|_\infty$. It should be noted here that it is computationally difficult to obtain $\|\mathbf{T}_{zd}(s)\|_\infty$ as compared to obtain a $\gamma > 0$ for which $\|\mathbf{T}_{zd}(s)\|_\infty < \gamma$ [9]. Therefore, in practice, the feedback gain matrix $\mathbf{G}_H$ is obtained by solving the optimization problem given as follows:

$$\begin{aligned} &\min_{\gamma}\ \gamma \\ &\text{s.t.}\ \ \|\mathbf{T}_{zd}(s)\|_\infty < \gamma \\ &\qquad \gamma > 0 \end{aligned} \tag{2.15}$$

Assuming (i) the pairs $(\mathbf{A}, \mathbf{B}_H)$ and $(\mathbf{A}, \mathbf{E})$ be stabilizable, (ii) the pair $(\mathbf{A}, \mathbf{W})$ be observable, (iii) $\mathbf{D}^T\mathbf{D} = \mathbf{I}$, and (iv) $\mathbf{D}^T\mathbf{W} = \mathbf{0}$; the constraint $\|\mathbf{T}_{zd}(s)\|_\infty < \gamma$ in Eq. (2.15) is satisfied if and only if, for a given $\gamma > 0$, there exists a solution $\mathbf{Y}$ of the ARE given as follows:

$$\mathbf{A}^T\mathbf{Y} + \mathbf{YA} - \mathbf{Y}\left(\mathbf{B}_H\mathbf{B}_H^T - \frac{1}{\gamma^2}\mathbf{EE}^T\right)\mathbf{Y} + \mathbf{W}^T\mathbf{W} = \mathbf{0} \tag{2.16}$$

where $\mathbf{Y} = \mathbf{Y}^T \geq \mathbf{0}$. If the optimal solution of the problem given by Eq. (2.15) be γ^*, then the corresponding feedback gain matrix is given by

$$\mathbf{G}_H^* = -\mathbf{B}_H^T\mathbf{Y} \tag{2.17}$$

where $\mathbf{Y}$ is the solution of the ARE given by Eq. (2.16) for $\gamma = \gamma^*$. Note that the feedback gain matrix $\mathbf{G}_H$ can also be obtained by solving an alternate optimization problem involving LMIs [24], however, not shown here to save space. Since the H_∞ technique is based on indirect minimization of $\|\mathbf{T}_{zd}(s)\|_\infty$, the resulting optimal closed-loop system will exhibit minimum response; hence, no alternate optimization formulation, which constrains the system response within certain user-prescribed limit, is required.

A comparison of the feedback gain matrices obtained via the LQR and H_∞ techniques indicates that the $\mathbf{G}_H^*$ is different from the $\mathbf{G}_L^*$ because the H_∞ technique accounts for the effect of $\mathbf{d}(t)$ whereas the LQR technique does not. Both $\mathbf{G}_H^*$ (see Eqs. (2.16)–(2.17)) and $\mathbf{G}_L^*$ (see Eqs. (2.8)–(2.9)) will be same if $\gamma \to \infty$ and $\rho = 1$. When $\|\mathbf{T}_{zd}(s)\|_\infty < \infty$, $\|\mathbf{z}(t)\|_2 < \infty$ for any $\|\mathbf{d}(t)\|_2 < \infty$, hence, $\|\mathbf{x}(t)\|_2 < \infty$ for any $\|\mathbf{d}(t)\|_2 < \infty$ implying that the closed-loop system associated with the H_∞ technique (see Eq. (2.13)) is stable. In this case, the closed-loop system given by Eq. (2.13) satisfies the objective of LQR technique, i.e., $\mathbf{x}(t \to \infty) \to 0$ for $\mathbf{d}(t) = 0$.

2.2.3 *Brief Review of MNQPEVA Technique*

The open-loop system given by Eq. (2.1) typically exhibits high dynamic response when some of the damped natural frequencies of the system are close to the dominant range of loading spectrum. The damped natural frequencies of the system are related to the eigenvalues λ associated with the quadratic pencil $\mathbf{P}_o(\lambda) = \left(\lambda^2\mathbf{M} + \lambda\mathbf{C} + \mathbf{K}\right)$. For an open-loop system with n dof, the set of eigenvalues denoted by $\{\lambda_i\}_{i=1}^{2n}$ can be obtained by solving the quadratic eigenvalue problem (QEP) $\mathbf{P}_o(\lambda)\mathbf{x} = \mathbf{0}$, where $\{\mathbf{x}^{(i)}\}_{i=1}^{2n}$ are the right eigenvectors of the system. Let $\{\lambda_i\}_{i=1}^{2p}$ with $2p \ll 2n$ be the set of problematic eigenvalues related to the set of damped natural frequencies which are close to the dominant range of loading spectrum. For vibration control of the open-loop system, the set of eigenvalues $\{\lambda_i\}_{i=1}^{2p}$ needs to be replaced by a suitably chosen set $\{\mu_i\}_{i=1}^{2p}$. The technique to replace the set $\{\lambda_i\}_{i=1}^{2p}$ by the set $\{\mu_i\}_{i=1}^{2p}$ is known as quadratic partial eigenvalue assignment (QPEVA) technique [5, 13, 27]. It should be noted at this point that, for large-scale systems (i.e., large n), only a small number of eigenvalues and eigenvectors can be computed using the state-of-the-art computational techniques (e.g., Jacobi–Davidson methods [28, 29]) or measured in a vibration laboratory [30–32]. Therefore, the computational and engineering challenges associated with QPEVA technique for AVC is to design a control system based only on the knowledge of the set of eigenvalues $\{\lambda_i\}_{i=1}^{2p}$ and the set of associated eigenvectors $\{x_{o_i}\}_{i=1}^{2p}$. In the recent past, few algorithms [10–12, 27] have been developed that can implement the QPEVA technique with only the knowledge of $\{\lambda_i\}_{i=1}^{2p}$ and $\{x_o^{(i)}\}_{i=1}^{2p}$. In addition, these algorithms [10–12, 27] ensure the *no-spillover property*, i.e., the rest of the eigenvalues $\{\lambda_i\}_{i=2p+1}^{2n}$ and the associated eigenvectors of the system remain unchanged even after the application of control force. The QPEVA technique, as developed in the literature [10], is presented in Sect. 2.2.3.1.

2.2.3.1 Traditional MNQPEVA Technique

The QPEVA technique typically assumes a control force of the form $\mathbf{Bu}(t)$, where $\mathbf{B}$ is a real-valued control matrix of dimension $n \times m$ with $m \leq n$ and the control input vector $\mathbf{u}(t) = \mathbf{F}^T\dot{\eta}(t) + \mathbf{G}^T\eta(t)$. The matrices $\mathbf{F}$ and $\mathbf{G}$ are real-valued feedback gain matrices of dimensions $n \times m$. With the application of the control force $\mathbf{Bu}(t)$, the governing equation of closed-loop system can be written as follows:

$$\mathbf{M}\ddot{\eta}(t) + \left(\mathbf{C} - \mathbf{BF}^T\right)\dot{\eta}(t) + \left(\mathbf{K} - \mathbf{BG}^T\right)\eta(t) = \mathbf{f}(t) \tag{2.18}$$

Using only the knowledge of $\{\lambda_i\}_{i=1}^{2p}$ and $\{x_o^{(i)}\}_{i=1}^{2p}$, the objective of QPEVA technique is to find the feedback matrices $\mathbf{F}$ and $\mathbf{G}$ for a given $\mathbf{B}$, such that the set of eigenvalues of the closed-loop system is $\{\{\mu_i\}_{i=1}^{2p}, \{\lambda_i\}_{i=2p+1}^{2n}\}$ with the eigenvectors $\{\mathbf{x}_o^{(i)}\}_{i=2p+1}^{2n}$ corresponding to $\{\lambda_i\}_{i=2p+1}^{2n}$ remain unchanged (i.e., no-spillover property is guaranteed). Assuming (i) $\{\lambda_i\}_{i=1}^{2p} \cap \{\mu_i\}_{i=1}^{2p} \cap \{\lambda_i\}_{i=2p+1}^{2n} = \phi$ (ii) $0 \notin \{\lambda_i\}_{i=1}^{2p}$, (iii) $\{\lambda_i\}_{i=1}^{2p}$ and $\{\mu_i\}_{i=1}^{2p}$ are closed under complex conjugation, and (iv) partial controllability of the pair $(\mathbf{P}_o(\lambda), \mathbf{B})$ with respect to $\{\lambda_i\}_{i=1}^{2p}$, the feedback matrices $\mathbf{F}$ and $\mathbf{G}$ satisfying the no-spillover property can be obtained as follows:

$$\begin{aligned} \mathbf{F}(\mathbf{\Gamma}) &= \mathbf{M}\mathbf{X}_{o_{2p}}\mathbf{\Lambda}_{o_{2p}}\mathbf{Z}^{-T}\mathbf{\Gamma}^T \\ \mathbf{G}(\mathbf{\Gamma}) &= -\mathbf{K}\mathbf{X}_{o_{2p}}\mathbf{Z}^{-T}\mathbf{\Gamma}^T \end{aligned} \tag{2.19}$$

where $\mathbf{\Lambda}_{o_{2p}} = diag\{\lambda_i\}_{i=1}^{2p}$, $\mathbf{\Lambda}_{c_{2p}} = diag\{\mu_i\}_{i=1}^{2p}$, $\mathbf{X}_{o_{2p}} = \left[\mathbf{x}_o^{(1)}, \mathbf{x}_o^{(2)}, \ldots, \mathbf{x}_o^{(2p)}\right]$, and $\mathbf{Z}$ is the unique solution of the *Sylvester equation* given by

$$\mathbf{\Lambda}_{o_{2p}}\mathbf{Z} - \mathbf{Z}\mathbf{\Lambda}_{c_{2p}} = -\mathbf{\Lambda}_{o_{2p}}\mathbf{X}_{o_{2p}}^T\mathbf{B}\mathbf{\Gamma} \tag{2.20}$$

In Eqs. (2.19) and (2.20), $\mathbf{\Gamma} = \{\gamma_i\}_{i=1}^{2p}$ is a parametric matrix of dimension $m \times 2p$, and the set $\{\gamma_i\}_{i=1}^{2p}$ is closed under complex conjugation in the same order as the set $\{\mu_i\}_{i=1}^{2p}$.

Exploiting the parametric nature of the feedback matrices **F** and **G** (see Eq. (2.19)), optimization problem has been formulated in literature [10] that results in feedback matrices with minimum norm. The technique to implement QPEVA with minimum norm feedback matrices is known as MNQPEVA technique, and the associated optimization problem is given by

$$\min_{\mathbf{\Gamma}} \left(\tfrac{1}{2}[\|\mathbf{F}(\mathbf{\Gamma})\|_F^2 + \|\mathbf{G}(\mathbf{\Gamma})\|_F^2]\right) \tag{2.21}$$

where $\|.\|_F$ denotes the Frobenius norm of a matrix.

2.2.3.2 Modified MNQPEVA Technique

The MNQPEVA formulation presented in Sect. 2.2.3.1 results in feedback matrices **F** and **G** with minimum norm for a chosen set $\{\mu_i\}_{i=1}^{2p}$. The dynamic responses (e.g., displacement, inter-story drift, velocity, acceleration, stress, etc.) of the closed-loop system given by Eq. (2.18) depend on the choice of $\{\mu_i\}_{i=1}^{2p}$. In engineering practice, manually choosing a set $\{\mu_i\}_{i=1}^{2p}$, which will ensure that the dynamic responses of the closed-loop system are within user-prescribe limit, can be challenging and might require iterations. As a way out, a nested optimization problem can be formulated that results in an optimal set $\{\mu_i\}_{i=1}^{2p}$ for which **F** and **G** have minimum norm and the dynamic responses of the closed-loop system are within user-prescribe limit. The outer optimization problem of the nested optimization scheme can be formulated as follows:

$$\begin{aligned} \min_{\mathbf{q}} \;& g(\mathbf{q}) \\ \text{s.t.} \;& y_i(\mathbf{q}) \leq y_{i_{cr}};\; i = 1, \ldots, n_y \\ & l_{q_j} \leq q_j \leq u_{q_j};\; j = 1, \ldots, 2p \end{aligned} \tag{2.22}$$

where $\mathbf{q}$ is the set of control input parameters associated with the set $\{\mu_i\}_{i=1}^{2p}$. The objective function $g(\mathbf{q})$ is obtained by solving an inner optimization problem given by

$$g(\mathbf{q}) = \min_{\mathbf{\Gamma}} \left(\frac{1}{2}[\|\mathbf{F}(\mathbf{q}, \mathbf{\Gamma})\|_F^2 + \|\mathbf{G}(\mathbf{q}, \mathbf{\Gamma})\|_F^2]\right) \tag{2.23}$$

Note that the optimization problem given in Eq. (2.23) is same as the traditional MNQPEVA problem but now expressed as a function of $\mathbf{q}$ (see Eq. (2.21)). In Eq. (2.22), the term $y_i(\mathbf{q})$ represents the ith response quantity of interest with the associated critical value given by $y_{i_{cr}}$. The terms l_{q_j} and u_{q_j} represent the lower and upper bounds, respectively, on the jth decision variable q_j.

Remark: Relative computational advantages/drawbacks of the LQR, H_∞, and MNQPEVA techniques are summarized below.

1. The matrices **M**, **C**, and **K** possess computationally exploitable properties, such as the symmetry, positive definiteness, sparsity, bandness, etc., which are assets for large-scale computing. The MNQPEVA technique works exclusively on the second-order model (see Eq. (2.18)), and hence can take full advantage of these computationally exploitable properties. The state-space based LQR and H_∞ techniques, on the other hand, require a transformation of the second-order model (see Eq. (2.1)) to a first-order one (see Eq. (2.2)) due to which matrix **A** loses all these computationally exploitable properties. Note that the symmetry of matrix **A** can be preserved by transforming the second-order model to the generalized state-space form, but not the definiteness [29, Sect. 11.9.3]. Additionally, if **M** is ill-conditioned, computation of the matrices **A** and **E** will be problematic.
2. The dimensions of matrices **M**, **C**, and **K**, and matrix products $\mathbf{BF}^T$, $\mathbf{BG}^T$ are $n \times n$ (see Eq. (2.18)) whereas the dimensions of matrices **A**, **E** and matrix products $\mathbf{B}_L\mathbf{G}_L$, $\mathbf{B}_H\mathbf{G}_H$ are $2n \times 2n$ (see Eqs. (2.10) and (2.13)). For large n, solving the dynamic equations associated with the LQR and H_∞ techniques (e.g., Eqs. (2.7), (2.10), and (2.13)) will be a formidable task even with the state-of-the-art large-scale matrix computation techniques.
3. The LQR and H_∞ techniques require solutions of AREs involving matrices of dimensions $2n \times 2n$ (see Eqs. (2.9) and (2.16)). If n is very large, it is difficult to obtain solutions of AREs as no computationally viable methods have still been developed for the solution of a very large ARE. The MNQPEVA technique, on the other hand, will not suffer computationally due to large n as it requires a solution of a Sylvester equation involving matrices of dimensions $2p \times 2p$ with $p \ll n$ (see Eq. (2.20)).
4. The LQR and H_∞ techniques ensure the stability of closed-loop systems by reassigning all the eigenvalues of the associated open-loop systems. In contrast, the MNQPEVA technique ensures the stability of a closed-loop system by reassigning only a few problematic eigenvalues to suitably chosen ones by the users. In addition, the MNQPEVA technique guarantees the no-spillover property by means of a sophisticated mathematical theory based on the orthogonal properties of the eigenvectors of the associated quadratic model [29, Sect. 11.9.1].

The computational advantages of the MNQPEVA technique make it a very suitable candidate for practical applications, such as vibration control of large-scale structures.

2.2.4 Numerical Comparison of LQR, H_∞, and MNQPEVA Techniques

A comparison of the MNQPEVA technique (see Sect. 2.2.3) with the LQR (see Sect. 2.2.1) and H_∞ (see Sect. 2.2.2) techniques is presented in this section using a 60 dof system (see Fig. 2.1). This 60 dof system is a simplified representation of a 2D frame of a 60-story steel building. The floor masses $m_i = 4 \times 10^5$ kg and the floor heights $h_i = 4$ m for $i = 1, \ldots, 60$. The distribution of the stiffness along the height of the system is presented in Table 2.1. Rayleigh type damping matrix with $\xi_{1,5} = 0.02$, where $\xi_{1,5}$ denote the damping ratios associated with the first and fifth modes of the system, is assumed for this example problem. The system is subjected to wind load that is typically expected in the west coast area of USA. The wind time-histories at different levels of the 60 dof system are simulated using the NatHaz online wind simulator [33, 34] with basic wind speed of 52 m/s and exposure category D for the system [35]. When subjected to the wind load, the open-loop system exhibits high dynamic responses which exceed the user-prescribed limits (see Table 2.2).

The comparison among the LQR, H_∞, and MNQPEVA techniques is based on two criteria—(i) *economy* and (iii) *computation time*. A technique is deemed as the most economical one if it requires the least actuator capacity for control of the same

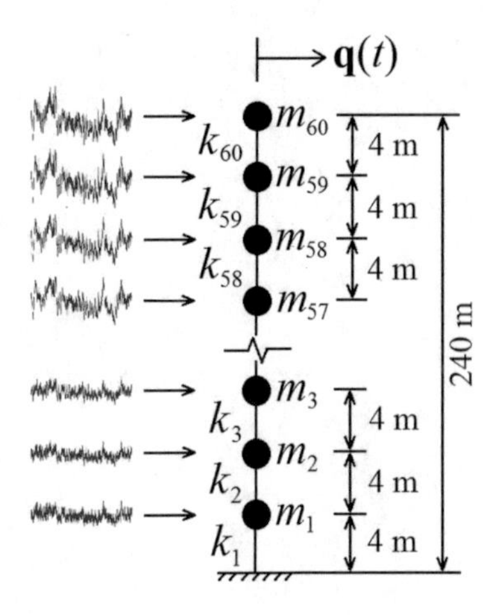

Fig. 2.1 Schematic representation of the 60 dof system subjected to wind load

Table 2.1 Distribution of the stiffness along the height of the 60 dof system

Range of dof	Stiffness (GN/m)	Range of dof	Stiffness (GN/m)	Range of dof	Stiffness (GN/m)	Range of dof	Stiffness (GN/m)
1–9	1.12	28–30	0.61	40–42	0.39	52–54	0.21
10–15	0.97	31–33	0.54	43–45	0.35	55–57	0.16
16–21	0.80	34–36	0.48	46–48	0.31	58–60	0.14
22–27	0.70	37–39	0.43	49–51	0.26		

open-loop system (viz., the 60 dof system) and simultaneously satisfy some safety criterion associated with the response of the closed-loop system. For this example problem, the safety criterion is based on the maximum displacement response and the maximum inter-story drift response of a system. A closed-loop system is deemed safe if (i) the maximum displacement response denoted by y_1 satisfies $y_1 \leq y_{1_{cr}} = 0.600$ m, and (ii) the maximum inter-story drift response denoted by y_2 satisfies $y_2 \leq y_{2_{cr}} = 0.0033$. The computation time associated with any control technique is defined as the time required by that technique to find the optimal feedback matrix (e.g., $\mathbf{G}_L$ for LQR; $\mathbf{G}_H$ for H_∞) or matrices (e.g., $\mathbf{F}$ and $\mathbf{G}$ for MNQPEVA). The comparison is presented in two stages. In the first stage, only the traditional formulations of the LQR, H_∞, and MNQPEVA techniques are compared with respect to the two criteria mentioned above. In the second stage, the modified LQR and modified MNQPEVA techniques are compared. For comparison purpose, the control matrices B_L, B_H, and B are chosen to be equivalent, i.e., (i) they satisfy $m_L = m_H = m = 2$, and (ii) they comply with the location of actuators at floor levels 5 and 60. Also, the matrices $\mathbf{W}$ and $\mathbf{D}$ are assumed as $\mathbf{W} = \left[\mathbf{I}_{2n\times 2n}, \mathbf{0}_{2\times 2n}\right]^T$ and $\mathbf{D} = \left[\mathbf{0}_{2n\times 2n}, \mathbf{I}_{2\times 2}\right]^T$, respectively, which satisfy the conditions $\mathbf{D}^T\mathbf{W} = \mathbf{0}$ and $\mathbf{D}^T\mathbf{D} = \mathbf{I}$. As mentioned earlier in Sect. 2.2.1.1, $\mathbf{Q} = \mathbf{W}^T\mathbf{W}$ is chosen in this example problem for the LQR technique. For comparison purpose, the results for the traditional LQR technique are obtained for two values of ρ (viz., $\rho = 1.0$ and $\rho = 0.5$). For MNQPEVA technique (both traditional and alternate formulations), only the first pair of eigenvalues $\{\lambda_{1,2}\}$ associated with the first damped natural frequency of the open-loop system are shifted. All the comparison results are presented in Table 2.2. Note that all computations in this section are performed in 32-bit MATLAB [36] using a single core in a computer with Intel(R) Core(TM)2 Duo processor having speed of 2 GHz and RAM of 3 GB.

It can be observed from Table 2.2 that the dynamic response of the 60 dof system can be reduced using all the three control techniques; however, the amount of reduction in response depends on the control technique adopted. Comparison of the traditional formulations of the LQR, H_∞, and MNQPEVA techniques (i.e., Stage-1) indicates that the LQR technique with $\rho = 1.0$, and the H_∞ technique cannot guarantee the safety of the system. Among the traditional formulations, the MNQPEVA technique emerges as the best technique because it is (i) more economic in terms of the actuator capacity required at floor levels 5 and 60 and (ii) computationally more efficient (see Table 2.2). Note that the traditional MNQPEVA technique has been implemented in this example problem by shifting only the first pair of eigenvalues of the system from $\{-0.0218 \pm 1.0917j\}$ to $\{-0.0800 \pm 1.1700j\}$, where $j = \sqrt{-1}$. The results of Stage-2 indicate that the modified MNQPEVA technique turns out to be the most economical one, however, at the cost of higher computational time (see Table 2.2). It should be remarked here that the difference in computational time for the different techniques presented in Sects. 2.2.1, 2.2.2 and 2.2.3 depends on several factors, for example, formulations of the optimization problems, size of the system defined by the degrees of freedom, and the underlying space on which the problem needs to be constructed (i.e., state-space based LQR and H_∞ problem, and physical-space based MNQPEVA problem). It can be concluded from the results presented

Table 2.2 Comparison of LQR, H_∞, and MNQPEVA techniques for a 60 dof system

Parameters for comparison	User-prescribed limit	Open-loop system	Closed-loop systems					
			Stage-1: Traditional				Stage-2: Modified	
			LQR with $\rho = 1$	LQR with $\rho = 0.5$	H_∞	MNQPEVA	LQR	MNQPEVA
y_1 (m)	0.6000	0.7952	0.6323	0.5926	0.6310	0.5748	0.6000	0.5885
y_2	0.0033	0.0042	0.0035	0.0033	0.0035	0.0033	0.0033	0.0033
Actuator capacity at floor 5 (MN)	–	–	0.0576	0.0884	0.0617	0.0668	0.0820	0.0628
Actuator capacity at floor 60 (MN)	–	–	0.8289	1.1141	0.8588	1.0605	1.0615	0.9975
Computation time (s)	–	–	0.1519	0.1537	87.5085	0.1277	38.4176	99.0121
Optimization algorithm	–	–	–	–	Interior-point	Quasi-Newton line search	Interior-point	Active-set

in Table 2.2 that the MNQPEVA technique performs better than the LQR and H_∞ techniques in terms of the economy and safety of the closed-loop systems, hence, justify the motivation for the development of a computationally effective stochastic MNQPEVA technique for economic and resilient design of closed-loop systems.

2.3 Control of Stochastic Systems Using MNQPEVA Technique

In this section, a variant of the modified MNQPEVA problem, termed as minimum norm quadratic partial eigenvalue assignment—minimum mass closed-loop system (MNQPEVA-MMCLS) problem, is presented first followed by a stochastic formulation of the MNQPEVA-MMCLS problem. The stochastic MNQPEVA-MMCLS problem is based on optimization under uncertainty (OUU). The optimal feedback matrices obtained by solving the stochastic MNQPEVA-MMCLS problem will lead to economic and resilient design of the stochastic structures. The computational challenge in solving the stochastic MNQPEVA-MMCLS problem is how to efficiently estimate a low probability of failure with high accuracy. An algorithm based on agglomerative hierarchical clustering technique (AHCT) and importance sampling (IS) scheme is presented next that can efficiently and accurately estimate very low probability of failure. Finally, the stochastic MNQPEVA-MMCLS technique is illustrated using a numerical example.

2.3.1 Stochastic Formulation of MNQPEVA-MMCLS Problem

The MNQPEVA-MMCLS problem minimizes the mass of the closed-loop system in addition to minimizing the norm of feedback matrices. The mass is minimized in order to reduce the material cost and inertia induced effects. Being a variant of the modified MNQPEVA problem, the deterministic MNQPEVA-MMCLS problem is also a nested optimization problem. This nested optimization scheme ensures both *economic design* and *safety* of the closed-loop system. The deterministic MNQPEVA-MMCLS problem, as developed in the literature [23], is given by

$$\begin{aligned} \min_{\mathbf{q}} \ & a\left(\frac{g(\mathbf{q})}{g_{target}}-1\right)^2+(1-a)\left(\frac{\mathscr{M}(\mathbf{q})}{\mathscr{M}_{avg}}\right)^2 \\ \text{s.t.} \ & y_i(\mathbf{q}) \le y_{i_{cr}};\ i=1,\ldots,n_y \\ & l_{q_j} \le q_j \le u_{q_j};\ j=1,\ldots,n_q \end{aligned} \tag{2.24}$$

where $\mathbf{q}$ is a vector of structural (material and geometric) and control input parameters, a is a positive real-valued weight coefficient, $\mathscr{M}(\mathbf{q})$ is the total mass of the closed-loop system for given $\mathbf{q}$, and $g(\mathbf{q})$ has the same form as given in Eq. (2.23). The terms g_{target} and $\mathscr{M}_{avg}$ in Eq. (2.24) are normalizing factors which are used to eliminate any bias due to difference in magnitude of the two terms while numerically carrying out the optimization scheme. In addition, g_{target} serves as a target value for $g(\mathbf{q})$. The terms $y_i(\mathbf{q})$, $y_{i_{cr}}$, l_{q_j}, u_{q_j}, n_y, and n_q in Eq. (2.24) are defined earlier in Sect. 2.2.3.2; however, $\mathbf{q}$ in Eq. (2.24) contains structural parameters in addition to the control input parameters related to the set $\{\mu_i\}_{i=1}^{2p}$.

The first step toward formulation of stochastic MNQPEVA-MMCLS problem is the characterization of various uncertainties, for example, *parametric uncertainty* [14] and *model uncertainty* [15], using the most suitable probabilistic model. The conventional parametric probabilistic models [14, 37, 38] can be used to characterize parametric uncertainties, whereas random matrix theory (RMT) based probabilistic models would be suitable for characterization of model uncertainties [15, 39–41]. Currently, there exists hybrid probabilistic formalism that can couple the conventional parametric model with the RMT-based model [42]. The stochastic MNQPEVA-MMCLS problem formulation, as developed in the literature [23], accounts for uncertainties in structural system parameters (e.g., material and geometric) and control input parameters by introducing a random vector $\mathbf{q}$, which collectively represent all random parameters associated with the structural system and control input. Using $\mathbf{q}$ and applying the concept of OUU [43], the stochastic MNQPEVA-MMCLS problem can be written as

$$\begin{aligned} \min_{\boldsymbol{\mu_q}} \ & \mathbb{E}\left[a\left(\frac{g(\mathbf{q})}{g_{target}}-1\right)^2+(1-a)\left(\frac{\mathscr{M}(\mathbf{q})}{\mathscr{M}_{avg}}\right)^2\right] \\ \text{s.t.} \ & P[y_i(\mathbf{q}) \le y_{i_{cr}}] = 1 - P_{f_{y_i}} \ge P_{y_i};\ i = 1, \ldots, n_y \\ & P[l_{q_j} \le \mathbf{q}_j \le u_{q_j}] \ge P_{\mathbf{q}_j};\ j = 1, \ldots, n_q \end{aligned} \tag{2.25}$$

where $\boldsymbol{\mu_q}$ is the vector of design variables representing the mean vector of $\mathbf{q}$. The terms P_{y_i} and $P_{\mathbf{q}_j}$ are the user-defined lowest probabilities to be satisfied for the ith constraint and the jth input bounds, respectively. Note that $(1 - P_{y_i})$ is the prescribed probability of failure for $y_i(\mathbf{q})$, where failure is defined by $y_i(\mathbf{q}) > y_{i_{cr}}$. The term $P_{f_{y_i}}$ denotes the current probability of failure for $y_i(\mathbf{q})$ given $\boldsymbol{\mu_q}$.

An OUU problem is typically solved after simplifying it to a *robust optimization* (RO) problem where the objective function and the constraints are expressed as weighted sum of mean and variance of respective quantities neglecting the higher order statistics [43–48]. The algorithms for solving RO typically assume statistical independence among the random input parameters and require a priori knowledge of the probability density functions (pdfs) of constraints and objective function for proper selection of *weight coefficients* for mean and variance. In RO, the probabilistic constraint associated with the ith random response $y_i(\mathbf{q})$ is satisfied by shifting the support of the pdf $p_{y_i(\mathbf{q})}$ of $y_i(\mathbf{q})$ to the left of $y_{i_{cr}}$ without changing the shape of $p_{y_i(\mathbf{q})}$ (see Fig. 2.2a). The constraint on $P_{f_{y_i}}$ can, however, be satisfied via a combination of change in shape and shift in support of $p_{y_i(\mathbf{q})}$ (see Fig. 2.2b) by considering the set of distribution parameters $\{\theta_k\}_{k=1}^{n_\theta}$ of the joint pdf $p_{\mathbf{q}}$ of $\mathbf{q}$ as the set of design variables for the MNQPEVA-MMCLS problem. The term n_θ denotes the number of distribution

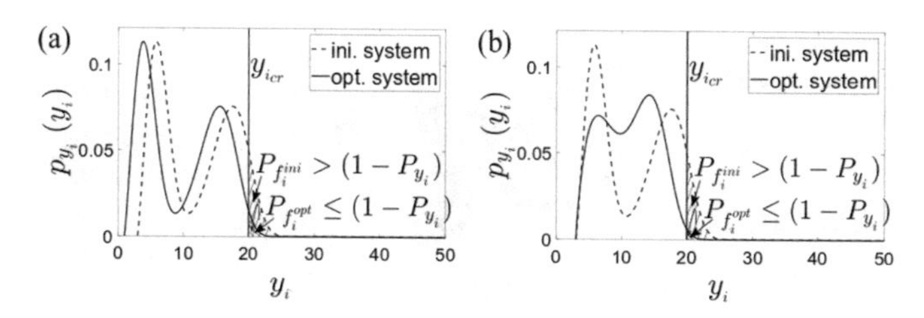

Fig. 2.2 Pictorial presentation of constraint satisfaction for probability of failure: **a** existing methods and **b** proposed method (adopted from [23])

parameters required to define the joint pdf $p_{\mathbf{q}}$. This idea can be implemented using families of pdfs for which the set of distribution parameters include shape parameters (e.g., Beta distribution). It should, however, be noted that the selection of the family of pdfs should be carried out with proper judgment so that the selected pdf complies with the manufacturing/construction specifications.

Using the idea of satisfying the constraint on $P_{f_{y_i}}$ via a combination of change in shape and shift in support of $p_{y_i(\mathbf{q})}$, the formulation of stochastic MNQPEVAP-MMCLS problem, as developed in [23], can be written as follows:

$$\begin{aligned} \min_{\{\theta_k\}_{k=1}^{n_\theta}} \quad & \mathbb{E}\left[a\left(\frac{g(\mathbf{q}|\{\theta_k\}_{k=1}^{n_\theta})}{g_{target}} - 1\right)^2 + (1-a)\left(\frac{\mathscr{M}(\mathbf{q}|\{\theta_k\}_{k=1}^{n_\theta})}{\mathscr{M}_{avg}}\right)^2\right] \\ \text{s.t.} \quad & P[y_i(\mathbf{q}|\{\theta_k\}_{k=1}^{n_\theta}) \leq y_{i_{cr}}] = 1 - P_{f_{y_i}} \geq P_{y_i};\ i = 1, \ldots, n_y \\ & l_{\theta_k} \leq \theta_k \leq u_{\theta_k};\ k = 1, \ldots, n_\theta \end{aligned} \tag{2.26}$$

where $g\left(\mathbf{q}|\{\theta_k\}_{k=1}^{n_\theta}\right)$ and $\mathscr{M}\left(\mathbf{q}|\{\theta_k\}_{k=1}^{n_\theta}\right)$ are same as mentioned earlier in the deterministic MNQPEVA-MMCLS problem formulation (see Eq. (2.24)), however, now expressed as functions of $\{\theta_k\}_{k=1}^{n_\theta}$. Note that, in accordance with the deterministic MNQPEVA-MMCLS problem, the stochastic MNQPEVA-MMCLS problem is also a nested optimization problem. In Eq. (2.26), the terms l_{θ_k} and u_{θ_k} represent the lower and upper bounds on the kth decision variable, respectively. The optimality of the solution of Eq. (2.26) depends on the accuracy of the estimate of $P_{f_{y_i}}\left(\{\theta_k\}_{k=1}^{n_\theta}\right), \forall i$. Efficient yet accurate estimation of $P_{f_{y_i}}\left(\{\theta_k\}_{k=1}^{n_\theta}\right), \forall i$ is computationally difficult because the estimate depends on the knowledge of failure domain $S_f^i = y_i(\mathbf{q}) \geq y_{i_{cr}}$ which might be disjointed and complicated in shape (see Fig. 2.3), and not known explicitly as a function of system parameters (for example, available only through large-scale finite element simulations). A way out from this computational difficulty is presented in the following section.

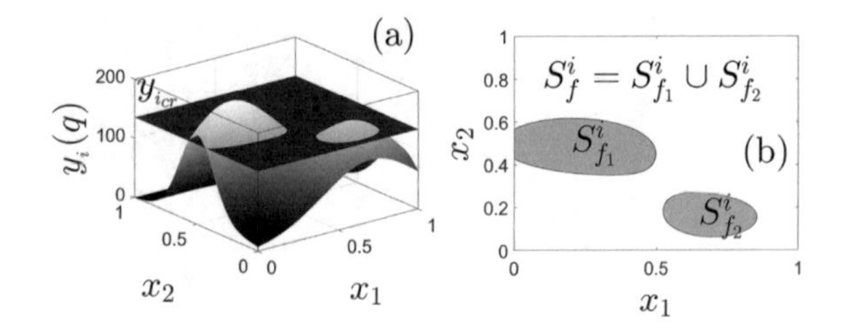

Fig. 2.3 Schematic representation of **a** variation of $y_i(\mathbf{q})$ with $\mathbf{q}$ and **b** disconnected S_f^i associated with $y_i(\mathbf{q})$ where $\mathbf{q} = [x_1, x_2]^T$ (adopted from [23])

2.3.2 Estimation of Probability of Failure

An algorithm developed in [23] for efficient yet accurate estimation of probability of failure P_f has been presented in this section. The algorithm is based on (i) AHCT for identification of disjointed and complicated shaped failure domain S_f and (ii) IS scheme for computation of P_f.
Unknown S_f can be identified efficiently by applying AHCT on digitally simulated failure samples as (i) unlike the k-means and other clustering techniques, the AHCT does not assume the failure samples to be independent and identically distributed and (ii) the time complexity of AHCT $\left(\mathcal{O}\left(N^3\right)\right)$ is much less compared to the time complexity of divisive hierarchical clustering technique $\left(\mathcal{O}\left(2^N\right)\right)$ for large sample size N [49, Sect. 14.3.12]. Based on certain distance measures among the available samples (e.g., Euclidean, Minkowski, Cosine, etc.) and among clusters (e.g., single linkage (SL), complete linkage (CL), average linkage (AL), etc.), the samples are sequentially grouped together in AHCT, which is pictorially depicted via a dendrogram [49, Sect. 14.3.12]. The efficiency of the identification process can be increased further by applying SL-based AHCT as (i) it has lesser time complexity $\left(\mathcal{O}\left(N^2\right)\right)$ as compared to the CL- and AL-based AHCTs $\left(\mathcal{O}\left(N^2 log(N)\right)\right)$ [50] and (ii) it is more stable and has better convergence criteria [51]. The algorithmic steps for identification of S_f are presented in Algorithm 1 (see Steps 1–2).

After S_f is identified, estimate of P_f can be obtained by simulating samples in S_f. Note that the accuracy of the estimate depends on the sample size in S_f. Towards this estimation process, IS scheme is preferred over the conventional Monte Carlo simulation (MCS) technique as MCS will require large number of samples in S to obtain sufficient number of samples in S_f. An IS estimate of an order statistic of $f(\mathbf{q})$ representing a function of the random vector $\mathbf{q}$ is obtained by first generating samples from the domain of interest S_f using an auxiliary pdf $g_{\mathbf{q}}(\mathbf{q})$ defined over S_f and then correcting for the bias using original pdf $p_{\mathbf{q}}(\mathbf{q})$ [52–54]. To ensure almost sure convergence of the IS scheme, the chosen $g_{\mathbf{q}}(\mathbf{q})$ should comply with (i) $\forall \mathbf{q} \in S_f$, $g_{\mathbf{q}}(\mathbf{q}) > 0$ if $p_{\mathbf{q}}(\mathbf{q}) > 0$ and (ii) $p_{\mathbf{q}}(\mathbf{q}) < k g_{\mathbf{q}}(\mathbf{q})$ with $k \gg 1$ [54]. Also, the IS estimator has finite variance when $\int_{S_f} f^2(\mathbf{q}) \frac{p_{\mathbf{q}}^2(\mathbf{q})}{g_{\mathbf{q}}(\mathbf{q})} d\mathbf{q} < \infty$ [54]. One should note here that the traditional IS scheme is restrictive as it requires the information of "exact" S_f to define the support of $g_{\mathbf{q}}(\mathbf{q})$. When exact S_f is unknown, the support of $g_{\mathbf{q}}(\mathbf{q})$ can be defined over a domain $S_S \supseteq S_f$ to employ the IS scheme. The IS estimate of $P[\mathbf{q} \in S_f]$ is given by

$$P[\mathbf{q} \in S_f] = \frac{1}{N_{S_S}} \sum_{i=1}^{N_{S_S}} \frac{p_{\mathbf{q}}(q^{(i)})}{g_{\mathbf{q}}(q^{(i)})} \mathbb{I}_{S_f} \tag{2.27}$$

where N_{S_S} is the number of samples generated within S_S. To obtain the estimate of P_f associated with a S_f composed of several disconnected parts, the IS scheme given by Eq. (2.27) needs to applied repeatedly over each disconnected failure domain (S_{f_j}) and summed over all j. The algorithmic steps to obtain IS estimate of P_f are presented in Algorithm 1 (see Steps 3–4).

Algorithm 1: Estimation of probability of failure

Input: (i) n-D Euclidean domain representing support S of $\mathbf{q}$, (ii) sample budget N_{ex} for domain exploration, (iii) failure criteria defined by $y_{i_{cr}}, \forall i$, (iv) tolerance ε, (v) sample budget N for IS scheme, and (vi) joint pdf $p_{\mathbf{q}}(\mathbf{q})$.

Step 1: Explore the failure domain $S_f \in S$ by first obtaining N_{ex} samples in S and then segregating the failure samples using the criteria $y_i > y_{i_{cr}}, \forall i$. For failure domain exploration without any bias, assume the elements $\mathbf{q}_j$ of $\mathbf{q}$ to be statistically independent and digitally simulate the N_{ex} samples using $\mathbf{q}_j \sim U[S_{min_{\mathbf{q}_j}}, S_{max_{\mathbf{q}_j}}], \forall j$ where $S_{min_{\mathbf{q}_j}}$ and $S_{max_{\mathbf{q}_j}}$ represent the possible minimum and maximum bounds on $\mathbf{q}_j$, respectively, to be chosen for numerical purpose.

Step 2: Identify n_{S_f} parts of a disjointed S_f by first obtaining a dendrogram using SL based AHCT and then slicing the dendrogram using a cutoff value associated with the normalized incremental height of the dendrogram.

Step 3: Using auxiliary pdfs $g^j_{\mathbf{q}}(\mathbf{q})$ for $j = 1, \ldots, n_{S_f}$; obtain a total of N new samples from the n-D boxes bounding the disjointed parts of S_f with tolerance ε. The sample size N_j associated with the j-th bounding box is proportional to the size of the box so that $\sum_{j=1}^{n_{S_f}} N_j = N$.

Step 4: Use the IS scheme $P_f = \sum_{j=1}^{n_{S_f}} \frac{1}{N_j} \sum_{i=1}^{N_j} f(q^{(i)}) \frac{p_{\mathbf{q}}(q^{(i)})}{g^j_{\mathbf{q}}(q^{(i)})} \mathbb{I}_{S_{f_j}}$ to estimate probability of failure.

Output: IS estimate of probability of failure P_f.

Example: Let $\mathbf{q} = [\mathbf{x}_1, \mathbf{x}_2]^T$ be a random vector with two statistically independent random variables $\mathbf{x}_1 \sim Beta\,(4, 3, 0, 1)$ and $\mathbf{x}_2 \sim Beta\,(6, 2, 0, 1)$. The failure domain S_f is assumed to be disconnected with 2 parts: $S_{f_1} = \{\mathbf{q} : \frac{(x_1-0.090)^2}{0.075^2} + \frac{(x_2-0.120)^2}{0.100^2} \leq 1\}$ and $S_{f_2} = \{\mathbf{q} : \frac{(x_1-0.900)^2}{0.075^2} + \frac{(x_2-0.070)^2}{0.050^2} \leq 1\}$ (see Fig. 2.4a). The true probability of failure for this problem is 3.763×10^{-6}. Using Algorithm 1 with (i) $S = [0, 1] \times [0, 1]$, (ii) $N_{ex} = 500$, (iii) failure criteria mentioned above (S_{f_1} and S_{f_2}), (iv) $\varepsilon = 0.1$, (v) $N = 600$, and (vi) $p_{\mathbf{q}}(\mathbf{q}) = p_{\mathbf{x}_1}(x_1)p_{\mathbf{x}_2}(x_2)$, the IS estimate of P_f is obtained as 3.696×10^{-6} with 1.77% error. Note that the cutoff value for the normalized incremental height of the dendrogram is taken as 0.1. For this problem,

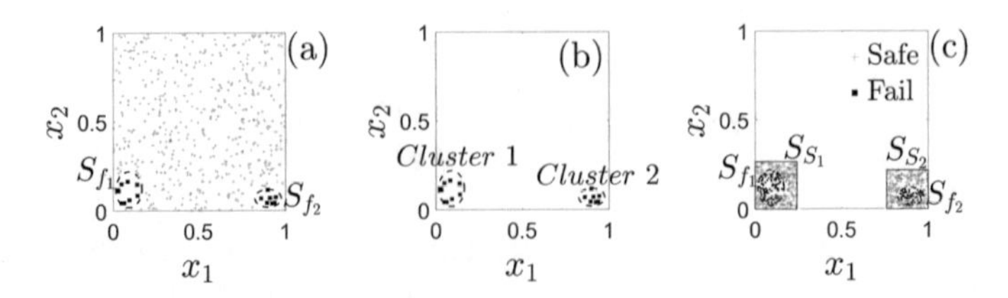

Fig. 2.4 Various attributes of the example problem: **a** domain exploration (Step 1), **b** failure domain identification (Step 2), and **c** sample generation from bounding boxes (Step 3) (adopted from [23])

Steps 1, 2, and 3 of Algorithm 1 are depicted in Fig. 2.4a, b, and c, respectively. A probabilistic convergence study conducted with 1000 different sets of $N_{ex} = 500$ exploratory samples indicates that the accuracy of Algorithm 1 increases significantly with sample budget N for IS scheme [23].

2.3.3 Numerical Illustration of Stochastic MNQPEVA-MMCLS Problem

The methodology presented in Sects. 2.3.1–2.3.2 for design of stochastic closed-loop system is numerically illustrated here using a 2D frame of a 4-story steel building (see Fig. 2.5a, adopted from [23]) subjected to the fault-normal component of ground acceleration recorded during the 1994 Northridge earthquake at the Rinaldi receiving station. The absolute maximum value of the ground acceleration record is scaled to 0.4 g where g is the acceleration due to gravity.

In this example, only the material properties, viz., density ρ and Young's modulus E, are assumed to be random to reduce the computation cost due to dimensionality. All other parameters are assumed to be deterministic and their values are $w = 2800$ kg/m, $\xi_1 = \xi_2 = 0.02$, $b_1 = 0.7754$ m, $h_1 = 0.3190$ m, $t_{f_1} = 0.0229$ m, $t_{w_1} = 0.0381$ m, $b_2 = 0.4922$ m, $h_2 = 0.3781$ m, $t_{f_2} = 0.0330$ m, $t_{w_2} = 0.0445$ m, $b_3 = 0.4826$ m, $h_3 = 0.3938$ m, $t_{f_3} = 0.0254$ m, $t_{w_3} = 0.0381$ m, $l_1 = 7.31$ m, $l_2 = 5.49$ m, and $l_3 = 3.66$ m, where w is the dead load, $\{\xi_i\}_{i=1}^{2}$ are the damping ratios associated

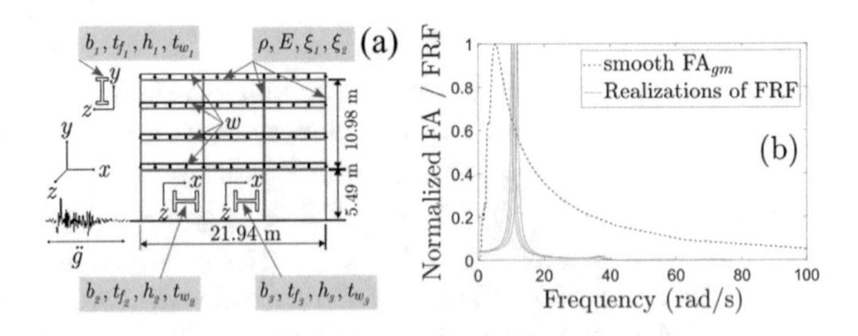

Fig. 2.5 Plots depicting **a** the 2D steel frame structure and **b** a few FRFs of the frame along with the normalized smooth FA of the ground motion (adopted from [23])

with the first two modes of vibration, and $\{b_i\}_{i=1}^3$, $\{h_i\}_{i=1}^3$, $\{t_{f_i}\}_{i=1}^3$, $\{t_{w_i}\}_{i=1}^3$, and $\{l_i\}_{i=1}^3$ are the geometric properties that represent the breadth, height, flange thickness, web thickness, and length of the I-sections, respectively, used as structural elements of the frame. It is assumed that $\boldsymbol{\rho} \sim Beta\left(\alpha_1, \beta_1, c_{l_1}, c_{u_1}\right)$, $\mathbf{E} \sim Beta\left(\alpha_2, \beta_2, c_{l_2}, c_{u_2}\right)$, and $\boldsymbol{\rho}$, $\mathbf{E}$ are statistically independent. The bounds of the distribution parameters $\left(\{\alpha_j\}_{j=1}^2, \{\beta_j\}_{j=1}^2, \{c_{l_j}\}_{j=1}^2, \{c_{u_j}\}_{j=1}^2\right)$ are presented in Table 2.3. An initial design of the stochastic 2D frame using the deterministic values mentioned earlier and assuming $\alpha_1 = 3, \beta_1 = 2, c_{l_1} = 7000\,\text{kg/m}^3, c_{u_1} = 8600\,\text{kg/m}^3, \alpha_2 = 2, \beta_2 = 3, c_{l_2} = 180$ GPa, and $c_{u_2} = 240$ GPa indicates that the fundamental damped natural frequency ω_{dn_1} of the structure lies within the dominant range of the spectrum of the ground motion (see Fig. 2.5b, adopted from [23]).

To reduce the vibration level of the structure using MNQPEVA-based AVC, $\{\lambda_{1,2}\}$ associated with ω_{dn_1} of the structure need to be replaced by new target eigenvalues $\{\mu_{1,2} = r \pm jm\}$ where $j = \sqrt{-1}$. For this purpose, the control matrix $\mathbf{B}$ is chosen as $\mathbf{B}_{100\times 2} = \begin{bmatrix} B_{1,1} = 1\; 0 \ldots 0 & 0 & 0 \ldots 0 \\ 0 & 0 \ldots 0\; B_{2,52} = 1 & 0 \ldots 0 \end{bmatrix}^T$ that comply with the placement of actuators at the roof and first floor of the structure. As mentioned earlier, control input parameters are plagued with various uncertainties which will propagate to $\{\mu_{1,2} = r \pm jm\}$, and therefore, $\{r = Re(\mu_i),\ m = Im(\mu_i), i = 1, 2\}$ have been assumed to be random with $\mathbf{r} \sim Beta\left(\alpha_3, \beta_3, c_{l_3}, c_{u_3}\right)$ and $\mathbf{m} \sim Beta\left(\alpha_4, \beta_4, c_{l_4}, c_{u_4}\right)$. The lower and upper bounds of the distribution parameters $\left(\{\alpha_j\}_{j=3}^4, \{\beta_j\}_{j=3}^4, \{c_{l_j}\}_{j=3}^4, \{c_{u_j}\}_{j=3}^4\right)$ are presented in Table 2.3.

In this example, the random variables $\boldsymbol{\rho}$, $\mathbf{E}$, $\mathbf{r}$, and $\mathbf{m}$ are assumed to be statistically independent. Introducing a random vector $\mathbf{q} = [\boldsymbol{\rho}, \mathbf{E}, \mathbf{r}, \mathbf{m}]^T$, we have $p_{\mathbf{q}}(\mathbf{q}) = p_{\boldsymbol{\rho}}(\rho) p_{\mathbf{E}}(E) p_{\mathbf{r}}(r) p_{\mathbf{m}}(m)$. Note that the set of design variables for this example is given by $\{\theta_k\}_{k=1}^{16} = \left\{\{\alpha_j\}_{j=1}^4, \{\beta_j\}_{j=1}^4, \{c_{l_j}\}_{j=1}^4, \{c_{u_j}\}_{j=1}^4\right\}$. For design, the maximum von Mises stress, denoted by $\sigma_{VM_{max}}$, is considered as the only response quantity y_1 of interest. Failure occurs when y_1 exceeds $\sigma_{yield} = 250$ MPa where σ_{yield} is the yield stress of steel. For this example, the domain of $\mathbf{q}$ obtained using the lower bound values of $\{c_{l_j}\}_{j=1}^4$ and the upper bound values of $\{c_{u_j}\}_{j=1}^4$ is explored using $N_{ex} = 50000$ samples and three disjointed parts of failure domain are detected using Algorithm 1. For design of stochastic closed-loop system using Eq. (2.26), a resilience level associated with $P_{y_1} = 0.9999$ is selected. The coefficient a is chosen as 0.5 to provide same weight to both the terms. For this example, the values of the normalization factors g_{target} and $\mathcal{M}_{avg}$ are assumed to be 8.3107×10^{13} and 42829, respectively. The optimization problem is solved in MATLAB [36] using genetic algorithm (GA) with 0.8 crossover fraction, 0.01 mutation rate, 1 elite count, 25 initial population, and tournament selection. Note that the probability of failure for the optimal closed-loop system $P_{f_{y_1}}^{opt}$ obtained by solving Eq. (2.26) is 0.0000 as compared to the probability of failure for the initial closed-loop system $P_{f_{y_1}}^{ini} = 0.0247$. For performance comparison, the distributions of $\sigma_{VM_{max}}$ of the closed-loop systems (in the form of normalized histograms obtained from 10000 samples) before and after optimization are presented in Fig. 2.6a. It can be observed from this figure that

Table 2.3 Lower and upper bounds of distribution parameters associated with pdfs of $\boldsymbol{\rho}$, **E**, **r**, and **m** (adopted from [23])

Parameter	$\boldsymbol{\rho}$				**E**				**r**				**m**			
Distribution parameter	α_1	β_1	c_{l_1} (kg/m^3)	c_{u_1} (kg/m^3)	α_2	β_2	c_{l_2} (GPa)	c_{u_2} (GPa)	α_3	β_3	c_{l_3}	c_{u_3}	α_4	β_4	c_{l_4} (rad/s)	c_{u_4} (rad/s)
Lower bound	0	0	7000	8280	0	0	180	228	0	0	−1.00	−0.52	0	0	16.0	28.8
Upper bound	∞	∞	7320	8600	∞	∞	192	240	∞	∞	−0.88	−0.40	∞	∞	19.2	32.0

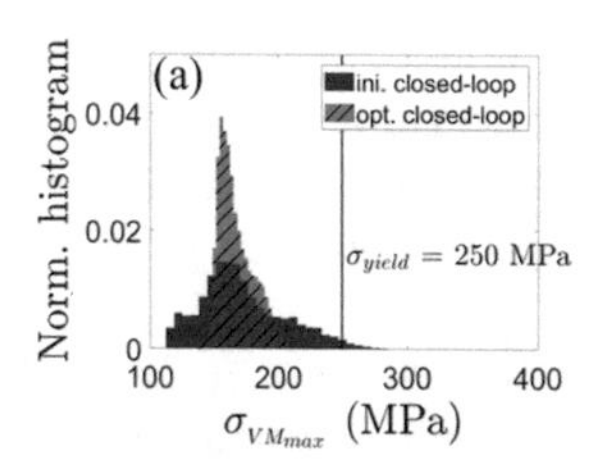

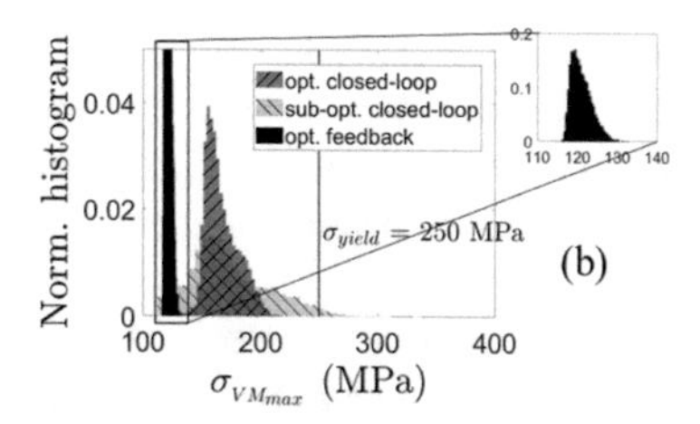

Fig. 2.6 Normalized histograms of **a** initial and optimal closed-loop systems and **b** optimal, sub-optimal closed-loop systems, and closed-loop system with optimal feedback (adopted from [23])

Table 2.4 Estimate of various statistics of $\sigma_{VM_{max}}$ for various stochastic systems obtained through solving various optimization problems (adopted from [23])

Statistics	$\sigma_{VM_{max}}$ for closed-loop systems			
	Initial	Optimal	Suboptimal	Optimal feedback
Mean	172.83	166.52	162.81	121.03
Standard deviation	34.62	14.03	29.32	2.59
Coeff. of variation	0.2003	0.0843	0.1801	0.0214

the optimal closed-loop systems are able to attain the required level of safety in the presence of uncertainties, whereas the initial closed-loop systems cannot. Also, it can be noted from Table 2.4 that the standard deviation of $\sigma_{VM_{max}}$ for the optimal closed-loop system is quiet less and hence good from design viewpoint.

A concern that might arise during the fabrication/construction of structural members is how to maintain the optimal probability distributions of $\boldsymbol{\rho}$ and $\mathbf{E}$ obtained by solving Eq. (2.26) as the state-of-the-art manufacturing process and/or construction technology are limited in their capabilities to produce material and geometric parameters with target distributions. Also, maintaining the optimal probability distributions of $\mathbf{r}$ and $\mathbf{m}$ might be difficult. To understand how the designed stochastic closed-loop system will behave under such circumstances, $\mathbf{q}_j \sim U(c_{l_j}^{opt}, c_{u_j}^{opt}), \forall j$ have been assumed (i.e., $\boldsymbol{\rho} \sim U(c_{l_1}^{opt}, c_{u_1}^{opt})$, $\mathbf{E} \sim U(c_{l_2}^{opt}, c_{u_2}^{opt})$, $\mathbf{r} \sim U(c_{l_3}^{opt}, c_{u_3}^{opt})$, and $\mathbf{m} \sim U(c_{l_4}^{opt}, c_{u_4}^{opt})$), and another 10000 samples of $\mathbf{q}$ are generated. Note that the terms $c_{l_j}^{opt}$ and $c_{u_j}^{opt}$ denote the optimal lower and upper bounds of the support of the random variable $\mathbf{q}_j$, respectively. The uniform distribution has been chosen here as it has maximum entropy and can account for the maximum variability within these bounds. A comparison of the normalized histograms of the optimal and the new sub-optimal closed-loop systems indicates that the mean of $\sigma_{VM_{max}}$ for both the cases is almost same while the standard deviation of $\sigma_{VM_{max}}$ for the suboptimal case is higher compared to the optimal counterpart (see Fig. 2.6b). The probability of failure for the suboptimal case $P_{f_{y_1}}^{subopt}$ turns out to be 0.0104 which exceeds the user-prescribed value. The suboptimal case, nevertheless, still represents a significant improvement over the initial closed-loop system in restricting the response (see Fig. 2.6b). This is practically very appealing since the proposed methodology can be confidently adapted in the design of active controlled system to account for the effects of uncertainties.

Since the state-of-the-art manufacturing process is currently limited in their capability to produce material and geometric parameters, and structural complexities with target optimal pdfs, the optimization problem given in Eq. (2.26) is solved again with $a = 1$ to exclude the contribution from $\mathcal{M}(\mathbf{q})$. This approach will provide the optimal distribution of feedback matrices only and, hence, will allow the current manufacturing technologies to embrace the design methodology presented in Sect. 2.3.1. The results for the $a = 1$ case are presented in Fig. 2.6b and Table 2.4. It is observed that the probability of failure for both $a = 1$ and $a = 0.5$ cases is 0.0000; however, the mean and standard deviation of $\sigma_{VM_{max}}$ for $a = 1$ case are much lesser compared to that of $a = 0.5$ case.

2.4 Conclusions

1. A brief review with emphasis on computational advantages and/or drawbacks of the state-space based LQR and H_∞ techniques and the physical-space based MNQPEVA technique is presented in Sect. 2.2. A numerical study of the three techniques indicates that the MNQPEVA technique is computationally efficient and require less actuator capacity (in turn, economic) as compared to the LQR and H_∞ techniques for design of optimal closed-loop systems (see Sect. 2.2.4).
2. A methodology for economic and resilient design of active controlled stochastic structural systems has been presented in Sect. 2.3.1. The methodology is based on a nested optimization scheme termed as stochastic MNQPEVA-MMCLS problem. In this nested optimization scheme, the outer optimization problem minimizes the mean of a combination of norm of feedback matrices and mass of the stochastic closed-loop system. The inner optimization problem is the MNQPEVA problem. The output of the stochastic MNQPEVA-MMCLS problem is a set of optimal parameters of the probability density functions of random material properties, geometric features, control input, etc. Following the methodology, a design example of control system for a stochastic 2D frame of a 4-story steel building is presented in Sect. 2.3.3.
3. The difficulty in numerical implementation of the methodology lies in accurate yet efficient estimation of low probability of failure. Furthermore,

the numerical implementation becomes significantly challenging since this probability of failure is typically associated with disjointed and complicated shaped failure domain. An algorithm based on hierarchical clustering technique and importance sampling scheme is presented in Sect. 2.3.2 that can mitigate the computational difficulty associated with the estimation of low probability of failure over a disjointed and complicated domain.

4. The output of the proposed methodology is a set of optimal parameters of the probability density functions of the controllable and manufacturable closed-system system properties. This is proposed with a vision that it is likely to create a new research direction in the field of manufacturing. This new direction will strive to enable the future manufacturing/fabrication technologies to produce/build structural materials, components, and control units following the target optimal distributions. The current manufacturing/fabrication techniques are, however, limited in their capacity to produce or build such optimal material, structural, and control systems. To address this issue, two alternative solutions are recommended in Sect. 2.3: (i) suboptimal closed-loop systems and (ii) closed-loop systems with optimal feedback matrices. From design viewpoint, the second way out is better than the first one as it ensures the required resilience level while leading to economic design (in terms of the energy required for the control purposes).

References

1. Billah, K., and R. Scanlan. 1991. Resonance, Tacoma Narrows bridge failure, and undergraduate physics textbooks. *American Journal of Physics* 59 (2): 118–124.
2. Dallard, P., A.J. Fitzpatrick, A. Flint, S. LeBourva, A. Low, R.M.R. Smith, and M. Willford. 2001. The London Millennium Footbridge. *The Structural Engineer* 79 (22): 17–33.
3. Anderson, B.D.O., and J.B. Moore. 1990. *Optimal control: Linear quadratic methods*. Englewood Cliffs, NJ: Prentice Hall.
4. Dorato, P., C. Abdallah, and V. Cerone. 1995. *Linear quadratic control: An introduction*. Englewood Cliffs, NJ: Prentice Hall.
5. Datta, B.N. 2004. *Numerical methods for linear control systems: Design and analysis*. San Diego: Elsevier Academic Press.
6. Francis, B.A., and J.C. Doyle. 1987. Linear control theory with an H_∞ optimality criterion. *SIAM Journal of Control and Optimization* 25: 815–844.
7. Doyle, J., K. Glover, P. Khargonekar, and B. Francis. 1989. State-space solutions to standard H_2 and H_∞ control problems. *IEEE Transactions on Automatic Control* AC-34: 831–847.
8. Kimura, H. 1996. *Chain-Scattering to H_∞ Control*. Boston: Birkhauser.
9. Zhou, K., J.C. Doyle, and K. Glover. 1996. *Robust and Optimal Control*. New Jersey: Prentice Hall.
10. Brahma, S., and B. Datta. 2009. An optimization approach for minimum norm and robust partial quadratic eigenvalue assignment problems for vibrating structures. *Journal of Sound and Vibration* 324 (3): 471–489.
11. Bai, Z.-J., B.N. Datta, and J. Wang. 2010. Robust and minimum norm partial quadratic eigenvalue assignment in vibrating systems: A new optimization approach. *Mechanical Systems and Signal Processing* 24 (3): 766–783.

12. Bai, Z.-J., M.-X. Chen, and B.N. Datta. 2013. Minimum norm partial quadratic eigenvalue assignment with time delay in vibrating structures using the receptance and the system matrices. *Journal of Sound and Vibration* 332 (4): 780–794.
13. Datta, B.N., and V. Sokolov. 2009. Quadratic inverse eigenvalue problems, active vibration control and model updating. *Applied and Computational Mathematics* 8 (2): 170–191.
14. Ghanem, R., and P.D. Spanos. 1991. *Stochastic finite elements: A spectral approach*. New York: Springer.
15. Soize, C. 2000. A nonparametric model of random uncertainties for reduced matrix models in structural dynamics. *Probabilistic Engineering Mechanics* 15 (3): 277–294.
16. Grandhi, R.V., I. Haq, and N.S. Khot. 1991. Enhanced robustness in integrated structural/control systems design. *AIAA Journal* 29 (7): 1168–1173.
17. Wang, S.-G., H.Y. Yeh, and P.N. Roschke. 2001. Robust control for structural systems with parametric and unstructured uncertainties. *Journal of Vibration and Control* 7 (5): 753–772.
18. Wang, S.-G., H.Y. Yeh, and P.N. Roschke. 2004. Robust control for structural systems with structured uncertainties. *Nonlinear Dynamics and Systems Theory* 4 (2): 195–216.
19. Wu, J.-C., H.-H. Chih, and C.-H. Chen. 2006. A robust control method for seismic protection of civil frame building. *Journal of Sound and Vibration* 294 (1–2): 314–328.
20. Dragan, V., T. Morozan, and A.-M. Stoica. 2006. *Mathematical methods in robust control of linear stochastic systems*. New York: Springer.
21. Du, H., N. Zhang, and F. Naghdy. 2011. Actuator saturation control of uncertain structures with input time delay. *Journal of Sound and Vibration* 330 (18–19): 4399–4412.
22. Yazici, H., R. Guclu, I.B. Kucukdemiral, and M.N. Alpaslan Parlakci. 2012. Robust delay-dependent H_∞ control for uncertain structural systems with actuator delay. *Journal of Dynamic Systems, Measurement, and Control* 134 (3): 031013-1–031013-15.
23. Das, S., K. Goswami, and B.N. Datta. 2016. Quadratic partial eigenvalue assignment in large-scale stochastic dynamic systems for resilient and economic design. *Mechanical Systems and Signal Processing* 72–73: 359–375.
24. Boyd, S., L. El Ghaoui, E. Feron, and V. Balakrishnan. 1994. *Linear Matrix Inequalities in System and Control Theory*. Philadelphia: SIAM.
25. Ge, M., M.-S. Chiu, and Q.-G. Wang. 2002. Robust PID controller design via LMI approach. *Journal of Process Control* 12: 3–13.
26. Inman, D. 2006. *Vibration with control*. Chichester: Wiley.
27. Datta, B.N., S. Elhay, and Y. Ram. 1997. Orthogonality and partial pole assignment for the symmetric definite quadratic pencil. *Linear Algebra and its Applications* 257: 29–48.
28. Sleijpen, G.L.G., and H.A.V.-D. Vorst. 2000. A Jacobi-Davidson iteration method for linear eigenvalue problems. *SIAM Review* 42 (2): 267–293.
29. Datta, B.N. 2010. *Numerical linear algebra and applications*, 387–483. Philadelphia: Society for Industrial and Applied Mathematics.
30. Ewins, D.J. 2009. *Modal testing: Theory practice and application*. New York: Wiley.
31. Maia, N.M.M., and J.M.M. Silva. 1997. *Theoretical and experimental modal analysis*. England: Research Studies Press Ltd.
32. McConnell, K.G., and P.S. Varoto. 2008. *Vibration testing: Theeory and practice*. New York: Wiley.
33. Kwon, D., A. Kareem. 2006. NatHaz on-line wind simulator (NOWS): Simulation of Gaussian multivariate wind fields. NatHaz Modelling Laboratory Report, University of Notre Dame. http://windsim.ce.nd.edu/.
34. Wittig, L.E., and A.K. Sinha. 1975. Simulation of multicorrelated random processes using the FFT algorithm. *The Journal of the Acoustical Society of America* 58 (3): 630–633.
35. ASCE. 2010. Minimum design loads for buildings and other structures. ASCE/SEI 7-10, American Society of Civil Engineers.
36. MATLAB, version 8.3.0.532 (R2014a), The MathWorks Inc., Natick, Massachusetts, 2014.
37. Papoulis, A., and S.U. Pillai. 2002. *Probability, random variables and stochastic processes*. New Delhi: Tata McGraw-Hill.
38. Jacod, J., and P. Protter. 2004. *Probability essentials*. New York: Springer.

39. Soize, C. 2001. Maximum entropy approach for modeling random uncertainties in transient elastodynamics. *Journal of the Acoustic Society of America* 109 (5): 1979–1996.
40. Das, S., and R. Ghanem. 2009. A bounded random matrix approach for stochastic upscaling. *SIAM Multiscale Modeling and Simulation* 8 (1): 296–325.
41. Das, S. 2012. New positive-definite random matrix ensembles for stochastic dynamical system with high level of heterogeneous uncertainties. In *Presented at SIAM conference on uncertainty quantification*, Raleigh, NC.
42. Ghanem, R., and S. Das. 2009. Hybrid representations of coupled nonparametric and parametric models for dynamic systems. *AIAA Journal* 47 (4): 1035–1044.
43. Padulo, M., and M.D. Guenov. 2011. Worst-case robust design optimization under distributional assumptions. *International Journal for Numerical Methods in Engineering* 88 (8): 797–816. http://dx.doi.org/10.1002/nme.3203.
44. Taguchi, G. 1986. Introduction to quality engineering: Designing quality into products and processes. Technical report. Tokyo: Asian Productivity Organization.
45. Phadke, M.S. 1989. *Quality engineering using robust design*. Englewood Cliffs, NJ: Prentice-Hall.
46. Box, G., and S. Jones. 1992. Designing products that are robust to the environment. *Total Quality Management and Business Excellence* 3 (3): 265–282.
47. Su, J., and J.E. Renaud. 1997. Automatic differentiation in robust optimization. *AIAA Journal* 35 (6): 1072–1079.
48. Park, G.J., T.H. Lee, K.H. Lee, and K.H. Hwang. 2006. Robust design: An overview. *AIAA Journal* 44 (1): 181–191.
49. Hastie, T., R. Tibshirani, and J. Friedman. 2009. *The elements of statistical learning: Data mining, inference, and prediction*. New York: Springer.
50. Müllner, D. 2011. Modern hierarchical, agglomerative clustering algorithms. arXiv:1109.2378 [stat.ML].
51. Carlsson, G., and F. Mémoli. 2010. Characterization, stability and convergence of hierarchical clustering methods. *Journal of Machine Learning Research* 11: 1425–1470.
52. Melchers, R.E. 1999. *Structural reliability analysis and prediction*. New York: Wiley.
53. Fishman, G. 2003. *Monte Carlo: Concepts, algorithms, and applications*. New York: Springer.
54. Robert, C.P., and G. Casella. 2004. *Monte Carlo statistical methods*. New York: Springer.

Chapter 3
Single-Time and Multi-Time Hamilton–Jacobi Theory Based on Higher Order Lagrangians

Savin Treanţă and Constantin Udrişte

Abstract This paper aims to present aspects of Hamilton–Jacobi theory via single-time and multi-time higher order Lagrangians, more precisely: Hamilton–Jacobi PDE, Hamilton–Jacobi system of PDEs, Hamilton–Jacobi divergence PDE, generating function, canonical momenta, change of variables in Hamiltonian and gauge transformation. The present work can be seen as a natural continuation of a recent paper (see [12]), where only multi-time Hamilton–Jacobi theory via second-order Lagrangians is considered. Over time, many researchers have been interested in the study of Hamilton–Jacobi equations. It is well known that the classical (single-time) Hamilton–Jacobi theory appeared in mechanics or in information theory from the desire to describe simultaneously the motion of a particle by a wave and the information dynamics by a wave carrying information. Thus, the Euler–Lagrange ODEs or the associated Hamilton ODEs are replaced by PDEs that characterize the generating function. Later, using the geometric setting of the k-osculator bundle (see [5, 8]), R. Miron and M. R. Roman studied the geometry of higher order Lagrange spaces, providing some applications in mechanics and physics. Also, O. Krupkova has investigated the Hamiltonian field theory in terms of differential geometry and local coordinate formulas (see [3]). The multi-time version of Hamilton–Jacobi theory has been extensively studied by many researchers in the last few years (see [1, 6, 7, 12, 15, 18]). In this paper, we develop our points of view (see the multi-time Lagrange–Hamilton–Jacobi theory—via first-order Lagrangians—formulated and studied by C. Udrişte and his collaborators, [18]), by developing the new concepts and methods (see, for instance, Hamilton–Jacobi divergence PDE) for a theory that involves single-time and multi-time higher order Lagrangians. This work can be used as a source for research problems and it should be of interest to engineers and applied mathematicians. For more contributions and various approaches about

S. Treanţă
Faculty of Applied Sciences, Department of Applied Mathematics, University "Politehnica" of Bucharest, Splaiul Independenţei 313, 060042 Bucharest, Romania
e-mail: savin_treanta@yahoo.com; savin.treanta@upb.ro

C. Udrişte (✉)
Faculty of Applied Sciences, Department of Mathematics-Informatics, University "Politehnica" of Bucharest, Splaiul Independenţei 313, 060042 Bucharest, Romania
e-mail: anet.udri@yahoo.com; udriste@mathem.pub.ro

A. Adhikari et al. (eds.), *Mathematical and Statistical Applications in Life Sciences and Engineering*, https://doi.org/10.1007/978-981-10-5370-2_3

different aspects of Lagrange-Hamilton dynamics and Hamilton-Jacobi theory, the reader is directed to [2, 4, 10, 11, 13, 14, 16, 17].

AMS Subject Classification: 70H03 · 70H05 · 70H20 · 70H50 · 49K15 · 49K20

3.1 Hamilton ODEs and Hamilton–Jacobi PDE

This section introduces Hamilton ODEs and Hamilton–Jacobi PDE involving single-time higher order Lagrangians.

Consider $k \geq 2$ a fixed natural number, $t \in [t_0, t_1] \subseteq R$, x: $[t_0, t_1] \subseteq R \to R^n$, $x = \left(x^i(t)\right)$, $i = \overline{1, n}$, and $x^{(a)}(t) := \frac{d^a}{dt^a} x(t)$, $a \in \{1, 2, \ldots, k\}$. We shall use alternatively the index a to mark the derivation or to mark the summation. The real C^{k+1}-class function $L\left(t, x(t), x^{(1)}(t), \ldots, x^{(k)}(t)\right)$, called *single-time higher order Lagrangian*, depends by $(k+1)n + 1$ variables.

Denoting

$$\frac{\partial L}{\partial x^{(a)i}}\left(t, x(t), x^{(1)}(t), \ldots, x^{(k)}(t)\right) = p_{ai}(t), \quad a \in \{1, 2, \ldots, k\},$$

the link $L = x^{(a)i} p_{ai} - H$ (with summation over the repeated indices!) changes the following simple integral functional

$$I(x(\cdot)) = \int_{t_0}^{t_1} L\left(t, x(t), x^{(1)}(t), \ldots, x^{(k)}(t)\right) dt \tag{P}$$

into

$$J(x(\cdot), p_1(\cdot), \ldots, p_k(\cdot)) \tag{P'}$$

$$= \int_{t_0}^{t_1} \left(x^{(a)i}(t) p_{ai}(t) - H(t, x(t), p_1(t), \ldots, p_k(t))\right) dt$$

and the (higher order) Euler–Lagrange ODEs,

$$\frac{\partial L}{\partial x^i} - \frac{d}{dt}\frac{\partial L}{\partial x^{(1)i}} + \frac{d^2}{dt^2}\frac{\partial L}{\partial x^{(2)i}} - \cdots + (-1)^k \frac{d^k}{dt^k}\frac{\partial L}{\partial x^{(k)i}} = 0, \quad i \in \{1, 2, \ldots, n\},$$

(no summation after k) written for (P'), are just the *higher order ODEs of Hamiltonian type*,

$$\sum_{a=1}^{k} (-1)^{a+1} \frac{d^a}{dt^a} p_{ai} = -\frac{\partial H}{\partial x^i}, \quad \frac{d^a}{dt^a} x^i = \frac{\partial H}{\partial p_{ai}}, \quad a \in \{1, 2, \ldots, k\}.$$

3.1.1 Hamilton–Jacobi PDE Based on Higher Order Lagrangians

Next, we shall describe Hamilton–Jacobi PDE based on higher order Lagrangians with single-time evolution variable.

Let us consider the real function $S\colon R \times R^{kn} \to R$ and the constant level sets $\Sigma_c\colon S\left(t, x, x^{(1)}, \dots, x^{(k-1)}\right) = c,\ k \geq 2$ a fixed natural number, where $x^{(a)}(t) := \dfrac{d^a}{dt^a}x(t),\ a = \overline{1, k-1}$. We assume that these sets are hypersurfaces in R^{kn+1}, that is the normal vector field satisfies

$$\left(\frac{\partial S}{\partial t}, \frac{\partial S}{\partial x^i}, \frac{\partial S}{\partial x^{(1)i}}, \dots, \frac{\partial S}{\partial x^{(k-1)i}}\right) \neq (0, \dots, 0).$$

Let $\tilde{\Gamma}\colon \left(t, x^i(t), x^{(1)i}(t), \dots, x^{(k-1)i}(t)\right),\ t \in R$, be a transversal curve to the hypersurfaces Σ_c. Then, the function $c(t) = S\left(t, x(t), x^{(1)}(t), \dots, x^{(k-1)}(t)\right)$ has nonzero derivative

$$\frac{dc}{dt}(t) = \frac{\partial S}{\partial t}\left(t, x(t), x^{(1)}(t), \dots, x^{(k-1)}(t)\right) \tag{3.1.1}$$

$$+ \frac{\partial S}{\partial x^i}\left(t, x(t), x^{(1)}(t), \dots, x^{(k-1)}(t)\right) x^{(1)i}(t)$$

$$+ \sum_{r=1}^{k-1} \frac{\partial S}{\partial x^{(r)i}}\left(t, x(t), x^{(1)}(t), \dots, x^{(k-1)}(t)\right) x^{(r+1)i}(t)$$

$$:= L\left(t, x(t), x^{(1)}(t), \dots, x^{(k)}(t)\right).$$

By computation, we obtain the *canonical momenta*

$$\frac{\partial L}{\partial x^{(a)i}}\left(t, x(t), x^{(1)}(t), \dots, x^{(k)}(t)\right) = \frac{\partial S}{\partial x^{(a-1)i}}\left(t, x(t), x^{(1)}(t), \dots, x^{(k-1)}(t)\right) := p_{ai}(t),$$

$a \in \{1, 2, \dots, k\}$. In these conditions, the relations

$$x^{(a)} = x^{(a)}\left(t, x, p_1, \dots, p_k\right), \quad a \in \{1, 2, \dots, k\},$$

become

$$x^{(a)} = x^{(a)}\left(t, x, \frac{\partial S}{\partial x}, \dots, \frac{\partial S}{\partial x^{(k-1)}}\right), \quad a \in \{1, 2, \dots, k\}.$$

On the other hand, the relation (3.1.1) can be rewritten as

$$-\frac{\partial S}{\partial t}\left(t, x(t), x^{(1)}(t), \dots, x^{(k-1)}(t)\right) \tag{3.1.2}$$

$$= \frac{\partial S}{\partial x^i}\left(t, x(t), x^{(1)}(t), \ldots, x^{(k-1)}(t)\right) x^{(1)i}\left(t, x^i, \frac{\partial S}{\partial x^i}(\cdot), \ldots, \frac{\partial S}{\partial x^{(k-1)i}}(\cdot)\right)$$

$$+ \sum_{r=1}^{k-1} \frac{\partial S}{\partial x^{(r)i}}\left(t, x(t), x^{(1)}(t), \ldots, x^{(k-1)}(t)\right) x^{(r+1)i}\left(t, x^i, \frac{\partial S}{\partial x^i}(\cdot), \ldots, \frac{\partial S}{\partial x^{(k-1)i}}(\cdot)\right)$$

$$- L\left(t, x(t), x^{(1)}(t), \ldots, x^{(k)}(t)\right).$$

Definition 3.1.1 The Lagrangian $L\left(t, x(t), x^{(1)}(t), \ldots, x^{(k)}(t)\right)$ is called super regular if the system

$$\frac{\partial L}{\partial x^{(a)i}}\left(t, x(t), x^{(1)}(t), \ldots, x^{(k)}(t)\right) = p_{ai}(t), \quad a \in \{1, 2, \ldots, k\},$$

defines the function of components

$$x^{(a)} = x^{(a)}(t, x, p_1, \ldots, p_k), \quad a \in \{1, 2, \ldots, k\}.$$

The super regular Lagrangian L enters in duality with the function of Hamiltonian type

$$H(t, x, p_1, \ldots, p_k)$$

$$= x^{(a)i}(t, x, p_1, \ldots, p_k) \frac{\partial L}{\partial x^{(a)i}}\left(t, x, \ldots, x^{(k)i}(t, x, p_1, \ldots, p_k)\right)$$

$$- L\left(t, x, x^{(1)i}(t, x, p_1, \ldots, p_k), \ldots, x^{(k)i}(t, x, p_1, \ldots, p_k)\right),$$

(*single-time higher order non-standard Legendrian duality*) or, shortly,

$$H = x^{(a)i} p_{ai} - L.$$

At this moment, we can rewrite (3.1.2) as *Hamilton–Jacobi PDE based on higher order Lagrangians*,

$$(H - J - hig.) \quad \frac{\partial S}{\partial t} + H\left(t, x^i, \frac{\partial S}{\partial x^i}, \frac{\partial S}{\partial x^{(1)i}}, \ldots, \frac{\partial S}{\partial x^{(k-1)i}}\right) = 0, \quad i = \overline{1, n}.$$

As a rule, this Hamilton–Jacobi PDE based on higher order Lagrangians is endowed with the initial condition

$$S\left(0, x, x^{(1)}, \ldots, x^{(k-1)}\right) = S_0\left(x, x^{(1)}, \ldots, x^{(k-1)}\right).$$

The solution $S\left(t, x, x^{(1)}, \ldots, x^{(k-1)}\right)$ is called the *generating function* of the canonical momenta.

Remark 3.1.2 Conversely, let $S\left(t, x, x^{(1)}, \ldots, x^{(k-1)}\right)$ be a solution of the Hamilton–Jacobi PDE based on higher order Lagrangians. We define

$$p_{ai}(t) = \frac{\partial S}{\partial x^{(a-1)i}}\left(t, x(t), x^{(1)}(t), \ldots, x^{(k-1)}(t)\right), \quad a \in \{1, 2, \ldots, k\}.$$

Then, the following link appears (see summation over the repeated indices!)

$$\int_{t_0}^{t_1} L\left(t, x(t), x^{(1)}(t), \ldots, x^{(k)}(t)\right) dt$$

$$= \int_{t_0}^{t_1} \left[x^{(a)i}(t) p_{ai}(t) - H\left(t, x^i(t), \frac{\partial S}{\partial x^i}(\cdot), \frac{\partial S}{\partial x^{(1)i}}(\cdot), \ldots, \frac{\partial S}{\partial x^{(k-1)i}}(\cdot)\right)\right] dt$$

$$= \int_\Gamma \frac{\partial S}{\partial x^{(a-1)i}} dx^{(a-1)i} + \frac{\partial S}{\partial t} dt = \int_\Gamma dS.$$

The last formula shows that the action integral can be written as a path independent curvilinear integral.

Theorem 3.1.3 *The generating function of the canonical momenta is solution of the Cauchy problem*

$$\frac{\partial S}{\partial t} + H\left(t, x^i, \frac{\partial S}{\partial x^i}, \frac{\partial S}{\partial x^{(1)i}}, \ldots, \frac{\partial S}{\partial x^{(k-1)i}}\right) = 0,$$

$$S\left(0, x, x^{(1)}, \ldots, x^{(k-1)}\right) = S_0\left(x, x^{(1)}, \ldots, x^{(k-1)}\right).$$

Theorem 3.1.4 *If*

$$L\left(t, x(t), x^{(1)}(t), \ldots, x^{(k)}(t)\right) = \frac{\partial S}{\partial t}\left(t, x(t), x^{(1)}(t), \ldots, x^{(k-1)}(t)\right)$$

$$+ \frac{\partial S}{\partial x^i}\left(t, x(t), x^{(1)}(t), \ldots, x^{(k-1)}(t)\right) x^{(1)i}(t)$$

$$+ \sum_{r=1}^{k-1} \frac{\partial S}{\partial x^{(r)i}}\left(t, x(t), x^{(1)}(t), \ldots, x^{(k-1)}(t)\right) x^{(r+1)i}(t)$$

is fulfilled and its domain is convex, then

$$\frac{\partial S}{\partial t} + H\left(t, x^i, \frac{\partial S}{\partial x^i}, \frac{\partial S}{\partial x^{(1)i}}, \ldots, \frac{\partial S}{\partial x^{(k-1)i}}\right)$$

is invariant with respect to the variable x.

Proof By direct computation, we get

$$\frac{\partial L}{\partial x^j}\left(t, x(t), x^{(1)}(t), \ldots, x^{(k)}(t)\right) = \frac{\partial^2 S}{\partial t \partial x^j}\left(t, x(t), x^{(1)}(t), \ldots, x^{(k-1)}(t)\right)$$

$$+ \frac{\partial^2 S}{\partial x^i \partial x^j}\left(t, x(t), x^{(1)}(t), \ldots x^{(k-1)}(t)\right) x^{(1)i}(t)$$

$$+ \sum_{r=1}^{k-1} \frac{\partial^2 S}{\partial x^{(r)i} \partial x^j}\left(t, x(t), x^{(1)}(t), \ldots, x^{(k-1)}(t)\right) x^{(r+1)i}(t),$$

equivalent with

$$- \frac{\partial H}{\partial x^j}\left(t, x(t), \frac{\partial S}{\partial x}(\cdot), \frac{\partial S}{\partial x^{(1)}}(\cdot), \ldots, \frac{\partial S}{\partial x^{(k-1)}}(\cdot)\right)$$

$$= \frac{\partial^2 S}{\partial t \partial x^j}\left(t, x(t), x^{(1)}(t), \ldots, x^{(k-1)}(t)\right)$$

$$+ \frac{\partial^2 S}{\partial x^i \partial x^j}\left(t, x(t), x^{(1)}(t), \ldots, x^{(k-1)}(t)\right) x^{(1)i}(t)$$

$$+ \sum_{r=1}^{k-1} \frac{\partial^2 S}{\partial x^{(r)i} \partial x^j}\left(t, x(t), x^{(1)}(t), \ldots, x^{(k-1)}(t)\right) x^{(r+1)i}(t),$$

or,

$$\frac{\partial}{\partial x^j}\left[\frac{\partial S}{\partial t} + H\left(t, x^i, \frac{\partial S}{\partial x^i}, \frac{\partial S}{\partial x^{(1)i}}, \ldots, \frac{\partial S}{\partial x^{(k-1)i}}\right)\right] = 0,$$

$$\frac{\partial S}{\partial t} + H\left(t, x^i, \frac{\partial S}{\partial x^i}, \frac{\partial S}{\partial x^{(1)i}}, \ldots, \frac{\partial S}{\partial x^{(k-1)i}}\right) = f(t, x^{(1)}(t), \ldots, x^{(k)}(t))$$

and the proof is complete.

Remark Suppose t is the time, $x = (x^i)$ is the vector of spatial coordinates, the function (operator) $H_1 = I$ is associated with the information as a measure of organization (synergy and purpose), the function (operator) $H_2 = H$ with the energy as a measure of movement, the function S^1 is the generating function for entropy, and S^2 is the generating function for action. A PDEs system of the type

$$\frac{\partial S^1}{\partial t} + H_1\left(t, x, \frac{\partial S^1}{\partial x}, \frac{\partial S^2}{\partial x}\right) = 0, \quad \frac{\partial S^2}{\partial t} + H_2\left(t, x, \frac{\partial S^1}{\partial x}, \frac{\partial S^2}{\partial x}\right) = 0$$

is called *physical control*. This kind of system can be written using the real vector function $S = (S^1, S^2)\colon R \times R^n \to R$.

3.2 Hamilton–Jacobi System of PDEs via Multi-Time Higher Order Lagrangians

In this section, we shall introduce Hamilton–Jacobi system of PDEs governed by higher order Lagrangians with multi-time evolution variable.

Let $S\colon R^m \times R^n \times R^{nm} \times R^{nm(m+1)/2} \times \cdots \times R^{[nm(m+1)\cdot\ldots\cdot(m+k-2)]/(k-1)!} \to R$ be a real function and the constant level sets,

$$\Sigma_c\colon S\left(t, x, x_{\alpha_1}, \ldots, x_{\alpha_1\ldots\alpha_{k-1}}\right) = c,$$

where $k \geq 2$ is a fixed natural number, $t = (t^1, \ldots, t^m) \in R^m$, $x_{\alpha_1} := \dfrac{\partial x}{\partial t^{\alpha_1}}, \ldots,$ $x_{\alpha_1\ldots\alpha_{k-1}} := \dfrac{\partial^{k-1} x}{\partial t^{\alpha_1}\ldots\partial t^{\alpha_{k-1}}}$. Here $\alpha_j \in \{1, 2, \ldots, m\}$, $j = \overline{1, k-1}$, $x = (x^1, \ldots, x^n) = \left(x^i\right)$, $i \in \{1, 2, \ldots, n\}$. We assume that these sets are submanifolds in $R^{m+n+\cdots+[nm(m+1)\cdot\ldots\cdot(m+k-2)]/(k-1)!}$. Consequently, the normal vector field must satisfy

$$\left(\frac{\partial S}{\partial t^\beta}, \frac{\partial S}{\partial x^i}, \frac{\partial S}{\partial x^i_{\alpha_1}}, \ldots, \frac{\partial S}{\partial x^i_{\alpha_1\ldots\alpha_{k-1}}}\right) \neq (0, \ldots, 0).$$

Let $\tilde{\Gamma}\colon \left(t, x^i(t), x^i_{\alpha_1}(t), \ldots, x^i_{\alpha_1\ldots\alpha_{k-1}}(t)\right)$, $t \in R^m$, be an m-sheet transversal to the submanifolds Σ_c. Then, the real function

$$c(t) = S\left(t, x(t), x_{\alpha_1}(t), \ldots, x_{\alpha_1\ldots\alpha_{k-1}}(t)\right)$$

has non-zero partial derivatives,

$$\begin{aligned} \frac{\partial c}{\partial t^\beta}(t) &= \frac{\partial S}{\partial t^\beta}\left(t, x(t), x_{\alpha_1}(t), \ldots, x_{\alpha_1\ldots\alpha_{k-1}}(t)\right) \\ &+ \frac{\partial S}{\partial x^i}\left(t, x(t), x_{\alpha_1}(t), \ldots, x_{\alpha_1\ldots\alpha_{k-1}}(t)\right) x^i_\beta(t) \\ + \sum_{\alpha_1\ldots\alpha_r; r=\overline{1,k-1}} &\frac{\partial S}{\partial x^i_{\alpha_1\ldots\alpha_r}}\left(t, x(t), x_{\alpha_1}(t), \ldots, x_{\alpha_1\ldots\alpha_{k-1}}(t)\right) x^i_{\alpha_1\ldots\alpha_r\beta}(t) \\ &:= L_\beta\left(t, x(t), x_{\alpha_1}(t), \ldots, x_{\alpha_1\ldots\alpha_k}(t)\right) \neq 0. \end{aligned} \quad (3.2.1)$$

For a fixed function $x(\cdot)$, let us define the *generalized multi-momenta* $p = (p^{\alpha_1\ldots\alpha_j}_{\beta,i})$, $i \in \{1, 2, \ldots, n\}$, $j \in \{1, 2, \ldots, k\}$, α_j, $\beta \in \{1, 2, \ldots, m\}$, by

$$p_{\beta,i}^{\alpha_1 \ldots \alpha_j}(t) := \frac{1}{n(\alpha_1, \alpha_2, \ldots, \alpha_j)} \frac{\partial L_\beta}{\partial x^i_{\alpha_1 \ldots \alpha_j}} \left(t, x(t), x_{\alpha_1}(t), \ldots, x_{\alpha_1 \ldots \alpha_k}(t)\right).$$

Remark 3.2.1 Here (see [9]),

$$n(\alpha_1, \alpha_2, \ldots, \alpha_k) := \frac{|\, 1_{\alpha_1} + 1_{\alpha_2} + \cdots + 1_{\alpha_k} \,|!}{(1_{\alpha_1} + 1_{\alpha_2} + \cdots + 1_{\alpha_k})!}$$

denotes the number of distinct indices represented by $\{\alpha_1, \alpha_2, \ldots, \alpha_k\}$, $\alpha_j \in \{1, 2, \ldots, m\}$, $j = \overline{1, k}$.

By computation, for $j = \overline{1, k}$ and $\dfrac{\partial S}{\partial x^i_{\alpha_0}} := \dfrac{\partial S}{\partial x^i}$, we get the non-zero components of p, namely,

$$p_{\alpha_j,i}^{\alpha_1 \ldots \alpha_{j-1} \alpha_j}(t) = \frac{1}{n(\alpha_1, \alpha_2, \ldots, \alpha_j)} \frac{\partial S}{\partial x^i_{\alpha_1 \ldots \alpha_{j-1}}} \left(t, x(t), x_{\alpha_1}(t), \ldots, x_{\alpha_1 \ldots \alpha_{k-1}}(t)\right).$$

Definition 3.2.2 The Lagrange 1-form $L_\beta\left(t, x(t), x_{\alpha_1}(t), \ldots, x_{\alpha_1 \ldots \alpha_k}(t)\right)$ is called super regular if the algebraic system

$$p_{\beta,i}^{\alpha_1 \ldots \alpha_j}(t) = \frac{1}{n(\alpha_1, \alpha_2, \ldots, \alpha_j)} \frac{\partial L_\beta}{\partial x^i_{\alpha_1 \ldots \alpha_j}} \left(t, x(t), x_{\alpha_1}(t), \ldots, x_{\alpha_1 \ldots \alpha_k}(t)\right)$$

defines the function

$$x^i_{\alpha_1} = x^i_{\alpha_1}(t, x, p^{\alpha_1}_{\alpha_1}, \ldots, p^{\alpha_1 \ldots \alpha_k}_{\alpha_k}),$$

$$\vdots$$

$$x^i_{\alpha_1 \ldots \alpha_k} = x^i_{\alpha_1 \ldots \alpha_k}(t, x, p^{\alpha_1}_{\alpha_1}, \ldots, p^{\alpha_1 \ldots \alpha_k}_{\alpha_k}).$$

In these conditions, the previous relations become

$$x^i_{\alpha_1} = x^i_{\alpha_1}\left(t, x, \frac{\partial S}{\partial x}, \ldots, \frac{1}{n(\alpha_1, \alpha_2, \ldots, \alpha_k)} \frac{\partial S}{\partial x_{\alpha_1 \ldots \alpha_{k-1}}}\right),$$

$$\vdots$$

$$x^i_{\alpha_1 \ldots \alpha_k} = x^i_{\alpha_1 \ldots \alpha_k}\left(t, x, \frac{\partial S}{\partial x}, \ldots, \frac{1}{n(\alpha_1, \alpha_2, \ldots, \alpha_k)} \frac{\partial S}{\partial x_{\alpha_1 \ldots \alpha_{k-1}}}\right).$$

On the other hand, the relation (3.2.1) can be rewritten as

$$
\begin{aligned}
&-\frac{\partial S}{\partial t^{\beta}}\left(t, x(t), x_{\alpha_1}(t), \ldots, x_{\alpha_1\ldots\alpha_{k-1}}(t)\right) \\
&= \frac{\partial S}{\partial x^{i}}\left(t, x(t), x_{\alpha_1}(t), \ldots, x_{\alpha_1\ldots\alpha_{k-1}}(t)\right) \\
&\cdot x^{i}_{\beta}\left(t, x, \frac{\partial S}{\partial x}(\cdot), \ldots, \frac{1}{n(\alpha_1, \alpha_2, \ldots, \alpha_k)} \frac{\partial S}{\partial x_{\alpha_1\ldots\alpha_{k-1}}}(\cdot)\right) \\
&+ \sum_{\alpha_1\ldots\alpha_r; r=\overline{1,k-1}} \frac{\partial S}{\partial x^{i}_{\alpha_1\ldots\alpha_r}}\left(t, x(t), x_{\alpha_1}(t), \ldots, x_{\alpha_1\ldots\alpha_{k-1}}(t)\right) \\
&\cdot x^{i}_{\alpha_1\ldots\alpha_r\beta}\left(t, x, \frac{\partial S}{\partial x}(\cdot), \ldots, \frac{1}{n(\alpha_1, \alpha_2, \ldots, \alpha_k)} \frac{\partial S}{\partial x_{\alpha_1\ldots\alpha_{k-1}}}(\cdot)\right) \\
&- L_{\beta}\left(t, x(t), x_{\alpha_1}(t), \ldots, x_{\alpha_1\ldots\alpha_k}(t)\right).
\end{aligned}
\tag{3.2.2}
$$

The super regular Lagrange 1-form L_β enters in duality with the following Hamiltonian 1-form,

$$
H_\beta\left(t, x, p^{\alpha_1}_{\alpha_1}, \ldots, p^{\alpha_1\ldots\alpha_k}_{\alpha_k}\right)
$$

$$
= \sum_{\alpha_1\ldots\alpha_j; j=\overline{1,k}} \frac{1}{n(\alpha_1, \alpha_2, \ldots, \alpha_j)} x^{i}_{\alpha_1\ldots\alpha_j}\left(t, x, p^{\alpha_1}_{\alpha_1}, \ldots, p^{\alpha_1\ldots\alpha_k}_{\alpha_k}\right)
$$

$$
\cdot \frac{\partial L_\beta}{\partial x^{i}_{\alpha_1\ldots\alpha_j}}\left(t, x, \ldots, x_{\alpha_1\ldots\alpha_k}(\cdot)\right)
$$

$$
- L_\beta\left(t, x, x_{\alpha_1}(t, x, p^{\alpha_1}_{\alpha_1}, \ldots, p^{\alpha_1\ldots\alpha_k}_{\alpha_k}), \ldots, x_{\alpha_1\ldots\alpha_k}(t, x, p^{\alpha_1}_{\alpha_1}, \ldots, p^{\alpha_1\ldots\alpha_k}_{\alpha_k})\right),
$$

(*multi-time higher order non-standard Legendrian duality*) or, shortly,

$$
H_\beta = x^{i}_{\alpha_1\ldots\alpha_j} p^{\alpha_1\ldots\alpha_j}_{\beta,i} - L_\beta.
$$

Now, we can rewrite (3.2.2) as *Hamilton–Jacobi system of PDEs based on higher order Lagrangians*

$$
(H - J - hig^{*}) \quad \frac{\partial S}{\partial t^{\beta}} + H_\beta\left(t, x, \frac{\partial S}{\partial x}, \ldots, \frac{\partial S}{\partial x_{\alpha_1\ldots\alpha_{k-1}}}\right) = 0, \quad \beta \in \{1, \ldots m\}.
$$

Usually, the Hamilton–Jacobi system of PDEs based on higher order Lagrangians is accompanied by the initial condition

$$
S\left(0, x, x_{\alpha_1}, \ldots x_{\alpha_1\ldots\alpha_{k-1}}\right) = S_0\left(x, x_{\alpha_1}, \ldots x_{\alpha_1\ldots\alpha_{k-1}}\right).
$$

The solution $S\left(t, x, x_{\alpha_1}, \ldots x_{\alpha_1\ldots\alpha_{k-1}}\right)$ is called the *generating function* of the generalized multi-momenta.

Remark 3.2.3 Conversely, let $S\left(t, x, x_{\alpha_1}, \dots x_{\alpha_1 \dots \alpha_{k-1}}\right)$ be a solution of the Hamilton–Jacobi system of PDEs based on higher order Lagrangians. We assume (the non-zero components of p)

$$p_{\alpha_j, i}^{\alpha_1 \dots \alpha_{j-1} \alpha_j}(t) := \frac{1}{n(\alpha_1, \alpha_2, \dots \alpha_j)} \frac{\partial S}{\partial x^i_{\alpha_1 \dots \alpha_{j-1}}} \left(t, x(t), x_{\alpha_1}(t), \dots x_{\alpha_1 \dots \alpha_{k-1}}(t)\right),$$

for $j = \overline{1, k}$ and $\dfrac{\partial S}{\partial x^i_{\alpha_0}} := \dfrac{\partial S}{\partial x^i}$.

Then, the following formula shows that the action integral can be written as a path independent curvilinear integral,

$$\int_{\Gamma_{t_0, t_1}} L_\beta \left(t, x(t), x_{\alpha_1}(t), \dots x_{\alpha_1 \dots \alpha_k}(t)\right) dt^\beta$$

$$= \int_{\Gamma_{t_0, t_1}} \left[x^i_{\alpha_1 \dots \alpha_j}(t) p_{\beta, i}^{\alpha_1 \dots \alpha_j}(t) - H_\beta \left(t, x, \frac{\partial S}{\partial x}(\cdot), \dots \frac{\partial S}{\partial x_{\alpha_1 \dots \alpha_{k-1}}}(\cdot)\right)\right] dt^\beta$$

$$= \int_\Gamma \sum_{\alpha_1 \dots \alpha_{j-1}; j=\overline{1,k}} \frac{1}{n(\alpha_1, \alpha_2, \dots \alpha_j)} \frac{\partial S}{\partial x^i_{\alpha_1 \dots \alpha_{j-1}}} dx^i_{\alpha_1 \dots \alpha_{j-1}} + \frac{\partial S}{\partial t^\beta} dt^\beta = \int_\Gamma dS.$$

Theorem 3.2.4 *The generating function of the generalized multi-momenta is solution of the Cauchy problem*

$$\frac{\partial S}{\partial t^\beta} + H_\beta \left(t, x, \frac{\partial S}{\partial x}, \dots, \frac{\partial S}{\partial x_{\alpha_1 \dots \alpha_{k-1}}}\right) = 0, \quad \beta \in \{1, \dots m\},$$

$$S\left(0, x, x_{\alpha_1}, \dots x_{\alpha_1 \dots \alpha_{k-1}}\right) = S_0 \left(x, x_{\alpha_1}, \dots x_{\alpha_1 \dots \alpha_{k-1}}\right).$$

3.3 Gauge Transformation and Moments for Higher Order Lagrangians

The classical Lagrangian dynamics is governed by second-order differential equations or second-order partial differential equations (see multi-time case) of Euler–Lagrange type with boundary conditions. The Euler–Lagrange ODEs (PDEs) solutions are called *extremals* or *critical points* of considered functionals (simple, multiple, curvilinear integrals). The integrating functions, named *Lagrange functions* or *Lagrangians*, are differentiable functions with vector argument.

On the other hand, the Hamiltonian dynamics is formulated using first-order differential equations or first-order partial differential equations (see multi-time case) arising from second-order Euler–Lagrange ODEs (PDEs). This transition is made using the *Legendre transformation*.

In this section, we shall study the relations which appear between two Lagrange functions joined by a transformation of gauge type.

The single-time case. Let us consider two single-time higher order Lagrangians,

$$L^{\zeta}\left(t, x(t), x^{(1)}(t), x^{(2)}(t), \ldots, x^{(k)}(t)\right), \quad \zeta = 1, 2,$$

with $t \in [t_0, t_1] \subset R$, $x(\cdot) \in R^n$, $k \geq 2$ a fixed natural number, joined by a transformation of *gauge* type (adding a total derivative), i.e.

$$L^2 = L^1 + \frac{d}{dt} f\left(t, x(t), x^{(1)}(t), x^{(2)}(t), \ldots, x^{(k-1)}(t)\right)$$

$$= L^1 + \frac{\partial f}{\partial t} + \frac{\partial f}{\partial x^j} x^{(1)j} + \frac{\partial f}{\partial x^{(1)j}} x^{(2)j} + \cdots + \frac{\partial f}{\partial x^{(k-1)j}} x^{(k)j}, \quad j = \overline{1, n}.$$

The summation over the repeated indices is assumed. Then, the corresponding moments p^1_{ai}, p^2_{ai}, $a = \overline{1, k}$, $i = \overline{1, n}$, satisfy the following relations

$$p^2_{ai} := \frac{\partial L^2}{\partial x^{(a)i}} = \frac{\partial L^1}{\partial x^{(a)i}} + \frac{d}{dt} \frac{\partial f}{\partial x^{(a)i}} + \frac{\partial f}{\partial x^{(a-1)i}}$$

$$= p^1_{ai} + \frac{d}{dt} \frac{\partial f}{\partial x^{(a)i}} + \frac{\partial f}{\partial x^{(a-1)i}}, \quad a = \overline{1, k-1},$$

$$p^2_{ki} := \frac{\partial L^2}{\partial x^{(k)i}} = \frac{\partial L^1}{\partial x^{(k)i}} + \frac{\partial f}{\partial x^{(k-1)i}} = p^1_{ki} + \frac{\partial f}{\partial x^{(k-1)i}}, \quad a = k.$$

The previous computations allow us to establish the following result.

Proposition 3.3.1 *Two single-time higher order Lagrangians, satisfying* $L^2 = L^1 + \frac{d}{dt} f\left(t, x(t), x^{(1)}(t), x^{(2)}(t), \ldots, x^{(k-1)}(t)\right)$, *where* L^2, L^1 *and* f *are considered* C^{k+1}*-class functions, produce the same Euler–Lagrange ODEs, i.e.*

$$\frac{\partial L^2}{\partial x^i} - \frac{d}{dt} \frac{\partial L^2}{\partial x^{(1)i}} + \frac{d^2}{dt^2} \frac{\partial L^2}{\partial x^{(2)i}} - \ldots + (-1)^k \frac{d^k}{dt^k} \frac{\partial L^2}{\partial x^{(k)i}}$$

$$= \frac{\partial L^1}{\partial x^i} - \frac{d}{dt} \frac{\partial L^1}{\partial x^{(1)i}} + \frac{d^2}{dt^2} \frac{\partial L^1}{\partial x^{(2)i}} - \cdots + (-1)^k \frac{d^k}{dt^k} \frac{\partial L^1}{\partial x^{(k)i}}, \quad i = \overline{1, n},$$

or

$$\sum_{r=1}^{k+1} (-1)^{r-1} \frac{d^{r-1}}{dt^{r-1}} \frac{\partial L^2}{\partial x^{(r-1)i}} = \sum_{r=1}^{k+1} (-1)^{r-1} \frac{d^{r-1}}{dt^{r-1}} \frac{\partial L^1}{\partial x^{(r-1)i}}, \quad i = \overline{1, n}.$$

Proof By a direct calculation, we get

$$\frac{\partial L^2}{\partial x^i} - \frac{d}{dt}\frac{\partial L^2}{\partial x^{(1)i}} + \frac{d^2}{dt^2}\frac{\partial L^2}{\partial x^{(2)i}} - \cdots + (-1)^k \frac{d^k}{dt^k}\frac{\partial L^2}{\partial x^{(k)i}}$$

$$= \sum_{r=1}^{k} (-1)^{r-1} \frac{d^{r-1}}{dt^{r-1}} \frac{\partial L^2}{\partial x^{(r-1)i}} + (-1)^k \frac{d^k}{dt^k}\frac{\partial L^2}{\partial x^{(k)i}}$$

$$= \frac{\partial L^2}{\partial x^i} + \sum_{r=2}^{k} (-1)^{r-1} \frac{d^{r-1}}{dt^{r-1}} \left(\frac{\partial L^1}{\partial x^{(r-1)i}} + \frac{d}{dt}\frac{\partial f}{\partial x^{(r-1)i}} + \frac{\partial f}{\partial x^{(r-2)i}} \right)$$

$$+ (-1)^k \frac{d^k}{dt^k} \left(\frac{\partial L^1}{\partial x^{(k)i}} + \frac{\partial f}{\partial x^{(k-1)i}} \right)$$

$$= \frac{\partial L^1}{\partial x^i} + \frac{d}{dt}\frac{\partial f}{\partial x^i} + \sum_{r=2}^{k} (-1)^{r-1} \frac{d^{r-1}}{dt^{r-1}} \frac{\partial L^1}{\partial x^{(r-1)i}} + (-1)^k \frac{d^k}{dt^k}\frac{\partial L^1}{\partial x^{(k)i}}$$

$$+ (-1)^k \frac{d^k}{dt^k}\frac{\partial f}{\partial x^{(k-1)i}} - \frac{d}{dt}\frac{\partial f}{\partial x^i} + (-1)^{k-1} \frac{d^k}{dt^k}\frac{\partial f}{\partial x^{(k-1)i}}$$

$$= \sum_{r=1}^{k} (-1)^{r-1} \frac{d^{r-1}}{dt^{r-1}} \frac{\partial L^1}{\partial x^{(r-1)i}} + (-1)^k \frac{d^k}{dt^k}\frac{\partial L^1}{\partial x^{(k)i}}$$

$$= \frac{\partial L^1}{\partial x^i} - \frac{d}{dt}\frac{\partial L^1}{\partial x^{(1)i}} + \frac{d^2}{dt^2}\frac{\partial L^1}{\partial x^{(2)i}} - \cdots + (-1)^k \frac{d^k}{dt^k}\frac{\partial L^1}{\partial x^{(k)i}}, \quad i = \overline{1, n}$$

and the proof is complete.

The multi-time case. Consider two multi-time higher order Lagrangians,

$$L^{\zeta} \left(t, x(t), x_{\alpha_1}(t), \ldots, x_{\alpha_1 \ldots \alpha_k}(t) \right), \quad \zeta = 1, 2,$$

that are joined by a transformation of *gauge* type (adding a total derivative), i.e.

$$L^2 = L^1 + D_{\eta} f^{\eta} \left(t, x(t), x_{\alpha_1}(t), \ldots, x_{\alpha_1 \ldots \alpha_{k-1}}(t) \right) \quad (3.3.1)$$

$$= L^1 + \frac{\partial f^{\eta}}{\partial t^{\eta}} + \frac{\partial f^{\eta}}{\partial x^j} x^j_{\eta} + \frac{\partial f^{\eta}}{\partial x^j_{\alpha_1}} x^j_{\alpha_1 \eta} + \frac{1}{n(\alpha_1, \alpha_2)} \frac{\partial f^{\eta}}{\partial x^j_{\alpha_1 \alpha_2}} x^j_{\alpha_1 \alpha_2 \eta}$$

$$+ \cdots + \frac{1}{n(\alpha_1, \ldots, \alpha_{k-1})} \frac{\partial f^{\eta}}{\partial x^j_{\alpha_1 \ldots \alpha_{k-1}}} x^j_{\alpha_1 \ldots \alpha_{k-1} \eta}, \quad \eta = \overline{1, m}, \quad j = \overline{1, n}.$$

Here $t = (t^1, \dots, t^m) \in \Omega_{t_0,t_1} \subset R^m$ (see Ω_{t_0,t_1} as the hyper parallelepiped determined by diagonal opposite points t_0, t_1 from R^m), $x_{\alpha_1}(t) := \frac{\partial x}{\partial t^{\alpha_1}}(t), \dots,$ $x_{\alpha_1 \dots \alpha_k}(t) := \frac{\partial^k x}{\partial t^{\alpha_1} \dots \partial t^{\alpha_k}}(t)$, $\alpha_j \in \{1, 2, \dots m\}$, $j = \overline{1,k}$, $x \colon \Omega_{t_0,t_1} \subset R^m \to R^n$, $x = \left(x^i\right)$, $i \in \{1, 2, \dots n\}$, and $n(\alpha_1, \alpha_2, \dots \alpha_k) = \frac{| 1_{\alpha_1} + 1_{\alpha_2} + \dots + 1_{\alpha_k} |!}{(1_{\alpha_1} + 1_{\alpha_2} + \dots + 1_{\alpha_k})!}$ (see [9]). The summation over the repeated indices is assumed.

The corresponding moments $p_{i1}^{\alpha_1 \dots \alpha_j}$, $p_{i2}^{\alpha_1 \dots \alpha_j}$, $j = \overline{1,k}$, $i = \overline{1,n}$, satisfy the following relations

$$p_{i2}^{\alpha_1 \dots \alpha_j} := \frac{\partial L^2}{\partial x^i_{\alpha_1 \dots \alpha_j}} = \frac{\partial L^1}{\partial x^i_{\alpha_1 \dots \alpha_j}} + \frac{\partial}{\partial x^i_{\alpha_1 \dots \alpha_j}} \left(D_\eta f^\eta\right)$$

$$= p_{i1}^{\alpha_1 \dots \alpha_j} + D_\eta \frac{\partial f^\eta}{\partial x^i_{\alpha_1 \dots \alpha_j}} + \frac{1}{n(\alpha_1, \dots, \alpha_{j-1})} \frac{\partial f^{\alpha_j}}{\partial x^i_{\alpha_1 \dots \alpha_{j-1}}}, \quad j = \overline{1, k-1},$$

$$p_{i2}^{\alpha_1 \dots \alpha_k} := \frac{\partial L^2}{\partial x^i_{\alpha_1 \dots \alpha_k}} = \frac{\partial L^1}{\partial x^i_{\alpha_1 \dots \alpha_k}} + \frac{1}{n(\alpha_1, \dots, \alpha_{k-1})} \frac{\partial f^{\alpha_k}}{\partial x^i_{\alpha_1 \dots \alpha_{k-1}}}$$

$$= p_{i1}^{\alpha_1 \dots \alpha_k} + \frac{1}{n(\alpha_1, \dots, \alpha_{k-1})} \frac{\partial f^{\alpha_k}}{\partial x^i_{\alpha_1 \dots \alpha_{k-1}}}, \quad j = k.$$

Taking into account the previous computations, we establish the following result.

Proposition 3.3.2 *Two multi-time higher order Lagrangians, satisfying* $L^2 = L^1 + D_\eta f^\eta \left(t, x(t), x_{\alpha_1}(t), \dots, x_{\alpha_1 \dots \alpha_{k-1}}(t)\right)$, *where* L^2, L^1 *and* f *are considered* C^{k+1}-*class functions, produce the same PDEs, i.e.*

$$\frac{\partial L^2}{\partial x^i} - D_{\alpha_1} \frac{\partial L^2}{\partial x^i_{\alpha_1}} + D^2_{\alpha_1 \alpha_2} \frac{\partial L^2}{\partial x^i_{\alpha_1 \alpha_2}} - D^3_{\alpha_1 \alpha_2 \alpha_3} \frac{\partial L^2}{\partial x^i_{\alpha_1 \alpha_2 \alpha_3}}$$

$$+ \dots + (-1)^k D^k_{\alpha_1 \alpha_2 \dots \alpha_k} \frac{\partial L^2}{\partial x^i_{\alpha_1 \alpha_2 \dots \alpha_k}}$$

$$= \frac{\partial L^1}{\partial x^i} - D_{\alpha_1} \frac{\partial L^1}{\partial x^i_{\alpha_1}} + D^2_{\alpha_1 \alpha_2} \frac{\partial L^1}{\partial x^i_{\alpha_1 \alpha_2}} - D^3_{\alpha_1 \alpha_2 \alpha_3} \frac{\partial L^1}{\partial x^i_{\alpha_1 \alpha_2 \alpha_3}}$$

$$+ \dots + (-1)^k D^k_{\alpha_1 \alpha_2 \dots \alpha_k} \frac{\partial L^1}{\partial x^i_{\alpha_1 \alpha_2 \dots \alpha_k}}, \quad i \in \{1, 2, \dots, n\},$$

(summation over the repeated indices!) or, shortly,

$$\sum_{r=0}^{k}(-1)^r D^r_{\alpha_1\alpha_2\ldots\alpha_r}\frac{\partial L^2}{\partial x^i_{\alpha_1\alpha_2\ldots\alpha_r}} = \sum_{r=0}^{k}(-1)^r D^r_{\alpha_1\alpha_2\ldots\alpha_r}\frac{\partial L^1}{\partial x^i_{\alpha_1\alpha_2\ldots\alpha_r}}, \quad i=\overline{1,n},$$

if and only if the total divergence of f is defined as

$$D_\eta f^\eta\left(t, x(t), x_{\alpha_1}(t), \ldots, x_{\alpha_1\ldots\alpha_{k-1}}(t)\right)$$

$$= \frac{\partial f^\eta}{\partial t^\eta} + \frac{\partial f^\eta}{\partial x^j}x^j_\eta + \frac{\partial f^\eta}{\partial x^j_{\alpha_1}}x^j_{\alpha_1\eta} + \frac{\partial f^\eta}{\partial x^j_{\alpha_1\alpha_2}}x^j_{\alpha_1\alpha_2\eta}$$

$$+\cdots+\frac{\partial f^\eta}{\partial x^j_{\alpha_1\ldots\alpha_{k-1}}}x^j_{\alpha_1\ldots\alpha_{k-1}\eta}, \quad \eta=\overline{1,m}, \quad j=\overline{1,n}.$$

Otherwise, (i.e. if the total divergence of f is defined as (3.3.1)) the following equality is true (i.e. L^2 and L^1 produce the same PDEs)

$$\sum_{r=0}^{k}(-1)^r D^r_{\alpha_1\ldots\alpha_r}\frac{\partial L^2}{\partial x^i_{\alpha_1\ldots\alpha_r}} = \sum_{r=0}^{k}(-1)^r D^r_{\alpha_1\ldots\alpha_r}\frac{\partial L^1}{\partial x^i_{\alpha_1\ldots\alpha_r}}, \quad i\in\{1,2,\ldots,n\},$$

if and only if

$$\sum_{r=2}^{k-1}(-1)^r D^{r+1}_{\alpha_1\ldots\alpha_r\eta}\frac{\partial f^\eta}{\partial x^i_{\alpha_1\ldots\alpha_r}}$$

$$=\sum_{r=3}^{k}(-1)^{r+1}\frac{1}{n(\alpha_1,\ldots,\alpha_{r-1})}D^r_{\alpha_1\ldots\alpha_{r-1}\alpha_r}\frac{\partial f^{\alpha_r}}{\partial x^i_{\alpha_1\ldots\alpha_{r-1}}}, \quad i\in\{1,2,\ldots,n\}.$$

Proof Direct calculation.

Corollary 3.3.3 *Let us consider that the relation (3.3.1) is verified. Then, L^2 and L^1 produce the same multi-time Euler–Lagrange PDEs, i.e.*

$$\sum_{r=0}^{k}(-1)^r\frac{1}{n(\alpha_1,\ldots,\alpha_r)}D^r_{\alpha_1\ldots\alpha_r}\frac{\partial L^2}{\partial x^i_{\alpha_1\ldots\alpha_r}}$$

$$=\sum_{r=0}^{k}(-1)^r\frac{1}{n(\alpha_1,\ldots,\alpha_r)}D^r_{\alpha_1\ldots\alpha_r}\frac{\partial L^1}{\partial x^i_{\alpha_1\ldots\alpha_r}}, \quad i\in\{1,2,\ldots,n\},$$

if and only if

$$\sum_{r=1}^{k-1}(-1)^r\frac{1}{n(\alpha_1,\ldots,\alpha_r)}D^{r+1}_{\alpha_1\ldots\alpha_r\eta}\frac{\partial f^\eta}{\partial x^i_{\alpha_1\ldots\alpha_r}}$$

$$= \sum_{r=2}^{k} (-1)^{r+1} \frac{1}{n(\alpha_1, \ldots, \alpha_r)} \frac{1}{n(\alpha_1, \ldots, \alpha_{r-1})} D^r_{\alpha_1 \ldots \alpha_{r-1} \alpha_r} \frac{\partial f^{\alpha_r}}{\partial x^i_{\alpha_1 \ldots \alpha_{r-1}}}, \quad i = \overline{1, n}.$$

Remark 3.3.4 The previous multi-time case takes into account the total divergence of f. As well, we can consider multi-time higher order Lagrangian 1-forms, $L^{\varepsilon}_{\zeta}\left(t, x(t), x_{\alpha_1}(t), \ldots, x_{\alpha_1 \ldots \alpha_k}(t)\right) dt^{\zeta}$, $\varepsilon = 1, 2$, and the transformation of *gauge* type becomes $L^2_{\zeta} = L^1_{\zeta} + D_{\zeta} f\left(t, x(t), x_{\alpha_1}(t), \ldots, x_{\alpha_1 \ldots \alpha_{k-1}}(t)\right)$, $\zeta = \overline{1, m}$.

The corresponding moments $p^{\alpha_1 \ldots \alpha_j}_{i\zeta,1}$, $p^{\alpha_1 \ldots \alpha_j}_{i\zeta,2}$, $j = \overline{1, k}$, $i = \overline{1, n}$, satisfy the following relations

$$p^{\alpha_1 \ldots \alpha_j}_{i\zeta,2} := \frac{\partial L^2_{\zeta}}{\partial x^i_{\alpha_1 \ldots \alpha_j}} = \frac{\partial L^1_{\zeta}}{\partial x^i_{\alpha_1 \ldots \alpha_j}} + \frac{\partial}{\partial x^i_{\alpha_1 \ldots \alpha_j}} \left(D_{\zeta} f\right) = p^{\alpha_1 \ldots \alpha_j}_{i\zeta,1}$$

$$+ D_{\zeta} \frac{\partial f}{\partial x^i_{\alpha_1 \ldots \alpha_j}} + \frac{1}{n(\alpha_1, \ldots, \alpha_p)} \frac{\partial f}{\partial x^i_{\alpha_1 \ldots \alpha_p}} \delta^{\alpha_{p+1} \ldots \alpha_j}_{\zeta}, \quad j = \overline{1, k-1}, \quad p = j - 1,$$

$$p^{\alpha_1 \ldots \alpha_k}_{i\zeta,2} := \frac{\partial L^2_{\zeta}}{\partial x^i_{\alpha_1 \ldots \alpha_k}} = \frac{\partial L^1_{\zeta}}{\partial x^i_{\alpha_1 \ldots \alpha_k}} + \frac{\partial}{\partial x^i_{\alpha_1 \ldots \alpha_k}} \left(D_{\zeta} f\right)$$

$$= p^{\alpha_1 \ldots \alpha_k}_{i\zeta,1} + \frac{1}{n(\alpha_1, \ldots, \alpha_{k-1})} \frac{\partial f}{\partial x^i_{\alpha_1 \ldots \alpha_{k-1}}} \delta^{\alpha_k}_{\zeta}, \quad j = k.$$

Using the previous relations and $\dfrac{\partial L^2_{\zeta}}{\partial x^i} = \dfrac{\partial L^1_{\zeta}}{\partial x^i} + D_{\zeta} \dfrac{\partial f}{\partial x^i}$ we establish the following result.

Proposition 3.3.5 *Two multi-time higher order Lagrangian* 1*-forms, satisfying* $L^2_{\zeta} = L^1_{\zeta} + D_{\zeta} f$, *where* L^2_{ζ}, L^1_{ζ} *and* f *are considered* C^{k+1}*-class functions, produce the same PDEs, i.e.*

$$\sum_{r=0}^{k} (-1)^r D^r_{\alpha_1 \alpha_2 \ldots \alpha_r} \frac{\partial L^2_{\zeta}}{\partial x^i_{\alpha_1 \alpha_2 \ldots \alpha_r}} = \sum_{r=0}^{k} (-1)^r D^r_{\alpha_1 \alpha_2 \ldots \alpha_r} \frac{\partial L^1_{\zeta}}{\partial x^i_{\alpha_1 \alpha_2 \ldots \alpha_r}}, \quad i = \overline{1, n},$$

if and only if

$$\sum_{r=2}^{k-1} (-1)^r D^{r+1}_{\alpha_1 \alpha_2 \ldots \alpha_r \zeta} \frac{\partial f}{\partial x^i_{\alpha_1 \alpha_2 \ldots \alpha_r}}$$

$$= \sum_{r=3}^{k} (-1)^{r+1} \frac{1}{n(\alpha_1, \ldots, \alpha_p)} D^r_{\alpha_1 \alpha_2 \ldots \alpha_r} \frac{\partial f}{\partial x^i_{\alpha_1 \alpha_2 \ldots \alpha_p}} \delta^{\alpha_{p+1} \ldots \alpha_r}_{\zeta}, \quad i = \overline{1, n}, \quad p = r - 1.$$

Proof Direct computation.

Corollary 3.3.6 *The multi-time higher order Lagrangian* 1*-forms,* L^2_ζ *and* L^1_ζ*, joined by a transformation of gauge type, produce the same multi-time Euler–Lagrange PDEs, i.e.*

$$\sum_{r=0}^{k}(-1)^r \frac{1}{n(\alpha_1,\ldots,\alpha_r)} D^r_{\alpha_1\ldots\alpha_r} \frac{\partial L^2_\zeta}{\partial x^i_{\alpha_1\ldots\alpha_r}}$$

$$= \sum_{r=0}^{k}(-1)^r \frac{1}{n(\alpha_1,\ldots,\alpha_r)} D^r_{\alpha_1\ldots\alpha_r} \frac{\partial L^1_\zeta}{\partial x^i_{\alpha_1\ldots\alpha_r}}, \quad i \in \{1,2,\ldots,n\},$$

if and only if

$$\sum_{r=1}^{k-1}(-1)^r \frac{1}{n(\alpha_1,\ldots,\alpha_r)} D^{r+1}_{\alpha_1\ldots\alpha_r\zeta} \frac{\partial f}{\partial x^i_{\alpha_1\ldots\alpha_r}}$$

$$= \sum_{r=2}^{k}(-1)^{r+1} \frac{1}{n(\alpha_1,\ldots,\alpha_r)} \frac{1}{n(\alpha_1,\ldots,\alpha_p)} D^r_{\alpha_1\ldots\alpha_r} \frac{\partial f}{\partial x^i_{\alpha_1\ldots\alpha_p}} \delta_\zeta^{\alpha_{p+1}\ldots\alpha_r}$$

$$i = \overline{1,n}, \quad p = r-1.$$

3.3.1 The Adding of the Dissipative Forces

The single-time case. Let us consider the function

$$R\left(t, x(t), x^{(1)}(t), \ldots, x^{(k)}(t)\right), \quad k \geq 1,$$

that determines the *generalized dissipative force* $-\dfrac{\partial R}{\partial x^{(k)i}}$. Such type of forces, for a fixed k, changes the ODEs of Hamiltonian type as

$$\sum_{a=1}^{k}(-1)^{a+1}\frac{d^a}{dt^a}p_{ai} = -\frac{\partial H}{\partial x^i} - \frac{\partial R}{\partial x^{(k)i}}, \quad \frac{d^a}{dt^a}x^i = \frac{\partial H}{\partial p_{ai}}.$$

We obtain

$$\frac{dH}{dt} = \frac{\partial H}{\partial x^i}x^{(1)i} + \frac{\partial H}{\partial p_{ai}}\frac{dp_{ai}}{dt} + \frac{\partial H}{\partial t}$$

$$= \left[\sum_{a=1}^{k}(-1)^a \frac{d^a}{dt^a}p_{ai} - \frac{\partial R}{\partial x^{(k)i}}\right]x^{(1)i} + x^{(a)i}\frac{dp_{ai}}{dt} + \frac{\partial H}{\partial t}$$

$$= \left(-\frac{\partial L}{\partial x^i} - \frac{\partial R}{\partial x^{(k)i}}\right) x^{(1)i} + x^{(a)i}\frac{dp_{ai}}{dt} + \frac{\partial H}{\partial t}$$

(summation over the repeated indices!) and $\frac{\partial H}{\partial t} = 0$ implies

$$\frac{dH}{dt} = 0 \Longleftrightarrow x^{(a)i}\frac{dp_{ai}}{dt} = \left(\frac{\partial L}{\partial x^i} + \frac{\partial R}{\partial x^{(k)i}}\right) x^{(1)i}.$$

The multi-time case. Let assume that the function

$$R\left(t, x(t), x_{\alpha_1}(t), \ldots, x_{\alpha_1\ldots\alpha_k}(t)\right), \quad k \geq 1,$$

determines the *generalized multi-time $\alpha_1 \ldots \alpha_k$-dissipative force* $-\frac{\partial R}{\partial x^i_{\alpha_1\ldots\alpha_k}}$, where $\alpha_1, \ldots \alpha_k \in \{1, 2, \ldots, m\}$ are fixed. The PDEs of Hamiltonian type becomes

$$\sum_{j=1}^{k}(-1)^{j+1} D^j_{\alpha_1\ldots\alpha_j} p_i^{\alpha_1\ldots\alpha_j} = -\frac{\partial H}{\partial x^i} - \frac{\partial R}{\partial x^i_{\alpha_1\ldots\alpha_k}},$$

$$x^i_{\alpha_1\ldots\alpha_j} = \frac{\partial H}{\partial p_i^{\alpha_1\ldots\alpha_j}}, \quad j = \overline{1,k}, \quad i = \overline{1,n}.$$

Here, $p_i^{\alpha_1\ldots\alpha_j} := \frac{1}{n(\alpha_1, \ldots, \alpha_j)}\frac{\partial L}{\partial x^i_{\alpha_1\ldots\alpha_j}}$, $i \in \{1, 2, \ldots, n\}$, $j \in \{1, 2, \ldots, k\}$, $\alpha_j \in \{1, 2, \ldots, m\}$. Computing the total derivative of H, we find

$$D_\zeta H = \frac{\partial H}{\partial x^i}\frac{\partial x^i}{\partial t^\zeta} + \sum_{j=1}^{k}\frac{\partial H}{\partial p_i^{\alpha_1\ldots\alpha_j}}\frac{\partial p_i^{\alpha_1\ldots\alpha_j}}{\partial t^\zeta} + \frac{\partial H}{\partial t^\zeta}$$

$$= \left(\sum_{j=1}^{k}(-1)^j D^j_{\alpha_1\ldots\alpha_j} p_i^{\alpha_1\ldots\alpha_j} - \frac{\partial R}{\partial x^i_{\alpha_1\ldots\alpha_k}}\right) x^i_\zeta$$

$$+ \sum_{j=1}^{k}\frac{\partial H}{\partial p_i^{\alpha_1\ldots\alpha_j}}\frac{\partial p_i^{\alpha_1\ldots\alpha_j}}{\partial t^\zeta} + \frac{\partial H}{\partial t^\zeta},$$

and $\frac{\partial H}{\partial t^\zeta} = 0$ implies

$$D_\zeta H = \left(-\frac{\partial R}{\partial x^i_{\alpha_1\ldots\alpha_k}} - \frac{\partial L}{\partial x^i}\right) x^i_\zeta + \sum_{j=1}^{k} x^i_{\alpha_1\ldots\alpha_j}\frac{\partial p_i^{\alpha_1\ldots\alpha_j}}{\partial t^\zeta}.$$

3.4 The Change of Variables in Hamiltonian and the Generating Function via Higher Order Lagrangians

The single-time case. Let $H = x^{(a)i} p_{ai} - L$ be the Hamiltonian and

$$\sum_{a=1}^{k}(-1)^{a+1}\frac{d^a}{dt^a}p_{ai}(t) = -\frac{\partial H}{\partial x^i}(x(t), p_1(t), \dots, p_k(t), t), \tag{3.4.1}$$

$$\frac{d^a}{dt^a}x^i(t) = \frac{\partial H}{\partial p_{ai}}(x(t), p_1(t), \dots, p_k(t), t), \quad i = \overline{1, n},$$

the associated ODEs. Let assume that we want to pass from our coordinates $(x^i, p_{1i}, \dots, p_{ki}, t)$ to the coordinates $(X^i, P_{1i}, \dots, P_{ki}, t)$ with the following change of variables (diffeomorphism)

$$X^\eta = X^\eta(x^i, p_{1i}, \dots, p_{ki}, t), \quad P_{1\eta} = P_{1\eta}(x^i, p_{1i}, \dots, p_{ki}, t),$$

$$\dots, P_{k\eta} = P_{k\eta}(x^i, p_{1i}, \dots, p_{ki}, t), \quad \eta \in \{1, 2, \dots, n\}.$$

Then, the Hamiltonian $H(x, p_1, \dots, p_k, t)$ changes in $K(X, P_1, \dots, P_k, t)$. The above change of variables is called *canonical transformation* if there is a Hamiltonian, $K(X, P_1, \dots, P_k, t)$, such that the associated ODEs

$$\sum_{a=1}^{k}(-1)^{a+1}\frac{d^a}{dt^a}P_{ai}(t) = -\frac{\partial K}{\partial X^i}(X(t), P_1(t), \dots, P_k(t), t),$$

$$\frac{d^a}{dt^a}X^i(t) = \frac{\partial K}{\partial P_{ai}}(X(t), P_1(t), \dots, P_k(t), t), \quad i = \overline{1, n},$$

and the ODEs (3.4.1) take place simultaneously. This thing is possible if the functions

$$x^{(a)i}(t)p_{ai}(t) - H(x(t), p_1(t), \dots, p_k(t), t)$$

and

$$X^{(a)i}(t)P_{ai}(t) - K(X(t), P_1(t), \dots, P_k(t), t)$$

differ by a total derivative $\frac{dW}{dt}\left(t, x(t), x^{(1)}(t), \dots, x^{(k-1)}(t)\right)$.

Lemma 3.4.1 *If the Lagrangians*

$$L_1 := x^{(a)i} p_{ai} - H,$$

$$L_2 := X^{(a)i} P_{ai} - K$$

produce the same Euler–Lagrange ODEs, then the change of variables

$$(x^i, p_{1i}, \ldots, p_{ki}, t) \hookrightarrow (X^i, P_{1i}, \ldots, P_{ki}, t), \quad i = \overline{1, n},$$

is a canonical transformation.

Proof Using Proposition 3.3.1, the result is obvious.

The function W is called the *(higher order) generating function* of the canonical transformation.

The multi-time case. Let $H = x^i_{\alpha_1 \ldots \alpha_j} p_i^{\alpha_1 \ldots \alpha_j} - L$ be the Hamiltonian and

$$\sum_{j=1}^{k} (-1)^{j+1} D^j_{\alpha_1 \ldots \alpha_j} p_i^{\alpha_1 \ldots \alpha_j}(t) = -\frac{\partial H}{\partial x^i}\left(x(t), p^{\alpha_1}(t), \ldots, p^{\alpha_1 \ldots \alpha_k}(t), t\right), \quad (3.4.2)$$

$$x^i_{\alpha_1 \ldots \alpha_j}(t) = \frac{\partial H}{\partial p_i^{\alpha_1 \ldots \alpha_j}}\left(x(t), p^{\alpha_1}(t), \ldots, p^{\alpha_1 \ldots \alpha_k}(t), t\right), \quad i = \overline{1, n},$$

the associated PDEs. The summation over the repeated indices is assumed. Let assume that we want to pass from our coordinates $\left(x^i, p_i^{\alpha_1}, \ldots, p_i^{\alpha_1 \ldots \alpha_k}, t\right)$ to the coordinates $\left(X^i, P_i^{\alpha_1}, \ldots, P_i^{\alpha_1 \ldots \alpha_k}, t\right)$ with the following change of variables (diffeomorphism)

$$X^\eta = X^\eta\left(x^i, p_i^{\alpha_1}, \ldots, p_i^{\alpha_1 \ldots \alpha_k}, t\right), \quad P_\eta^{\alpha_1} = P_\eta^{\alpha_1}\left(x^i, p_i^{\alpha_1}, \ldots p_i^{\alpha_1 \ldots \alpha_k}, t\right),$$

$$\ldots, P_\eta^{\alpha_1 \ldots \alpha_k} = P_\eta^{\alpha_1 \ldots \alpha_k}\left(x^i, p_i^{\alpha_1}, \ldots, p_i^{\alpha_1 \ldots \alpha_k}, t\right), \quad \eta \in \{1, 2, \ldots, n\}.$$

Then, the Hamiltonian $H\left(x, p^{\alpha_1}, \ldots, p^{\alpha_1 \ldots \alpha_k}, t\right)$ changes in

$$K\left(X, P^{\alpha_1}, \ldots, P^{\alpha_1 \ldots \alpha_k}, t\right).$$

The above change of variables is called *canonical transformation* if there is a Hamiltonian, $K\left(X, P^{\alpha_1}, \ldots, P^{\alpha_1 \ldots \alpha_k}, t\right)$, such that the associated PDEs

$$\sum_{j=1}^{k} (-1)^{j+1} D^j_{\alpha_1 \ldots \alpha_j} P_i^{\alpha_1 \ldots \alpha_j}(t) = -\frac{\partial K}{\partial X^i}\left(X(t), P^{\alpha_1}(t), \ldots, P^{\alpha_1 \ldots \alpha_k}(t), t\right),$$

$$X^i_{\alpha_1 \ldots \alpha_j}(t) = \frac{\partial K}{\partial P_i^{\alpha_1 \ldots \alpha_j}}\left(X(t), P^{\alpha_1}(t), \ldots, P^{\alpha_1 \ldots \alpha_k}(t), t\right), \quad i = \overline{1, n},$$

and the PDEs (3.4.2) take place simultaneously. This thing is possible if the functions

$$x^i_{\alpha_1 \ldots \alpha_j}(t) p_i^{\alpha_1 \ldots \alpha_j}(t) - H\left(x(t), p^{\alpha_1}(t), \ldots, p^{\alpha_1 \ldots \alpha_k}(t), t\right)$$

and

$$X^i_{\alpha_1\ldots\alpha_j}(t)P_i^{\alpha_1\ldots\alpha_j}(t) - K\left(X(t), P^{\alpha_1}(t), \ldots, P^{\alpha_1\ldots\alpha_k}(t), t\right)$$

differ by a total divergence $D_\zeta W^\zeta\left(x(t), x_{\alpha_1}(t), \ldots, x_{\alpha_1\ldots\alpha_{k-1}}(t), t\right)$, $\zeta = \overline{1,m}$, and

$$\sum_{r=1}^{k-1}(-1)^r \frac{1}{n(\alpha_1,\ldots,\alpha_r)} D^{r+1}_{\alpha_1\ldots\alpha_r\zeta} \frac{\partial W^\zeta}{\partial x^i_{\alpha_1\ldots\alpha_r}}$$

$$= \sum_{r=2}^{k}(-1)^{r+1} \frac{1}{n(\alpha_1,\ldots,\alpha_r)} \frac{1}{n(\alpha_1,\ldots,\alpha_{r-1})} D^r_{\alpha_1\ldots\alpha_{r-1}\alpha_r} \frac{\partial W^{\alpha_r}}{\partial x^i_{\alpha_1\ldots\alpha_{r-1}}}, \quad i = \overline{1,n}.$$

Lemma 3.4.2 *If the Lagrangians*

$$L_1 := x^i_{\alpha_1\ldots\alpha_j} p_i^{\alpha_1\ldots\alpha_j} - H,$$

$$L_2 := X^i_{\alpha_1\ldots\alpha_j} P_i^{\alpha_1\ldots\alpha_j} - K$$

produce the same multi-time Euler–Lagrange PDEs [see $L_2 = L_1 + D_\zeta W^\zeta$,

$$\sum_{r=1}^{k-1}(-1)^r \frac{1}{n(\alpha_1,\ldots,\alpha_r)} D^{r+1}_{\alpha_1\ldots\alpha_r\zeta} \frac{\partial W^\zeta}{\partial x^i_{\alpha_1\ldots\alpha_r}}$$

$$= \sum_{r=2}^{k}(-1)^{r+1} \frac{1}{n(\alpha_1,\ldots,\alpha_r)} \frac{1}{n(\alpha_1,\ldots,\alpha_{r-1})} D^r_{\alpha_1\ldots\alpha_{r-1}\alpha_r} \frac{\partial W^{\alpha_r}}{\partial x^i_{\alpha_1\ldots\alpha_{r-1}}}, \quad i = \overline{1,n}\ ],$$

then the change of variables

$$\left(x^i, p_i^{\alpha_1}, \ldots, p_i^{\alpha_1\ldots\alpha_k}, t\right) \hookrightarrow \left(X^i, P_i^{\alpha_1}, \ldots, P_i^{\alpha_1\ldots\alpha_k}, t\right), \quad i = \overline{1,n},$$

is a canonical transformation.

Proof Using Corollary 3.3.3, the result is obvious.

The vector function W is called the *(higher order) multi-time generating function* of the canonical transformation.

3.5 Hamilton–Jacobi Divergence PDE Based on Higher Order Lagrangians

This section aims to present Hamilton–Jacobi divergence PDE involving multi-time higher order Lagrangians.

As in the previous sections, we start with the function $S\colon R^m \times R^n \times R^{nm} \times R^{nm(m+1)/2} \times \cdots \times R^{[nm(m+1)\cdot\ldots\cdot(m+k-2)]/(k-1)!} \to R^m$ and the constant level sets,

$$\Sigma_c\colon S^\beta\left(t, x, x_{\alpha_1}, \ldots, x_{\alpha_1\ldots\alpha_{k-1}}\right) = c^\beta, \quad \beta = \overline{1,m},$$

where $k \geq 2$ is a fixed natural number, $t = (t^1, \ldots, t^m) \in R^m$, $x_{\alpha_1} := \dfrac{\partial x}{\partial t^{\alpha_1}}, \ldots,$ $x_{\alpha_1\ldots\alpha_{k-1}} := \dfrac{\partial^{k-1} x}{\partial t^{\alpha_1}\ldots\partial t^{\alpha_{k-1}}}$. Here $\alpha_j \in \{1, 2, \ldots, m\}$, $j = \overline{1, k-1}$, $x = (x^1, \ldots, x^n) = \left(x^i\right)$, $i \in \{1, 2, \ldots, n\}$. We assume that these sets are submanifolds in $R^{m+n+\cdots+[nm(m+1)\cdot\ldots\cdot(m+k-2)]/(k-1)!}$, that is the normal vector fields

$$\left(\frac{\partial S^\beta}{\partial t^\gamma}, \frac{\partial S^\beta}{\partial x^i}, \frac{\partial S^\beta}{\partial x^i_{\alpha_1}}, \ldots, \frac{\partial S^\beta}{\partial x^i_{\alpha_1\ldots\alpha_{k-1}}}\right)$$

are linearly independent.

Consider $\tilde{\Gamma}\colon \left(t, x^i(t), x^i_{\alpha_1}(t), \ldots, x^i_{\alpha_1\ldots\alpha_{k-1}}(t)\right)$ an m-sheet transversal to the submanifolds Σ_c. Then, the vector function

$$c(t) = S\left(t, x(t), x_{\alpha_1}(t), \ldots, x_{\alpha_1\ldots\alpha_{k-1}}(t)\right)$$

has non-zero total divergence,

$$\begin{aligned} Div(c) &= \frac{\partial c^\beta}{\partial t^\beta}(t) = \frac{\partial S^\beta}{\partial t^\beta}\left(t, x(t), x_{\alpha_1}(t), \ldots, x_{\alpha_1\ldots\alpha_{k-1}}(t)\right) \\ &+ \frac{\partial S^\beta}{\partial x^i}\left(t, x(t), x_{\alpha_1}(t), \ldots, x_{\alpha_1\ldots\alpha_{k-1}}(t)\right) x^i_\beta(t) \\ &+ \sum_{\alpha_1\ldots\alpha_r; r=\overline{1,k-1}} \frac{\partial S^\beta}{\partial x^i_{\alpha_1\ldots\alpha_r}}\left(t, x(t), x_{\alpha_1}(t), \ldots, x_{\alpha_1\ldots\alpha_{k-1}}(t)\right) x^i_{\alpha_1\ldots\alpha_r\beta}(t) \\ &:= L\left(t, x(t), x_{\alpha_1}(t), \ldots, x_{\alpha_1\ldots\alpha_k}(t)\right) \neq 0. \end{aligned} \tag{3.5.1}$$

For a fixed function $x(\cdot)$, let us define the *generalized multi-momenta* $p = (p_i^{\alpha_1\ldots\alpha_j})$, $i \in \{1, 2, \ldots, n\}$, $j \in \{1, 2, \ldots, k\}$, $\alpha_j \in \{1, 2, \ldots, m\}$, by

$$p_i^{\alpha_1}(t) := \frac{1}{n(\alpha_1)} \frac{\partial L}{\partial x^i_{\alpha_1}}\left(t, x(t), x_{\alpha_1}(t), \ldots, x_{\alpha_1\ldots\alpha_k}(t)\right),$$

$$\vdots$$

$$p_i^{\alpha_1\ldots\alpha_k}(t) := \frac{1}{n(\alpha_1, \alpha_2, \ldots, \alpha_k)} \frac{\partial L}{\partial x^i_{\alpha_1\ldots\alpha_k}}\left(t, x(t), x_{\alpha_1}(t), \ldots, x_{\alpha_1\ldots\alpha_k}(t)\right).$$

By a direct computation, for $j = \overline{1, k}$ and $\frac{\partial S^\beta}{\partial x^i_{\alpha_0}} := \frac{\partial S^\beta}{\partial x^i}$, we get

$$p_i^{\alpha_1 \ldots \alpha_{j-1}\alpha_j}(t) = \frac{1}{n(\alpha_1, \alpha_2, \ldots, \alpha_j)} \frac{\partial S^{\alpha_j}}{\partial x^i_{\alpha_1 \ldots \alpha_{j-1}}} \left(t, x(t), x_{\alpha_1}(t), \ldots, x_{\alpha_1 \ldots \alpha_{k-1}}(t)\right).$$

We accept that the previous relations define a Legendre duality.

Definition 3.5.1 The multi-time higher order Lagrangian

$$L\left(t, x(t), x_{\alpha_1}(t), \ldots, x_{\alpha_1 \ldots \alpha_k}(t)\right)$$

is called super regular if the algebraic system

$$p_i^{\alpha_1 \ldots \alpha_j}(t) = \frac{1}{n(\alpha_1, \alpha_2, \ldots, \alpha_j)} \frac{\partial L}{\partial x^i_{\alpha_1 \ldots \alpha_j}} \left(t, x(t), x_{\alpha_1}(t), \ldots, x_{\alpha_1 \ldots \alpha_k}(t)\right)$$

defines the function

$$x^i_{\alpha_1} = x^i_{\alpha_1}(t, x, p^{\alpha_1}, \ldots, p^{\alpha_1 \ldots \alpha_k}),$$

$$\vdots$$

$$x^i_{\alpha_1 \ldots \alpha_k} = x^i_{\alpha_1 \ldots \alpha_k}(t, x, p^{\alpha_1}, \ldots, p^{\alpha_1 \ldots \alpha_k}).$$

In these conditions, the previous relations become

$$x^i_{\alpha_1} = x^i_{\alpha_1}\left(t, x, \frac{\partial S^{\alpha_1}}{\partial x}, \ldots, \frac{1}{n(\alpha_1, \alpha_2, \ldots, \alpha_k)} \frac{\partial S^{\alpha_k}}{\partial x_{\alpha_1 \ldots \alpha_{k-1}}}\right),$$

$$\vdots$$

$$x^i_{\alpha_1 \ldots \alpha_k} = x^i_{\alpha_1 \ldots \alpha_k}\left(t, x, \frac{\partial S^{\alpha_1}}{\partial x}, \ldots, \frac{1}{n(\alpha_1, \alpha_2, \ldots, \alpha_k)} \frac{\partial S^{\alpha_k}}{\partial x_{\alpha_1 \ldots \alpha_{k-1}}}\right).$$

On the other hand, the relation (3.5.2) can be rewritten as

$$-\frac{\partial S^\beta}{\partial t^\beta}\left(t, x(t), x_{\alpha_1}(t), \ldots, x_{\alpha_1 \ldots \alpha_{k-1}}(t)\right) \tag{3.5.2}$$

$$= \frac{\partial S^\beta}{\partial x^i}\left(t, x(t), x_{\alpha_1}(t), \ldots, x_{\alpha_1 \ldots \alpha_{k-1}}(t)\right)$$

$$\cdot x^i_\beta\left(t, x, \frac{\partial S^{\alpha_1}}{\partial x}(\cdot), \ldots, \frac{1}{n(\alpha_1, \alpha_2, \ldots, \alpha_k)} \frac{\partial S^{\alpha_k}}{\partial x_{\alpha_1 \ldots \alpha_{k-1}}}(\cdot)\right)$$

$$+ \sum_{\alpha_1 \dots \alpha_r; r=\overline{1,k-1}} \frac{\partial S^{\beta}}{\partial x^i_{\alpha_1 \dots \alpha_r}} \left(t, x(t), x_{\alpha_1}(t), \dots, x_{\alpha_1 \dots \alpha_{k-1}}(t)\right)$$

$$\cdot x^i_{\alpha_1 \dots \alpha_r \beta} \left(t, x, \frac{\partial S^{\alpha_1}}{\partial x}(\cdot), \dots, \frac{1}{n(\alpha_1, \alpha_2, \dots, \alpha_k)} \frac{\partial S^{\alpha_k}}{\partial x_{\alpha_1 \dots \alpha_{k-1}}}(\cdot)\right)$$

$$- L\left(t, x(t), x_{\alpha_1}(t), \dots, x_{\alpha_1 \dots \alpha_k}(t)\right).$$

The super regular Lagrangian L and the function $H\ (t, x, p^{\alpha_1}, \dots, p^{\alpha_1 \dots \alpha_k})$ present the following duality

$$H\ (t, x, p^{\alpha_1}, \dots, p^{\alpha_1 \dots \alpha_k})$$

$$= \sum_{j=1}^{k} \frac{1}{n(\alpha_1, \alpha_2, \dots, \alpha_j)} x^i_{\alpha_1 \dots \alpha_j} \left(t, x, p^{\alpha_1}, \dots, p^{\alpha_1 \dots \alpha_k}\right) \frac{\partial L}{\partial x^i_{\alpha_1 \dots \alpha_j}} \left(t, x, \dots, x_{\alpha_1 \dots \alpha_k}(\cdot)\right)$$

$$- L\left(t, x, x_{\alpha_1}(t, x, p^{\alpha_1}, \dots, p^{\alpha_1 \dots \alpha_k}), \dots, x_{\alpha_1 \dots \alpha_k}(t, x, p^{\alpha_1}, \dots, p^{\alpha_1 \dots \alpha_k})\right),$$

(*multi-time higher order non-standard Legendrian duality*) or, shortly,

$$H = x^i_{\alpha_1 \dots \alpha_j} p_i^{\alpha_1 \dots \alpha_j} - L.$$

The relation (3.5.2) can be rewritten as *Hamilton–Jacobi divergence PDE based on higher order Lagrangians*

$$(H - J - div^*)\ \frac{\partial S^{\beta}}{\partial t^{\beta}} + H\left(t, x, \frac{\partial S}{\partial x}, \dots, \frac{\partial S}{\partial x_{\alpha_1 \dots \alpha_{k-1}}}\right) = 0, \quad \beta \in \{1, \dots, m\}.$$

Initial conditions for Hamilton–Jacobi divergence PDE based on higher order Lagrangians are usually of the following form

$$S^{\beta}\left(0, x, x_{\alpha_1}, \dots, x_{\alpha_1 \dots \alpha_{k-1}}\right) = S_0^{\beta}\left(x, x_{\alpha_1}, \dots, x_{\alpha_1 \dots \alpha_{k-1}}\right).$$

The solution $\left(S^{\beta}\left(t, x, x_{\alpha_1}, \dots, x_{\alpha_1 \dots \alpha_{k-1}}\right)\right)$ is called the *generating function* of the generalized multi-momenta.

Remark 3.5.2 Consider $\left(S^{\beta}\left(t, x, x_{\alpha_1}, \dots, x_{\alpha_1 \dots \alpha_{k-1}}\right)\right)$ a solution of the previous Hamilton–Jacobi divergence PDE based on higher order Lagrangians and define

$$p_i^{\alpha_1 \dots \alpha_{j-1} \alpha_j}(t) = \frac{1}{n(\alpha_1, \alpha_2, \dots, \alpha_j)} \frac{\partial S^{\alpha_j}}{\partial x^i_{\alpha_1 \dots \alpha_{j-1}}} \left(t, x(t), x_{\alpha_1}(t), \dots, x_{\alpha_1 \dots \alpha_{k-1}}(t)\right),$$

for $j = \overline{1, k}$. The following link is satisfied

$$\int_{\Omega} L\left(t, x(t), x_{\alpha_1}(t), \ldots, x_{\alpha_1 \ldots \alpha_k}(t)\right) dt^1 \cdots dt^m$$

$$= \int_{\Omega} \left[x^i_{\alpha_1 \ldots \alpha_j}(t) p_i^{\alpha_1 \ldots \alpha_j}(t) - H\left(t, x, \frac{\partial S}{\partial x}(\cdot), \ldots, \frac{\partial S}{\partial x_{\alpha_1 \ldots \alpha_{k-1}}}(\cdot)\right)\right] dt^1 \cdots dt^m$$

$$= \int_{\Omega} \frac{\partial c^{\beta}}{\partial t^{\beta}}(t) dt^1 \cdots dt^m = \int_{\partial \Omega} \delta_{\beta\eta} c^{\beta}(t) n^{\eta}(t) d\sigma.$$

The last formula shows that the action multiple integral depends only on the boundary values of $c(t)$.

Theorem 3.5.3 *The generating function of the generalized multi-momenta is solution of the Cauchy problem*

$$\frac{\partial S^{\beta}}{\partial t^{\beta}} + H\left(t, x, \frac{\partial S}{\partial x}, \ldots, \frac{\partial S}{\partial x_{\alpha_1 \ldots \alpha_{k-1}}}\right) = 0, \quad \beta \in \{1, \ldots, m\},$$

$$S^{\beta}\left(0, x, x_{\alpha_1}, \ldots, x_{\alpha_1 \ldots \alpha_{k-1}}\right) = S_0^{\beta}\left(x, x_{\alpha_1}, \ldots, x_{\alpha_1 \ldots \alpha_{k-1}}\right).$$

References

1. Cardin, F., and C. Viterbo. 2008. Commuting Hamiltonians and Hamilton-Jacobi multi-time equations. *Duke Mathematical Journal* 144 (2): 235–284.
2. Ibragimov, N.Y. 2006. Integrating factors, adjoint equations and Lagrangians. *Journal of Mathematical Analysis and Applications* 318 (2): 742–757.
3. Krupkova, O. 2000. Hamiltonian field theory revisited: A geometric approach to regularity. In *Steps in differential geometry, proceedings of the colloquium on differential geometry*, 25–30 July, Debrecen, Hungary.
4. Lebedev, L.P., and M.J. Cloud. 2003. The calculus of variations and functional analysis with optimal control and applications in mechanics. *World Scientific, Series A* 12.
5. Miron, R. 1997. The geometry of higher order lagrange spaces. Applications to Mechanics and Physics. Kluwer, FTPH no. 82.
6. Motta, M., and F. Rampazzo. 2006. Nonsmooth multi-time Hamilton-Jacobi systems. *Indiana University Mathematics Journal* 55 (5): 1573–1614.
7. Rochet, J.C. 1985. The taxation principle and multitime Hamilton-Jacobi equations. *Journal of Mathematical Economics* 14 (2): 113–128.
8. Roman, M.R. 2001. Higher order Lagrange spaces. Applications. PhD thesis, University of Iassy.
9. Saunders, D.J. 1989. *The geometry of jet bundles*. Cambridge Univ Press.
10. Treanţă, S., and C. Udrişte. 2013. Optimal control problems with higher order ODEs constraints. *Balkan Journal of Geometry Applications* 18 (1): 71–86.
11. Treanţă, S. 2014. Optimal control problems on higher order jet bundles. In *BSG Proceedings 21, The international conference "differential geometry—dynamical systems", DGDS-2013*, vol. 21, 181–192, Oct 10–13, 2013, Bucharest-Romania.

12. Treanţă, S. 2014. On multi-time Hamilton-Jacobi theory via second order Lagrangians. *University Politehnica of Bucharest Scientific Bulletin, Series A: Applied Mathematics and Physics* 76 (3): 129–140.
13. Treanţă, S., and C. Vârsan. 2014. Linear higher order PDEs of Hamilton-Jacobi and parabolic type. *Mathematical Reports* 16 (66), 2, 319–329.
14. Treanţă, S.. 2014. PDEs of Hamilton-Pfaff type via multi-time optimization problems. *University Politehnica of Bucharest Scientific Bulletin, Series A: Applied Mathematics and Physics* 76 (1): 163–168.
15. Udrişte, C., and L. Matei. 2008. *Lagrange-Hamilton Theories (in Romanian), Monographs and Textbooks*, vol. 8. Bucharest: Geometry Balkan Press.
16. Udrişte, C., and I. Ţevy. 2007. Multi-time Euler-Lagrange-Hamilton theory. *WSEAS Transactions on Mathematics* 6 (6): 701–709.
17. Udrişte, C., and I. Ţevy. 2007. Multi-time Euler-Lagrange dynamics. In *Proceedings of the 7-th WSEAS international conference on systems theory and scientific computation*, 66–71.
18. Udrişte, C., L. Matei, and I. Duca. 2009. Multitime Hamilton-Jacobi theory. In *Proceedings of the 8-th WSEAS international conference on applied computer and applied computational science*, 509–513.

Part II
Statistics

Chapter 4
On Wavelet-Based Methods for Noise Reduction of cDNA Microarray Images

Tamanna Howlader, S. M. Mahbubur Rahman and Yogendra Prasad Chaubey

Abstract Denoising is recognized as one of the mandatory preprocessing tasks in microarray image analysis. Sparse representations of image pixels are commonly exploited to develop efficient image denoising algorithms. Existing approaches to transform image pixels into sparse representations require computationally demanding optimization techniques or a huge amount of prior knowledge to learn the kernels. Nevertheless, due to the mathematical elegancy, different types of multiresolution analysis, in particular, the variants of wavelet transforms such as the discrete wavelet transform, stationary wavelet transform, and complex wavelet transform have been employed successfully to develop many high-performance microarray array image denoising algorithms. This article presents a review of the sequential development of the wavelet-based methods for microarray image denoising. The useful and well-known properties of wavelet coefficients have led to the development of these algorithms by exploiting the statistical nature of the coefficients of the image and noise. The objective of this article is to summarize the key features of these algorithms and provide constructive analysis through categorization and comparison. The surveyed methods are discussed with respect to algorithmic issues such as the type of wavelet transforms used, statistical models employed, computational complexity, and denoising performance metrics.

Keywords cDNA microarray image · Gene expression · Noise reduction
Wavelet transform

T. Howlader (✉)
Institute of Statistical Research and Training, University of Dhaka,
Dhaka 1000, Bangladesh
e-mail: tamanna@isrt.ac.bd

S. M. M. Rahman
Department of Electrical and Electronic Engineering, University of Liberal
Arts Bangladesh, Dhaka 1209, Bangladesh
e-mail: mahbubur.rahman@ulab.edu.bd

Y. P. Chaubey
Department of Mathematics and Statistics, Concordia University,
1455 de Maisonneuve Blvd. West, Montreal, QC H3G 1M8, Canada
e-mail: chaubey@alcor.concordia.ca

A. Adhikari et al. (eds.), *Mathematical and Statistical Applications in Life Sciences and Engineering*, https://doi.org/10.1007/978-981-10-5370-2_4

4.1 Introduction

DNA microarray imaging technology has led to significant advances in genomic research and may be hailed as one of the greatest discoveries of the century. By allowing scientists to measure the expression levels of thousands of genes simultaneously, the technology has elucidated our understanding of how genes function, regulate, and interact [23, 43]. It has, therefore, found numerous applications in clinical diagnosis, plant biotechnology, drug discovery, and gene discovery. Although various microarray platforms exist, this article is concerned with the two-channel complementary DNA (cDNA) microarray, which measures the relative expressions of a set of genes under treatment and control conditions. The microarray experiment is a complex process that may be briefly summarized as follows. First, messenger RNA are extracted separately from treatment and control samples and converted to cDNA. The cDNA from the treatment and control samples are tagged with fluorescent green (Cy3) and red dyes (Cy5), respectively. The tagged samples are hybridized onto a solid support bearing sequences from known genes (probes) at specified locations called spots. Following hybridization, the array is scanned at two different wavelengths to generate two 16-bit digital images. These images may be superimposed to obtain a combined false-color image as shown in Fig. 4.1. A gene is differentially expressed if the intensity of the spot corresponding to that gene differs between the red and green channel images. A variety of summary statistics for each spot in each channel are reported such as the mean, median, and total intensity values. Relative gene expression is measured by the expression ratio and the reciprocal transformation or logarithmic transformation of the expression ratio [19]. The latter,

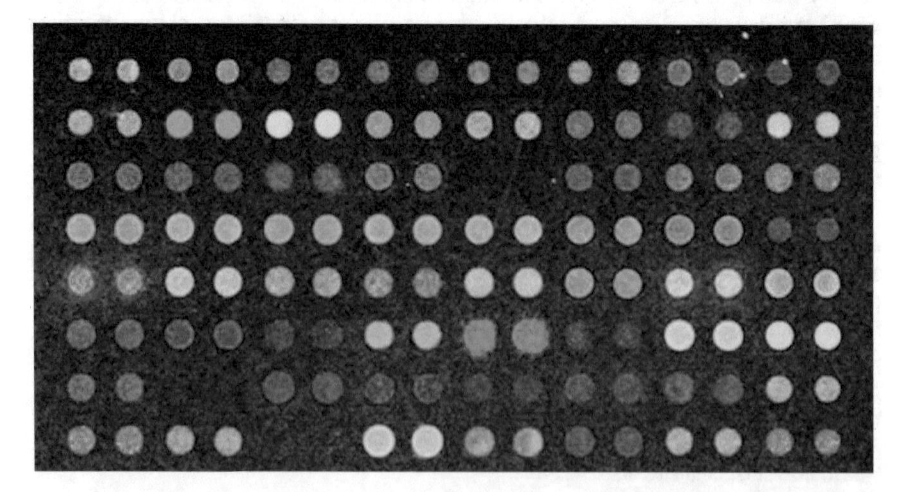

Fig. 4.1 A combined false-color image for cDNA microarray [57]. Spots expressed more in channel one appear red in the combined image whereas spots expressed more in channel two appear green. Yellow spots indicate similar levels of expression in both channels. Dark spots are expressed low in both channels

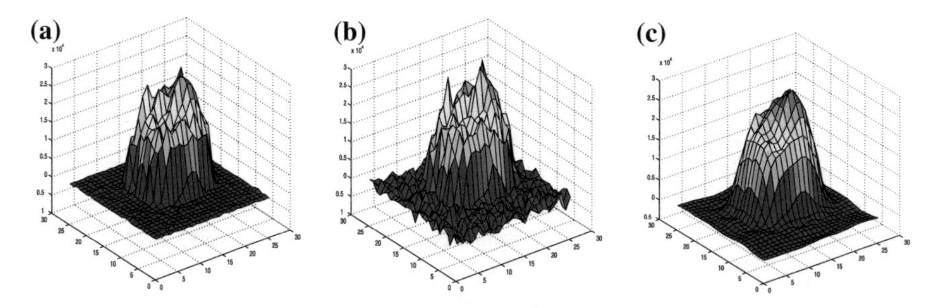

Fig. 4.2 3-D representation of a spot. **a** Original and **b** Noisy spot. **c** Denoised spot obtained using the noise reduction technique NeighCoeff [3]

commonly referred to as the log-intensity ratio, is the most widely used measure of gene expression in cDNA microarray experiments. This summary statistic is later used in downstream statistical analysis. For a thorough description of microarray experiments and subsequent statistical analysis, readers are referred to [35, 56].

Simple as it may seem, the step of extracting gene expression measurements from the images is actually quite tricky because the images are often noisy. Noise is caused by random processes associated with digital imaging [43] and several error-prone steps in the experiments [33]. Examples of noise that corrupt microarray images are photon noise, dark current noise, electronic noise, quantization noise [29, 61], hybridization noise, and dust on the microarray surface [60]. The noise produces unwanted artifacts and spots that are irregular in shape, size, and position [9]. This impedes gridding and accurate segmentation of spots which in turn leads to inaccurate estimation of gene expression measurements. Thus, noise removal from cDNA microarray images is a crucial preprocessing step that minimizes the likelihood of erroneous biological conclusions. Figure 4.2 shows the 3D visualization of a typical noise-free spot in a microarray image, and its noisy and denoised versions. It is desirable to have a denoising technique that reduces the noise significantly with minimum distortion with respect to the noise-free image.

There have been primarily two approaches for denoising in microarray experiments. The first is to estimate the experimental error via replications and to use ANOVA methods to account for additional sources of variation when estimating gene expression [25, 54]. The second approach is to denoise the microarray image using filtering techniques so as to obtain an approximate noise-free image from which relatively accurate gene expression measurements may be obtained. This review paper is concerned with the second approach. Although commercially available image processing softwares are available for image analysis, these employ low-level noise reduction techniques, such as the median filter, and are often inadequate. Some research works have found that the various impairments in microarray images can be described mathematically using additive or multiplicative noise models [55]. The noise characteristics in such models are described using statistical distributions such as the Gaussian [12, 29], Poisson, [2] and exponential distributions [10]. The noise may or may not be independent of the unknown true image. Interestingly, common noise models such as, electronic noise and quantization noise can be mathematically remodeled as the additive white Gaussian noise (AWGN) [42], which is one of the reasons why the AWGN is so important.

A survey of the vast literature on image denoising reveals that most methods can be broadly classified into pixel-based and transform-based methods [37]. Early methods for noise removal from microarray images were implemented in the pixel domain. For example, one approach consisted of estimating the noise-free image by subtracting a noise image from the original noisy image where the noise image was obtained by constructing masks of the artifacts [38]. Other approaches involved the use of center-weighted vector median filters [31] and order-statistic filters [29]. Further examples include the studies by [30, 49]. An advantage of pixel-based methods is that they are simpler to implement in general. However, research on the denoising of natural images has revealed that methods developed using an appropriate transform domain yield better results. Among the various transforms used, the wavelet-like transforms such as the discrete wavelet transform (DWT) [32], stationary wavelet transform (SWT), complex wavelet transform (CWT) [26], steerable pyramid transform [17], ridgelet transform [4], curvelet transform [5], contourlet transform [11], and directionlet transform [53] have shown significant success in the denoising of natural images. In general, different types of wavelet transforms host many attractive features such as the space-frequency localization, high energy compaction, high directional selectivity, and flexibility in choosing suitable basis functions [32, 48]. Moreover, the wavelet transform allows multiresolution analysis to be performed so that images may be denoised more efficiently by processing in more than one resolution. These factors have motivated the development of highly successful denoising algorithms based on different types of wavelet transforms applied not only for the natural images (see [40, 41]), but also for the microarray images (see [33, 48, 51, 54]). In the literature, the approach of sparse representation of image pixels has also been adopted for denoising of natural images. The methods of this approach include the block matching and 3D filtering [8] and the weighted encoding with sparse nonlocal regularization [24]. The sparse representation-based noise reduction methods are computationally expensive due to adoption of intense iterative optimization techniques of training patches or images to obtain the basis filters. On the other hand, the wavelet-like transforms are computationally efficient and mathematically elegant due to the well-established choice of the multiscale basis functions. Considering the fact that the spots maintain regular shapes in a microarray image and computational efficiency is desirable for processing huge size database of genetic experiments, the wavelet-based denoising techniques are preferred to the sparse-based techniques in general.

This article provides a summary of the noise models, wavelet-like transforms, and statistical estimation techniques used in the denoising of microarray images and a narrative review of several studies in the field. These studies are examined qualitatively with respect to several characteristics, namely, the type of transform used, noise model, the statistical models employed, performance measures used for evaluation and databases. By investigating how wavelet-based microarray image denoising methods have evolved over the years, this paper identifies the gaps in previous studies and outlines steps that may be taken to further enhance the denoising of microarray images using wavelets or wavelet-like transforms.

The paper is organized as follows. Section 4.2 presents a brief review of common degradation models of images due to noise. The preliminaries of wavelet transform and its evolution over the recent past are given in Sect. 4.3. Section 4.4 summarizes the statistical approaches used in wavelet-based microarray image denoising. Section 4.5 looks at the trends in research while Sect. 4.6 concludes with a summary of the major observations made in this paper and directions for future research.

4.2 Degradation Models

A microarray experiment consists of a series of complicated steps involving electrical, optical, and chemical processes that depend on multiple random factors. Consequently, there are many sources of error that show up as noise in the resulting images. A denoising algorithm is based on certain assumptions regarding the characteristics of the noise and the mechanism by which this noise corrupts the image pixels. These assumptions are expressed mathematically through a noise or degradation model that describes the statistical nature of the noise component through a probability density function (PDF) or probability mass function (PMF). Common noise distributions include the Gaussian, Rayleigh, Gamma, Uniform, Poisson, exponential PDFs or impulse-type PMFs. Let $I_n(x, y)$, $I(x, y)$, and $n(x, y)$ be the intensity values of noisy image, noise-free image, and noise, respectively, at the spatial location (x, y) $(x \in 1, 2, \ldots, X)$ $(y \in 1, 2, \ldots, Y)$ of a cDNA microarray image of size $(X \times Y)$. The common noise models that have been used in the context of microarray images are briefly described below:

Model 1: The additive white Gaussian noise (AWGN) model is given by

$$I_n(x, y) = I(x, y) + n(x, y) \tag{4.1}$$

where the noise samples $n(x, y)$ are independent of the image and distributed as independently and identically distributed (i.i.d.) zero-mean Gaussian $\mathcal{N}(0, \sigma_n)$. Photon noise, dust on the glass slide and electronic noise are examples of additive noise [52]. The common approaches for removing AWGN from images include the Wiener filter [18], wavelet thresholding [14, 15], Bayesian estimation [20, 52], sparse coding, or dictionary learning [8, 24]. It is interesting to note that it is possible to re-express many nonadditive and non-Gaussian noise models as the additive Gaussian noise using mathematical transformations [42]. Moreover, the assumption of AWGN often leads to tractable mathematical solutions which is why many of the denoising algorithms for microarray images are based on this assumption (e.g., [20, 21, 48, 51, 54, 62]).

Model 2:
The multiplicative white Gaussian noise (MWGN) model is given by

$$I_n(x, y) = I(x, y) \cdot n_1(x, y) + n_2(x, y) \tag{4.2}$$

where multiplicative noise $n_1(x, y)$ and additive noise $n_2(x, y)$ are samples from two independent zero-mean Gaussian distributions, $\mathcal{N}(0, \sigma_{n1})$ and $\mathcal{N}(0, \sigma_{n2})$, respectively, such that $\sigma_{n1} \gg \sigma_{n2}$ and as a result, the additive part can be ignored. An example of multiplicative noise is detector noise [52]. In denoising images corrupted by the MWGN, the homomorphic approach is used, which converts the multiplicative model to additive form by ignoring the additive component. The logarithm of Gaussian samples, often referred to as the "speckles", are assumed to follow the Fisher Tippet (also know as the generalized extreme value) distribution or Rayleigh distribution. [16] showed that the Rician Inverse Gaussian distribution statistically models the multiscale representation of speckles better than the traditional Rayleigh distribution. [52] proposed a wavelet-based denoising method for microarray images that accounts for both additive and multiplicative noise components to make the spot area more homogeneous and distinctive from its local background.

Model 3:
The microarray image may contain outliers or artifacts that are isolated, discrete, and random in nature and are best described using impulse noise (IN) models. The most common form of the IN model is the salt and pepper noise model, in which the probabilities of a pixel being corrupted by one of two gray levels of noise are equal. If the probability of corruption is ρ and the gray levels of noise are $d_{\min}$ and $d_{\max}$, then the degraded image is given by

$$I_n(x, y) = \begin{cases} d_{\min} & \text{with probability } \rho/2 \\ d_{\max} & \text{with probability } \rho/2 \\ I(x, y) & \text{with probability } 1 - \rho \end{cases} \tag{4.3}$$

The usual approach for removing impulsive noise is to use order statistic filters such as median filter or adaptive median filter, both of which, perform very well. There have been several studies on IN removal from microarray images in the pixel domain [31, 50] as well as in the wavelet domain [1, 34].

Model 4:
The mixed noise model best describes noise contamination of microarray images when the noise-free image is simultaneously degraded by the AWGN and IN. This may occur, for instance, when the foreground and background pixels are contaminated by thermal noise or photon noise and the image contains isolated discrete image artifacts [28, 30]. The degraded image in such a case is given by

$$I_n(x, y) = \begin{cases} d_{\min} & \text{with probability } \rho/2 \\ d_{\max} & \text{with probability } \rho/2 \\ I(x, y) + n(x, y) & \text{with probability } 1 - \rho \end{cases} \quad (4.4)$$

where $n(x, y)$ are the samples from $\mathcal{N}(0, \sigma_n)$. The general approach for removing mixed noise is a two-step procedure. In the first step, the image is preprocessed by order statistic filter to remove the impulse noise, and then successful algorithms for removal of AWGN are applied in the second step. Special filters such as the alpha-trimmed mean filter [39] or bilateral filter [59] also provide satisfactory performance in dealing with the problem of reducing mixed noise in images.

4.3 Wavelets for Denoising

The problem of image denoising is to recover an image $I(x, y)$ from the observed image $I_n(x, y)$, which is distorted by noise $n(x, y)$ such that recovered image has minimum distortion with respect to the noise-free image. The classical image denoising techniques are based on filtering and are implemented in the spatial domain, examples being spatial averaging, order statistic filters, and morphological filtering. However, such denoising techniques are known to cause blurring and other undesirable effects on the denoised version of the images [55]. Since its inception, wavelets have shown a significant success in denoising by transforming 1D signal in terms of multiscale coefficients which are sparse as well as very compactly represented. Due to sparse and compact nature of wavelet coefficients, the denoising can be performed by suitably eliminating the noise components from the coefficients. Nevertheless, research has continued in the recent past to improve certain properties of wavelet transforms to tackle signals with high dimensions such as 2D image signal. In addition to the properties of sparsity and coding efficiency of a basis function of wavelet transformation, the directional selectivity of basis function has been extensively studied for the wavelet transformation of images. The development of different types of wavelet transforms such as the complex wavelet and a family of wavelet transforms including the steerable pyramid, ridgelet, curvelet, contourlet, and directionlet was motivated by the need for better directional selectivity. In a generic sense, the wavelet family with selective directional features in the coefficients are often referred to as the X-lets. This section provides an overview of the types of wavelets that are used in microarray image denoising techniques.

4.3.1 Discrete Wavelet Transform

Let $g(i, j)$, $f(i, j)$, and $v(i, j)$ be the wavelet coefficients of the noisy image, noise-free image, and noise, respectively, at the spatial location (i, j) $(i \in 1, 2, \ldots, M)$

Fig. 4.3 Tiling of space-frequency plane (x-ω_x) for 1D continuous wavelet transform

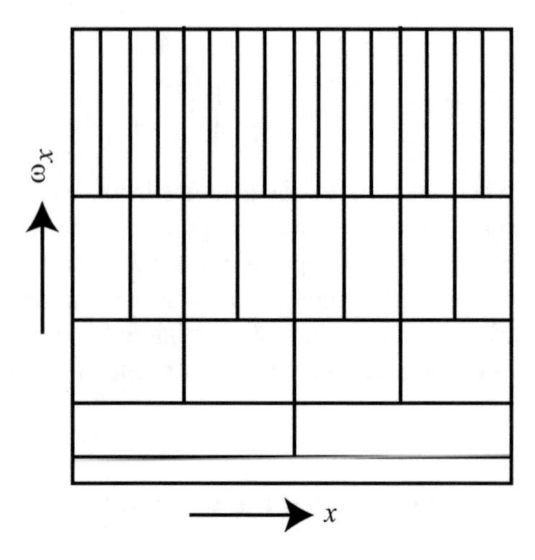

$(j \in 1, 2, \ldots, N)$ of a subband of size $(M \times N)$ for a microarray image. Here, the subband refers to groups into which the wavelet coefficients are clustered according to different levels or orientations. Figure 4.3 shows a conceptual tiling of space-frequency plane, i.e., (x, ω_x)-plane, for continuous wavelet transform, where each partition represents a subband. In case of 2D signal, the noise-free image $I(x, y)$ can be expressed in terms of discrete wavelet transform (DWT) as [32]

$$
\begin{aligned}
I(x, y) = {} & \frac{1}{\sqrt{MN}} \sum_{x=1}^{X} \sum_{y=1}^{Y} f_J^A(i, j)\{2^{J/2}\phi(2^J i - x)\phi(2^J j - y)\} + \\
& \frac{1}{\sqrt{MN}} \sum_{l=1}^{J} \Bigg[\sum_{x=1}^{X} \sum_{y=1}^{Y} f_l^H(x, y)\{2^l \psi(2^l i - x)\phi(2^l j - y)\} + \\
& \sum_{x=1}^{X} \sum_{y=1}^{Y} f_l^V(x, y)\{2^l \phi(2^l i - x)\psi(2^l j - y)\} + \\
& \sum_{x=1}^{X} \sum_{y=1}^{Y} f_l^D(x, y)\{2^l \psi(2^l i - x)\psi(2^l j - y)\} \Bigg]
\end{aligned}
\tag{4.5}
$$

where ϕ and ψ are the real-valued scaling and wavelet functions, respectively. Different types of wavelet transforms can be obtained by choosing one of the available scaling and wavelet functions such as the Haar, Daubechies, Symlet, and Gabor for decomposition. The decimated DWT is nonredundant and this feature makes it attractive for fast and efficient image denoising. The DWT, in spite of its good performance, has two important limitations: it is shift variant and has poor directional selectivity.

4.3.2 Stationary Wavelet Transform

The SWT is a redundant transform that has a desirable property of being shift-invariant, which shows a better performance in denoising. Due to shift-invariance property, the coefficients do not change due to shifted version of the original signal. As a result, similar edges in images are restored well in a denoising technique using SWT. The SWT coefficients are calculated by the same procedure as the DWT, except that downsampling is avoided to account for all possible shifts. The SWT is also called the overcomplete representation, shift-invariant form, or non-decimated form of the DWT. Other examples of redundant wavelet transforms include the double-density wavelet transforms [44].

4.3.3 Complex Wavelet Transform

Both the DWT and SWT possess the drawback of having poor directional selectivity. This means that the transform coefficients of these wavelets capture only three directional features in the 2D signal, namely, the horizontal (0°), vertical (90°) and diagonal features (45°). The CWT is a redundant transform having complex valued scaling and wavelet functions that capture six directional features, namely, −15°, −45°, −75°, 15°, 45°, and 75° of an image. Therefore, the CWT has better directional selectivity as compared to both the decimated DWT and SWT. Implementation details regarding the CWT may be found in [26, 27, 45].

4.3.4 X-let Transform

The scaling and wavelet basis functions of the DWT and CWT are isotropic in nature due to the fact that same length filters are applied to two dimensions, namely, x- and y-axis of an image, and at the same time decimation strategy does not change with the directions. Anisotropic basis functions are generated in the family of X-let transforms such as in the steerable pyramid [17], ridgelet [4], curvelet [5], contourlet [11], and directionlet [53] transforms by adopting different implementation strategies in the filtering and decimation stages. In other words, the X-let transform can be implemented by synthesizing different types of directional filter bank and by adopting lattice-based convolution operation and sub-sampling mechanism. Figure 4.4 shows a typical tiling in the 2D frequency plane (ω_x-ω_y) using pseudopolar support to form anisotropic basis functions. It is seen from this figure that an arbitrary set of directionally selective subbands can be obtained by designing suitable anisotropic basis functions in the multiscale nature of the X-let transform. Figure 4.5 shows a conceptual approximation of the curved edge of a circle representing a synthetic spot in a microarray image using both the isotropic and anisotropic basis functions. It

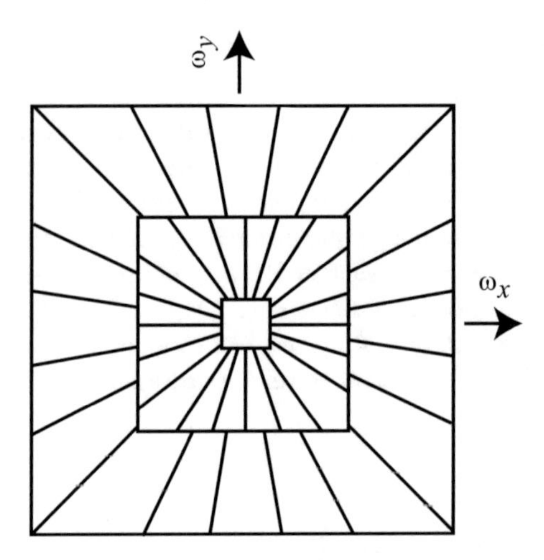

Fig. 4.4 Tiling with pseudopolar support in the two-dimensional frequency plane (ω_x-ω_y) in discrete X-let transform

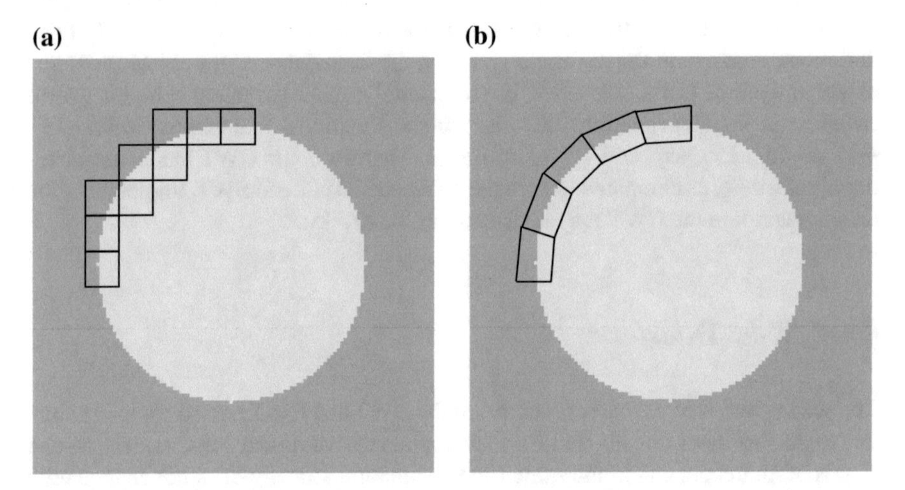

Fig. 4.5 A synthetic spot in microarray image with a curve-like edge, which is schematically represented by space-frequency rectangles of two types of basis functions, viz., isotropic and anisotropic, of the X-let transform. **a** A large number of significant coefficients are required for the isotropic basis functions to represent the curve-like edge. **b** On the other hand, a few significant coefficients are sufficient to represent the curve by the anisotropic basis functions

is evident from this figure that the directionally selective anisotropic basis function requires a significantly less number of coefficients as compared to that required for the isotropic basis functions. It is due to such high compaction efficiency, the reconstruction error of a denoised microarray image obtained by a method using the X-let transform is expected to be lower than that obtained by employing the traditional wavelet transforms.

4.4 Wavelet-Based Statistical Methods

Wavelet denoising falls within the realm of nonparametric estimation and functional data analysis, where the goal is to recover or estimate a function of interest based on sampled data that are contaminated with noise. In image denoising, the unknown function of interest is the noise-free image. Noise reduction using wavelet transforms involves three major steps: a linear forward wavelet transform, modification of the wavelet coefficients according to some rule, and a linear inverse wavelet transform using modified coefficients. The second step involves the methods that have been developed along two main lines: thresholding or nonlinear shrinkage functions and Bayesian estimation.

4.4.1 Wavelet Thresholding

The concepts of "parsimony" and "sparsity" are central to many of the problems arising in statistics and signal processing. Wavelet transforms enable signals to be represented with a high degree of sparsity which implies that only a few significant coefficients in a subband contain information about the underlying image, while insignificant values can be attributed to the noise. It is this property that makes wavelet thresholding or shrinkage successful in denoising. The idea of wavelet thresholding or shrinkage is to modify each coefficient of the subband by using a thresholding or shrinkage function, which shrinks the coefficients in magnitude towards zero. Removing the small coefficients then removes most of the noise. Mathematically, wavelet coefficients are estimated using a hard- or soft-thresholding rule for a threshold T as given below:

Hard-thresholding [14]: $\hat{f} = g \cdot \mathbf{1}(|g| > T)$
Soft-thresholding [14]: $\hat{f} = \mathrm{sgn}(g) \cdot \max(0, |g| - T)$

Although hard-thresholding can preserve edge information better than soft-thresholding, it often creates discontinuities in the processed image for which soft-thresholding is often preferred for microarray image denoising [43]. Several authors have proposed different choices for the optimal threshold T. Some of the commonly used thresholds are given below:

- Universal threshold in VisuShrink method [13]: $T = \sigma_n\sqrt{2\log(MN)}$.
- Threshold in translation invariant denoising method [7]: $T = \sigma_n\sqrt{2\ln(MN\log_2(MN))}$.
- Sure threshold in SureShrink method [15]: $T = \arg\min_{0\leq T\leq\sqrt{2\log(MN)}}\left[MN - 2\cdot\#\{k : |\frac{g_k}{\sigma_n}| \leq T\} + \sum_{k=1}^{MN}\{\min(|\frac{g_k}{\sigma_n}|, T)\}^2\right]$.
- Threshold in BayesShrink method [6]: $T = \sigma_n^2/\sigma_f$, where σ_f is the standard deviation of noise-free subband coefficients.

The thresholds used in various denoising methods may be global (as in VisuShrink [13]), subband-adaptive (as in BayesShrink [6] and SureShrink [15]) or spatially adaptive (as in NeighCoeff [3]). Statistical thresholding functions have also been designed considering PDFs for the noise-free coefficients. For instance, [22] has proposed the following rule

$$\hat{f} = \text{sgn}(g) \cdot \max\left(0, |g| - \sigma_n^2 |\Omega(g)|\right) \tag{4.6}$$

where $\Omega(z) = -\frac{\mathrm{d}}{\mathrm{d}z}\left[\log(p_Z(z))\right]$ is the score function of z. Different shrinkage formulas are obtained for different choices of the PDF z in (4.6). For example, [46] have obtained a shrinkage rule by using the bivariate Laplacian distribution in (4.6) to model the inter-scale dependencies of the noise-free coefficients. Due to its simplicity and effectiveness, the wavelet thresholding approach has been used to denoise microarray images in a number of studies (e.g., [1, 34, 54, 62]).

4.4.2 Bayesian Wavelet Denoising

Following the thresholding approach, researchers developed statistical models for natural images as well as their multiscale transformed coefficients, and utilized these models as tools for designing new wavelet-based denoising algorithms. The basic idea is to capture the sparseness and statistical nature of the wavelet transform coefficients by modeling them with *prior* probability distributions. Then the problem can be expressed as the estimation of noise-free coefficients using this a priori information with Bayesian estimation techniques. Standard Bayesian estimators that have been used include the maximum a posteriori (MAP), minimum mean squared error (MMSE), and minimum mean absolute error (MMAE) estimators [3, 36].

Let $g(i, j)$, $f(i, j)$, and $v(i, j)$ be the samples of the random variables $\boldsymbol{G}$, $\boldsymbol{F}$, and $\boldsymbol{V}$, which represent noisy coefficients, noise-free coefficients, and noise coefficients of the image, respectively. Joint PDFs have been used to model the nonlinear dependency between the coefficients at a particular location in a given subband and the coefficient at the corresponding location in a coarser subband (inter-scale dependency) [47, 58]. In the context of cDNA microarray images, statistical models have also been used to model the correlation between the coefficients in the corresponding subbands of the red and green channel images at the same location (inter-channel dependency) [20, 21]. Hence, we denote the joint PDFs of the random variables of two subbands by $p_{\boldsymbol{G}}(\boldsymbol{g})$, $p_{\boldsymbol{F}}(\boldsymbol{f})$, and $p_{\boldsymbol{V}}(\boldsymbol{v})$ by considering the inter-scale or inter-channel dependency of the cDNA microarray image.

In order to remove AWGN, several studies have obtained shrinkage functions by maximizing the posterior joint density function $p_{\boldsymbol{F}|\boldsymbol{G}}(\boldsymbol{f}|\boldsymbol{g})$. This yields the MAP estimator, which is given by

$$\begin{aligned}\hat{f}(g) &= \arg\max_{f} p_{F|G}(f|g) \\ &= \arg\max_{f} \left[p_{G|F}(g \mid f) \cdot p_F(f)\right] \\ &= \arg\max_{f} \left[\ln(p_V(g-f)) + \ln(p_F(f))\right]\end{aligned} \tag{4.7}$$

Alternative shrinkage functions for AWGN have been obtained by taking the mean of the posterior PDF yielding the Bayes least squares (BLS) estimator as

$$\hat{f}(g) = \int p_{F|G}(f|g) f \mathrm{d}f \tag{4.8}$$

In either case, the posterior PDF is derived from joint PDF of the image wavelet coefficients $p_F(f)$ using Bayes' rule:

$$p_{F|G}(f|g) = \frac{p_v(g-f)p_F(f)}{\int p_v(g-f)p_F(f)\mathrm{d}f} \tag{4.9}$$

When microarray images are denoised in the DWT or CWT domain, the real-valued noise coefficients are modeled as bivariate Gaussian (BG) distribution [20] while magnitude values of the complex coefficients are modeled as bivariate Rayleigh (BR) distribution [21]. In order to take into account the intrascale dependency of the coefficients as well to obtain closed-form expressions for the MAP and BLS estimators, $p_F(f)$ has been chosen as locally adaptive BG distribution both for the real-valued wavelet coefficients as well as magnitude of the complex coefficients [20, 21]. The pixel dependent variance and covariance of BG distribution are estimated using locally adaptive window-based MAP (LAWMAP) estimator (see [36]). The PDF $p_F(f)$ for the subband coefficients are also modeled in terms of complex Gaussian scale mixture (CGSM) to obtain the BLS estimator. However, this estimator fails to provide a closed-form expression, although the Jeffrey's noninformative prior has been used to statistically model the scales of CGSM PDF (see [51]).

4.5 Research Trends

This section examines the trends in research on wavelet-based microarray image denoising by reviewing key papers in the field. These papers are listed chronologically in Table 4.1 along with a brief summary of their notable features. In particular, this section provides a critical discussion of these papers with respect to important algorithmic issues including the noise models, type of wavelets, and statistical approaches used in the papers along with the performance evaluation methodology and computational complexity of the methods presented there.

Noise models: As Table 4.1 reveals, the AWGN is the most common noise model employed in studies of microarray image denoising. There are several reasons for

Table 4.1 Overview of wavelet-based denoising of microarray images

References	Noise model	Type of wavelet **or complexity**	Statistical techniques	Performance evaluation
[54]	• AWGN	• SWT • Complexity: $\mathcal{O}(N)$	• Soft-threshold • Hard-threshold • SURE-threshold	• UQI of pixels • No information of database
[1]	• AWGN • IN	• TI-wavelet (cycle-spinning) • Complexity: $\mathcal{O}(N \log N)$	• Soft-threshold • Hard-threshold • TI-median for shifts	• MSE and MAE of pixels • Databases used: Stanford Yeast and MicroZip
[52]	• AWGN • MWGN	• SWT • Complexity: $\mathcal{O}(N)$	• Bayesian MAP • Heavy-tailed Laplacian PDF for signal • Interscale dependency of wavelet is considered	• CV from pixels of spots and background • ROC of spot detection • No information of database
[34]	• AWGN • IN	• DWT • Complexity: $\mathcal{O}(N)$	• Median and Wiener filters • Soft threshold • Hard threshold • Preprocessing by spatial filter is highlighted	• PSNR and SNR of pixels • Database used: Stanford Yeast
[20]	• AWGN	• DWT • Complexity: $\mathcal{O}(wN)$	• Bayesian MAP estimator • Locally-adaptive BG PDF for signal and noise • Exponential distribution for local variances • Correlation between channels is highlighted	• PSNR and MAE of pixels • Log-intensity ratio of spots • Database used: Stanford Yeast and SIECR

(continued)

Table 4.1 (continued)

References	Noise model	Type of wavelet **or complexity**	Statistical techniques	Performance evaluation
[62]	• AWGN	• DMWT • Complexity: $\mathcal{O}(N)$	• Modified soft threshold • Modified hard threshold • Strength of multiwavelet is exploited	• PSNR, IF, UQI, and PQM of pixels • Database used: Keck Lab
[21]	• AWGN	• CWT • Complexity: $\mathcal{O}(wN)$	• BLS and MAP estimators • Locally-adaptive BG and BR PDFs for signal and noise, respectively • Correlation between channels and directional properties of wavelets are highlighted	• PSNR and MAE of pixels • Log-intensity ratio of spots • Database used: Stanford Yeast
[48]	• AWGN	• X-let (Curvelet, Contourlet, Steerable Pyramid, and Shearlet) • Complexity: $\mathcal{O}(N)$	• Bayes-threshold • Highlights the performance of different directional wavelets	• PSNR, SSIM, and EPI of pixels • No information of database
[51]	• AWGN	• CWT • Steerable Pyramid • Complexity: $\mathcal{O}(wN)$	• BLS estimator • Locally-adaptive CGSM PDF for signal and noise • Statistical model of complex wavelets is highlighted	• PSNR and SSIM of pixels • Database used: Stanford Yeast

this. First, the source noise, such as photon noise and dust on the slides are additive in nature [52]. Secondly, the assumption of Gaussian distributed noise often leads to mathematically tractable solutions compared to other noise distributions. Finally, other common noise models can be mathematically remodeled as AWGN [42]. For instance, [52] assumed that degradation occurred according to the MWGN model given in (4.2). In their study, the model was transformed to an additive one by ignoring the additive component and then taking logarithmic transformation. Other studies have evaluated the performance of wavelet-based denoising techniques on microarray images corrupted by salt and pepper noise [34] and mixed noise, i.e., combination of IN and AWGN [1].

Type of wavelet: Early studies on microarray image denoising recognized the importance of the shift-invariance or translation-invariance property of the wavelet transform in representing spots and other structural features of the image. For instance, [1] pointed out that DWT-based thresholding methods suffer from pseudo-random Gibbs phenomenon at points of discontinuity, which leads to oversmoothing of the edges and loss of image details. Thus, to avoid artifacts in the denoised image, some studies on microarray image denoising have used redundant transforms such as the SWT [52, 54] while others have employed cycle spinning [7] to "average" out translation invariance [1]. However, it is to be noted that both approaches achieve shift-invariance but at the expense of increased computation time relative to the DWT. This is an issue that needs to be taken into consideration when working with high-dimensional data. There have been some studies on DWT-based microarray image denoising. For example, [34] carried out a comparative study of spatial filtering methods and DWT thresholding methods when applied to microarray images and concluded that the latter was more efficient for removing AWGN. [20] proposed a DWT-based denoising algorithm for removing AWGN from cDNA microarray images taking into the account the correlation between the DWT coefficients of the red and green channel images. In a later study, [62] used the undecimated discrete multiwavelet transform (DMWT), which is a sparser representation of signals than the DWT and possesses useful properties such as the redundancy, orthogonality, symmetry, and higher order approximation of the multiwavelet filters. The authors showed that thresholding based on the undecimated DMWT yields better results compared to the SWT and DWT. However, none of these transforms possess good directional selectivity, which is a useful property in the context of microarray image denoising for better representation of the circular edges of spots. This motivated studies involving wavelet transforms with better directional selectivity, such as the methods based on the CWT [21, 51], and the curvelet, contourlet, shearlet, and steerable pyramid [48]. In a recent study by [48], directional transforms such as the CWT, shearlet, and steerable pyramid were found to perform better than the DWT and SWT when hard-thresholding was used with a global threshold.

Statistical methods: From Table 4.1, it can be seen that most studies have used wavelet thresholding to remove AWGN [1, 34, 48, 54, 62] while some studies have derived Bayesian estimators for denoising [20, 21, 51]. In addition, order statistic filters, such as the median filter, have been used to remove IN in the wavelet domain [1, 34]. The PDF has emerged as a powerful statistical tool for developing Bayesian thresholds or Bayesian estimators in image denoising. In the context of microarray denoising, PDFs or prior functions for the noise-free wavelet coefficients have been used in the methods proposed by [20, 21, 51, 52]. For instance, [52] assume that the SWT coefficients are statistically dependent within each subband and model the coefficients with the heavy-tailed Laplacian PDF. They also consider the dependency between the coefficients in adjacent scales. However, in microarray denoising, there is another source of dependency between transform coefficients that cannot be ignored. It is well known that significant correlations exist between the coefficients of the red and green channel images of cDNA microarrays at the same spatial location known as inter-channel correlation [1, 20]. As a consequence, inferior results may be obtained if the images are processed separately by ignoring the inter-channel dependency. To take this correlation into account, [20] consider the bivariate Gaussian distribution as the joint PDF for the DWT coefficients of the red and green channel images at a given location. In a later study, [21] proposed a CWT-based denoising method that models the magnitude components of CWT coefficients at a given location in the subbands of both channels using a locally i.i.d. bivariate Gaussian PDF. Following the work of [21, 51] also consider the joint information in both channels. But, instead of using the magnitude components of the coefficients, they model the CWT coefficients of the channel images jointly using the CGSM model. As the two-channel images are produced from the same microarray slide, a significant noise correlation is also expected. Hence, these studies have also used joint PDFs to model the correlation between the noise coefficients in the two channels. For example, [21] have used the bivariate Rayleigh distribution for the magnitude components of the noise coefficients in the two channels, whereas [51] have used the bivariate zero-mean complex Gaussian distribution to model the complex-valued noise coefficients. These locally adaptive prior functions and PDFs for the noise coefficients are used to derive the Bayesian MAP or BLS estimator for noise-free image coefficients.

Performance evaluation: There appears to be little consensus among researchers regarding which performance indices to use as indicated by the variety of performance measures used by different studies. Moreover, in the absence of common reference data sets, direct comparison of the denoising performance across studies is not always meaningful. From Table 4.1, it is evident that the most popular index for evaluating microarray image denoising performance is the peak-signal-to-noise ratio (PSNR) [20, 34, 51]. Other image quality measures that have been used are the mean absolute error (MAE) [1, 20], signal-to-noise ratio (SNR) [34], structural similarity (SSIM) [48, 51], universal quality index (UQI) [54, 62], image fidelity (IF) [62], edge preserving index (EPI) [48], and perceptual quality measure (PQM) [62]. The above indices assess denoising performance by measuring the noise content, visual quality, or preservation of structural features in the denoised image. In an alternative approach, [52] have used the coefficient of variation (CV) to measure the homogeneity of low-intensity spots in the denoised image and the receiver operating characteristics (ROC) curve to determine how well their method discriminates between detectable and non-detectable spots. However, for a more thorough assessment, one should investigate the efficacy of the denoising method by measuring the accuracy of the gene expression measurements derived from the denoised images or by observing its effects on downstream analysis such as clustering. Very few studies have considered this approach. For instance, [20, 21] have calculated the MAE of log-intensity ratios estimated from denoised images to determine the efficacy of their denoising methods.

Computational complexity: The computational complexity of a denoising algorithm determines the time required to obtain the denoised image. Since thousands of genes need to be examined simultaneously, algorithms with low computation times yet good denoising performance are preferred. Computational complexity of the wavelet-based microarray denoising algorithms are determined by several factors such as the type of wavelet transform used, number of parameters to be estimated, whether the method is subband-adaptive or locally adaptive, and whether direct calculation, numerical integration or iterative methods are required in estimation. For instance, redundant transforms and transforms with greater directional selectivity often have higher computational complexity. Again, subband-adaptive techniques that estimate parameters from the entire subband generally require less computation time than locally adaptive techniques. Thus, a tradeoff needs to be made between estimation accuracy and mathematical tractability in high-dimensional applications such as microarray image denoising. Table 4.1 outlines the computational complexity of the statistical methods used in each of the studies. It is evident that the locally adaptive methods (e.g., [20, 21, 51]) with $\mathcal{O}(wN)$ computations are more complex than the other methods, where w denotes the window size. Among the locally adaptive methods, those with closed-form solutions (e.g., [20, 21]) generally require less computational time and are preferred to methods requiring numerical integration and iterative solutions.

4.6 Conclusion

Since the raw data of cDNA microarray experiments are a pair of red and green channel images, the reliability of biological conclusions drawn from microarray experiments relies heavily on the quality of these images. In spite of microarray experiments being conducted with extreme care, the resulting images are far from ideal and this makes extracting accurate gene expression measurements challenging. This paper has reviewed the latest developments in the field of wavelet-based microarray image denoising. Certain trends in these developments have emerged such as the increasing use of near shift-invariant directional transforms such as the CWT, curvelet, and steerable pyramid as opposed to stationary wavelet transforms. Where previous studies have denoised the red and green channel images independently, recent research has focused more on joint estimation of the noise-free coefficients for both the channels by taking into consideration the noise correlation. In general, wavelet thresholding methods are simple to implement and require less time, but the Bayesian wavelet methods often deliver better denoising results with an expense of computational load. In the absence of benchmark data for comparisons and a consensus regarding which performance indicators to use, it is difficult to comment on performance across studies. A potential drawback of microarray denoising studies is that the true nature of the noise is never known. The same microarray slide may be contaminated by multiple noise types, and thus the AWGN model assumed by the majority of studies is an oversimplified version of reality. Nevertheless, denoising performance of the wavelet-based methods have improved over the years, although most of the commercial image analysis softwares are yet to incorporate sophisticated algorithms. Future studies on microarray denoising should incorporate the effects on quality of gene expression measurements and downstream analysis such as detection of differentially expressed genes and cluster analysis. Apart from wavelets, other types of sparse representations such as those obtained from learning-based algorithms including the nonlocal means, dictionary learning or convolutional neural network could be the subject of future research to design high-performance microarray denoising methods.

References

1. Adjeroh, D.A., Y. Zhang, and R. Parthe. 2006. On denoising and compression of DNA microarray images. *Pattern Recognition* 39: 2478–2493.
2. Balagurunathan, Y., E.R. Dougherty, Y. Chen, M.L. Bittner, and J.M. Trent. 2002. Simulation of cDNA microarrays via a parameterized random signal model. *Journal of Biomedical Optics* 7 (3): 507523.
3. Cai, T., and B. Silverman. 2001. Incorporating information on neighboring coefficients into wavelet estimation. *Sankhya: The Indian Journal of Statistics* 63: 127–148.
4. Candès, E.J., and D.L. Donoho. 1999. Ridgelets: A key to higher-dimensional intermittency? *Philosophical Transactions of the Royal Society A* 357 (1760): 2495–2509.
5. Candès, E.J., and D.L. Donoho. 2004. New tight frames of curvelets and optimal representations of objects with piecewise C^2 singularities. *Communications on Pure and Applied Mathematics* 57 (2): 219–266.
6. Chang, S.G., B. Yu, and M. Vettereli. 2000. Adaptive wavelet thresholding for image denoising and compression. *IEEE Transactions on Image Processing* 9 (9): 1532–1546.
7. Coifman, R.R., and D.L. Donoho. 1995. Translation-invariant de-noising. In *Wavelets and statistics*, ed. A. Antoniadis, and G. Oppenheim. Berlin: Springer.
8. Dabov, K., A. Foi, V. Katkovnik, and K. Egiazarian. 2007. Image denoising by sparse 3D transform-domain collaborative filtering. *IEEE Transactions on Image Processing* 16 (8): 2080–2095.
9. Daskalakis, A., D. Cavouras, P. Bougioukos, S. Kostopoulos, D. Glotsos, I. Kalatzis, G.C. Kagadis, C. Argyropoulos, and G. Nikiforidis. 2007. Improving gene quantification by adjustable spot-image restoration. *Bioinformatics* 23 (17): 2265–2272.
10. Davies, S.W., and D.A. Seale. 2005. DNA microarray stochastic model. *IEEE Transactions on Nanobioscience* 4: 248–254.
11. Do, M.N., and M. Vetterli. 2005. The contourlet transform: An efficient directional multiresolution image representation. *IEEE Transactions on Image Processing* 14 (12): 2091–2106.
12. Donald, A.A., Y. Zhang, and R. Parthe. 2006. On denoising and compression of DNA microarray images. *Pattern Recognition* 39: 2478–2493.
13. Donoho, D.L. 1995. Denoising by soft-thresholding. *IEEE Transactions on Information Theory* 41 (3): 613–627.
14. Donoho, D.L., and I.M. Johnstone. 1994. Ideal spatial adaptation by wavelet shrinkage. *Biometrika* 81 (3): 425–455.

15. Donoho, D.L., and I.M. Johnstone. 1995. Adapting to unknown smoothness via wavelet shrinkage. *Journal of the American Statistical Association* 90 (432): 1200–1224.
16. Eltoft, T. 2005. The Rician Inverse Gaussian distribution: A new model for non-Rayleigh signal amplitude statistics. *IEEE Transactions on Image Processing* 14 (11): 1722–1735.
17. Freeman, W.T., and E.H. Adelson. 1991. The design and use of steerable filters. *IEEE Transations on Pattern Analysis and Machine Intelligence* 13 (9): 891–906.
18. Gonzalez, R.C., and R.E. Woods. 2002. *Digital image processing*, 2nd ed. Singapore: Pearson.
19. Grant, R.P. 2004. *Computational genomics: Theory and application*, 1st ed. NJ: Taylor & Francis.
20. Howlader, T., and Y.P. Chaubey. 2009. Wavelet-based noise reduction by joint statistical modeling of cDNA microarray images. *Journal of Statistical Theory and Practice* 3 (2): 349–370.
21. Howlader, T., and Y.P. Chaubey. 2010. Noise reduction of cDNA microarray images using complex wavelets. *IEEE Transactions on Image Processing* 19 (8): 1953–1967.
22. Hyverinen, A. 1999. Sparse code shrinkage: Denoising of nongaussian data by maximum likelihood estimation. *Neural Computation* 11 (7): 1739–1768.
23. Ishwaran, H., and J.S. Rao. 2003. Detecting differentially expressed genes in microarrays using Bayesian model selection. *Journal of the American Statistical Association* 98: 438–455.
24. Jiang, J., L. Zhang, and J. Yang. 2014. Mixed noise removal by weighted encoding with sparse nonlocal regularization. *IEEE Transations on Image Processing* 23 (6): 2651–2662.
25. Kerr, M.K., M. Martin, and G. Churchill. 2000. Analysis of variance for gene expression microarray data. *Journal of Computational Biology* 7 (6): 819–837.
26. Kingsbury, N.G. 1999. Image processing with complex wavelets. *Philosophical Transactions of the Royal Society A* 357 (1760): 2543–2560.
27. Kingsbury, N.G. 2001. Complex wavelets for shift invariance analysis and filtering of signals. *Applied and Computational Harmonic Analysis* 10 (3): 234–253.
28. Lukac, R. 2014. Microarray image restoration and noise filtering. In *Microarray image and data analysis: Theory and practice*, ed. L. Rueda, 171–194. CRC Press.
29. Lukac, R., K.N. Plataniotis, B. Smolka, and A.N. Venetsanopoulos. 2004. A multichannel order-statistic technique for cDNA microarray image processing. *IEEE Transactions on Nanobioscience* 3: 272–285.
30. Lukac, R., K.N. Plataniotisa, B. Smolkab, and A.N. Venetsanopoulos. 2005. cDNA microarray image processing using fuzzy vector filtering framework. *Fuzzy Sets and Systems* 152: 17–35.
31. Lukac, R., and B. Smolka. 2003. Application of the adaptive center-weighted vector median framework for the enhancement of cDNA microarray images. *International Journal of Applied Mathematics and Computer Science* 13 (3): 369–383.
32. Mallat, S. 1999. *A wavelet tour of signal processing*, 2nd ed. San Diego, CA: Academic Press.
33. Mastriani, M., and A.E. Giraldez. 2006. Microarrays denoising via smoothing of coefficients in wavelet domain. *International Journal of Biomedical Sciences* 1: 7–14.
34. Mastrogianni, A., E. Dermatas, and A. Bezerianos. 2008. Microarray image denoising using spatial filtering and wavelet transformation. In *Proceedings of international federation of medical and biological engineering, Singapore: International conference on biomedical engineering*, 594–597.
35. McLachlan, G.J., K. Do, and C. Ambroise. 2004. *Analyzing microarray gene expression data*, 1st ed. NJ: Wiley.
36. Mihçak, M.K., I. Kozintsev, K. Ramchandran, and P. Moulin. 1999. Low-complexity image denoising based on statistical modeling of wavelet coefficients. *IEEE Signal Processing Letters* 6 (12): 300–303.
37. Motwani, M.C., M.C. Gadiya, R.C. Motwani, and F. Harris. 2004. Survey of image denoising techniques. In *Proceedings of global signal processing expo and conference*, Santa Clara, CA, 27–30.
38. O'Neill, P., G.D. Magoulas, and X. Liu. 2003. Improved processing of microarray data using image reconstruction techniques. *IEEE Transactions on Nanobioscience* 2: 176–183.
39. Peterson, S.R., Y.H. Lee, and S.A. Kassam. 1988. Some statistical properties of alpha-trimmed mean and standard type M filters. *IEEE Transactions on Acoustics, Speech, and Signal Processing* 36 (5): 707–713.

40. Portilla, J., V. Strela, M.J. Wainwright, and E.P. Simoncelli. 2003. Image denoising using scale mixtures of Gaussians in the wavelet domain. *IEEE Transactions on Image Processing* 12 (11): 1338–1351.
41. Rahman, S.M.M., O. Ahmad, and M.N.S. Swamy. 2008. Bayesian wavelet-based image denoising using the Gauss-Hermite expansion. *IEEE Transactions on Image Processing* 17 (10): 1755–1771.
42. Rangayyan, R.M., M. Ciuc, and F. Faghih. 1998. Adaptive-neighborhood filtering of images corrupted by signal-dependent noise. *Appl. Opt.* 37: 4477–4487.
43. Rueda, L. 2014. *Microarray image and data analysis: Theory and practice*, 1st ed. Boca Raton, FL: CRC Press.
44. Selesnick, I.W. 2001. The double density DWT. In *Wavelets in signal and image analysis: From theory to practice*. Kluwer.
45. Selesnick, I.W., R.G. Baraniuk, and N.G. Kingsbury. 2005. The dual-tree complex wavelet transform. *IEEE Signal Processing Magazine* 22 (6): 123–151.
46. Şendur, L., and I.W. Selesnick. 2002. Bivariate shrinkage functions for wavelet-based denoising exploiting interscale dependency. *IEEE Transactions on Signal Processing* 50 (11): 2744–2756.
47. Şendur, L., and I.W. Selesnick. 2002. Bivariate shrinkage with local variance estimation. *IEEE Signal Processing Letters* 9 (12): 438–441.
48. Shams, R., H. Rabbani, and S. Gazor. 2014. A comparison of x-lets in denoising cDNA microarray images. In *Proceedings of IEEE international conference on acoustics, speech, and signal processing*, 2862–2866. IEEE Signal Processing Society, Florence, Italy.
49. Smolka, B., R. Lukac, and K. Plataniotis. 2006. Fast noise reduction in cDNA microarray images. In *Proceedings of Biennial symposium on communications*, Kingston, ON, Canada, 348–351.
50. Smolka, B., and K. Plataniotis. 2005. Ultrafast technique of impulsive noise removal with application to microarray image denoising. In *Proceedings of international conference on image analysis and recognition*, vol. 3656, 990–997. Toronto, Canada.
51. Srinivasan, L., Y. Rakvongthai, and S. Oraintara. 2014. Microarray image denoising using complex Gaussian scale mixtures of complex wavelets. *IEEE Journal of Biomedical and Health Informatics* 18 (4): 1423–1430.
52. Stefanou, H., T. Margaritis, D. Kafetzopoulos, K. Marias, and P. Tsakalides. 2007. Microarray image denoising using a two-stage multiresolution technique. In *Proceedings of IEEE international conference on bioinformatics and biomedicine*, 383–389. IEEE Computer Society, Freemont, CA.
53. Velisavljević, V., B. Lozano, M. Vetterli, M., and P.L. Dragotti. 2006. Directionlets: anisotropic multidirectional representation with separable filtering. *IEEE Transactions on Image Processing* 15 (7): 1916–1933.
54. Wang, X.H., R.S.H. Istepanian, and Y.H. Song. 2003. Microarray image enhancement by denoising using stationary wavelet transform. *IEEE Transactions on Nanonbioscince* 2 (4): 184–189.
55. Wei, D., and A.C. Bovik. 2000. Wavelet denoising for image enhancement. In *Handbook of image and video processing*, ed. A.C. Bovik. NY: Academic Press.
56. Wit, E., and J. McClure. 2004. *Statistics for microarrays: Design, analysis and inference*, 1st ed. England: Wiley.
57. Zhang, A. 2006. *Advanced analysis of gene expression microarray data*, 1st ed. Singapore: World Scientific.
58. Zhang, L., P. Bao, and X. Wu. 2005. Multiscale LMMSE-based image denoising with optimal wavelet selection. *IEEE Transactions on Circuits and Systems for Video Technology* 15 (4): 469–481.
59. Zhang, M., and B.K. Gunturk. 2008. Multiresolution bilateral filtering for image denoising. *IEEE Transactions on Image Processing* 17 (12): 2324–2333.

60. Zhang, W., I. Shmulevich, and J. Astola. 2004. *Microarray quality control*, 1st ed. NJ: Wiley.
61. Zhang, X.Y., F. Chen, Y. Zhang, S.C. Agner, M. Akay, Z. Lu, M.M.Y. Waye, and S.K. Tsui. 2002. Signal processing techniques in genomic engineering. *Proceedings of the IEEE* 90 (12): 1822–33.
62. Zifan, A., M.H. Moradi, and S. Gharibzadeh. 2010. Microarray image enhancement by denoising using decimated and undecimated multiwavelet transforms. *Signal, Image and Video Processing* 4 (2): 177–185.

Chapter 5
A Transformation for the Analysis of Unimodal Hazard Rate Lifetimes Data

Kobby Asubonteng, Govind S. Mudholkar and Alan Hutson

Abstract The family of distributions introduced by [34] is the best known, best understood, most extensively investigated, and commonly employed model used for lifetimes data analysis. A variety of software packages are available to simplify its use. Yet, as is well known, the model is appropriate only when the hazard rate is monotone. However, as suggested in an overview by [23], the software packages may be usefully employed by transforming data when exploratory tools such as TTT transform or nonparametric estimates indicate unimodal, bathtub or J-shaped hazard rates, which are also commonly encountered in practice. Mudholkar et al. [22] discussed the details of one such transformation relevant for the bathtub case. In this paper, specifics of another transformation which is appropriate when data exploration indicates a unimodal hazard rate is discussed. The details of parameter estimation and hypothesis testing are considered in conjunction with earlier alternatives and illustrated using examples from the fields of biological extremes and finance.

Keywords Weibull distribution · Exponentiated Weibull · Generalized Weibull Lifetimes data · Maximum likelihood · Transformation

MSC: 62F03 · 62F10 · 62P20 · 62P20

K. Asubonteng (✉)
AstraZeneca Pharmaceuticals, Gaithersburg, MD, USA
e-mail: asowusu77@gmail.com

G. S. Mudholkar
Department of Statistics and Biostatistics, University of Rochester, Rochester, NY, USA
e-mail: mudholkarg@gmail.com

A. Hutson
Department of Biostatistics, University at Buffalo, Buffalo, NY, USA
e-mail: ahutson@buffalo.edu

A. Adhikari et al. (eds.), *Mathematical and Statistical Applications in Life Sciences and Engineering*, https://doi.org/10.1007/978-981-10-5370-2_5

5.1 Introduction

The well-known Weibull model used in survival and reliability studies is known to be inappropriate when exploratory tools such as TTT transform, Gini index plot or non-parametric graphical estimates indicate a non-monotone hazard rate, in which case some specialized model is employed. However, widely available Weibull software packages, in conjunction with data transformations can be used to analyze unimodal, bathtub-shaped, as well as a broader spectrum of monotone hazard rates. This point was outlined and illustrated in a paper by [23].

Bathtub-hazard rates arise in several areas such as demographic life tables and actuarial risk analysis. A classic example corresponding to the bathtub-hazard rate assumes decreasing hazard due to infant mortality in early life and increasing hazard due to eventual aging have been considered since the earliest studies of demographical life tables and actuarial risk analysis (see Fig. 5.1 for the shape of a bathtub-hazard rate). The details of the use of the transformation,

$$g(x,\eta) = \left(\frac{x}{1-\eta x}\right), \qquad \max(x) < 1/\eta,\ \eta \geq 0, \tag{5.1}$$

which transforms data to a Weibull distribution, can be used in this case, e.g., in the case of modeling bath-shaped data see [22]. Note that η is a transformation parameter, the value of $\eta = 0$ implies no transformation is needed.

Unimodal hazard rates, although not as common as bathtub-shaped hazard rates, also appear in many areas of applications of lifetime data analysis. An example of a unimodal hazard rate is the case of organ transplantation. For example, in the case of heart transplantation the hazard rate increases due to the body adapting to a new heart and then decreases as the patient accepts the transplant. This feature is common in the area of biomedical sciences. However, the general phenomena may be expected in the areas of finance as "*initial public offering*" and "*speculative bubbles*." To analyze lifetime data with assumed unimodal hazard rates, commonly employed models include the following models: log-logistic, log-normal, and inverse Gaussian distributions. Note, however, these models have limitations (see; [11, 23]). Moreover, these models do not easily accommodate the use of goodness-of-fit methodology, which is possible with the two Weibull families proposed by [24–27]. Towards this end, we propose a flexible transformational approach, which allows one to employ standard software and is described below.

An effective statistical model should be practical and sufficiently comparable to familiar models in order to be easily motivated. The model should be simple enough to be analytically tractable, yet general in scope to be comprehensive in practice. The data transformation

$$g(x,\theta) = \left(\frac{x^2}{\theta + x}\right), \qquad \theta \geq 0, \tag{5.2}$$

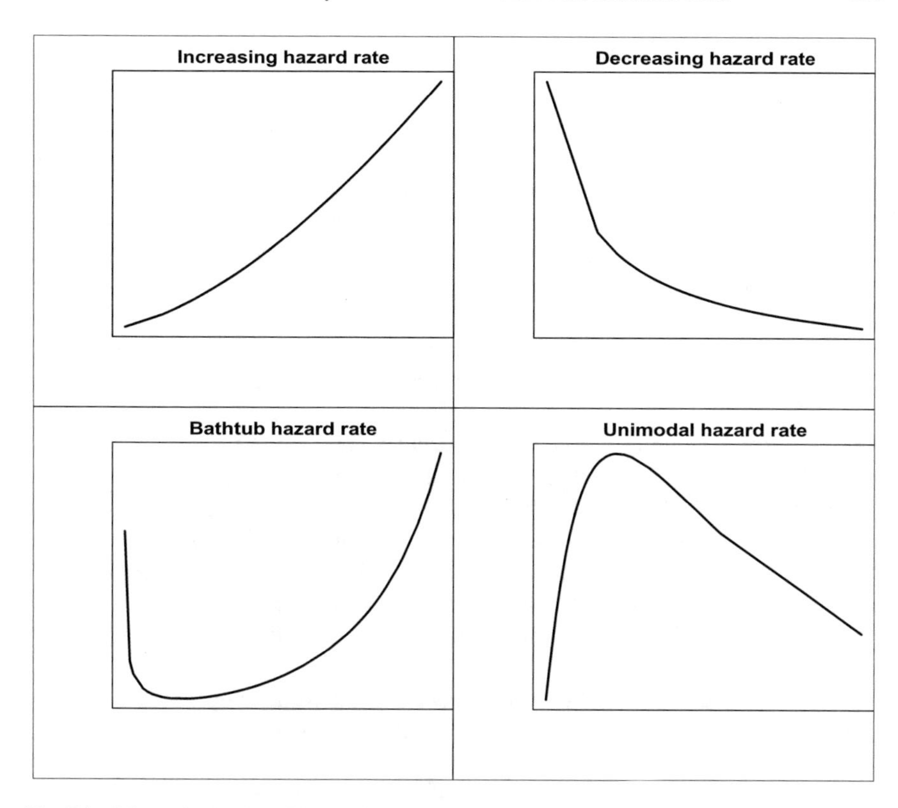

Fig. 5.1 Schematic display of four different hazard rates

to the Weibull family has several software packages available for its implementation. The richness of the included hazard functions meets the requirements practicality and generalizability. Note that θ is a transformation parameter, the value of $\theta = 0$ implies no transformation is needed.

A schematic plot of four different hazard shapes (increasing hazard rate, decreasing hazard rate, bathtub-hazard rate, and unimodal hazard rate) are shown in Fig. 5.1.

In this paper, we present a model based on the use of transforming lifetime data for modeling and analyzing unimodal hazard rates to the Weibull family. In Sect. 5.2 we present the detailed distributional properties of the transformation family in (5.2). In Sect. 5.3 we discuss parameter estimation using the likelihood method. Simulation studies are presented in Sect. 5.4. An application of the method is presented in Sect. 5.5, as well as carrying out some comparative studies. Conclusions are made in Sect. 5.5.

5.2 The Power Transformation

Transformation can be used in different contexts in statistical community. Other well-known transformations in statistics are [10] Z-transformation of the correlation coefficient, Fisher's square root transform of the χ^2 variable and many others, which was introduced to approximate the percentiles and probabilities of the χ^2 distribution; see also [3, 32]. The square root transformation is variance stabilizing and the cube root transformation is approximately symmetrizing. Transformations of these types are used for approximating sampling or probability distributions. However, transformations are also used for adherence of the data to the assumptions (e.g., normality and linearity) of the statistical methodology of interest.

In this paper, we are interested in transformations of data in order to obtain reasonable agreement with some standard model (Weibull model) which is convenient for analysis of data. Earliest of such data transformation is Simon Newcomb's [29] (nineteenth century) log transformation used for pulling in the long right tail of skew data in order to achieve approximate normality. However, the power transformations proposed by [4] is best known and is used to handle deviations of assumptions such as normality, additivity, homoscedasticity, and linearity in linear model theory. An analogous transformation approach for the case of lifetime data analysis can be useful.

A typical set of lifetime data can be presented as n pairs of independent identically distributed random variables $(X_i,\ \delta_i),\ \ i = 1, 2, \ldots, n$, where

$$X_i = \min(T_i,\ C_i) \quad \text{and} \quad \delta_i = \begin{cases} 1, & \text{if } T_i \leq C_i, \ \text{(uncensored)}, \\ 0, & \text{if } C_i < T_i, \ \text{(right-censored)}, \end{cases} \tag{5.3}$$

T_i is the lifetime and C_i the censoring time and δ_i the censoring indicator. Detailed discussion of different types of censoring can be found in [14, 15]. More discussion of survival analysis with several new illustrative examples appears in "Handbook of Statistics," Advances in Survival Analysis by [2].

Suppose that the data are $(X_i, \delta_i),\ \ i = 1, 2, \ldots, n$, as described in (5.3), suppose also that there exists a parameter θ as defined in (5.2) such that the transformed data $(y_i, \delta_i),\ \ i = 1, 2, \ldots, n$, are distributed as Weibull (σ, α) with shape and scale parameters α and σ, respectively. The probability density function $f(t)$ of the Weibull distribution with shape and scale parameters α and σ is given by

$$f(t) = (\alpha/\sigma)\,(t/\sigma)^{\alpha-1} \exp\left[-t/\sigma\right]^{\alpha},\ \sigma > 0,\ \alpha > 0,\ \ t > 0. \tag{5.4}$$

The transformation given in (5.2) is proposed when the shape of a lifetime data on the basis of empirical hazard function or empirical TTT transform plot indicate unimodal or increasing or decreasing hazard rate.

Useful Conditions: Properties of the transformation at (5.2):

1. The range of the transformation is 0 to ∞. This corresponds to the support of the Weibull distribution.

2. The identity transformation is a special case. Thus, no transformation is needed when the parameter θ is equal to 0.
3. The transformation should be invertible.

Translation of Weibull Results: The original observations x can be derived from (5.2) as follows:

$$x = \left\{ y + \sqrt{y^2 + 4\theta\, y} \right\} /2, \tag{5.5}$$

where only the positive solution of x is to be considered, since x cannot be negative and y represents the transformed Weibull compatible data.

The transformed data, $y_i = g(x_i, \theta)$, with respect to the hazard shape assumptions described previously satisfy the Weibull (σ, α) model assumptions. In addition, we may easily derive the corresponding survival and hazard functions.

The survival function of the original observations corresponding to the transformation $g(x, \theta)$ is written as,

$$S(x) = \exp\left[- \left\{ \frac{1}{\sigma} \left(\frac{x^2}{x+\theta} \right) \right\}^{\alpha} \right], \quad \sigma > 0,\ \alpha > 0, \theta \geq 0,\ x > 0. \tag{5.6}$$

Once the survival function is obtained, the density function, $f(x)$, follows straightforward as the derivative the derivative of $F(x) = 1 - S(x)$. The hazard function is $h(x) = f(x)/(1 - F(x))$. The density and hazard functions in terms of original observations are given by

$$f(x) = \frac{\alpha}{\sigma} \left\{ \frac{1}{\sigma} \left(\frac{x^2}{x+\theta} \right) \right\}^{\alpha-1} \exp\left[- \left\{ \frac{1}{\sigma} \left(\frac{x^2}{x+\theta} \right) \right\}^{\alpha} \right] \frac{(x^2 + 2\theta x)}{(x+\theta)^2}, \tag{5.7}$$

and

$$h(x) = \frac{\alpha}{\sigma} \left(\frac{1}{\sigma} \right) \frac{x^{2(\alpha-1)}}{(x+\theta)^{\alpha+1}} (x^2 + 2\theta x), \tag{5.8}$$

respectively.

Let (X_i, δ_i), $i = 1, 2, \ldots, n$, be the original lifetime data as described in (5.3), and let $y_i = g(x_i, \theta)$ denote the transformed observations. The hazard function in (5.8) assumes different shapes depending on the parameter values. The nature of the hazard functions is summarized in the following theorem:

Theorem 5.1 *Suppose there exists* θ, *such that* $g(x_i, \theta) \sim$ Wiebull(σ, α), $i = 1, 2, \ldots, n$. *Then, the hazard function* $h(x)$ *is (a) monotone increasing if* $\alpha > 1$, *(b) unimodal if* $0.5 < \alpha < 1$ *and (c) monotone decreasing for* $0 < \alpha < 0.5$.

See Table 5.1 for the summary of Theorem 5.1.

Proof See Appendix.

Table 5.1 Hazard rate classification

Hazard rate	Transformation
Shape	$g(x,\theta)$
Increasing	$\alpha \geq 1$
Unimodal	$0.5 < \alpha < 1$
Decreasing	$0 < \alpha \leq 0.5$

5.3 Statistical Inference

The methods of estimation and the construction of approximate confidence intervals for the transformation parameter θ and the Weibull scale and shape parameters σ and α, respectively is discussed in this section.

5.3.1 Maximum Likelihood Estimation

The analysis of lifetime data modeled by the new transformation in (5.2) can be performed using likelihood methods, e.g. See [5, 13, 15, 31]. The basic ideas for likelihood are outlined in many books, including Chap. 2 of [6]. A reasonable comprehensive account of the likelihood methods has been given by [16–19, 30]. The method of maximum likelihood estimation in well-behaved models is generally one of the most efficient and well-understood approaches and will be the method that we have chosen to employ in our model estimation procedure.

The likelihood function of the transformed observations can be expressed as

$$\begin{aligned}\mathcal{L}(\alpha,\sigma,\theta,y) &= \prod_{i=1}^{n}\{h(y_i)\}^{\delta_i}\,S(y_i)\\ &= \prod_{i=1}^{n}\left\{\frac{\alpha}{\sigma}\left(\frac{y_i}{\sigma}\right)^{\alpha-1}\right\}^{\delta_i}\exp\left(-\left(\frac{y_i}{\sigma}\right)^{\alpha}\right),\end{aligned}\tag{5.9}$$

where the $y_i's$ are the transformed observations and δ_i is 1 if the ith event time is observed and 0 if censored.

The likelihood to the original observations is achieved by multiplying (5.9) by the Jacobian of the transformation as follows:

$$\mathcal{L}(\alpha,\sigma,\theta;x) = \prod_{i=1}^{n}\left\{\frac{\alpha}{\sigma}\left(\frac{g(x_i,\theta)}{\sigma}\right)^{\alpha-1}\right\}^{\delta_i}\exp\left(-\left(\frac{g(x_i,\theta)}{\sigma}\right)^{\alpha}\right)|\mathbf{J}\,(\theta;\mathbf{x}_i)|\,,\tag{5.10}$$

where $|\mathbf{J}(\theta; \mathbf{x}_i)| = (x_i^2 + 2\theta x_i)/(x_i + \theta)^2$ and $g(x_i, \theta)$ is the transformation defined in (5.2). The log-likelihood function of (5.10) is then given by

$$\ell(\alpha, \sigma, \theta, x) = d \log\left(\frac{\alpha}{\sigma}\right) + (\alpha - 1)\sum_{i=1}^{n} \delta_i \log\left(\frac{g(x_i, \theta)}{\sigma}\right) - \sum_{i=1}^{n}\left(\frac{g(x_i, \theta)}{\sigma}\right)^{\alpha} + \\ + \sum_{i=1}^{n} \log|\mathbf{J}(\theta; \mathbf{x}_i)|, \tag{5.11}$$

where d is the number of uncensored observations and $|\mathbf{J}(\theta; \mathbf{x}_i)|$, the Jacobian of the transformation is defined above.

Estimates of the parameters of the model are obtained by maximizing the logarithm of the likelihood function in (5.11). Equation (5.11) is nonlinear in the three parameters, the solution of the nonlinear equation can be obtained using one of many numerical maximization routines.

Confidence Intervals: The asymptotic distribution of the maximum likelihood estimates can be used to construct approximate confidence intervals for the individual transformation parameter θ and Weibull parameters σ and α, based on the approximate multivariate normality of the maximum likelihood estimates. A variety of confidence intervals may be constructed. A notable exception is the likelihood ratio test confidence region by [21], which is based on an asymptotic chi-squared distribution. Cox and Hinkley [6] provided an explicit proof that Wald and likelihood ratio confidence intervals or regions are asymptotically equivalent.

5.3.2 Simulation Study

We conducted simulation studies to examine the small-sample performance of the proposed transformation model using a Monte Carlo experiment. We have seen that using the transformation $y = g(x, \theta)$ in (5.2) leads to a Weibull model fit for the transformed data y_i, $i = 1, \ldots, n$, which then translates directly to the distribution function $F(x)$, the survival function $S(x)$ and the density function $f(x)$ of the original random variable. Clearly, this helps us to obtain the quantile function and simulate samples for the lifetime values in the original problem.

Monte Carlo Experiment and Results: The performance of the maximum likelihood estimators for the transformation model is first evaluated. These evaluations are conducted by generating 10,000 random samples of sizes $n \in \{20, 30, 40, 50, 100, 500\}$ from the quantile function, given by:

$$Q_u(x) = \frac{v + \sqrt{v^2 + 4\theta v}}{2}, \tag{5.12}$$

where

$$v = \sigma \{-\log(1-u)\}^{1/\alpha} \quad (5.13)$$

and u is a uniformly distributed random variable in (0, 1). It may be noted that in (5.13), we have admitted only the positive solution of x.

We varied the choices of the parameters σ, α, and θ based on the shapes of the hazard function (5.8) and based on Theorem 5.1 in Sect. 5.2. For each simulated sample, the likelihood method discussed in Sect. 5.3 is implemented to obtain the MLE's of the parameters in the model. The 10,000 estimated MLE's are then averaged. The MLE's were computed using "nlminb in R Project for Statistical Computing." The bias and standard errors of the estimators for each parameter value were then calculated from their simulated values.

Note that we have three hazard shapes that may be considered; (i) $\alpha > 1$, for increasing hazard rate, (ii) $1/2 < \alpha < 1$, for unimodal hazard rate and (iii) $0 < \alpha < 1/2$ for decreasing hazard rate. However, the focus of this paper is on unimodal hazard rates. The hazard function from a random sample generated from the true parameter values based on the largest sample size (i.e., $n = 500$) is plotted and compared with the hazard function plot obtained from the simulated average value of the 10,000 MLE's for $n = 500$. The plot examines the closeness of the MLE estimates to their true values. The parameters σ and θ are taken arbitrarily, but α is selected according to Theorem 5.1 of Sect. 5.2, which states that the hazard function $h(x)$, is unimodal for $1/2 < \alpha < 1$.

Unimodal hazard function: For the unimodal hazard rate, we set $\sigma = 25.000$, $\alpha = 0.800$ and $\theta = 5.000$. These parameters are considered the true values from which the random samples were generated. The results are presented in Table 5.2.

Table 5.2 summarizes the results from 10,000 replications for different samples of sizes n. The column labeled "Average MLEs" gives the average of the estimated MLEs. The standard errors of the estimates are represented "(Se)." The column

Table 5.2 An Empirical comparison of the true parameter values and their Monte Carlo estimates for samples of sizes n, standard errors and bias from the simulated values included

n	σ average MLEs[a] (Se) Bias	α average MLEs[b] (Se) Bias	θ average MLEs[c] (Se) Bias
20	26.943 (0.0817) 1.943	0.925 (0.0020) 0.125	3.768 (0.0380) −1.232
30	26.873 (0.0688) 1.873	0.899 (0.0016) 0.099	3.853 (0.0389) −1.147
40	26.659 (0.0611) 1.659	0.884 (0.0014) 0.084	3.973 (0.0386) −1.027
50	26.674 (0.0577) 1.674	0.875 (0.0013) 0.075	3.956 (0.0384) −1.044
100	26.325 (0.0465) 1.325	0.852 (0.0010) 0.052	4.284 (0.0371) −0.716
150	26.149 (0.0422) 1.149	0.839 (0.0009) 0.039	4.409 (0.0367) −0.591
500	25.380 (0.0310) 0.380	0.815 (0.0006) 0.015	5.063 (0.0325) 0.063

[a] σ estimate, based on 10,000 MLEs, true parameter value of $\sigma = 25.000$
[b] α estimate, based on 10,000 MLEs, true parameter value of $\alpha = 0.800$
[c] θ estimate, based on 10,000 MLEs, true parameter value of $\theta = 5.000$

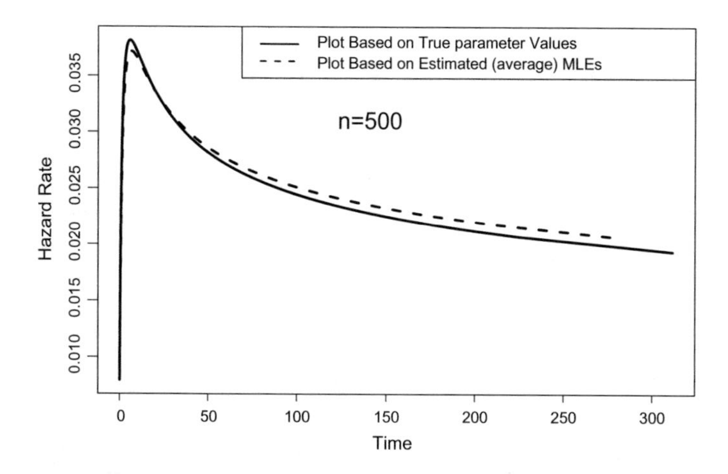

Fig. 5.2 Simulated hazard function corresponding to true values of $\sigma = 25,\ \alpha = 0.8,\ \theta = 5.0$ and estimated MLEs $\hat{\sigma} = 25.38,\ \hat{\alpha} = 0.82,\ \hat{\theta} = 5.06$

labeled "Bias" is computed as the difference between the average MLEs and the true parameter values.

Figure 5.2 displays a comparison of the hazard function plotted by using the true parameter values $\sigma = 25,\ \alpha = 0.800,$ and $\theta = 5.00$ and the hazard function plotted by the estimated MLEs $\hat{\sigma} = 25.38,\ \hat{\alpha} = 0.82,\ \hat{\theta} = 5.06$ for the largest sample size $n = 500$ from Table 5.2. From Fig. 5.2 and Table 5.2, it is seen that, the bias and standard errors decreases as sample size increases and also the estimators of the parameters converge to their true values as the sample size increases. The Monte Carlo experiment conducted above evaluates the performance of the estimators by observing the values of the standard errors and biases. The results from the experiment indicate that the estimators from the proposed transformation method perform well in estimating the model parameters.

In the second stage of the simulation study, we investigate the coverage probabilities of the model parameters. Performance of the transformation model is evaluated using the 95% coverage probability. The bootstrap percentile method based on empirical distribution, e.g., See [8], is used in this simulation experiment. For the specifics of the problems of bootstrap interval estimation see the review by [7]. The interval estimation is repeated I times (I replications) and the true level (coverage probability) of an interval is estimated by the proportion of times among the I replications when the true value belonged to the interval. The simulation sample size I is 1000, the bootstrap sample size B is set to 500 and $n \in \{(20, 30, 40, 50, 100, 150)\}$ with the experiment having the same specifications and associated parameter values (true parameters) as defined previously in the first simulation study. The simulation sample size I is different from the bootstrap sample size B, the simulation sample size is for the purpose of testing the accuracy of the bootstrap percentile confidence interval.

Table 5.3 Estimated coverage probabilities with samples of sizes n and nominal 0.95, based on 1000 replications and bootstrap sample $B = 500$ for model parameters $\sigma = 25.000$, $\alpha = 0.800$, and $\theta = 5.000$

n	Coverage probability for σ	Coverage probability for α	Coverage probability for θ
20	0.965	0.850	0.932
30	0.970	0.900	0.930
40	0.974	0.913	0.921
50	0.969	0.918	0.943
100	0.968	0.937	0.930
150	0.950	0.950	0.945

Table 5.4 Arm A survival times (in days) of 51 head-and-neck cancer patients, + means censored

7, 34, 42, 63, 64, 74+, 83, 84,91, 108, 112, 129, 133, 133, 139, 140, 140, 146, 149, 154, 157, 160, 160, 165, 173, 176, 185+, 218, 225, 241, 248, 273, 277, 279+, 297, 319+, 405, 471, 420, 440, 523, 523+, 583, 594, 1101, 1116+, 1146, 1226+, 1349+, 1412+, 1417

The results from Tables 5.3 shows that the empirical coverage probabilities are quite accurate and close to the nominal 95% as the sample size increases, this indicates that the proposed method performs stably and leads to very satisfactory coverage probabilities.

5.4 Examples

Practical examples will be presented in this section to show the usefulness of the proposed methodology.

Example 5.1 In this example, a clinical trial dataset involving survival times (in days) of head-and-neck cancer patients given in Table 5.4 studied by [9] is discussed for studying the effectiveness of the proposed model. The data is analyzed using the new model and compared with existing models for lifetime data. Nine patients were lost-to-follow-up and were regarded as censored. Data were reanalyzed by [26] using the exponentiated Weibull model and further studied in [27] by the generalized Weibull model.

The empirical TTT transform plot and the empirical hazard plot in Fig. 5.3 indicate a unimodal shape hazard rate for data in Table 5.4, e.g., See [1] for detail discussion of TTT plot.

Inference about the model parameters: Maximum likelihood estimates of the model parameters, along with their standard errors and the corresponding 95% confidence intervals based on large sample theory of the likelihood ratio test are reported in Table 5.5.

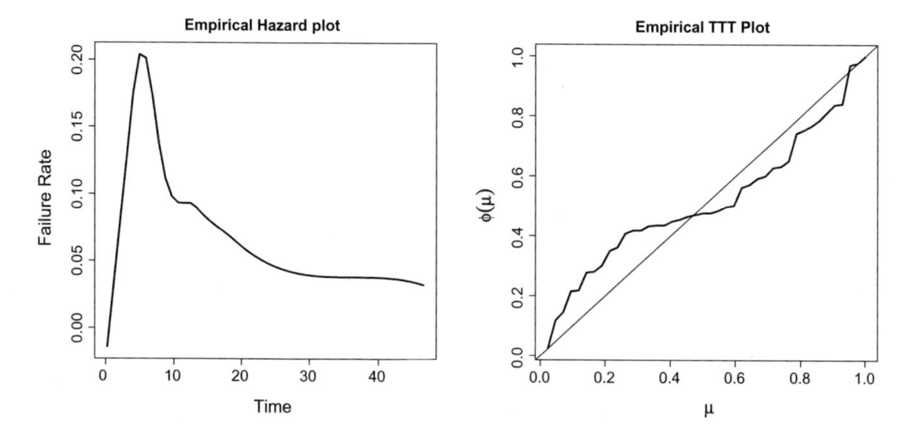

Fig. 5.3 The empirical TTT and hazard plots of Arm A data

Table 5.5 Estimates for [9] arm A data

MLE estimates	Standard error	95% confidence interval
$\hat{\sigma} = 11.0500$	0.4136	(10.2393, 11.8607)
$\hat{\alpha} = 0.7602$	0.0171	(0.7267, 0.7937)
$\hat{\theta} = 2.6548$	0.3253	(2.0172, 3.2924)

The individual hypothesis tested for θ corresponding to the Weibull fit is given is given by;

$$H_0 : \theta = 0, \text{ versus } H_1 : \theta \neq 0. \tag{5.14}$$

The 95% confidence interval for θ is (2.0172, 3.2924) from Table 5.5, this shows that $\theta \neq 0$, implying that we can apply the proposed transformation to the data.

Weibull Goodness-of-Fit Test: The choice of the transformation does not guarantee, however, that, the transformed observations have an approximate Weibull distribution. A Weibull goodness-of-fit test is necessary to ensure that we have achieved our goal by using the transformation model and also whether or not the transformation is valid given the data and the model. The presence of censoring makes Pearson's chi-square goodness-of-fit statistic inappropriate to assess the suitability of the Weibull model because the censoring times cannot be put in any of the class intervals since we do not know their exact lifetimes, hence the likelihood ratio statistic is used to test the adequacy of a Weibull model as sub-model of the exponentiated Weibull family mentioned in the previous sections.

The log-likelihood function for the exponentiated Weibull family is shown in (5.15) as:

$$\ell(\alpha, \lambda, \sigma; y) = \sum_{i=1}^{n} \delta_i \log h(y_i) + \sum_{i=1}^{n} \log S(y_i), \tag{5.15}$$

where $h(y_i)$ and $S(y_i)$ are respectively the hazard and survival functions associated with the exponentiated Weibull family (see; [26]). The null hypothesis, $H_0 : \lambda = 1$, corresponds to the Weibull sub-model of the exponentiated Weibull model. In terms of the maximum likelihood (ML) estimates, the likelihood ratio statistic for H_0 is

$$\Lambda = \frac{L(\alpha_w, \lambda = 1, \sigma_w)}{L(\alpha_{ML}, \lambda_{ML}, \sigma_{ML})}, \tag{5.16}$$

where α_w, and σ_w are the estimates for the reduced model (Weibull model) and α_{ML}, λ_{ML} and σ_{ML} are the maximum likelihood estimates for the full model (exponentiated Weibull).

Under the null hypothesis, $-2\log(\Lambda)$ follows a χ^2 distribution with 1 degree of freedom. The values of the likelihood ratio statistics and their corresponding p-values for testing the Weibull goodness-of-fit hypotheses for Arm A data are, $-2\log(\Lambda) = 7.619$, with p-value $= 0.0058$ for the original data and $-2\log(\Lambda) = 3.1150$, with p-value $= 0.0800$ for the transformed data.

Weibull model QQ-plots for both the original and transformed observations are obtained by plotting the logarithm of the ordered lifetimes against the logarithm of the Weibull theoretical quantiles.

The Q-Q plots in Fig. 5.4 suggest a less satisfactory Weibull fit for the original data, but Weibull fit for the transformed data appears to be almost ideal. This is in agreement with the p-values from the goodness-of-fit test as the p-value for transformed data was slightly greater than 0.05. Hence the assumption of the transformation model is satisfied. The competing model fits appear in Fig. 5.5, it displays a comparison of the fitted hazard function of Arm A data by the transformation model, generalized Weibull, exponentiated Weibull and Weibull models.

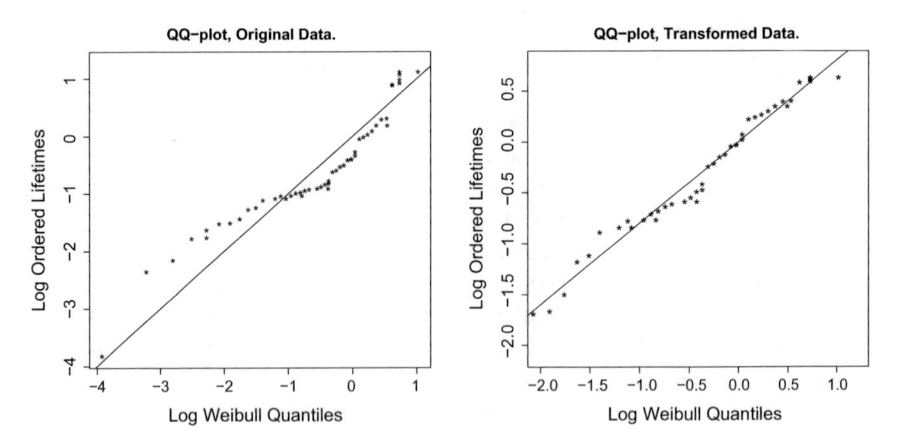

Fig. 5.4 QQ-plots for the original Arm A data and its transformed version. The straight lines are for assessing linearity of the QQ-plots

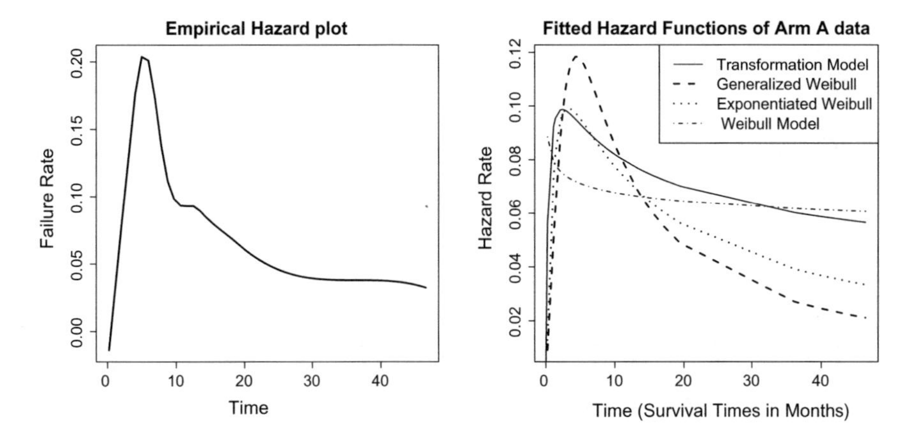

Fig. 5.5 Comparison of the empirical hazard rate and the hazard rates of four model fits for Arm A Data

Table 5.6 Annual flood discharge rates (1935–1973), (rate in ft^3/s) of the Floyd River at James, Iowa

1460 4050 3570 2060 1300 1390 1720 6280 1360 7440 5320 1400 3240 2710 4520 4840 8320 13900 71500 6250 2260 318 1330 970 1920 15100 2870 20600 3810 726 7500 7170 2000 829 17300 4740 13400 2940 5660

It is seen from the fitted hazard plots and goodness-of-fit tests that the Weibull model is inadequate for fitting this unimodal shape hazard rate data. However, the proposed transformation model provides a very satisfactory unimodal hazard fit to Arm A data and it competes very well with the existing models.

Example 5.2 The data consist of 39 consecutive annual flood discharge rates (1935–1973), (Rate in ft^3/s) of the Floyd River at James, Iowa, Table 5.6. The flood rates of rivers, which obviously are the extremes, have significant economic, social, political, and engineering implications. For example, consider the case of the 1993 Mississippi River floods. Hence modeling of flood data and analyses involving predictions such as 50 or 1000 year maxima constitute an important application of the extreme value theory. Mudholkar and Hutson [28] used the exponentiated Weibull family to analyze the flood data which had already been examined earlier by the [33]. We further study this flood data applying the new transformation method and make comparisons using the fitted hazard functions by various models.

The empirical TTT transform and hazard plots in Fig. 5.6 shows a unimodal shape hazard rate for the flood river data in Table 5.6.

Inference about the model parameters: Maximum likelihood estimates of the model parameters are reported in Table 5.7, along with standard errors based on large sample theory of the likelihood ratio test, and the corresponding 95% confidence interval.

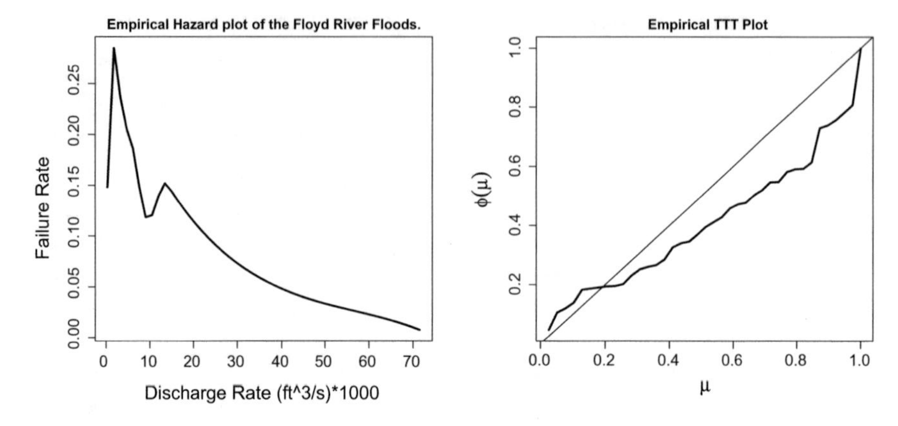

Fig. 5.6 The Empirical TTT transform and hazard plots for the Floyd River data

Table 5.7 Estimates for Floyd River data

MLE estimates	Standard error	95% confidence interval
$\hat{\sigma} = 3.3570$	0.2846	(2.7992, 3.9148)
$\hat{\alpha} = 0.6549$	0.0200	(0.6157, 0.6941)
$\hat{\theta} = 3.7968$	0.6890	(2.4464, 5.1472)

The individual hypothesis tested for θ is given by;

$$H_0 : \theta = 0, \text{ versus } H_1 : \theta \neq 0. \tag{5.17}$$

The 95% confidence interval for θ is (2.4464, 5.1472); see Table 5.7, the interval excludes 0.

Weibull Goodness-of-Fit Test: Weibull goodness-of-fit test is performed to test the appropriateness of the transformation model proposed in this paper.

The Q-Q plots in Fig. 5.7 suggest an inadequacy Weibull fit for the original data; whereas the Weibull fit for the transformed data indicates an improved fit. This inadequacy of the Weibull model for the original data and improvement of the fit by the transformation model is confirmed by Pearson's chi-square and Anderson-Darling's goodness-of-fit tests. Pearson's chi-square goodness-of-fit test for the Weibull fit are as follows: original data has a p-value of 0.0224 whiles the transformed data has a p-value of 0.2001. For Anderson-Darling's test, the p-value is 0.0076 for the original data whereas the p-value corresponding to the transformed data is 0.2027. Both test's results support that Weibull model assumptions are improved when the original data is transformed by the transformation family in (5.2).

Plots of the fitted hazard function by different models are shown in Fig. 5.8. It is clear from the figure that the fit by the transformation method is superior to the Weibull model fit in terms of the hazard function plot. Also, we note that, the

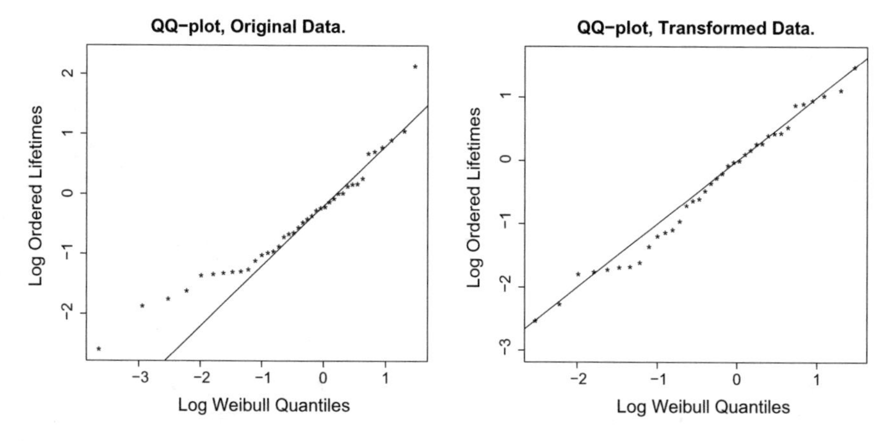

Fig. 5.7 QQ-plots for the original flood data and its transformed version. The straight lines are for assessing linearity of the QQ-plots

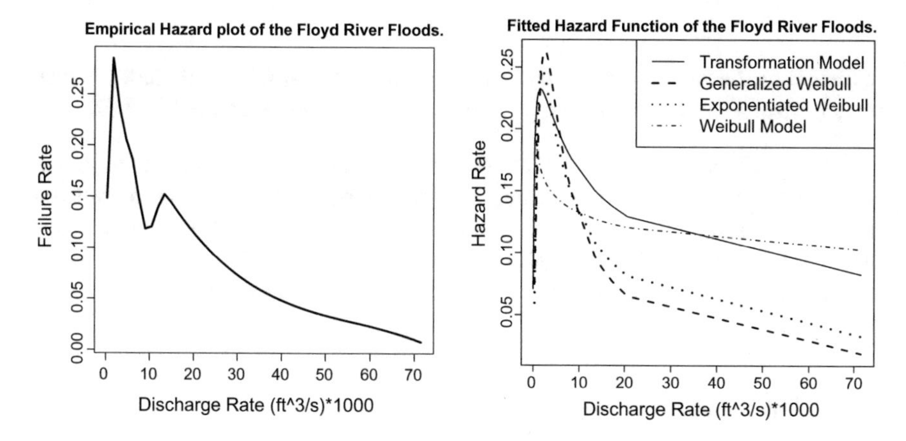

Fig. 5.8 Comparison of the empirical hazard rate and the hazard rates of four model fits for the Floyd River data

transformation method performs well when compared with the other competitors. The forgoing observations suggest that the transformation model yields very accurate results and is also very flexible.

Example 5.3 Rational Bubbles, NYSE Portfolio Econometric Duration Analysis: This example employs the innovative transformation method to illustrate the behavior of *speculative bubbles* in security prices and to also shows how the traditional model log-logistic accommodates only narrow spectrum of unimodal hazard rates. Speculative bubbles is a term often used to describe continual market over valuation followed by market collapse [11]. The stock returns on the NYSE rational bubbles were first analyzed by [12, 20], log-logistic model was used. The data were later studied by [11]. We also apply the new transformation model suitable for analyzing

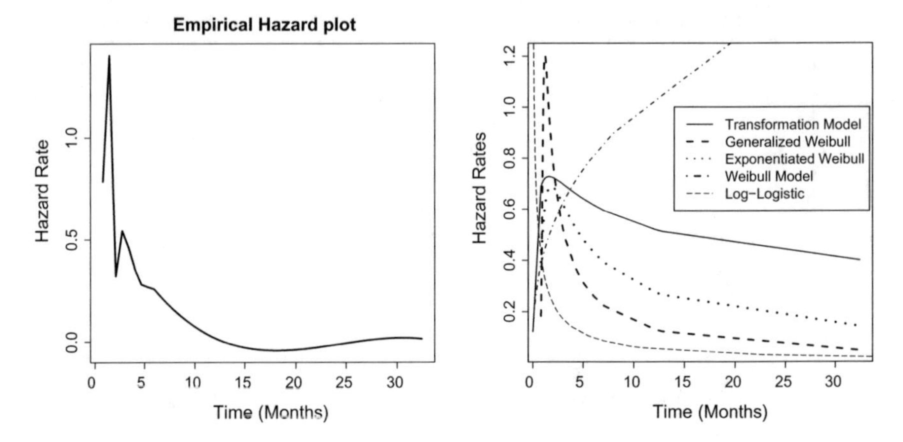

Fig. 5.9 Comparison of the empirical hazard rate and the hazard rates of five model fits for the Runs of abnormally positive returns, NYSE portfolio data

unimodal shape hazard rates to the data. A comparison of the profile hazards rates by empirical hazard function and five different models are shown in Fig. 5.9.

From Fig. 5.9, it can be seen that, log-logistic is not able to depict the unimodal shape of the hazard plot as indicated by the empirical hazard plot. However, the transformation model and the two Weibull extension models are able to bring out the unimodal shape of the plot. This example emphasizes that the log-logistic model can accommodate only a narrow spectrum of unimodal hazard rates.

5.5 Conclusions

In this paper, we have explored the use of data-transformation technique for examining lifetime data with unimodal shape hazard rate. These types of data are commonly found in biomedical areas and also in such areas of finance as initial public offering and speculative bubbles. We have also demonstrated the usefulness of the proposed method using examples. The transformation is shown to transform the data from a family of distributions with assumed hazard rates, such as unimodal, successfully to the Weibull model. As can be seen from the numerical examples, the transformation approach is easy to use and it seems to be more effective in application as compared with competing models. Hence, the new method serves as a practical alternative for modeling unimodal hazard rate data.

Appendix A

Proof of Theorem 1. The hazard function is given by:

$$h(x)=\frac{\alpha}{\sigma}\left(\frac{1}{\sigma}\right)\frac{x^{2(\alpha-1)}}{(x+\theta)^{\alpha+1}}(x^2+2\theta x). \tag{5.18}$$

Since logarithm is a monotone function, we may consider $\log h(x)$ instead of $h(x)$. We have

$$\log h(x)=(\alpha-1)\log\left(\frac{x^2}{x+\theta}\right)+\log(x^2+2\theta x)-2\log(x+\theta)+C, \tag{5.19}$$

where C is independent of x. Then

$$\begin{aligned}\ell'_{h(x)}=\frac{d}{dx}(\log h(x))&=\frac{(\alpha-1)(x+2\theta)}{x(x+\theta)}+\frac{2\theta^2}{x(x+\theta)(x+2\theta)}\\&=\frac{1}{x(x+\theta)}\left\{(\alpha-1)(x+2\theta)+\frac{2\theta^2}{x+2\theta}\right\}.\end{aligned} \tag{5.20}$$

- (a) For $\alpha\geq 1$, the sign of (5.20) is positive for all positive values of x, hence $\log h(x)$ is increasing and hence $h(x)$ is also increasing and (a) is proved.
- (b) $1/2<\alpha<1$: The proof of (b) is more involved, and requires additional machinery. It amounts to proving, roughly speaking that, the hazard function $h(x)$ is unimodal if and only if (5.20) has opposite signs at zero and ∞ and has one and only one zero over $0<x<\infty$. For critical point, the derivative of $\log h(x)$ is equal to zero, this means (5.20) is equal to zero and hence

$$\left\{(\alpha-1)(x+2\theta)+\frac{2\theta^2}{x+2\theta}\right\}=0. \tag{5.21}$$

Simplifying (5.21) gives the quadratic equation

$$\begin{aligned}&(\alpha-1)(x+2\theta)^2+2\theta^2=0\\ \Leftrightarrow\ & x^2+4\theta x+4\theta^2+\frac{2\theta^2}{(\alpha-1)}=0\\ \Leftrightarrow\ & x^2+4\theta x+4\theta^2-\frac{2\theta^2}{(1-\alpha)}=0.\end{aligned} \tag{5.22}$$

Equation (5.22) is solved by taking only the positive part of the solution, since x is positive, we then obtain

$$x^*=\theta\left\{-2+\sqrt{2/(1-\alpha)}\right\}, \tag{5.23}$$

hence the derivative of $\log h(x)$ has only one solution x^*.
For $\log h(x)$ to have an interior extreme point over $0 < x < \infty$, the critical point x^* has to be positive, and hence $-2 + \sqrt{2/(1-\alpha)}$ should be greater than zero, this implies that $1/2 < \alpha < 1$. Thus when $1/2 < \alpha < 1$, the derivative of $\log h(x)$ has only one zero and hence $\log h(x)$ has a turning point and therefore $h(x)$ has a turning point. Next, we show that the turning point is maximum by showing that the derivative of $\log h(x)$ has a positive sign at zero and a negative sign at ∞. If we let x approaches 0, then we have

$$\begin{aligned}\lim_{x\to 0}\left\{\frac{1}{x(x+\theta)}\left[(\alpha-1)(x+2\theta)+\frac{2\theta^2}{x+2\theta}\right]\right\} &= \frac{1}{0}\left[(\alpha-1)(2\theta)+\theta\right]\\ &= \frac{\theta}{0}\left[2(\alpha-1)+1\right]\\ &= +\infty. \end{aligned} \tag{5.24}$$

We let x goes to ∞ in the next step.

$$\begin{aligned}\ell'_{h(x)} &= \lim_{x\to\infty}\left\{\frac{1}{x(x+\theta)}\left[(\alpha-1)(x+2\theta)+\frac{2\theta^2}{x+2\theta}\right]\right\}\\ &= \lim_{x\to\infty}\left\{\frac{1}{x(x+\theta)}\left[(\alpha-1)(x+2\theta)\right]\right\},\\ &= \lim_{x\to\infty}\left\{\frac{(\alpha-1)}{2x}\right\}, \text{ by L'Hospital's Rule}\\ &= -(0) \text{ since } \alpha < 1. \end{aligned} \tag{5.25}$$

We have shown that the derivative of $\log h(x)$ has only one zero and also changes sign from $(+)$ to $(-)$ over $0 < x < \infty$ when $1/2 < \alpha < 1$. This shows that $\log h(x)$ has a maximum turning point and hence $h(x)$ is unimodal.

- (c) $0 < \alpha \leq 1/2$, the proof of (c) is straight forward, for $0 < \alpha \leq 1/2$, (5.20) has no zero over $0 < x < \infty$ and hence no turning point and therefore $\log h(x)$ is monotone. Following the steps in (5.24) and (5.25), we see that the derivative of $\log h(x)$ does not change signs and (5.20) is negative in both cases. Thus $\log h(x)$ is decreasing and hence $h(x)$ is a decreasing hazard function.

References

1. Aarset, M.V. 1987. How to identify bathtub hazard rate. *IEEE Transactions on Reliability* 36: 106–108.
2. Balakrishnan, N., and C.R. Rao. 2004. Advances in survival analysis. *Handbook of statistics*, vol. 23. Amsterdam: North-Holland.
3. Bartlett, M.S. 1947. The use of transformations. *Biometrics* 3: 39–52.
4. Box, G.E.P., and D.R. Cox. 1964. An analysis of transformations. *Journal of the Royal Statistical Society, Series B* 26: 211–243.

5. Cox, D.R., and D. Oakes. 1984. *Analysis of survival data*. London: Chapman & Hall.
6. Cox, D.R., and D.V. Hinkley. 1974. *Theoretical statistics*. London: Chapman & Hall.
7. Diciccio, T.J., and J.P. Romano. 1988. A review of bootstrap confidence intervals. *Journal of Royal Statistical Society B* 50: 338–354.
8. Efron, B. 1987. Better bootstrap confidence intervals. *Journal of the American Statistical Association* 82: 171–185.
9. Efron, B. 1988. Logistic regression, survival analysis and the Kaplan-Meier curve. *Journal of the American Statistical Association* 83: 414–425.
10. Fisher, R.A. 1915. Frequency distribution of the values of the correlation coefficient in samples of an indefinitely large population. *Biometrika* 10: 507–521.
11. Harman, Y.S., and T.W. Zuehlke. 2007. Nonlinear duration dependence in stock market cycles. *Review of Financial Economics* 16: 350–362.
12. Heckman, J.J., and S. Burton. 1984. Econometric duration analysis. *Journal of Econometrics* 24: 63–132.
13. Kalbfleisch, J.D., and R.L. Prentice. 1980. *The statistical analysis of failure data*. New York: Wiley.
14. Klein, J.P., and M.L. Moeschberger. 2003. *Survival analysis, techniques for censored and truncated data*, 2nd ed. New York: Springer.
15. Lawless, J.F. 1982. *Statistical methods and model for lifetime data*. New York: Wiley.
16. Le Cam, L. 1986. *Asymptotic methods in statistical decision theory*. New York: Springer.
17. Le Cam, L. 1990. Maximum likelihood: An introduction. *International Statistical Institute (ISI)* 58: 153–171.
18. Le Cam, L., and G. Lo Yang. 2000. *Asymptotics in statistics: Some basic concepts*, 2nd ed. New York: Springer.
19. Lehmann, E.L., and G. Casella. 1998. *Theory of point estimation*, 2nd ed. New York: Springer.
20. McQueen, G., and S. Thorley. 1994. Bubbles, stock returns, and duration dependence. *Journal of Financial and Quantitative Analysis* 29: 379–401.
21. Meeker, W.Q., and L.A. Escobar. 1995. Assessing influence in regression analysis with censored data. *Biometrics* 48: 50728.
22. Mudholkar, G.S., K.O. Asubonteng, and D.A. Hutson. 2009. Transformation for Weibull model analysis of bathtub failure rate data in reliability analysis. *Statistical Methodology* 6: 622–633.
23. Mudholkar, G.S., and K.O. Asubonteng. 2010. Data-transformation approach to lifetimes data analysis: An overview. *Journal of Statistical Planning and Inference* 140: 2904–2917.
24. Mudholkar, G.S., and D.K. Srivastava. 1993. Exponentiated Weibull family for analyzing bathtub failure rate data. *IEEE Transactions on Reliability* 42: 299–302.
25. Mudholkar, G.S., and G.D. Kollia. 1994. Generalized Weibull family: A structural analysis. *Communication Statistics-Theory and Methods* 23: 1149–1171.
26. Mudholkar, G.S., D.K. Srivastava, and M. Freimer. 1995. Exponentiated Weibull family: A reanalysis of the bus motor failure data. *Technometrics* 37: 436–445.
27. Mudholkar, G.S., D.K. Srivastava, and G. Kollia. 1996. A generalization of Weibull distribution with application to the analysis of survival data. *Journal of the American Statistical Association* 91: 1575–1583.
28. Mudholkar, G.S., and D.A. Hutson. 1996. The exponentiated Weibull family: Some properties and a flood data application. *Communication Statistics—Theory and Methods* 25: 3059–3083.
29. Newcomb, S. 1881. Note on the frequency of use of the different digits in natural numbers. *American Journal of Mathematics* 4: 39–40.
30. Pawitan, Y. 2001. *In all likelihood: Statistical modeling and inference using likelihood method*. New York: Oxford University Press.
31. Rao, C.R. 1973. *Linear statistical inference and its application*. New York: Wiley.
32. Terrell, G.R. 2003. The Wilson-Hilfety transformation is locally saddlepoint. *Biometrika* 445–453.
33. United States Water Resources Council. 1977. Guidelines For determining flood flow frequency. Hydrology Committee. Washington, D.C.: Water Resources Council.
34. Weibull, W. 1939. Statistical theory of the strength of materials. *Ingenioor Vetenskps Akademiens Handlingar* 151: 1–45.

Chapter 6
The Power M-Gaussian Distribution: An R-Symmetric Analog of the Exponential-Power Distribution

Saria Salah Awadalla, Govind S. Mudholkar and Ziji Yu

Abstract The mode-centric M-Gaussian distribution, which may be considered a fraternal twin of the Gaussian distribution, is an attractive alternative for modeling non-negative, unimodal data, which are often right-skewed. In this paper, we aim to expand upon the existing theory and utility of R-symmetric distributions by introducing a three-parameter generalization of the M-Gaussian distribution, namely the Power M-Gaussian distribution. The basic distributional character of this R-symmetric analog of the exponential-power distribution will be studied extensively. Estimation of the mode, dispersion, and kurtosis parameters will be developed based on both moments and maximum likelihood methods. Simulation and real data examples will be used to evaluate the model.

6.1 Introduction

The family of exponential-power distributions, also known as the θ-generalized normal, has been proposed and extensively studied as a robust alternative to the Gaussian model for data analysis. It was first introduced by Subbotin [24] and later investigated by several authors including Box [3], Diananda [7], and Turner [25]. Box and Tiao [4] also used it in their study of the robustness of the Bayesian version of normal theory. The exponential-power distribution denoted by θ-N(μ, α, θ) has density function

S. S. Awadalla, (✉)
Division of Epidemiology and Biostatistics, UIC School
of Public Health (SPH-PI), Chicago, IL 60612-4394, USA
e-mail: saria@uic.edu

G. S. Mudholkar
Department of Statistics and Biostatistics, University of Rochester,
Rochester, NY 14612, USA
e-mail: mudholkarg@gmail.com

Z. Yu
Biostatistics Department, Jazz Pharmaceuticals,
3180 Porter Drive, Palo Alto, CA 94304, USA
e-mail: ziji.yu@jazzpharma.com

A. Adhikari et al. (eds.), *Mathematical and Statistical Applications in Life Sciences and Engineering*, https://doi.org/10.1007/978-981-10-5370-2_6

$$f(x;\mu,\alpha,\theta)=\frac{\theta}{2\alpha\Gamma(1/\theta)}\exp\left\{-\left(\frac{|x-\mu|}{\alpha}\right)^{\theta}\right\},\quad x,\mu \text{ real}, \alpha>0,\theta>0, \tag{6.1}$$

where μ and α are the location and dispersion parameters, respectively, and θ is referred to in Box and Tiao [4] as the kurtosis parameter. Refer to the recent article by Mineo and Ruggieri [17] for a more thorough introduction and a useful software package.

Remark 6.1 The θ-N(μ,α,θ) distribution reduces to the normal distribution if $\theta=2$ and to the Laplace distribution if $\theta=1$. Also, in the limit as $\theta\to\infty$, it converges to the uniform density on the interval $(\mu-\alpha,\mu+\alpha)$.

The Gaussian distribution, although commonly used and well developed, can be restrictive in practice when studying populations that are non-negative and highly right-skewed. Both data transformations and the use of generalized distributions such as the power exponential are effective remedies but only in the close neighborhood of normality. In this paper, we develop a generalization of the recently introduced M-Gaussian distribution by Mudholkar et al. [20], which may be regarded as the R-symmetric twin of the normal distribution. The M-Gaussian, which is right-skewed, unimodal, and R-symmetric about its mode μ, is defined by its density function:

$$f(x;\mu,\sigma)=\sqrt{\frac{2}{\pi\sigma^2}}\exp\left\{-\frac{1}{2\sigma^2}\left(\frac{\mu^2}{x}-x\right)^2\right\},\quad x\geq 0,\mu>0,\sigma>0, \tag{6.2}$$

where μ is the population mode and σ^2 is the harmonic variance. The M-Gaussian distribution presents many properties and inferential methods surrounding the mode that are analogous to those of its Gaussian counterpart and its mean. Many of these similarities, which are referred to as the G-MG analogies, have been discussed in Mudholkar et al. [20]. In this paper, however, we introduce the Power M-Gaussian distribution and study its attributes and properties.

This paper is structured as follows: in Sect. 6.2, the notion of R-symmetry and the basic properties of the M-Gaussian distribution are reviewed. Section 6.3 contains the definition and derivation of the Power M-Gaussian distribution as well as its basic properties. Section 6.4 is given to the estimation of the parameters of the Power M-Gaussian as well as the development of finite and asymptotic results, both analytically and using empirical studies. In Sect. 6.5, the practical value of the model is illustrated with two real data scenarios. A discussion of miscellaneous properties is given in Sect. 6.6 along with the concluding remarks.

6.2 R-Symmetry and the M-Gaussian Distribution

Reciprocal symmetry is to non-negative random variables as symmetry is to real-valued random variables. It encompasses the relatively well-known log-symmetry property: a random variable X is log-symmetric if $\log X$ is symmetric. More recently, however, Mudholkar and Wang [18] introduced another type of reciprocal symmetry, which they termed R-symmetry, that describes an equality involving the density function of non-negative distributions. Specifically, a random variable is R-symmetric about an R-center θ if

$$f(x) = f\left(\theta^2/x\right) \quad \text{or} \quad f(x/\theta) = f(\theta/x), \quad \theta \geq 0. \tag{6.3}$$

The class of R-symmetric distributions includes both unimodal and multimodal densities; if $f(x)$ is unimodal, however, then θ is the unique mode parameter. Thus the mode, which connotes the most likely value and has the highest probability content neighborhoods, is also the natural centrality parameter of the unimodal R-symmetric distributions.

The relationships between unimodality, symmetry, and convolutions have been studied by a number of prominent statisticians and mathematicians including Khintchine [15] and Wintner [28], whose contributions are well known. A more comprehensive discussion of these results as well as analogous developments in the context of R-symmetry can be found in Chaubey et al. [6] and Mudholkar and Wang [19]. Jones [12, 13] and Jones and Arnold [14] discuss the relationships between symmetry, R-symmetry and log-symmetry, and present distributions that exhibit both types of reciprocal symmetries, including the log-normal and its powers, which they refer to as *doubly symmetric* distributions.

Moment Relationship. [18] show that if a random variable $X \geq 0$ is R-symmetric about $\theta > 0$, then the following moment relationship holds true:

$$\mathbb{E}\left[\left(\frac{X}{\theta}\right)^{r}\right] = \mathbb{E}\left[\left(\frac{X}{\theta}\right)^{-(r+2)}\right], \quad r \in \mathbb{R}. \tag{6.4}$$

This is analogous to the vanishing odd-ordered central moments of symmetric distributions, including the normal family. In practical terms, the relationship in (6.4) provides a simple path to mode estimation (see Sect. 4.1) and, hence, R-symmetry holds promise of a mode-based inference regime.

M-Gaussian Distribution. Among the class of R-symmetric distributions, the M-Gaussian distribution is pivotal and, in the context of mode-based inference, it shares many similarities with the Gaussian model in terms of properties and methodology surrounding the mean. The M-Gaussian is defined by its density given in (6.2), where $\mu = (EX^{-2})^{-1/2}$ is the mode and $\sigma^2 = EX^2 - (EX^{-2})^{-1}$ is the harmonic variance.

The parallels between the M-Gaussian and Gaussian distributions, which provides a convenient framework for modeling right-skewed, unimodal, and non-negative data, may be due to the intrinsic links of their respective density functions. In particular, the M-Gaussian density may be derived from a Gaussian parent distribution by using either the product method due to Mudholkar and Wang [18] or the more general Cauchy-Schlömilch transformation described in Baker [2]. Mudholkar et al. [20] provide many inferential similarities between the Gaussian and M-Gaussian distributions, which they term *G-MG analogies*, including methods for testing equality of one, two, or k modes that also involve Student's t and F distributions.

The M-Gaussian distribution is also related to the well-known Inverse Gaussian (IG) distribution, where if $Y \sim IG(\nu, \lambda)$, then $X = 1/\sqrt{Y}$ is $MG(\nu^{-2}, \lambda^{-1})$. The IG distributions, which originated from the studies of Brownian motion, has seen increased popularity in practical applications since its introduction to the statistical literature through the works of [9, 26], and many others; for a comprehensive anthology, we refer to the monographs by [21, 22]. As a result of this one-to-one correspondence between the M-Gaussian and IG distributions, the former inherits many of the established inference methods of the IG family, particularly those analogous to the normal paradigm. However, these similarities are more striking and intuitive in the M-Gaussian framework where the parameter of interest is the mode because of the physical transparency and clarity of R-symmetry; a detailed discussion of the relationship between IG and its root reciprocal distribution is provided in Awadalla [1].

6.3 The Power M-Gaussian Distribution

The M-Gaussian distribution with mode μ and dispersion parameter σ^2 plays a central role in the class of R-symmetric distributions. In this section, we present the *Power M-Gaussian distribution* (P-MG(μ, σ^2, θ)), which generalizes the M-Gaussian distribution while retaining the R-symmetry property. As such, the P-MG family, which has a wide range of density shapes, may better accommodate the disparate class of right-skewed data while still exploiting the mode as the focal point of inferential methods.

The development of the P-MG distribution is in part based on Baker's [2] application of the Cauchy-Schlömilch transformation on a special case of the power exponential density given in (6.1), assuming $\mu = 0$ and $\alpha = 1$, to obtain:

$$f(x; b, c, \theta) = \frac{c\theta}{2\,\Gamma(1/\theta)} \exp\left\{-\frac{1}{2}|cx - b/cx|^{\theta}\right\} 1_{\{x \geq 0\}}, \quad b \geq 0\,, c > 0,\ \theta > 0. \tag{6.5}$$

This results in a generalization of the MG(μ, σ^2) distribution, which corresponds to the particular case $\theta = 2$, $b = \mu^2/\sigma^2$, $c = 1/\sigma^2$. Baker also showed that distributions obtained in this manner have many desirable properties and relations with the parent distributions. However, unlike the M-Gaussian, this generalization cannot be easily transformed to obtain the Generalized Inverse Gaussian (GIG) distribution.

Now we present an alternative R-symmetric analog of the exponential-power distribution obtained through the product method used by [18]. Specifically, applying the product method to θ-N$(0, 1, \theta)$ in (6.1) yields the density kernel

$$f(x) \propto \exp\left\{-\left(x^{\theta} + x^{-\theta}\right)\right\} 1_{\{x \geq 0\}}, \quad \theta > 0. \tag{6.6}$$

That the integral $\int_0^\infty f(x)dx$ is finite follows from the property of the modified Bessel function of the second kind discussed in [27]; see also [11]. This leads to the Power M-Gaussian distribution (P-MG) defined below.

Definition 6.1 A random variable X is said to be P-MG(μ, σ^2, θ) distributed if its PDF is

$$f(x;\mu,\sigma,\theta) = \frac{\theta}{2\mu K_{1/\theta}\left(1/\sigma^2\right)} \exp\left\{-\frac{1}{2\sigma^2}\left((\mu/x)^\theta + (x/\mu)^\theta\right)\right\} 1_{\{x\geq 0\}}, \quad \mu > 0,\ \sigma > 0,\ \theta > 0, \tag{6.7}$$

where $K_\gamma(\cdot)$ is the modified Bessel function of the second kind.

Alternative parameterizations of the P-MG(μ, σ^2, θ) distribution may also be considered in order to facilitate different applications. For instance, the density given above may be expressed as

$$f_X(x;\chi,\psi,\theta) = \frac{\theta\chi^{1/2\theta}}{2\psi^{1/2\theta} K_{1/\theta}(\sqrt{\psi\chi})} \exp\left\{-\frac{1}{2}\left(\chi x^\theta + \psi x^{-\theta}\right)\right\} 1_{\{x\geq 0\}}, \quad \chi > 0,\ \psi > 0,\ \theta > 0, \tag{6.8}$$

where $\mu = (\psi/\chi)^{1/2\theta}$ and $\sigma^2 = 1/\sqrt{\chi\psi}$. This parameterization is convenient in the simulation study presented in Sect. 4.3 since it directly relates to the more well-established GIG distribution for which software packages exists. In particular, if $Y \sim$ GIG(χ, ψ, θ) with density

$$f_Y(y;\chi,\psi,\theta) = \frac{\chi^{1/2\theta}}{2\psi^{1/2\theta} K_{1/\theta}(\sqrt{\psi\chi})} y^{1/\theta-1} \exp\left\{-\frac{1}{2}\left(\chi y + \frac{\psi}{y}\right)\right\} 1_{\{y\geq 0\}}, \quad \chi > 0,\ \psi > 0,\ \theta > 0, \tag{6.9}$$

then $X = Y^{1/\theta} \sim$ P-MG(χ, ψ, θ) with PDF given in (6.8). However, the primary appeal of the density form given in (6.7) is that the mode is naturally represented by μ and it is not confounded within the Bessel function, making it easier to derive an estimator for it. Furthermore, as will be shown later, parametric functions such as skewness and kurtosis are location-free using the parametrization in (6.7).

Proposition 6.1 *If $X \sim$ P-MG(μ, σ^2, θ) with PDF given by (6.7) then (i) X is R-symmetric about μ, and (ii) μ is the population mode.*

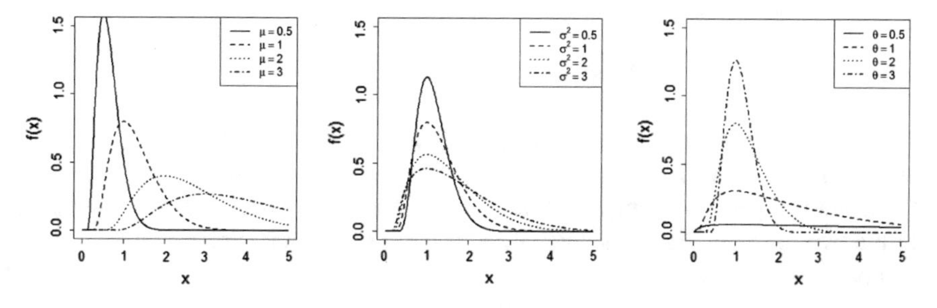

Fig. 6.1 Density functions of P-MG(μ, σ^2, θ) for different values of μ, σ^2 and θ

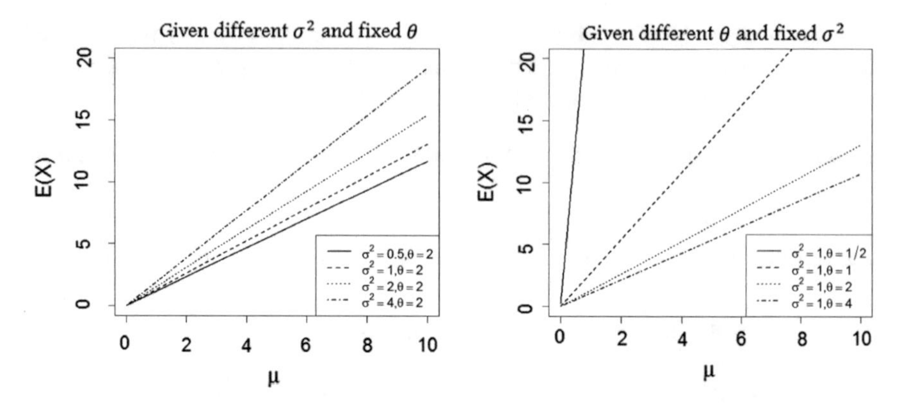

Fig. 6.2 Expectation of P-MG(μ, σ^2, θ) as a function of σ^2, μ and θ

Proof (i) Substituting μ^2/x for x in (6.7) we get $f(\mu^2/x) = f(x)$. (ii) Based on the derivatives of $f(x)$ given in (6.7) with respect to x, it is easy to show analytically that $x = \mu$ is the solution of $f'(x) = 0$ and $f''(\mu) < 0$.

The P-MG(μ, σ^2, θ) distribution, which is R-symmetric for all values of μ, σ^2 and θ in the parameter domain, has a wide range of density shapes. Figure 6.1, which illustrates a selection of parameter combinations, clarifies the role of μ as the centrality parameter, σ^2 as the dispersion parameter and θ as the kurtosis parameter.

We concern the remainder of this section with the basic moment properties of the Power M-Gaussian distribution.

Moment Properties. If $X \sim$ P-MG(μ, σ^2, θ) then the r-th raw moment, $r = 1, 2, \ldots$, is given by

$$\mu_r' = \mathbb{E}\left(X^r\right) = \frac{\mu^r K_{(1+r)/\theta}(\sigma^{-2})}{K_{1/\theta}(\sigma^{-2})}, \tag{6.10}$$

and, based on (6.4), we have that $\mu_{-r}' = \mathbb{E}\left(X^{-r}\right) = \mu_{r-2}'/\mu^{2r-2}$. Hence, the mean is $\mathbb{E}(X) = \mu\ K_{2/\theta}(\sigma^{-2})\big/K_{1/\theta}(\sigma^{-2})$ and $\mathbb{E}(X) \leq \mu$ based on the properties of the Bessel function. Also, given that Bessel functions satisfy $K_\nu(\cdot) = K_{-\nu}(\cdot)$, if we take $r = -2$ in (6.10) we have that $\mathbb{E}X^{-2} = \mu^{-2}$ and

$$\text{Mode}(X) = \mu = (\mathbb{E}X^{-2})^{-1/2}. \tag{6.11}$$

The relationship between mean and mode is illustrated in Fig. 6.2 for different σ^2 and θ values. It can be seen that the relationship between μ_1' and μ is approximately linear with slopes increasing as values of σ^2 increase and θ decrease. A comparison of the two panes in Fig. 6.2 suggests that θ has a more drastic effect on the slopes compared to σ^2.

The next four raw moments of X, $\mu_r' = \mathbb{E}[X^r]$, are given by

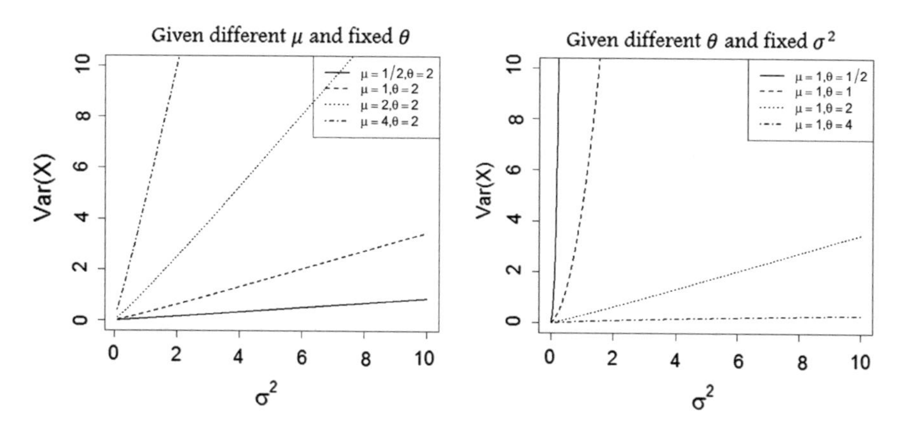

Fig. 6.3 Variance μ_2 of P-MG(μ, σ^2, θ) versus σ^2 for select values of μ and θ

$$\begin{aligned} \mu_2' &= \mu^2 K_{3/\theta}(\sigma^{-2})/K_{1/\theta}(\sigma^{-2}), \\ \mu_3' &= \mu^3 K_{4/\theta}(\sigma^{-2})/K_{1/\theta}(\sigma^{-2}), \\ \mu_4' &= \mu^4 K_{5/\theta}(\sigma^{-2})/K_{1/\theta}(\sigma^{-2}), \\ \mu_5' &= \mu^5 K_{6/\theta}(\sigma^{-2})/K_{1/\theta}(\sigma^{-2}). \end{aligned} \tag{6.12}$$

The variance is given by

$$Var(X) = \frac{\mu^2}{K_{1/\theta}(\sigma^{-2})} \left\{ K_{3/\theta}(\sigma^{-2}) - \frac{K_{2/\theta}(\sigma^{-2})^2}{K_{1/\theta}(\sigma^{-2})} \right\}. \tag{6.13}$$

As in the case of expectation discussed above, in Fig. 6.3 we illustrate the relationship between the population variance in (6.13) and the dispersion parameter σ^2 for a selection of μ and θ values. It can be seen that over the considered range of parameters, as σ^2 increases, the variance also increases. Also, we observe that for fixed σ^2 and θ, $Var(X)$ increases with μ and for fixed σ^2 and μ, $Var(X)$ decreases with θ.

The coefficients of skewness and kurtosis denoted by $\sqrt{\beta_1}$ and β_2, respectively, are given by

$$\sqrt{\beta_1} = \frac{\mu_3' - 3\mu_1'\mu_2' + 2(\mu_1')^3}{\left(\sqrt{Var(X)}\right)^3} \text{ and } \beta_2 = \frac{\mu_4' - 4\mu_1'\mu_3' + 6(\mu_1')^2\mu_2' - 3(\mu_1')^4}{(Var(X))^3}, \tag{6.14}$$

were the raw moments and variance are given in (6.12) and (6.13). In each quantity, the numerator terms have modes raised to the powers of 3 and 4, corresponding to the power of the mode in the denominator. As a result, both skewness and kurtosis are location-free parameters in the sense that they are not affected by the values of μ.

The behaviors of $\sqrt{\beta_1}$ and β_2 with respect to different values of σ^2 and θ are illustrated in Fig. 6.4, from which we observe that $\sqrt{\beta_1}$ is a monotonically increasing

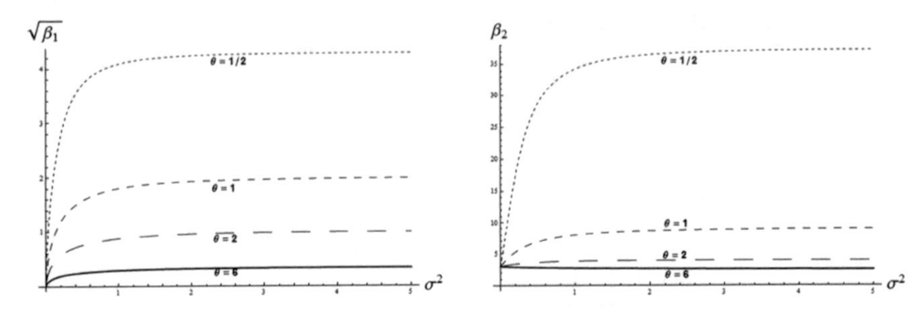

Fig. 6.4 The coefficients of skewness (left) and kurtosis (right) of P-MG(μ, σ^2, θ) as functions of σ^2 and θ values

function of σ^2 and also decreasing with respect to θ. The relationship between the coefficient of kurtosis and θ is more pronounced. We can observe that for $\theta = 1/2, 1, 2$, β_2 is monotonically increasing as σ^2 increases, much in the same way as $\sqrt{\beta_1}$. However, for $\theta = 6$ the kurtosis measure decreases with σ^2. The impact of θ on β_2 is not unexpected: as $\theta \to 2$, kurtosis converges to 0 for all σ^2; as θ increases (or decreases), then kurtosis increases (decreases) with increasing σ^2.

6.4 Estimation

In this section, the method of moment and maximum likelihood estimators of the mode μ and dispersion parameter σ^2 of the P-MG(μ, σ^2, θ) distribution, and their properties are studied analytically and empirically. The parameter θ, however, cannot be readily estimated in the same way and its MLE is considered later. These estimation procedures are used to estimate the parameters μ, σ^2 and θ in different scenarios and their performances are evaluated in an expansive simulation study. For the specified purposes of this section, let $x_1, x_2, \ldots, x_n$ be a random sample from a P-MG(μ, σ^2, θ) population with PDF given in (6.7).

6.4.1 *Moment-Method Estimation*

In this section, we provide method of moment estimators of the mode μ and dispersion parameter σ^2, given that the value of θ is already known.

Estimation of μ. By taking $r = 0$ in (6.4) and replacing the population moments with its sample counterparts can we obtain a simple moment estimator of the population mode μ as follow:

$$\bar{\mu} = \left(\frac{n}{\sum_{i=1}^{n} x_i^{-2}} \right)^{\frac{1}{2}}. \tag{6.15}$$

Remark 6.2 In the case of the M-Gaussian distribution, the moment estimator of μ also coincides with its MLE.

The asymptotic distribution of $\bar{\mu}$ in (6.15) for an arbitrary R-symmetric population is considered in the following theorem.

Theorem 6.1 *If $\mathbb{E}(X^r) < \infty$ for $r = \pm 2$, then we have, as $n \to \infty$,*

$$\sqrt{n}\ (\bar{\mu} - \mu) \to_d N\left(0, \frac{1}{4\tau^2}\right), \tag{6.16}$$

where $\bar{\mu}$ is defined in (6.15) and $\tau^2 = \mathbb{E}(X^2) - 1/\mathbb{E}(X^{-2})$.

Proof Using the Central Limit Theorem and Mann-Wald (delta) method, it follows that

$$\sqrt{n}(\bar{\mu} - \mu) \to_d N\left(0, \frac{Var(X^{-2})}{4(\mathbb{E}X^{-2})^3}\right). \tag{6.17}$$

Because X is an R-symmetric random variable, from (6.4) we have $\theta^{-6}\mathbb{E}X^2 = \mathbb{E}X^{-4}$ and consequently

$$\frac{Var(X^{-2})}{4(\mathbb{E}X^{-2})^3} = \frac{\mathbb{E}X^{-4} - (\mathbb{E}X^{-2})^2}{4(\mathbb{E}X^{-2})^3} = \frac{\mathbb{E}X^2\theta^{-6} - \theta^{-4}}{4\theta^{-6}} = \frac{\tau^2}{4}. \tag{6.18}$$

Thus, the moment estimator $\bar{\mu}$ is a consistent estimator of μ and its large sample result may be used in hypothesis testing procedures involving the mode.

Estimation of σ^2. A class of moment estimators of dispersion parameter σ^2 can be derived using the recurrence relationship of modified Bessel functions of the second kind:

$$K_{\nu-1}(\lambda) - K_{\nu+1}(\lambda) = -2\nu\lambda^{-1}K_\nu(\lambda), \quad \nu \in \mathbb{R}, \lambda \neq 0. \tag{6.19}$$

The above relationship is considered by [22] in the context of deriving moment recurrences of Inverse Gaussian populations. In this aspect of the section, we use (6.19) to derive a relationship between σ^2 and moments of P-MG(μ, σ^2, θ).

Theorem 6.2 *If $X \sim$ P-MG(μ, σ^2, θ), we have:*

$$\sigma^2 = -\frac{\theta}{2(r+1)\mu'_r} \left(\mu^\theta \mu'_{r-\theta} - \mu^{-\theta}\mu'_{r+\theta}\right), \quad r = 1, 2, 3 \ldots, \tag{6.20}$$

with $\mu'_r = \mathbb{E}(X^r)$.

Proof Let $\nu = (r+1)/\theta$, $\lambda = 1/\sigma^2$ and multiply (6.19) by $\mu^r / K_{1/\theta}(\sigma^{-2})$ to get

$$\frac{\mu^\theta\ \mu^{r-\theta}\ K_{(r-\theta+1)/\theta}(\sigma^{-2})}{K_{1/\theta}(\sigma^{-2})} - \frac{\mu^{r+\theta}\ K_{(r+\theta+1)/\theta}(\sigma^{-2})}{\mu^\theta\ K_{1/\theta}(\sigma^{-2})} = -\frac{2(r+1)\sigma^2}{\theta}\frac{\mu^r\ K_{(r+1)/\theta}(\sigma^{-2})}{K_{1/\theta}(\sigma^{-2})}. \tag{6.21}$$

Given that

$$\mu'_r = \mu^r\ K_{(r+1)/\theta}(\sigma^{-2}) / K_{1/\theta}(\sigma^{-2}),$$

Equation (6.21) reduces to the moment relationship

$$\mu'_r = -\frac{\theta}{2\sigma^2(r+1)}\left(\mu^\theta \mu'_{r-\theta} - \mu^\theta \mu'_{r+\theta}\right), \tag{6.22}$$

where the parameter μ is the mode. A simple algebraic manipulation completes the proof.

Hence, by taking $r = 0$ in (6.20) we get the simple relationship

$$\sigma^2 = -\frac{\theta}{2}\left(\mu^\theta \mu'_{-\theta} - \mu^{-\theta}\mu'_\theta\right), \tag{6.23}$$

which leads to the following moment estimator of σ^2 for known θ,

$$V = -\frac{\theta}{2}\left(\bar{\mu}^\theta m'_{-\theta} - \bar{\mu}^{-\theta} m'_\theta\right), \tag{6.24}$$

which is obtained by replacing the population moment in (6.23) by its sample counterparts.

The estimation of θ, which cannot be obtained in closed form using similar mechanic, will be considered in the next section.

6.4.2 Maximum Likelihood Estimation

Method of moment estimators of μ and σ^2 when θ is known have been discussed in Sect. 4.1. However, it is desirable to consider the maximum likelihood estimation because of its associated properties such as its asymptotic efficiency and consistency.

Let $x_1, x_2, \ldots, x_n$ be a random sample from P-MG(μ, σ^2, θ), then the log-likelihood function is given by

$$L(\mu, \sigma, \theta) = n\left\{\log\theta - \log 2 - \log\left(K_{1/\theta}(\sigma^{-2})\right) - \log\mu\right\} - \frac{1}{2\sigma^2\mu^\theta}\sum_{i=1}^n x_i^\theta - \frac{\mu^\theta}{2\sigma^2}\sum_{i=1}^n x_i^{-\theta}. \tag{6.25}$$

The MLEs, denoted as $\hat{\mu}$, $\hat{\sigma}^2$ and $\hat{\theta}$, of the respective parameters μ, σ^2, and θ, can be obtained by maximizing the log-likelihood in (6.25) for the following scenarios:

Case I: MLE of μ when (σ^2, θ) known. A closed form MLE $\hat{\mu}$ can be obtained by maximizing the log-likelihood in (6.25) when (θ, σ^2) are assumed to be known and fixed. Specifically it is given by

$$\hat{\mu} = \left(\frac{\sqrt{n^2\sigma^4 + \theta^2 \left(\sum_{i=1}^n x_i^{\theta}\right) \left(\sum_{i=1}^n x_i^{-\theta}\right)} - n\sigma^2}{\theta \sum_{i=1}^n x_i^{-\theta}} \right)^{1/\theta}. \quad (6.26)$$

Case II: MLE of (μ, σ^2) when θ known. Closed form expressions other than for **Case I** are not readily available, and thus we employ a numerical maximization of the log-likelihood equation. Specially, the maximization procedure used is the quasi Newton-Raphson method described independently by [5, 8, 10, 23]. The optimization method used, however, is susceptible to the choice of the starting values. In this scenario, starting values of μ and σ^2 can be taken to be their moment estimators $\bar{\mu}$ and V in (6.15) and (6.24), respectively.

Case III: MLE of (μ, σ^2, θ). This case presents the most realistic scenario in a practical sense. As in **Case II**, no closed form expression for the MLEs are available, and thus we employ the quasi Newton-Raphson method described earlier. Here, we tackle the issue of appropriate starting values using the following approach: first, let $\mu_0 = \bar{\mu}$; second, assume $\theta_0 = 2$, which corresponds to the M-Gaussian distribution, and estimate $\sigma_0^2 = V$ according to (6.24). With these values in hand, the log-likelihood in (6.25) is maximized with respect to all the parameters simultaneously. It should be noted that the choice of θ_0 when in the neighborhood of 2 does not appear to substantially impact the estimates in simulation studies; moreover, varying θ_0 has almost no impact on the mode estimate.

6.4.3 A Simulation Experiment

In this section, the performances of the method of moment estimators and maximum likelihood estimators are evaluated using a Monte Carlo experiment with 2000 replications of random samples generated from several Power M-Gaussian populations with different parameters and sample sizes. For each sample, the parameters are estimated using the estimation procedures introduced in Sects. 4.1 and 4.2 and are reported along with their simulation standard errors. Specifically, the simulation experiment concerns the following 4 cases:

i. **Simulation results for method of moment estimators of μ and σ^2 with known θ**. The moment estimators $\bar{\mu}$ and V defined in (6.15) and (6.24), respectively, of μ and σ^2 are evaluated empirically for various combinations of the parameters of P-MG(μ, σ^2, θ) and sample sizes $n = 10, 20, 30, 50$ by a Monte Carlo experiment of 2000 replications. A selection of results of the simulation are displayed in Table 6.1. The results show that the method of moment estimators exhibit relatively minor upward biases for μ and downward biases for σ^2. The

Table 6.1 Method of moment estimators of the mode and dispersion of P-MG(μ, σ^2, θ) given in (6.15) and (6.24) for known θ; 2000 Monte Carlo replications

n	P-MG(1, 1, 1)				P-MG(1, 2, 2)				P-MG(2, 2, 4)			
	$\hat{\mu}$	s.e.	V	s.e.	$\hat{\mu}$	s.e.	$\hat{\sigma}^2$	s.e.	$\hat{\mu}$	s.e.	$\hat{\sigma}^2$	s.e.
10	1.27	0.07	0.807	0.10	1.08	0.02	1.80	0.50	2.03	0.01	1.87	0.51
20	1.15	0.03	0.89	0.04	1.04	0.01	1.90	0.16	2.02	0.004	1.95	0.18
30	1.11	0.01	0.92	0.024	1.03	0.003	1.93	0.09	2.01	0.002	1.98	0.10
50	1.07	0.006	0.96	0.01	1.02	0.001	1.97	0.04	2.01	0.00	1.99	0.04

variance of the estimator decreases with respect to n and is relatively small. The relatively small biases and variability justify their use as starting points in the other cases below.

ii. **Simulation results for MLE of μ with known (σ^2, θ).** Table 6.2 contains results of a simulation study aimed at evaluating the MLE of μ given fixed values of σ^2 and θ. The details of the experiment are similar to those described in **Case I**. From the results it seems that $\hat{\mu}$ exhibits small downward bias and is also more efficient.

iii. **Simulation results for MLE** of **μ and σ^2 with known θ**. When θ is known, the simulation result aimed at evaluating the MLE of μ and σ^2 are displayed in Table 6.3. If we compare this result with those displayed in Table 6.1, we can reasonably conclude that the results of MLE are fairly better than the method of moment estimators of μ and σ^2 for the case θ is known.

iv. **Simulation results for MLE of μ, σ^2, *and* θ**. The results displayed in Table 6.4 show that for both distributions examined, the mode estimates are reasonable and comparable to mode estimates when the harmonic variance or shape parameter are known. This result is reassuring because it suggests that even though we are dealing with a three-dimensional optimization problem, the mode estimation process, which is of primary interest, is not compromised. We also observe that estimates of both σ^2 and θ are within 10% of the target parameter. Additionally, we used the *Jackknife* procedure to estimate the standard error of $\hat{\theta}$ and, consequently, its asymptotic confidence interval. Using this result, we show that coverage probability of the $\hat{\theta}$ is reasonable even for a moderate sample size. However, we do note that as θ approaches 1, the coverage probability is less than desirable.

Table 6.2 Performance of the maximum likelihood estimator of mode given in (6.26) with known σ^2 and θ; 2000 Monte Carlo replications

n	P-MG(1, 1, 1)		P-MG(1, 2, 2)		P-MG(2, 2, 4)	
	$\hat{\mu}$	s.e.	$\hat{\mu}$	s.e.	$\hat{\mu}$	s.e.
10	1.03	0.07	1.00	0.03	2.00	0.03
20	1.02	0.03	1.00	0.01	2.00	0.01
30	1.02	0.02	1.00	0.01	2.00	0.01
50	1.01	0.01	1.00	0.01	2.00	0.01

Table 6.3 The performance of the maximum likelihood estimators $\hat{\mu}$, $\hat{\sigma}^2$ with known θ; 2000 Monte Carlo replications

n	P-MG(1, 1, 1)				P-MG(1, 2, 2)				P-MG(2, 2, 4)			
	$\hat{\mu}$	s.e.	V	s.e.	$\hat{\mu}$	s.e.	$\hat{\sigma}^2$	s.e.	$\hat{\mu}$	s.e.	$\hat{\sigma}^2$	s.e.
10	1.20	0.01	0.99	0.03	1.08	0.01	1.79	0.03	2.04	0.00	1.77	0.02
20	1.10	0.01	1.00	0.01	1.04	0.00	1.90	0.02	2.02	0.00	1.89	0.02
30	1.07	0.01	1.00	0.01	1.03	0.00	1.93	0.02	2.01	0.00	1.92	0.01
50	1.03	0.00	1.02	0.01	1.02	0.00	1.97	0.01	2.01	0.00	1.96	0.01

Table 6.4 The mean, bias, and standard error of the maximum likelihood estimators $\hat{\mu}$, $\hat{\sigma}^2$ and $\hat{\theta}$ of the P-MG(μ, σ^2, θ) distribution based on 2000 Monte Carlo replications. Coverage probabilities of the jackknife confidence interval of θ is given

n	$\hat{\mu}$	s.e.	Bias	$\hat{\sigma}^2$	s.e.	Bias	$\hat{\theta}$	s.e.	Bias	Coverage P
P-MG(1, 1, 1)										
10	1.19	0.51	0.19	1.59	0.24	0.24	1.39	0.55	0.39	0.876
20	1.09	0.35	0.09	1.53	0.18	0.53	1.24	0.38	0.24	0.849
30	1.04	0.28	0.04	1.51	0.15	0.51	1.19	0.34	0.19	0.830
50	1.00	0.21	0.00	1.49	0.12	0.49	1.14	0.29	0.14	0.814
P-MG(1, 2, 2)										
10	1.08	0.23	0.08	1.92	0.13	0.08	2.35	0.66	0.35	0.922
20	1.04	0.16	0.04	1.89	0.09	0.11	2.12	0.37	0.12	0.939
30	1.03	0.14	0.03	1.88	0.08	0.12	2.07	0.30	0.07	0.928
50	1.02	0.10	0.02	1.86	0.06	0.14	2.01	0.22	0.01	0.925
P-MG(2, 2, 4)										
10	2.03	0.19	0.03	2.14	0.06	0.14	4.75	1.23	0.75	0.910
20	2.02	0.13	0.02	2.12	0.04	0.12	4.40	0.70	0.40	0.909
30	2.02	0.11	0.02	2.11	0.04	0.11	4.28	0.52	0.28	0.923
50	2.01	0.08	0.01	2.10	0.03	0.10	4.16	0.39	0.16	0.931

Table 6.5 The CEO salaries, mercury level and calcium level data used for the practical illustration of Power M-Gaussian models

Name of the data set	Data
Mercury level (parts per million)	0.01 0.06 0.11 0.12 0.13 0.14 0.15 0.15 0.15 0.17 0.21 0.23 0.23 0.23 0.24 0.30 0.30 0.30 0.30 0.36 0.37 0.39 0.40 0.44 0.44 0.45 0.45 0.46 0.46 0.48 0.52 0.52 0.55 0.59 0.61 0.67 0.69 0.73 0.77 0.79 0.80 0.82 0.83 0.90 0.94 1.04 1.06 1.12 1.16 1.19 1.29
Calcium level (mg/l)	0.5 0.6 0.8 0.9 1.0 1.4 1.6 1.7 1.8 1.9 1.9 1.9 2.2 2.2 2.6 2.9 3.4 3.5 4.1 4.1 5.2 5.2 7.7 8.1 9.1 9.6 11.5 12.0 12.7 12.8 13.9 14.8 15.3 19.4 19.4 22.5 23.1 24.1 24.9 34.5 37.3 40.1 44.4 44.5 54.1 56.3 57.5 65.4 71.5 84.4 85.4 89.6

6.5 Applications to Real Data

In order to assess the applicability of the Power M-Gaussian distribution, we considered two real data sets that represent different ends of the tail-length (kurtosis) spectrum. The data for which the results are: (i) the mercury levels of sea bass; (ii) the calcium levels of certain lakes. The full data are presented in Table 6.5.

Here, we model these data using the M-Gaussian, the Power M-Gaussian, and the log-normal distributions, and compare the performances of the three models. In the cases of the Power M-Gaussian distribution, we use the simulation method discuss when all three parameters are assumed unknown. For the M-Gaussian, we use the MLE's described in [20], which yielded similar values to the MLE when $\theta = 2$ is known, which was described in the previous section. The results are discussed below.

6.5.1 *Results: Mercury and Calcium Levels from the Sea Bass Study*

A study of largemouth bass in 53 different Florida lakes is conducted by [16] in order to examine factors that may influence the level of mercury contamination in the fish. The collected water samples were from the surface of the middle of each lake in August, 1990 and then again in March, 1991. For each lake, the pH levels, amount of chlorophyll, alkalinity, and calcium were recorded. Then, they sampled bass fish from each lake and proceeded to measure the age and mercury concentration in the muscle tissue. In this illustration, we consider the average mercury levels of the fish and the calcium levels of the lakes as two univariate data sets. For each sample, the necessary parameters for the M-Gaussian, Power M-Gaussian, and log-normal families are estimated to obtain model fits (Figs. 6.5 and 6.6).

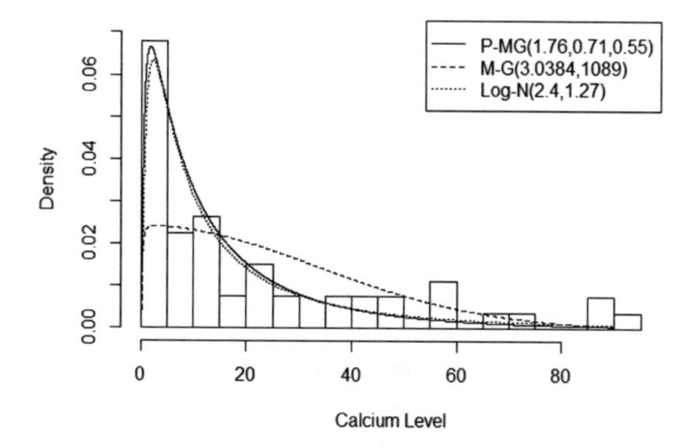

Fig. 6.5 The Power M-Gaussian, M-Gaussian, and log-normal models are fit to the calcium data described in Table 6.5; kurtosis = 0.613

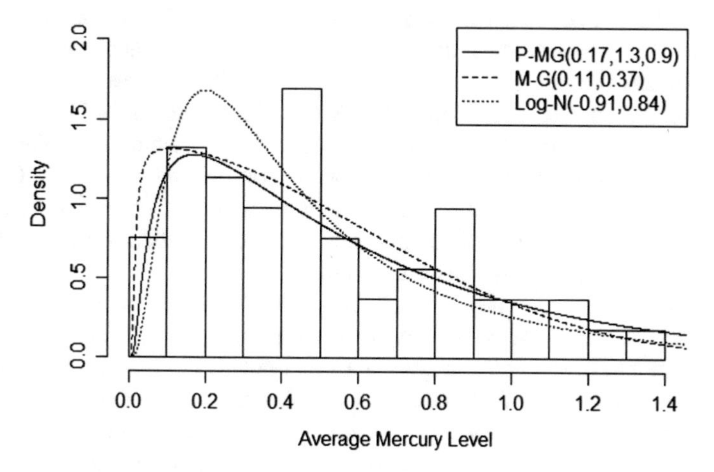

Fig. 6.6 The Power M-Gaussian, M-Gaussian, and log-normal models are fit to the mercury data described in Table 6.5; kurtosis = −0.631

The results of the fits to the mercury level data as well as the calcium level data are illustrated in Table 6.5. In the case of the mercury level, which demonstrates a heavy tail distribution (excess kurtosis = −0.631), the limitations of the M-Gaussian and log-normal are visible at the right-tail. We can see that for both these distributions the extreme value probabilities are under-estimated. On the other hand, the calcium data suggests that the two-parameter M-Gaussian is not ideal for light-tailed distributions (kurtosis = 0.613). In both cases, however, the Power M-Gaussian provides reasonable flexibility to accommodate fluctuations in tail lengths.

When focusing on the region around the modes, both data results show that modal estimates are relatively similar between all three distributions. However, the M-Gaussian underestimates the mode, and more so in the calcium data. However, it should be noted that in both cases $\theta \neq 0$, suggesting that M-Gaussian may not be ideal.

6.6 Conclusion

Unlike the distributions used for modeling the commonly encountered non-negative and right-skewed data, for example, Gamma, log-normal, Weibull, and Inverse Gaussian distributions, the R-symmetric M-Gaussian distribution is sometimes a more preferable model especially because it offers a systematic path to inferences regarding the mode of right-skewed population. The M-Gaussian distribution is also analytically convenient because it shares many similarities with the ubiquitous Gaussian distribution in terms of the mathematical properties and inference methodologies. In this paper, we present a generalization of the M-Gaussian distribution, namely the Power M-Gaussian distribution, by adding a kurtosis parameter into the M-Gaussian distribution. This family allows for right tails that are either heavier than M-Gaussian (when $\theta < 2$) or lighter than M-Gaussian (when $\theta > 2$). The density function is derived using the Mudholkar-Wang product method from the PDF of exponential-power distribution. It is also related to the generalized Inverse Gaussian distribution through a one-to-one transformation. Parameter estimations via maximum likelihood and the method of moments have been studied and the usefulness of the model is illustrated by real case studies.

In this paper, the properties and uses of the Power M-Gaussian distribution are only briefly sketched. Besides the practical benefits of the new distribution that can be fitted to the right-skewed non-negative data, other potentially important applications are in order. There's a natural need of developing the multivariate version of the model as well as the extensions to the cases, where the data indicate only a near M-Gaussian population or a M-Gaussian population shifted by a nonzero real left threshold parameter.

References

1. Awadalla, S.S. 2012. *Some contributions to the theory and applications of R-symmetry*. Ph.D. thesis, Department of Computational Biology, University of Rochester, Rochester, NY, USA.
2. Baker, R. 2008. Probabilistic applications of the Schlömilch transformation. *Communications in Statistics - Theory and Methods*. 37: 2162–2176.
3. Box, G.E.P. 1953. A note on regions for tests of kurtosis. *Biometrika* 40: 465–468.
4. Box, G.E.P., G.C. Tiao. 1973. *Bayesian inference in statistical analysis*. Wiley Online Library.
5. Broyden, C.G. 1970. The convergence of a class of double-rank minimization algorithms 1. general considerations. *IMA Journal of Applied Mathematics* 6: 76–90.
6. Chaubey, Y.P., G.S. Mudholkar, and M.C. Jones. 2010. Reciprocal symmetry, unimodality and Khintchine's theorem. *Proceedings of the Royal Society of London A* 466: 2079–2096.
7. Dianandа, P.H. 1949. Note on some properties of maximum likelihood estimates. *Mathematical Proceedings of the Cambridge Philosophical Society* 45: 536–544.

8. Fletcher, R. 1970. A new approach to variable metric algorithms. *The Computer Journal* 13: 317–322.
9. Folks, J.L., and R.S. Chhikara. 1978. The inverse Gaussian distribution and its statistical application—a review. *Journal of the Royal Statistical Society Series B* 40: 263–289.
10. Goldfarb, D. 1970. A family of variable metric methods derived by variational means. *Mathematics of Computation* 24: 23–26.
11. Gradshtein, I.S., I.M. Ryzhik. 2007. *Table of integrals, series and products*, 7th ed. Academic Press.
12. Jones, M.C. 2010. Distributions generated by transformations of scale using an extended Schlomilch transformation. *Sankhya A: The Indian Journal of Statistics* 72: 359–375.
13. Jones, M.C. 2012. Relationships between distributions with certain symmetries. *Statistical and Probability Letters* 82: 1737–1744.
14. Jones, M.C., and B.C. Arnold. 2012. Distributions that are both log-symmetric and R-symmetric. *Electronic Journal of Statistics* 2: 1300–1308.
15. Khintchine, A.Y. 1938. On unimodal distributions. *Izvestiya Nauchno-Issledovatel'skogo Instituta Matematiki i Mekhaniki* 2: 1–7.
16. Lange, T.R., H.E. Royals, and L.L. Connor. 1993. Influence of water chemistry on mercury concentration in largemouth bass from Florida lakes. *Transactions of the American Fisheries Society* 122: 74–84.
17. Mineo, A.M., and M. Ruggieri. 2005. A software tool for the exponential power distribution: The normalp package. *Journal of Statistical Software* 12 (4): 1–24.
18. Mudholkar, G.S., and H. Wang. 2007. IG-symmetry and R-symmetry: Interrelations and applications to the inverse Gaussian theory. *Journal of Statistical Planning and Inference* 137: 3655–3671.
19. Mudholkar, G.S., and H. Wang. 2007. Product-Convolution of R-symmetric unimodal distributions: An analogue to Wintner's Theorem. *Journal of Statistical Theory and Practice* 4: 803–811.
20. Mudholkar, G.S., Z. Yu, and S.S. Awadalla. 2015. The mode-centric M-Gaussian distribution: A model for right skewed data. *Statistics & Probability Letters* 107: 1–10.
21. Seshadri, V. 1994. *The Inverse Gaussian distribution: A case study in exponential families*. Oxford University Press.
22. Seshadri, V. 1999. *The inverse Gaussian distribution: Statistical theory and applications*. Springer.
23. Shanno, D.F. 1970. Conditioning of quasi-Newton methods for function minimization. *Mathematics of Computation* 24: 647–656.
24. Subbotin, M.T. 1923. On the law of frequency of error. *Matematicheskii Sbornik* 31 (2): 296–301.
25. Turner, M.E. 1960. 150. Note: On heuristic estimation methods. *Biometrics*. 16: 299–301.
26. Tweedie, M.C.K. 1947. Functions of a statistical variate with given means, with special reference to Laplacian distributions. *Mathematical Proceedings of the Cambridge Philosophical Society* 43: 41–49.
27. Watson, G.N. 1958. *A treatise on the theory of Bessel functions*. Cambridge Press.
28. Wintner, A. 1938. *Asymptotic distributions and infinite convolutions*. Edwards Brothers.

Chapter 7
Stochastic Volatility Models (SVM) in the Analysis of Drought Periods

Jorge Alberto Achcar, Roberto Molina de Souza and Emílio Augusto Coelho-Barros

Abstract In the last few years, very atypical behavior of rain precipitation has been observed globally that may be attributed to climate changes. In this chapter, we approach the analysis of rain precipitation for a large city in Brazil: Campinas located in the southeast region of Brazil, São Paulo State, considering the time series of SPI (standard precipitation Index) measures (1, 3, 6, and 12-month timescales) ranging from January 01, 1947 to May 01, 2011. The present authors have previously used nonhomogeneous Poisson process approach (Achcar et al. Environ Ecol Stat 23:405–419, 2016, [1]) to analyze this data set. However, the analysis in this chapter uses a simpler methodology based on recently introduced SV (stochastic volatility) model (Ghysels, Statistical methods on finance, 1996, [9]) under a Bayesian approach. An excellent fit of the model for the data set is seen that shows some periods of great volatility, confirming atypical behavior for the rain precipitation.

7.1 Introduction

With the meteorological changes observed throughout the world, rainfall indices indicate places with large amounts of rain, as well as places with great periods of drought. In Brazil, large amounts of rainfall can be observed in the extreme regions of the country, in the South and in the North, where part of the Amazon Forest is located, while the regions of great drought are the central and northeastern regions of the country. There are two popular indices used to monitor droughts. The first one is the usual Palmer Drought Severity Index (PDSI). This index is a measure of dryness based on recent precipitation and temperature [19]. The other index known

J. A. Achcar (✉)
Medical School, University of São Paulo, Ribeirão Preto, SP, Brazil
e-mail: achcar@fmrp.usp.br

J. A. Achcar
Department of Social Medicine, FMRP University of São Paulo,
Av. Bandeirantes 3900, Monte Alegre Ribeirão Preto, SP 14049-900, Brazil

R. Molina de Souza · E. A. Coelho-Barros
Federal Technological University of Paraná, Cornélio Procópio, PR, Brazil

A. Adhikari et al. (eds.), *Mathematical and Statistical Applications in Life Sciences and Engineering*, https://doi.org/10.1007/978-981-10-5370-2_7

as the Standardized Precipitation Index (SPI) has been recently introduced in the literature by [16, 17] that has been extensively used as a good alternative to monitor droughts. This index can also be used for rainy periods, but it is not a forecasting tool of droughts. Some climatologists have used this index to evaluate periods of drought (see, for example, [4, 12, 15]).

Considering some climatic factors, [16] originally calculated the SPI for 3, 6, 12, 24, and 48-month timescales. The calculation of the SPI index is performed using the cumulative probability of a precipitation that occurs in a climatic season. An asymmetric distribution (gamma distribution, for example) is then used, estimating its parameters from maximum likelihood methods [6]. Therefore, the probability of rainfall being less than or equal to the rainfall median is approximately 0.5 for a specific area. Basically, low probability values are related to drought events, while high probability values are related to extremely humid periods.

The SPI index is obtained from a transformation of the obtained cumulative probability into a standard normal random variable Z. The probability that the rainfall is less than or equal to a given rainfall amount will be the same as the probability that the new variate is less than or equal to the corresponding Z value of that rainfall amount. A classification system introduced by McKee et al. [16] (see Table 7.1) is used to define drought intensities obtained from the SPI. They also defined the criteria for a drought event for different timescales.

In this chapter, we focus on the SPI measures (1, 3, 6 and 12-month timescales) for Campinas (Brazil), a large industrial city located in the southeast region of Brazil, São Paulo State, for January 01, 1947 to May 01, 2011. The data set is available at the URL http://www.ciiagro.sp.gov.br/ciiagroonline/Listagens/SPI/LspiLocal.asp.

Figure 7.1 gives the time series plots for the SPI-1, SPI-3, SPI-6 and SPI-12 in Campinas for the period January 01, 1947 to May 01, 2011. From these plots it is observed very atypical values of SPI (less than −2.0) indicating severely dry period from the 600*th* to the 620*th* months that corresponds to the period ranging from December, 1996 to August, 1998.

Table 7.1 SPI values

2.0+	Extremely wet
1.5 to 1.99	Very wet
1.0 to 1.49	Moderately wet
−0.99 to 0.99	Near normal
−1.0 to −1.49	Moderately dry
−1.5 to −1.99	Severely dry
−2 and less	Extremely dry

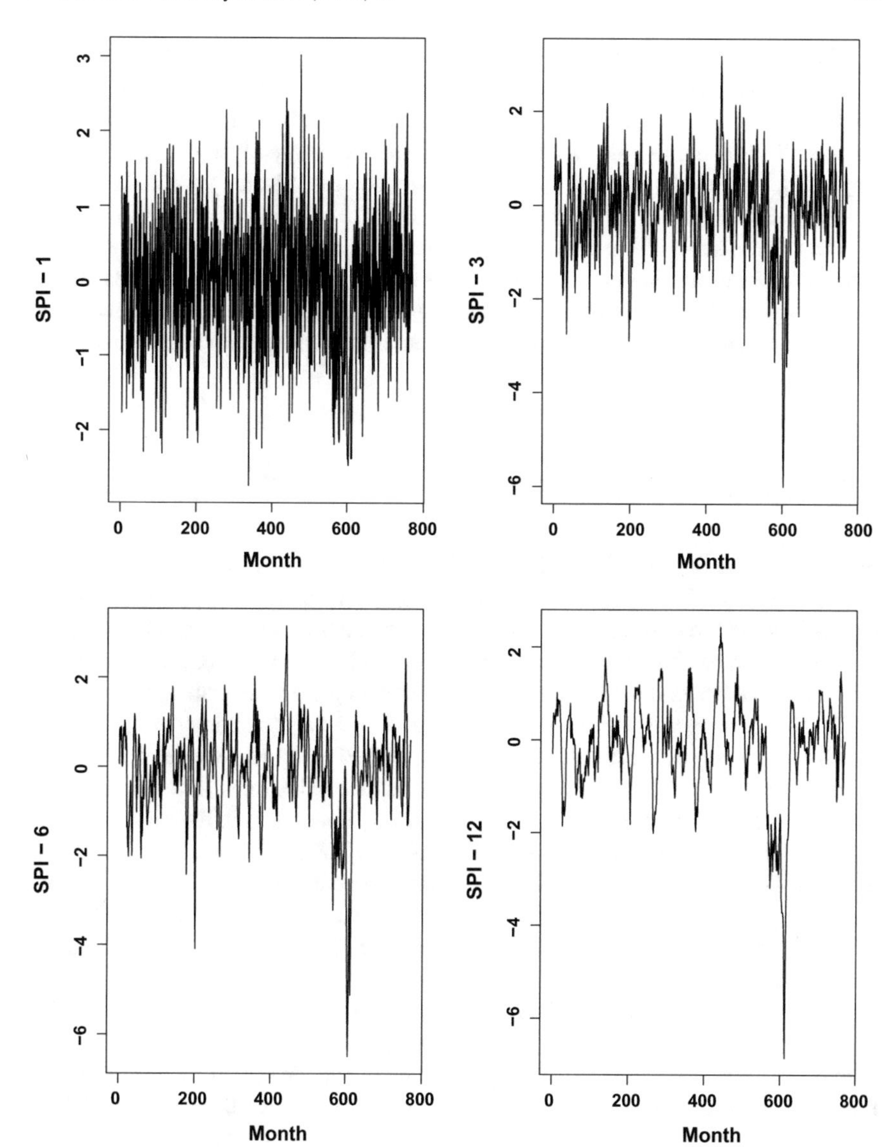

Fig. 7.1 Campinas SPI measures

The present authors have previously used non-homogeneous Poisson process approach (Achcar et al. [1]) to analyze this data set. The analysis in this chapter, however, follows a simpler methodology based on recently introduced SV (stochastic volatility) model [9, 14, 18]. Using a test for ARCH specification introduced by Engle [7], the null hypothesis (no ARCH effects) was rejected ($p < 0.01$) for the four time series (SPI-1, SPI-3, SPI-6, and SPI-12).

The organization of the rest of the chapter is as follows. Section 7.2 introduces stochastic volatility models and Sect. 7.3 presents a Bayesian formulation of this model. Section 7.4 gives the details of the Bayesian analysis for the SPI time series of Campinas and the final Sect. 7.5 presents some concluding remarks and discussion of the results.

7.2 Stochastic Volatility Models

Stochastic volatility models (SVM) have been extensively used to analyze financial time series (see [5]) as a powerful alternative for existing autoregressive models such as ARCH (autoregressive conditional heteroscedastic) introduced by Engle [7] and the generalized autoregressive conditional heteroscedastic (GARCH) models introduced by Bollerslev [3] but rarely used in ecological or climate applications.

For formalizing the setting of the SVM, let $N \geq 1$ be a fixed integer that records the observed data (in our case it will represent the SPI measurements in each month). Also, let $Y_j(t), t = 1, 2, \ldots, N; j = 1, \ldots, K$ indicate the times series recording of the four SPI measurements (1, 3, 6 and 12-month timescales) in the tth month, $t = 1, 2, \ldots, N$. Here $N = 770$ months, $K = 4$, and $Y_1(.)$, $Y_2(.)$, $Y_3(.)$ and $Y_4(.)$ represent $SPI - 1$, $SPI - 3$, $SPI - 6$ and $SPI - 12$ measurements respectively.

In the presence of heteroscedasticity, that is, variances of $Y_j(t)$ depending on the time t, assume that the time series $Y_j(t), t = 1, 2, \ldots, N; j = 1, \ldots, K$, can be written as,

$$Y_j(t) = \sigma_j(t)\, \varepsilon_j(t) \tag{7.1}$$

where $\varepsilon_j(t)$ is a noise considered to be independent and identically distributed with a normal distribution $N\left(0, \sigma_\varepsilon^2\right)$ and $\sigma_j(t)$ is the square root of the variance of (7.1) (as an identification restriction, we will assume $\sigma_\varepsilon = 1$). Observe that we are assuming that $Y_j(t)$ behaves like the square root of its conditional second moment perturbed by a random quantity. We also assume $\sigma_j(t) = \exp\left[h_j(t)\right]$, where $h_j(t)$ is considered to be a latent variable that will be assumed to have an $AR(1)$ structure for the data set considered here as described below: for $t = 1, 2, \ldots, N; j = 1, \ldots, K$, assume

$$h_j(1) = \mu_j + \zeta_j(1), \ t = 1 \tag{7.2}$$
$$h_j(t) = \mu_j + \phi_j\left[h_j(t-1) - \mu_j\right] + \zeta_j(t), t = 2, 3, \ldots, N$$

where $\zeta_j(t)$ is a noise with a Normal distribution $N\left(0, \sigma_{j\zeta}^2\right)$. The quantities $\sigma_{j\zeta}^2$, μ_j and $\phi_j, j = 1, 2, 3, 4$ are unknown parameters that must be estimated.

7.3 A Bayesian Formulation of the Model

In this study, Bayesian methods using Markov chain Monte Carlo (MCMC) methods (see for example, [8] or [21]) are considered to analyze the data-set assuming SVM.

For a Bayesian analysis of the SV model defined in (7.2), let us assume that the prior distributions for the parameters μ_j, ϕ_{vj} and $\sigma_{j\zeta}^2$, $v = 1, 2; j = 1, 2, 3, 4$ are respectively given by, a Normal $N(0, a_j)$ distribution, a Beta(b_j, c_j) distribution and a Gamma(d_j, e_j) distribution, where Beta(b, c) denotes a Beta distribution with mean $\frac{b}{(b+c)}$ and variance $\frac{bc}{[(b+c)^2(b+c+1)]}$ and Gamma(d, e) denotes a Gamma distribution with mean $\frac{d}{e}$ and variance $\frac{d}{e^2}$. The hyperparameters a_j, b_j, c_j, d_j, and e_j are considered to be known and are specified later.

7.4 A Bayesian Analysis of the Campinas SPI Data

Let us assume the model introduced in Sect. 7.2 with all hyperparameters a_j, b_j, c_j, d_j and e_j assumed to be equal to one (approximately non-informative priors).

In Table 7.2, we have the posterior summaries of interest (Monte Carlo estimates of the posterior mean, posterior standard deviation, and 95% credible interval) assuming model defined by (7.1) and (7.2) considering 2,000 generated Gibbs samples. The Gibbs samples were generated using the JAGS software [20] taking every 50th sample to have approximately uncorrelated samples and after a "burn-in-sample" of size 50,000 to eliminate the effect of the initial values of the parameters.

In Fig. 7.2 we have the plots of the square roots of the estimated volatilities for the time series SPI-1, SPI-3, SPI-6, and SPI-12. From these plots, we observe large and atypical volatilities for the period ranging from the 600th to the 620th months which corresponds to the period ranging from December, 1996 to August, 1998. That is, we observe a substantial variability of the SPI measures in this period of 2 years with alarming consequences (indication of a severely dry period).

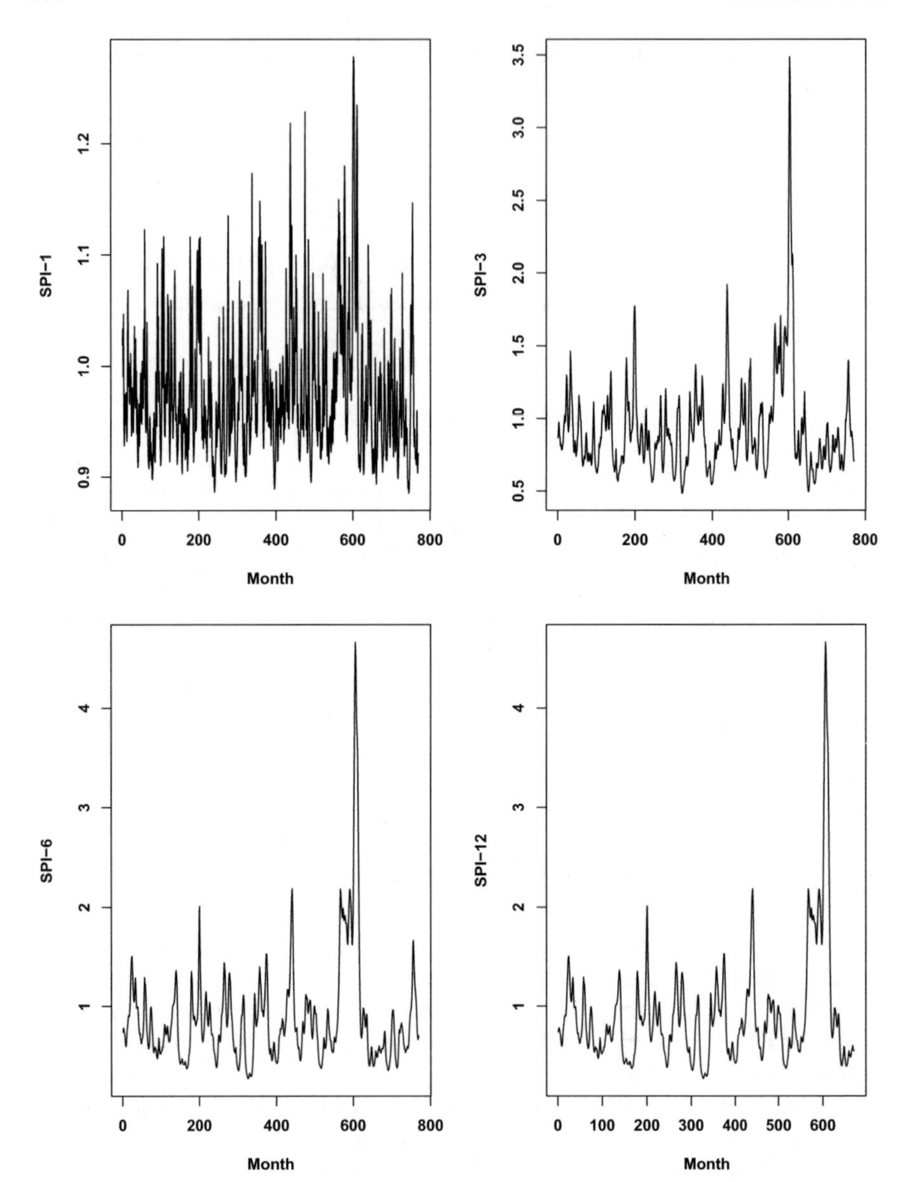

Fig. 7.2 Square roots of SPI volatilities against months

Table 7.2 Posterior summaries

	Posterior mean	Standard deviation	95% Cred. Interval
μ_1	−0.0956	0.0599	(−0.2145; 0.0199)
μ_2	−0.3446	0.1167	(−0.5776; −0.1180)
μ_3	−0.5883	0.1930	(−0.9786; −0.2171)
μ_4	−0.9197	0.3141	(−1.5518; −0.2973)
ϕ_1	0.3666	0.1776	(0.0351; 0.6821)
ϕ_2	0.8220	0.0418	(0.7335; 0.8967)
ϕ_3	0.8990	0.0232	(0.8503; 0.9409)
ϕ_4	0.9448	0.0146	(0.9159; 0.9717)
ζ_1	7.0186	1.9578	(4.0083; 11.5022)
ζ_2	4.4458	1.1325	(2.6710; 7.1073)
ζ_3	3.9367	0.0812	(2.5969; 5.8146)
ζ_4	4.1434	0.6970	(2.9819; 5.6982)

7.5 Concluding Remarks

Usually, the Palmer Drought Severity Index (PDSI) and the Standardized Precipitation Index (SPI) are the best known and used worldwide in order to monitor a drought.

According to [10] the PDSI is a quantifier of the severity of a drought, and a single index value is used to evaluate drought. The index is calculated based on a time series of at least 30 years of air temperature and precipitation data, in the monthly scale. It is interesting to point out that [19] developed the PDSI as a meteorological drought indicator without, however, specifying what time scale (memory) the index considers in its analysis. The PDSI is criticized by some climatologists (see for example, [2, 11, 13, 16]).

In Fig. 7.3, we have the plot of the Palmer Drought Severity Index (PDSI) for Campinas ranging from January 01, 1970 to May 01, 2011. From this plot, we also observe that the period tanging from the 300th month (01/01/1995) to 350th month (12/31/1998) has an atypical drought period, a result similar to the one obtained using the SPI-1 index (see Fig. 7.1).

The Standardized Precipitation Index (SPI) has many advantages when compared to the Palmer Drought Severity Index (PDSI) as pointed out by many climatologists since it quantifies the precipitation deficit for different timescales. These timescales reflect the impact of drought on the availability of the different water resources. Soil moisture conditions respond to precipitation anomalies on a relatively short scale; groundwater, streamflow, and reservoir storage reflect the longer term precipitation anomalies. In this way, many climatologists are using the SPI index in place of the PDSI index, although the statistical modeling approach based on time series SVM presented here could be easily extended to the PDSI index.

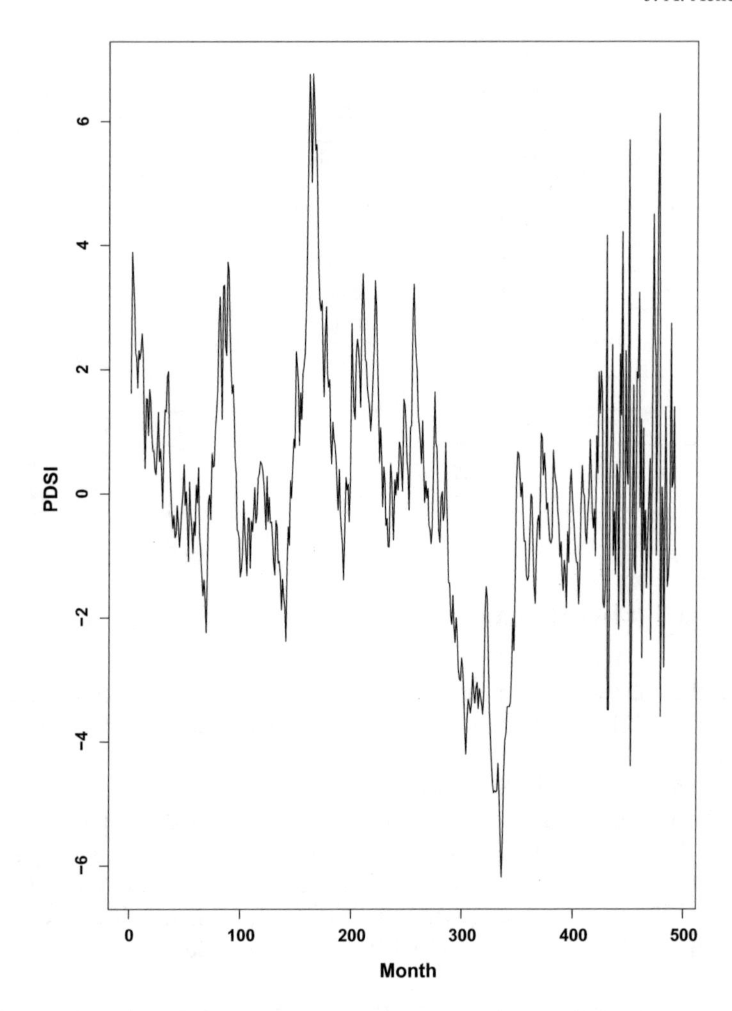

Fig. 7.3 PDSI against months for Campinas (January 01, 1970 to May 01, 2011)

Other structures of SVM could also be considered to analyze SPI measures, for example, considering autoregressive model $AR(L)$ structures with L larger than 1 to get better fit of the model for the data. The use of a Bayesian approach with MCMC (Markov Chain Monte Carlo) methods and existing freely available software like OpenBugs or JAGS could simplify the computational task to get the posterior summaries of interest. The choice of a better model could be made using some existing Bayesian discrimination criteria as the Deviance Information Criterion (DIC) criterion [22].

Using this family of SVMs we could possibly relate the time periods with atypical drought to some covariates (for example, the sea temperature in equatorial Pacific

Ocean like El Niño by unusually warm temperatures or La Niña by unusually cool temperatures) which could be affecting the climate of the world, or even other causes showing atypical extremely wet or extremely dry periods.

References

1. Achcar, J.A., E.A. Coelho-Barros, and R.M. Souza. 2016. Use of non-homogeneous Poisson process (NHPP) in presence of change-points to analyze drought periods: a case study in Brazil. *Environmental and Ecological Statistics* 23 (3): 405–419.
2. Alley, W.M. 1984. The Palmer drought severity index: Limitations and assumptions. *Journal of Applied Meteorology* 23: 1100–1109.
3. Bollerslev, T. 1986. Generalized autoregressive conditional heteroskedasticity. *Journal of Econometrics* 31: 307–327.
4. Chortaria, C., C.A. Karavitis, and S. Alexandris. Development of the SPI drought index for Greece using geo-statistical methods. In *Proceedings of BALWOIS 2010 internation conference* 2010.
5. Danielsson, J. 1994. Stochastic volatility in asset prices: Estimation with simulated maximum likelihood. *Journal of Econometrics* 61: 375–400.
6. Edwards, D.C. 1997. *Characteristics of 20th century drought in the united states at multiple time scales*. DTIC Document: Technical report.
7. Engle, R.F. 1982. Autoregressive conditional heteroscedasticity with estimates of the variance of united kingdom inflation. *Econometrica* 50 (4): 987–1007.
8. Gelfand, A.E., and A.F.M. Smith. 1990. Sampling-based approaches to calculating marginal densities. *Journal of the American Statistical Association* 85 (410): 398–409.
9. Ghysels, E. 1996. Stochastic volatility. In *Statistical methods on finance*: North-Holland.
10. Guttman, N.B. 1998. Comparing the palmer drought index and the standardized precipitation index1. *Journal of the American Water Resources Association* 34 (1): 113–121.
11. Hayes, M.J., M.D. Svoboda, D.A. Wilhite, and O.V. Vanyarkho. 1999. Monitoring the 1996 drought using the standardized precipitation index. *Bulletin of the American Meteorological Society* 80 (3): 429–438.
12. Karavitis, C.A., S. Alexandris, D.E. Tsesmelis, and G. Athanasopoulos. 2011. Application of the standardized precipitation index (spi) in Greece. *Water* 3 (3): 787–805.
13. Karl, T.R. 1986. The sensitivity of the palmer drought severity index and Palmer's Z-index to their calibration coefficients including potential evapotranspiration. *Journal of Applied Meteorology* 25 (1): 77–86.
14. Kim, S., and N. Shephard. 1998. Stochastic volatility: likelihood inference and comparison with arch models. *Review of Economic Studies* 65: 361–393.
15. Livada, I., and V.D. Assimakopoulos. 2007. Spatial and temporal analysis of drought in Greece using the standardized precipitation index (spi). *Theoretical and applied climatology* 89 (3–4): 143–153.
16. McKee, T.B., N.J. Doesken, and J. Kleist. The relationship of drought frequency and duration to time scales. In *Proceedings of the 8th conference on applied climatology*, vol. 17, 179–183. American Meteorological Society Boston, MA, USA, 1993.
17. McKee, T.B., N.J. Doesken, and J. Kleist. Drought monitoring with multiple time scales. In *Ninth conference on applied climatology. 1995 Boston: American Meteorological Society Boston*.
18. Meyer, R., and T. Yu. 2000. Bugs for a bayesian analysis of stochastic volatility models. *Econometrics Journal* 3: 198–215.
19. Palmer, W.C. 1965 Meteorological drought, weather bureau research paper no. 45. Washington, DC: US Department of Commerce 1965.

20. Yu-Sung, S., and Y. Masanao. *R2jags: Using R to Run 'JAGS'*, 2015. R package version 0.5-6.
21. Smith, A.F.M., and G.O. Roberts. 1993. Bayesian computation via the Gibbs sampler and related Markov chain Monte Carlo methods. *Journal of the Royal Statistical Society. Series B. Methodological* 55(1):3–23 .
22. Spiegelhalter, D.J., N.G. Best, B.P. Carlin, and A. Van Der Linde. 2002. Bayesian measures of model complexity and fit. *Journal of the Royal Statistical Society: Series B (Statistical Methodology)* 64 (4): 583–639.

Chapter 8
Nonparametric Estimation of Mean Residual Life Function Using Scale Mixtures

Sujit K. Ghosh and Shufang Liu

Abstract It is often of interest in clinical trials and reliability studies to estimate the remaining lifetime of a subject or a device given that it survived up to a given period of time, that is commonly known as the so-called *mean residual life function (mrlf)*. There have been several attempts in literature to estimate the mrlf nonparametrically ranging from empirical estimates to more sophisticated smooth estimation. Given the well known one-to-one relation between survival function and mrlf, one can plug-in any known estimates of the survival function (e.g., Kaplan–Meier estimate) into the functional form of mrlf to obtain an estimate of mrlf. In this chapter, we present a scale mixture representation of mrlf and use it to obtain a smooth estimate of the mrlf under right censoring. Asymptotic properties of the proposed estimator are also presented. Several simulation studies and a real data set are used for investigating the empirical performance of the proposed method relative to other well-known estimates of mrlf. A comparative analysis shows computational advantages of the proposed estimator in addition to somewhat superior statistical properties in terms of bias and efficiency.

8.1 Introduction

Let T be a positive valued random variable that represents the lifetime of a subject. For example, T could represent the time until a patient dies due to a terminal disease or it could also represent the time until an equipment fails or it could also represent the time until a stock value exceeds or proceeds a given threshold value. Next, let $F(t) = \Pr[T \leq t]$ be the cumulative distribution function (cdf). Notice that $F(0) = 0$ as $T > 0$ with probability 1.

In survival analysis, it is customary to work with the survival function (sf), defined as $S(t) = 1 - F(t) = \Pr[T > t]$. For the rest of the development, we assume that T has a finite expectation, i.e., $E(T) = \int_0^\infty t dF(t) = \int_0^\infty S(t)dt < \infty$.

S. K. Ghosh (✉) · S. Liu
Department of Statistics, NC State University, 2311 K. Stinson Drive, Raleigh, NC 27695-8203, USA
e-mail: sujit.ghosh@ncsu.edu

A. Adhikari et al. (eds.), *Mathematical and Statistical Applications in Life Sciences and Engineering*, https://doi.org/10.1007/978-981-10-5370-2_8

Definition 8.1 The **mean residual life function (mrlf)** of a lifetime random variable T with a finite expectation is defined as

$$m(t) \equiv E[T - t|T > t] = \begin{cases} \int_t^\infty \frac{S(u)}{S(t)} du & \text{if } S(t) > 0, \\ 0 & \text{otherwise}, \end{cases} \quad (8.1)$$

where $S(t)$ denotes the survival function associated with T.

From above definition, it is clear that an mrlf provides a measure of the average remaining/residual lifetime of a subject given that the subject has survived beyond time t. The mrlf can play a very useful role in many fields of applied sciences such as biomedical studies, reliability models, actuarial sciences and economics where the goal is often to characterize the residual life expectancy.

A related function that is often used in such studies is known as the *hazard function*, which is defined as $h(t) = -\frac{d \log S(t)}{dt}$ (assuming that the sf, $S(t)$ is differentiable). A hazard function can be interpreted as the instantaneous risk of failure given that the subject has survived up to at least time t.

Sometimes, in applied sciences the mrlf can serve as a more useful tool than the hazard function, because the mrlf has a direct interpretation in terms of average long-term behavior. For example, patients in a clinical trial might be more interested to know how many more years they are expected to survive given that they began a treatment at a certain time ago as compared to their instantaneous risk of dying given that they have started the treatment at a given time (Elandt-Johnson and Johnson [6]). In an industrial reliability study, researchers prefer the use of the mrlf to that of the hazard function, because they could determine the optimal maintaining and replacing time for a device based on the mrlf [3]. In economics, Kopperschmidt and Potter [16] gave an example of applying the mrlf in market research. In the social sciences, Morrison [21] had used an increasing mrlf to model the lifelength of wars and strikes. A variety of applications of the mrlf can be found in Guess and Proschan [9].

Although $m(t)$ and $h(t)$ have different interpretations in practice, they are related to each other by a one-to-one map, in the sense that one can be obtained from the other provided that they are well-defined (see Lemma 8.1 in the Appendix). However, Guess and Proschan [9] pointed out that it is possible for the mrlf to exist but for the hazard function not to exist (e.g., the standard Cantor ternary function), and also it is possible for the hazard function to exist but for the mrlf not to exist (e.g., $S(t) = 1 - \frac{2}{\pi} \arctan(t)$. It is well known that under mild regularity conditions (see Theorem 8.3 in the Appendix, due to Hall and Wellner [12]), the mrlf completely determines the distribution via the well-known inversion formula:

$$S(t) = \frac{m(0)}{m(t)} \exp\left(-\int_0^t \frac{1}{m(u)} du\right). \quad (8.2)$$

Notice that $m(0) = E(T)$ is assumed to be finite.

8.1.1 Inference Based on Completely Observed Data

Let T_i denote the survival time of the i-th subject for $i = 1, 2, \ldots, n$ subjects. If all the realizations of $\{T_i : i = 1, \ldots, n\}$ are completely observed independently and identically (iid) from distribution with survival function $S(t)$, we denote the data set as $\mathcal{D}_0 = \{T_i : i = 1, 2, \ldots, n\}$. We can easily obtain an estimate of the mrlf, $m(t)$ as defined in (8.1) either based on a parametric model (e.g., Gamma, Weibull, Log-normal etc.) or nonparametrically as follows:

$$\hat{m}_e(t) = \frac{\sum_{i=1}^{n}(T_i - t)\mathbb{I}(T_i > t)}{\sum_{i=1}^{n}\mathbb{I}(T_i > t)} = \int_t^{\infty}\frac{\hat{S}(u)}{\hat{S}(t)}du, \quad \text{for } t \in [0, T_{(n)}), \tag{8.3}$$

where $\mathbb{I}(\cdot)$ denotes the indicator function, such that $\mathbb{I}(A) = 1$ if the statement A is correct otherwise $\mathbb{I}(A) = 0$. Further, $T_{(n)} = \max_{1\le i\le n} T_i$ denotes the largest observed time and $\hat{S}(t)$ denotes the empirical survival function estimate given by $\hat{S}(t) = \sum_{i=1}^{n}\mathbb{I}(T_i > t)/n$. Notice that to be consistent with the definition of $m(t)$, if $t \ge T_{(n)}$, we define $\hat{m}_e(t) = 0$.

The empirical mrlf $\hat{m}_e(t)$ has been shown to be asymptotically unbiased, uniformly strongly consistent, and under mild regularity conditions, it converges in distribution to a Gaussian process [26]. Although $\hat{m}_e(t)$ has good asymptotic properties, it is a discontinuous estimate of $m(t)$. Consequently, smooth estimation of the mrlf has been developed.

There are different approaches to obtain smooth estimators of $m(t)$ in the literature. Essentially, all the methods derive the smooth estimators by smoothing empirical survival function $\hat{S}(\cdot)$ and then plug that in the Eq. (8.3) to obtain a smoothed estimator.

Abdous and Berred [1] had adopted the classical kernel smoothing method to estimate m(t) for complete observed data using the local linear fitting technique. Chaubey and Sen [4] had used the so-called Hille's theorem [13] to smooth the survival functions in the numerator and denominator in the expression of $m(t)$ in (8.3). Ruiz and Guillamon [23] had estimated the survival function in the numerator in $m(t)$ by a recursive kernel estimate and used the empirical survival function to estimate the denominator in (8.3). To reduce the bias of the basic kernel density estimator, Swanepoel and Van Graan [24] introduced a new kernel density function estimator based on a nonparametric transformation of complete data. In this chapter, we present scale mixture to smooth $\hat{m}_e(t)$ directly instead of first obtaining a smooth estimate of $\hat{S}(\cdot)$ (see [19]).

8.1.2 Inference Based on Right-Censored Data

Sometimes we may not be able to observe survival times of all subjects completely within a given study period. In many biomedical applications, especially in clinical trials, right-censored data are very common, because some patients might be lost to follow-up or might die from other causes, or might be alive at the end of the period of study. Therefore, estimating $m(t)$ based on right-censored data is necessary in many practical scenarios.

Let C_i denote the censoring time of the i-th subject, i.e., we only observe $X_i = \min\{T_i, C_i\}$ and the indicator of censoring $\Delta_i = \mathbb{I}(C_i > T_i)$ for $i = 1, \ldots, n$. In such situations, the observed data set is given by $\mathcal{D}_1 = \{(X_i, \Delta_i) : i = 1, 2, \ldots, n\}$. We assume that (T_i, C_i) are independent and identically distributed (iid) from the joint distribution of (T, C) and further we assume that T is independent of C, which is often referred to as noninformative censoring, i.e., the censoring mechanism does not influence or influenced by the survival time. When observations are censored the nonparametric estimation of $m(t)$ has also been studied extensively. It can be seen from (8.1) that the mrlf has a disadvantage for its high dependence on the tail behavior of the survival function. Therefore it is hard to estimate $m(t)$ with greater precision, especially when no parametric forms are assumed for the underlying distribution of T.

If the underlying distribution is assumed to arise from a parametric family, then it will be relatively easier to estimate $m(t)$ by method of maximum likelihood. Tsang and Jardine [25], Lai et al. [18] obtained estimates of $m(t)$ based on a 2-parameter Weibull distribution model, while Agarwal and Kalla [2], Kalla et al. [14], and Gupta and Lvin [11] obtained estimates based on a Gamma distribution model. Gupta and Bradley [10] studied $m(t)$ when T_i's were assumed to belong to the Pearsonian family of distributions. However, it is obvious that the parametric assumptions seriously dictates the shape and character of the mrlf which, in case of an incorrect specification, is undesirable, especially when prediction is of interest. So many studies have focussed on using nonparametric estimation procedures to estimate $m(t)$.

Ghorai et al. [8] first used the classical product-limit estimator $\hat{S}(t)$ of Kaplan and Meier [15] of $S(t)$ into (8.3) to obtain the estimate of $m(t)$ under the assumption of right censoring and also established the consistency and asymptotic normality of the estimator. However as in the case of complete data, the Ghorai et al. [8] estimator of the mrlf for censored data, is also a discontinuous estimate of $m(t)$ and hence a smoothed estimator is desirable.

Kulasekara [17] used smoothed estimate of $\hat{S}(\cdot)$ in the numerator and the denominator of the expression of $m(t)$ in (8.3) for both complete and censored data; and also established the asymptotic consistency and normality of his estimator. In a simulation study, Kulasekera [17] also demonstrated that the kernel based estimators often have much smaller mean squared error (MSE) than the empirical estimator. Consequently, the kernel estimators are more efficient compared to the empirical estimators.

In this chapter, we present a scale mixture approach (see Liu [19]) to directly obtain a smooth estimator of $m(t)$ for both complete data and censored data. In addition, we also present an extension of the method of Chaubey and Sen [4] for complete data to obtain a smooth estimate based on right-censored data which is essentially same as the methodology of Chaubey and Sen [5] which also provides asymptotic properties for the censored case. In Sect. 8.2, we present the mrlf estimator using scale mixture and then present the asymptotic properties of the proposed mrlf. The proofs of the results along with computational details are presented in the appendices. In Sect. 8.3, we present a simulation study to evaluate the performance of the proposed mrlf, the empirical mrlf, and the smooth mrlf (Chaubey and Sen [5]). In Sect. 8.4, we compare the performance of the three mrlf estimators based on a real data set. Finally, in Sect. 8.5, we present some discussion and directions for further extensions.

8.2 Scale Mixtures of the MRLF

The basic approach to obtain a smooth estimate of $m(t)$ directly is based on the following result:

Theorem 8.1 *Let $m(t)$ be an mrlf as defined in (8.1). Then*

(a) $\frac{m(t\theta)}{\theta}$ *is also a mrlf for any* $\theta > 0$*; and*
(b) $\int_0^\infty \frac{m(t\theta)}{\theta}\pi(\theta)d\theta$ *is a mrlf for any density* $\pi(\cdot)$ *on* $[0, \infty)$.

Proof Notice that, for $\theta > 0$,

$$\frac{m(t\theta)}{\theta} = E[T - t\theta|T > t\theta]\frac{1}{\theta} = E\left[\frac{T}{\theta} - t\middle|\frac{T}{\theta} > t\right].$$

Hence $\frac{m(t\theta)}{\theta}$ is the mrlf of $\frac{T}{\theta}$ and (a) is proved. Next,

$$\int_0^\infty \frac{m(t\theta)}{\theta}\pi(\theta)d\theta = E_\pi\left[E\left[\frac{T}{\theta} - t\middle|\frac{T}{\theta} > t\middle|\theta\right]\right] = E\left[\frac{T}{\theta} - t\middle|\frac{T}{\theta} > t\right]$$

Hence, $\int_0^\infty \frac{m(t\theta)}{\theta}\pi(\theta)d\theta$ is the mrlf of $\frac{T}{\theta}$ where conditional distribution of $\frac{T}{\theta}$ given θ has mrlf $\frac{m(t\theta)}{\theta}$ and the marginal distribution of θ has density $\pi(\cdot)$. This completes the proof of Theorem 8.1. □

We now use the above result to develop a class of smooth estimators of $m(t)$, based on the empirical estimate $\hat{m}_e(t)$ as defined in (8.3) with $\hat{S}(\cdot)$ replaced by the Kaplan–Meier estimate when the data is right censored. Our proposed class of estimators is given by

$$\hat{m}_m(t) = \int_0^\infty \frac{\hat{m}_e(t\theta)}{\theta}\pi_n(\theta)\, d\theta, \tag{8.4}$$

where $\pi_n(\theta)$ is to be chosen suitably so that we obtain a consistent estimate of $m(t)$. In general, it can be shown that if we choose $\pi_n(\cdot)$ that satisfies the following two conditions: (a) $E_{\pi_n}[T_n^{-1}] = 1$, and (b) $T_n \xrightarrow{p} 1$ as $n \to \infty$ where $T_n \sim \pi_n$, then the estimator proposed in (8.4) will be consistent. However, in this article we will focus on a specific choice of π_n and from now on we would use the density of a Gamma distribution with mean $(1 + k_n)/k_n$ and variance $(1 + k_n)/k_n^2$, denoted by $Ga(k_n + 1, \frac{1}{k_n})$, where k_n will be chosen suitably (as a function of n) which will be used to establish desired asymptotic properties of the smoothed estimator. In other words, we use the following choice of π_n:

$$\pi_n(\theta) \equiv \pi(\theta|k_n) = \frac{k_n^{k_n}}{\Gamma(k_n)}\theta^{k_n}e^{-k_n\theta}\mathbb{I}(\theta > 0).$$

One advantage of the above choice of the mixing density is that it provides a closed form expression for $\hat{m}_m(\cdot)$ which is based on the following closed form expression of $\hat{m}_e(t)$ for the censored case:

$$\hat{m}_e(t) = \begin{cases} \frac{\sum_{j=l+1}^{n} X_j w_j}{\sum_{j=l+1}^{n} w_j} - t, & \text{if } X_l \le t < X_{l+1}, l = 0, 1, \ldots, n-1, \\ 0 & \text{if } t \ge X_n, \end{cases} \tag{8.5}$$

where we assume that $0 \stackrel{def}{=} X_0 < X_1 \le \ldots \le X_n < X_{n+1} \stackrel{def}{=} \infty$ are ordered observed values of the data, $w_j = \hat{S}(X_j) - \hat{S}(X_j-)$ and $\hat{S}(\cdot)$ denotes the Kaplan–Meier (KM) estimate. Notice that $w_j = \hat{S}(X_j) - \hat{S}(X_j-) = 1/n$ for complete data. It can be shown that (for details see Appendix)

$$\begin{aligned} \hat{m}_m(t) &= \int_0^\infty \hat{m}_e(u) f\left(u \middle| k_n, \frac{t}{k_n}\right) du \\ &= \sum_{l=0}^{n-1} \frac{\sum_{j=l+1}^{n} X_j w_j}{\sum_{j=l+1}^{n} w_j} \left[F\left(X_{l+1} \middle| k_n, \frac{t}{k_n}\right) - F\left(X_l \middle| k_n, \frac{t}{k_n}\right) \right] \\ &\quad - tF\left(X_n \middle| k_n + 1, \frac{t}{k_n}\right), \end{aligned} \tag{8.6}$$

where $F(\cdot|k_n, \frac{t}{k_n})$ is the cdf of $\text{Ga}(k_n, \frac{t}{k_n})$. We will use the expression (8.6) to compute our proposed estimator. From the expression (8.6) it is obvious that $\hat{m_m}(t)$ is a smooth estimator and is a valid mrlf for any t and n.

Next we state the asymptotic property of our proposed estimator $\hat{m}_m(t)$:

Theorem 8.2 *Suppose* $\{(X_1, \Delta_1), \ldots, (X_n, \Delta)\}$ *denotes the set of observed data obtained under random right censoring from a distribution with mrlf* $m(t)$*. Then,*

(a) for each $t > 0$*, the estimator* $\hat{m}_m(t)$ *converges in probability to* $m(t)$*; and*
(b) the process $\{\sqrt{n}(\hat{m}_m(t) - m(t)) : t \in (0, \infty)\}$ *converges weakly to a Gaussian process with mean identically zero and covariance function* $\sigma(s, t)$ *given by,*

$$\sigma(s,t) = \frac{1}{S(s)S(t)}\int_t^\infty u^2 dF(u) - \frac{1}{S(t)}\left(\int_t^\infty u dF(u)\right)^2, \quad 0 \le s \le t < \infty$$

for complete data and

$$\sigma(s,t) = \frac{1}{S(s)S(t)} \int_t^{\infty} \frac{\phi^2(\nu)}{(S(\nu)G(\nu))^2} d\widetilde{H}(\nu), \quad 0 \le s \le t < \infty,$$

where $\phi(t) = \int_t^{\infty} S(u)du$, $G(t) = Pr[C > t]$, *and* $\widetilde{H}(t) = Pr[\Delta_1 = 1, X_1 \le t]$ *for censored data.*

The proof of the above theorem depends on the use of Feller approximation lemma which establishes the asymptotic equivalence of $\hat{m}_m(t)$ with $\hat{m}_e(t)$. The details of the proof is given in the Appendix. Although asymptotically the estimators $\hat{m}_m(t)$ and $\hat{m}_e(t)$ have the same limiting distribution, the finite sample properties of $\hat{m}_m(t)$ can be superior to that of $\hat{m}_e(t)$ and some other existing smooth estimators of $m(t)$ (see the Appendix for further details). Next, we explore the finite sample properties of the scale mixture estimator using simulated data sets and comparing the performance with other estimators.

8.3 A Simulation Study

Given the complicated nature of the estimator, it is not possible to derive the exact finite sample mean squared error (MSE) of the proposed estimator. Thus, following other similar work in the literature a thorough simulation study was carried out instead to explore the empirical properties of the estimator. In order to compare different estimates for censored data an extended version of smooth estimation procedures of Chaubey and Sen [4] was used for our comparative empirical analysis. In our simulation study we included the following estimators: (i) empirical mrlf $\hat{m}_e(t)$ (emrlf); (ii) the scale mixture mrlf $\hat{m}_m(t)$(mmrlf), and (iii) the smooth mrlf $\hat{m}_s(t)$ (smrlf) following the work of Chaubey and Sen [4].

In this chapter, we present only a subset of the full version of the simulation studies presented in Liu [19] for a sample size of $n = 100$ each repeated $N = 1000$ times:

(i) True data generating distribution: We used a Weibull distribution (denoted by Wei(2, 2)), with both the shape and scale parameter set at 2. The emrlf, smrlf, and mmrlf are evaluated at 20 quantiles ranging between 0.01 qunatile to 0.90 quantile of this distribution.
(ii) Censoring distribution: We used the Exponential distribution with the scale parameter λ to obtain on average censoring rates of 0% ($\lambda = \infty$), 20% ($\lambda = 7.63$), 40% ($\lambda = 3.22$), and 60% ($\lambda = 1.67$)

(iii) Performance measures: We report the following measures to compare the three estimators:
(a) Pointwise (additive) bias: $\hat{B}(t) = \frac{\sum_{i=1}^{N} \hat{m}_i(t)}{N} - m(t)$,
(b) Pointwise (relative) bias: $\frac{\hat{B}(t)}{m(t)}$,
(c) Pointwise mean squared error (MSE): $\bar{\hat{m}}(t))^2 + (\bar{\hat{m}}(t) - m(t))^2$ and
(d) Relative efficiencies: $\widehat{RE}_{12}(t) = \frac{\widehat{MSE}_1(t)}{\widehat{MSE}_2(t)}$.

In this study, we compare the efficiencies of the proposed mmrlf and smrlf with respect to emrlf and report $\frac{\widehat{MSE}_{emrlf}(t)}{\widehat{MSE}_{mmrlf}(t)}$ and $\frac{\widehat{MSE}_{emrlf}(t)}{\widehat{MSE}_{smrlf}(t)}$ evaluated at the selected quantiles of the data generating distribution.

In computing the mmrlf we used the sequence $k_n = n^{1.01}$ following the asymptotic normality result obtained in Theorem 8.2. Other possibilities include the use of cross-validation methods that is not pursued here.

The results of the simulation study are presented in Figs. 8.1, 8.2, 8.3 and 8.4 which provide a graphical summary of the results for the targeted censoring rates of

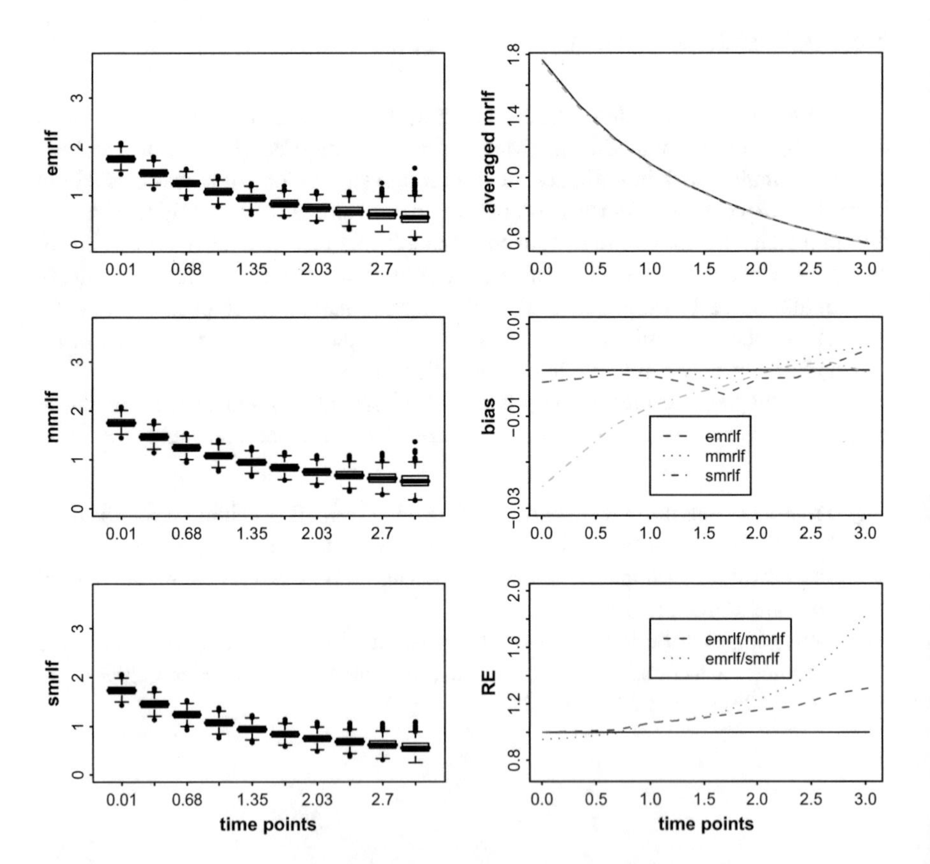

Fig. 8.1 Estimated emrlf, mmrlf, and smrlf under 0% censoring rate. For details see Sect. 8.3

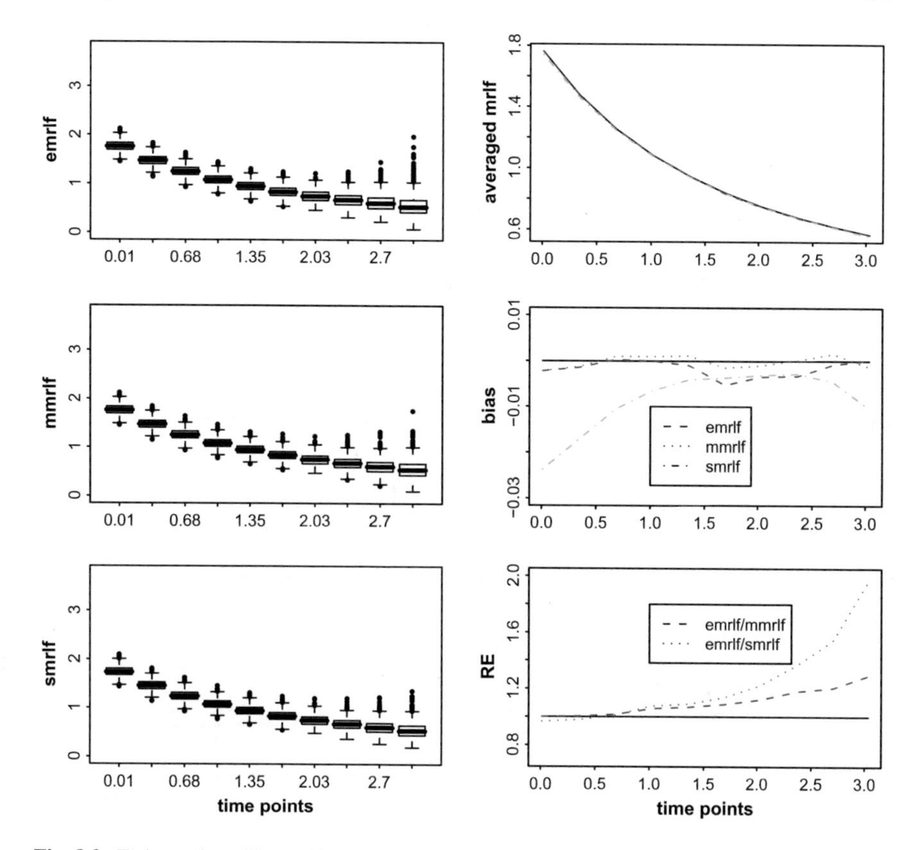

Fig. 8.2 Estimated emrlf, mmrlf, and smrlf under 20% censoring rate. For details see Sect. 8.3

0%, 20%, 40%, and 60%, respectively. In each of these four figures, the first column presents the boxplots of estimated mrlf using three estimates each evaluated at 20 selected quantiles of the generating distribution. Large variations near the tail part of the distribution is clearly visible which is expected as there are less number of observed values from the tails of the distribution and such variability increases with censoring rates as well. The second column in each of the four figures present the average (over 1000 Monte Carlo repetitions) values of estimated mrlf using three methods along with the true mrlf; the pointwise bias (as defined above) and the pointwise relative efficiencies (as defined above). Clearly, in all scenarios, all three estimates are nearly unbiased across all censoring rates, though the biases are larger (but still not statistically significant) near the tails of the distributions.

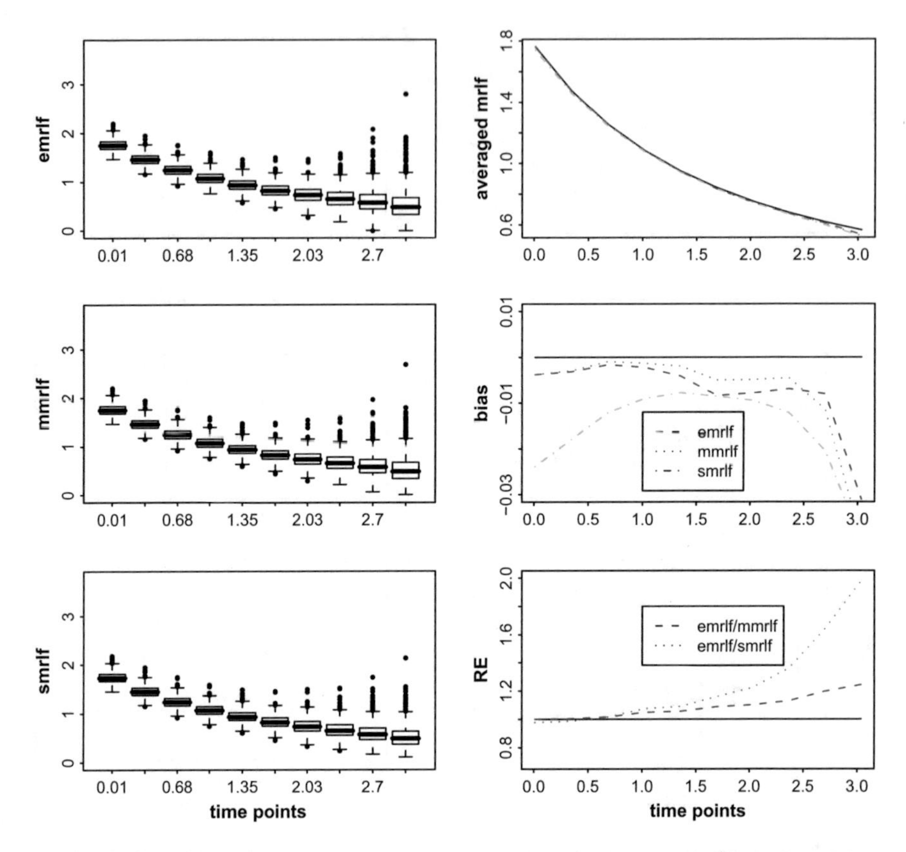

Fig. 8.3 Estimated emrlf, mmrlf, and smrlf under 40% censoring rate. For details see Sect. 8.3

We also report the numerical values of the biases and relative efficiencies in Tables 8.1, 8.2, 8.3 and 8.4 for each of the censoring rates of 0, 20, 40, and 60%. Clearly, the emrlf has the largest variation and the smrlf seems to have the least variation at the tails compared to mmrlf. However, it turns out that relative biases of smrlf are statistically significant (P-value < 0.05) for all time points smaller than 1.92 (the 0.33 quantile of the Weibull distribution). Generally, mmrlf has smaller biases than emrlf, though none of the biases from emrlf or mmrlf are statistically significant. In terms of relative efficiency, mmrlf is uniformly better than emrlf across all 20 time points while the smrlf is less efficient for high density regions but more efficient for tail part of the distributions compared to emrlf and smrlf. The reason for smrlf to have better performance at tail ends might be due to the fact that the number

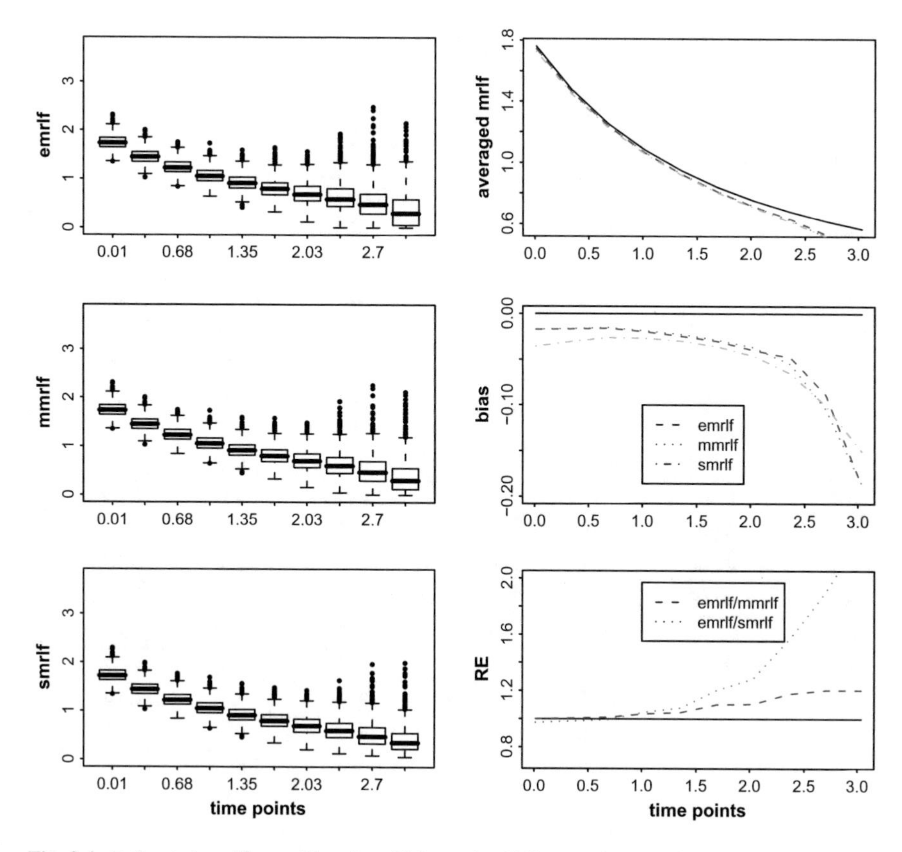

Fig. 8.4 Estimated emrlf, mmrlf, and smrlf for under 60% censoring rate. For details see Sect. 8.3

of the observations used to calculate mmrlf and emrlf decreases at tail ends, while the number of the observation used to calculate smrlf stays the same. Overall, we find that mmrlf is a definitely better estimator compared to emrlf and a competitive estimator to smrlf for complete data. Similar conclusions can also be made for censored data scenario and the reader is referred to find more details and more results reported in Liu [19].

Table 8.1 Relative biases and efficiencies of estimated mrlf's under 0% censoring rate. For details see Sect. 8.3

Time	$\frac{\widehat{B}_{emrlf}(t)}{m(t)}$	$\frac{\widehat{B}_{mmrlf}(t)}{m(t)}$	$\frac{\widehat{B}_{smrlf}(t)}{m(t)}$	$\frac{\widehat{MSE}_{emrlf}(t)}{\widehat{MSE}_{mmrlf}(t)}$	$\frac{\widehat{MSE}_{emrlf}(t)}{\widehat{MSE}_{smrlf}(t)}$	$\frac{\widehat{MSE}_{smrlf}(t)}{\widehat{MSE}_{mmrlf}(t)}$
0.010	−0.001	−0.001	−0.014	1.000	0.947	1.056
0.169	−0.002	−0.001	−0.014	1.003	0.961	1.044
0.328	−0.001	−0.001	−0.013	1.014	0.970	1.045
0.488	−0.001	−0.001	−0.011	1.015	0.992	1.024
0.647	−0.001	0.000	−0.010	1.012	0.987	1.025
0.806	−0.001	0.000	−0.009	1.037	1.021	1.015
0.965	−0.001	0.000	−0.008	1.056	1.056	1.000
1.124	−0.002	0.000	−0.007	1.067	1.069	0.998
1.284	−0.001	0.000	−0.006	1.064	1.067	0.997
1.443	−0.004	−0.001	−0.005	1.096	1.099	0.998
1.602	−0.004	−0.002	−0.005	1.091	1.102	0.990
1.761	−0.004	−0.002	−0.004	1.159	1.198	0.967
1.920	−0.004	−0.001	−0.002	1.162	1.226	0.948
2.080	−0.002	0.001	−0.001	1.155	1.244	0.928
2.239	0.001	0.002	0.001	1.182	1.309	0.903
2.398	−0.003	0.003	0.002	1.186	1.354	0.876
2.557	−0.001	0.005	0.003	1.261	1.490	0.846
2.716	0.000	0.007	0.003	1.248	1.541	0.810
2.876	0.008	0.009	0.001	1.256	1.643	0.765
3.035	0.008	0.009	−0.001	1.312	1.852	0.708

On average the MCSE is about 0.004

In addition to above moderate sample size ($n = 100$) simulation study, given that our results are based on asymptotic theory, we also explored the performance of emrlf, mmrlf, and smrlf for a simulation study for data with a much larger sample size of $n = 5000$ under the same set of scenario as earlier. Unfortunately, we were not able to carry out the full simulation study (with 1000 MC reps) for the smrlf as the computation of smrlf involves large sums with combinatorial expressions both in the numerator and denominator (see (8.10)), requiring huge computing resources. On the other hand, both emrlf and mmrlf were relatively easy to compute within a reasonable amount of time. In Table 8.5, we provide the relative efficiency of emrlf to mmrlf for the censoring rates of 0, 20, 40, and 60%. To our surprise, it appears that the mmrlf seems still more efficient than emrlf for very large data sets, despite the fact that asymptotically they have the same limit distributions.

Table 8.2 Relative biases and efficiency of estimated mrlf's under 20% censoring rate. For details see Sect. 8.3

Time	$\frac{\widehat{B}_{emrlf}(t)}{m(t)}$	$\frac{\widehat{B}_{mmrlf}(t)}{m(t)}$	$\frac{\widehat{B}_{smrlf}(t)}{m(t)}$	$\frac{\widehat{MSE}_{emrlf}(t)}{\widehat{MSE}_{mmrlf}(t)}$	$\frac{\widehat{MSE}_{emrlf}(t)}{\widehat{MSE}_{smrlf}(t)}$	$\frac{\widehat{MSE}_{smrlf}(t)}{\widehat{MSE}_{mmrlf}(t)}$
0.010	−0.001	−0.001	−0.013	1.000	0.966	1.036
0.169	−0.001	−0.001	−0.013	1.002	0.977	1.026
0.328	−0.001	−0.001	−0.012	1.010	0.981	1.030
0.488	0.000	0.000	−0.010	1.013	1.007	1.006
0.647	0.000	0.001	−0.009	1.010	1.002	1.008
0.806	0.000	0.001	−0.007	1.035	1.038	0.998
0.965	0.000	0.001	−0.006	1.052	1.067	0.986
1.124	−0.001	0.001	−0.005	1.057	1.077	0.981
1.284	0.001	0.001	−0.005	1.063	1.084	0.981
1.443	−0.001	0.001	−0.004	1.083	1.105	0.980
1.602	−0.002	−0.001	−0.004	1.083	1.117	0.969
1.761	−0.005	−0.002	−0.004	1.124	1.187	0.947
1.920	−0.005	−0.002	−0.004	1.152	1.240	0.929
2.080	−0.005	−0.001	−0.004	1.143	1.253	0.912
2.239	−0.002	0.000	−0.004	1.160	1.308	0.887
2.398	−0.006	0.000	−0.004	1.177	1.374	0.857
2.557	−0.002	0.002	−0.005	1.222	1.486	0.822
2.716	−0.005	0.003	−0.008	1.178	1.517	0.777
2.876	0.002	0.003	−0.012	1.237	1.722	0.718
3.035	0.000	−0.002	−0.018	1.292	1.963	0.658

On average the MCSE is about 0.004

Thus, over all, based on both moderate and very large sample size simulation scenarios that we have reported above, we find the performance of mmrlf very satisfactory both in terms of computational and statistical efficiency compared to emrlf and smrlf.

8.4 Application to Melanoma Study

For the purpose of empirical illustration, we present an analysis by applying our proposed method to the data set given in Ghorai et al. [8]. In addition, we present analysis based on the empirical mrlf method and Chaubey and Sen's [4] method. The data set contains 68 observations which correspond to the survival times (in weeks) of 68 patients with melanoma and were originally obtained by the Central Oncology Group with headquarters at the University of Wisconsin–Madison. The data set has about 58.8% censoring, meaning that the study ended before an event was observed

Table 8.3 Relative biases and efficiency of estimated mrlf's under 40% censoring rate. For details see Sect. 8.3

Time	$\frac{\widehat{B}_{emrlf}(t)}{m(t)}$	$\frac{\widehat{B}_{mmrlf}(t)}{m(t)}$	$\frac{\widehat{B}_{smrlf}(t)}{m(t)}$	$\frac{\widehat{MSE}_{emrlf}(t)}{\widehat{MSE}_{mmrlf}(t)}$	$\frac{\widehat{MSE}_{emrlf}(t)}{\widehat{MSE}_{smrlf}(t)}$	$\frac{\widehat{MSE}_{smrlf}(t)}{\widehat{MSE}_{mmrlf}(t)}$
0.010	−0.002	−0.002	−0.014	1.000	0.977	1.024
0.169	−0.002	−0.002	−0.013	1.004	0.990	1.014
0.328	−0.002	−0.002	−0.012	1.006	0.986	1.020
0.488	−0.002	−0.001	−0.011	1.014	1.013	1.001
0.647	−0.002	−0.001	−0.010	1.004	1.001	1.002
0.806	−0.002	−0.001	−0.009	1.021	1.025	0.996
0.965	−0.002	−0.001	−0.008	1.040	1.061	0.980
1.124	−0.004	−0.001	−0.008	1.047	1.077	0.973
1.284	−0.002	−0.002	−0.008	1.060	1.091	0.971
1.443	−0.004	−0.003	−0.009	1.070	1.110	0.964
1.602	−0.006	−0.005	−0.010	1.069	1.126	0.949
1.761	−0.009	−0.007	−0.011	1.110	1.193	0.930
1.920	−0.010	−0.007	−0.012	1.107	1.212	0.913
2.080	−0.009	−0.006	−0.013	1.113	1.246	0.893
2.239	−0.008	−0.006	−0.015	1.161	1.346	0.862
2.398	−0.011	−0.007	−0.019	1.104	1.345	0.820
2.557	−0.009	−0.011	−0.025	1.171	1.515	0.773
2.716	−0.019	−0.020	−0.034	1.178	1.623	0.726
2.876	−0.028	−0.038	−0.049	1.160	1.712	0.678
3.035	−0.055	−0.070	−0.071	1.243	1.977	0.628

On average the MCSE is about 0.005

for about 40 patients. The entire data set is given below separated by observed and censored cases:

Uncensored observations: 16, 44, 55, 67, 73, 76, 80, 81, 86, 93, 100, 108, 114, 120, 125, 129, 134, 140, 147, 148, 151, 152, 181, 190, 193, 213, 215.

Censored observations: 13, 14, 19, 20, 21, 23, 25, 26, 27, 31, 32, 34, 37, 38, 40, 46, 50, 53, 54, 57, 57, 59, 60, 65, 66, 70, 85, 90, 98, 102, 103, 110, 118, 124, 130, 136, 138, 141, 194, 234.

The estimated mrlf using the three methods (emrlf, smrl and mmrlf) are presented in Fig. 8.5. The first plot on the leftmost corner presents all three estimated curves overlaid for visual comparison showing the overall similarity of the estimates for this data set. The other three plots present the estimated curves separately along with pointwise 95% bootstrap based confidence intervals. As expected, the emrlf provides a rather non-smooth estimate compared to the other two methods. Moreover

Table 8.4 Relative biases and efficiency of estimated mrlf's under 60% censoring rate. For details see Sect. 8.3

Time	$\frac{\widehat{B}_{emrlf}(t)}{m(t)}$	$\frac{\widehat{B}_{mmrlf}(t)}{m(t)}$	$\frac{\widehat{B}_{smrlf}(t)}{m(t)}$	$\frac{\widehat{MSE}_{emrlf}(t)}{\widehat{MSE}_{mmrlf}(t)}$	$\frac{\widehat{MSE}_{emrlf}(t)}{\widehat{MSE}_{smrlf}(t)}$	$\frac{\widehat{MSE}_{smrlf}(t)}{\widehat{MSE}_{mmrlf}(t)}$
0.010	−0.010	−0.010	−0.020	1.000	0.974	1.027
0.169	−0.010	−0.010	−0.021	1.003	0.980	1.023
0.328	−0.011	−0.011	−0.021	1.007	0.986	1.022
0.488	−0.011	−0.011	−0.020	1.010	0.988	1.023
0.647	−0.013	−0.012	−0.021	1.005	0.987	1.018
0.806	−0.014	−0.013	−0.022	1.022	1.014	1.008
0.965	−0.017	−0.016	−0.024	1.020	1.026	0.994
1.124	−0.022	−0.019	−0.027	1.043	1.063	0.981
1.284	−0.023	−0.022	−0.030	1.046	1.073	0.975
1.443	−0.028	−0.026	−0.034	1.030	1.074	0.959
1.602	−0.033	−0.031	−0.039	1.092	1.174	0.930
1.761	−0.039	−0.037	−0.046	1.088	1.201	0.906
1.920	−0.047	−0.044	−0.054	1.095	1.242	0.882
2.080	−0.055	−0.052	−0.065	1.102	1.300	0.848
2.239	−0.058	−0.065	−0.081	1.114	1.394	0.799
2.398	−0.081	−0.087	−0.102	1.132	1.531	0.739
2.557	−0.110	−0.124	−0.131	1.162	1.711	0.680
2.716	−0.155	−0.176	−0.168	1.206	1.921	0.628
2.876	−0.233	−0.246	−0.213	1.196	2.066	0.579
3.035	−0.332	−0.329	−0.266	1.203	2.295	0.524

On average the MCSE is about 0.006

it is clearly evident that emrlf vanishes at the largest time point, while mmrlf and smrlf can take positive values beyond the largest censored observation. In practice, the smooth estimators are preferred as they can also provide estimates beyond the observed data range. In terms of 95% pointwise confidence intervals, the smrlf seems to have wider intervals compared to mmrlf showing slight efficiency gain, but such differences are not statistically significant.

8.5 Discussion

A common approach to obtain smooth estimator of mrlf is to use Eq. (8.1) by first obtaining a smooth estimator of the survival function and then calculating the appropriate functional of the survival function. Our proposed scale mixture method provides an alternative strategy in order to smooth the empirical estimate $\hat{m}_e(t)$ directly

Table 8.5 Efficiency of mmrlf for a sample size of 5000. For details see Sect. 8.3

	$\widehat{MSE}_{emrlf}(t)/\widehat{MSE}_{mmrlf}(t)$			
Time	Censoring rate			
	0%	20%	40%	60%
0.010	1.000	1.000	1.000	1.000
0.169	1.000	1.000	1.000	0.999
0.328	0.999	0.999	0.999	1.000
0.488	1.003	1.003	1.002	1.002
0.647	1.002	1.002	1.003	1.000
0.806	1.006	1.005	1.005	1.003
0.965	1.000	1.002	1.002	1.002
1.124	1.010	1.012	1.007	1.005
1.284	1.010	1.008	1.008	1.007
1.443	1.011	1.011	1.012	1.007
1.602	1.013	1.011	1.006	1.002
1.761	1.014	1.012	1.011	1.013
1.920	1.018	1.024	1.016	1.008
2.080	1.020	1.015	1.015	1.014
2.239	1.020	1.022	1.019	1.016
2.398	1.023	1.032	1.029	1.015
2.557	1.034	1.044	1.039	1.031
2.716	1.039	1.036	1.027	1.029
2.876	1.031	1.021	1.025	1.038
3.035	1.034	1.028	1.037	1.039

to obtain a closed form of our proposed estimate $\hat{m}_m(t)$ for both complete and right-censored data (8.6).

Our simulation studies indicate that $\hat{m}_m(t)$ is more efficient estimator compared to $\hat{m}_e(t)$ even for much larger samples and also has computational advantage relative to the Chaubey and Sen's [4] estimator $\hat{m}_s(t)$. However, we have also noticed that more moderately sized samples, the smrlf has better performances near the tail of the distributions compared to the mmrlf and hence there might be an opportunity to combine these two estimators that enjoys better efficiencies than either of the two estimators.

Another line of research in this area is to extend the mrlf estimation in the presence of predictor variables. Essentially, this amounts to modeling conditional mrlf given a vector of baseline covariates. Several parametric and semi-parametric models have appeared in the literature, however McLain and Ghosh [20] points out several limitations of the semi-parametric models and presents nonparametric regression models that provide valid conditional mrlf (in terms of Hall and Wellner [12] characterization) in the presence of baseline predictor variables.

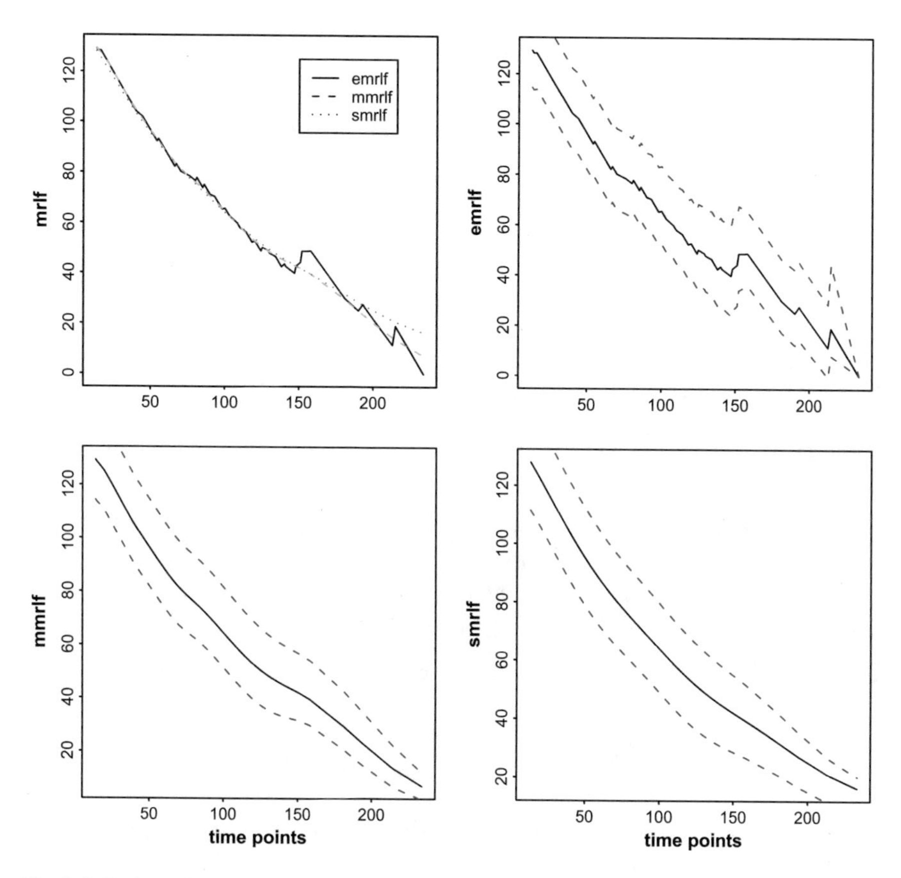

Fig. 8.5 Estimated mrlf's and 95% Bootstrap based pointwise confidence bands for the Melanoma Study. For details see Sect. 8.4

Appendix

A: Characterization of MRLF

Lemma 8.1 *Let $h(t)$ be the hazard function of a lifetime random variable T. Then the mrlf, $m(t)$ of T is differentiable and is obtained by solving the following differential equation:*

$$m'(t) + 1 = m(t)h(t) \quad \textit{for all } t > 0, \tag{8.7}$$

where $m'(\cdot)$ denotes the derivative of $m(\cdot)$.

Proof From (8.1), it follows that $m(t)S(t) = \int_t^\infty S(u)du$. The result follows by differentiating both sides of the previous identity with respect to (wrt) t and using the definition of $h(t) = -S'(t)/S(t)$.

It thus follows (8.7) that given $h(t)$ we can obtain

$$m(t) = \int_t^{\infty} \exp\left\{-\int_t^u h(v)dv\right\} du, \tag{8.8}$$

and given $m(t)$ we can obtain

$$h(t) = \frac{m'(t) + 1}{m(t)}. \tag{8.9}$$

Also under mild regularity conditions, an mrlf completely determines the distribution as can be seen by the following characterization result:

Theorem 8.3 (Hall-Wellner 1981) Let $m\colon \mathbb{R}^+ \to \mathbb{R}^+$ be a function that satisfies the following conditions:

(i) $m(t)$ is right continuous and $m(0) > 0$;
(ii) $e(t) \equiv m(t) + t$ is non-decreasing;
(iii) if $m(t-) = 0$ for some $t = t_0$, then $m(t) = 0$ on $[t_0, \infty)$;
(iv) if $m(t-) > 0$ for all t, then $\int_0^{\infty} 1/m(u)du = \infty$.

Let $\tau \equiv \inf\{t : m(t-) = 0\} \leq \infty$, and define

$$S(t) = \frac{m(0)}{m(t)} \exp\left\{-\int_0^t \frac{1}{m(u)} du\right\}.$$

Then $F(t) = 1 - S(t)$ is a cdf on $\mathbb{R}^+$ with $F(0) = 0$ and $\tau = \inf\{t : F(t) = 1\}$, finite mean $m(0)$ and mrlf $m(t)$.

Proof See Hall and Wellner (1981), p. xxx.

B: Chaubey-Sen's (1999, 2008) Estimator

Given a sample of n iid positive values random variables, $T_i \overset{iid}{\sim} F(\cdot)$ for $i = 1, \ldots, n$, the empirical survival function S_n is defined by

$$S_n(t) = \frac{1}{n} \sum_{i=1}^{n} \mathbb{I}(T_i > t)$$

Define a set of nonnegative valued Poisson weights as

$$w_k(t\lambda_n) = e^{-t\lambda_n} \frac{(t\lambda_n)^k}{k!}, \quad k = 0, 1, 2, \ldots,$$

where $\lambda_n = n/T_{(n)}$ and $T_{(n)} = \max_{1\leq i\leq n} T_i$. Notice that λ_n is chosen data-dependent, which makes the weight function stochastic. A smoothed empirical survival function can be obtained as

$$\tilde{S}_n(t) = \sum_{k\geq 0} S_n\left(\frac{k}{\lambda_n}\right) w_k(t\lambda_n).$$

Plugging the smoothed empirical survival function into (8.3), the smooth estimator of the mrlf is given by

$$\tilde{m}_n(t) = \frac{1}{\lambda_n}\frac{\sum_{k=0}^{n}\sum_{r=0}^{k}((t\lambda_n)^{(k-r)}/(k-r)!)S_n(k/\lambda_n)}{\sum_{(k=0)}((t\lambda_n)^k/k!)S_n(k/\lambda_n)}. \tag{8.10}$$

Chaubey and Sen (1999) proved that $\tilde{m}_n(t)$ is a consistent estimator of $m(t)$ and $\lambda_n^{1/2}(\tilde{m}_n(t) - m(t)) \xrightarrow{d} N\left(0, \frac{m(t)}{S(t)}\right)$ pointwise. Later Chaubey and Sen (2008) extended their methodology for the censored case and derived the asymptotic properties.

C: The Details of the Calculation of $\hat{m}_m(t)$

$\hat{m}_m(t)$, the smooth estimator of $m(t)$ for censored data (complete data are special case of censored data where weight function $w_j = \frac{1}{n}$), can be calculated with a closed form. The details of the calculation are given here.

$$\hat{m}_m(t) = \int_0^\infty \hat{m}_e(u) f\left(u\middle|k_n, \frac{t}{k_n}\right)du = \sum_{l=0}^{n-1}\int_{X_l}^{X_{l+1}} \hat{m}_e(u) f\left(u\middle|k_n, \frac{t}{k_n}\right)du$$

$$= \sum_{l=0}^{n-1}\left[\frac{\sum_{j=l+1}^{n} X_j w_j}{\sum_{j=l+1}^{n} w_j}\int_{X_l}^{X_{l+1}} f\left(u\middle|k_n, \frac{t}{k_n}\right)du - \frac{\Gamma(k_n+1)}{\Gamma(k_n)}\frac{t}{k_n}\int_{X_l}^{X_{l+1}}\frac{u^{k_n}\left(\frac{t}{k_n}\right)^{k_n+1}}{\Gamma(k_n+1)}e^{-(\frac{t}{k_n})u}du\right]$$

$$= \sum_{l=0}^{n-1}\left[\frac{\sum_{j=l+1}^{n} X_j w_j}{\sum_{j=l+1}^{n} w_j}\int_{X_l}^{X_{l+1}} f\left(u\middle|k_n, \frac{t}{k_n}\right)du - t\int_{X_l}^{X_{l+1}} f\left(u\middle|k_n+1, \frac{t}{k_n}\right)du\right]$$

$$= \sum_{l=0}^{n-1}\frac{\sum_{j=l+1}^{n} X_j w_j}{\sum_{j=l+1}^{n} w_j}\left[F\left(X_{l+1}\middle|k_n, \frac{t}{k_n}\right) - F\left(X_l\middle|k_n, \frac{t}{k_n}\right)\right]$$

$$-\sum_{l=0}^{n-1} t\left[F\left(X_{l+1}\middle|k_n+1, \frac{t}{k_n}\right) - F\left(X_l\middle|k_n+1, \frac{t}{k_n}\right)\right]$$

$$= \sum_{l=0}^{n-1}\frac{\sum_{j=l+1}^{n} X_j w_j}{\sum_{j=l+1}^{n} w_j}\left[F\left(X_{l+1}\middle|k_n, \frac{t}{k_n}\right) - F\left(X_l\middle|k_n, \frac{t}{k_n}\right)\right]$$

$$-t\left[F\left(X_n\middle|k_n+1, \frac{t}{k_n}\right) - F\left(X_0\middle|k_n+1, \frac{t}{k_n}\right)\right]$$

$$= \sum_{l=0}^{n-1}\frac{\sum_{j=l+1}^{n} X_j w_j}{\sum_{j=l+1}^{n} w_j}\left[F\left(X_{l+1}\middle|k_n, \frac{t}{k_n}\right) - F\left(X_l\middle|k_n, \frac{t}{k_n}\right)\right] - tF\left(X_n\middle|k_n+1, \frac{t}{k_n}\right),$$

where $w_j = \hat{S}(X_j) - \hat{S}(X_j-)$ and $\hat{S}(\cdot)$ is the KM estimate.

D: Proof of Theorem 8.2

(a) Proof of consistency

First we prove part (i) of Theorem 8.2 by showing that $\hat{m}_m(t)$ is pointwise consistent for estimating $m(t)$. The main tool to prove consistency is based on the following well known approximation result originally due to Feller [7], p. xxx but extended by Petrone and Veronese [22] for a wider application:

Lemma 8.2 Feller Approximation Lemma *(Petrone and Veronese [22]): Let $g(\cdot)$ be a bounded and right continuous function on $\mathbb{R}$ for each t. Let $Z_k(t)$ be a sequence of random variables for each t such that $\mu_k(t) \equiv E[Z_k(t)] \to t$ and $\sigma_k^2(t) \equiv Var[Z_k(t)] \to 0$ as $k \to \infty$. Then*

$$E[g(Z_k(t))] \to g(t) \;\; \forall t.$$

First, notice that by definition, $\hat{m}_e(\cdot)$ is a right continuous function on $[0, T_{(n)}]$ and $\hat{m}_e(t) = 0$ for $t > T_{(n)}$ and hence $\hat{m}_e(\cdot)$ is a bounded function on $[0, \infty)$.

Let $Z_n(t) \sim Ga(k_n, \frac{t}{k_n})$ for $t > 0$, where $Ga(k_n, \frac{t}{k_n})$ denotes a Gamma distribution with mean $\mu_n(t) = t$ and variance $\sigma_n^2(t) = \frac{t^2}{k_n}$ and the density function is given by

$$f_{k_n,t}(z) = f\left(z \middle| k_n, \frac{t}{k_n}\right) = \left(\frac{k_n}{t}\right)^{k_n} \frac{1}{\Gamma(k_n)} z^{k_n - 1} e^{-\frac{k_n z}{t}}.$$

It easily follows that we can write our scale mixture estimator as

$$\begin{aligned} \hat{m}_m(t) &= \int_0^\infty \frac{\hat{m}_e(t\theta)}{\theta} \pi(\theta|k_n) d\theta \\ &= \int_0^\infty \hat{m}_e(u) f\left(u \middle| k_n, \frac{t}{k_n}\right) du \\ &= E[\hat{m}_e(Z_n(t))], \end{aligned} \tag{8.11}$$

Thus, by Feller approximation result in Lemma 8.2 it follows that $E[m(Z_n(t))]$ converges (pointwise) to $m(t)$ if we choose the sequence k_n such that $k_n \to \infty$ as $n \to \infty$. Next, by the consistency of $\hat{m}_e(t)$ and Dominated Convergence Theorem it follows that $E[\hat{m}_e(Z_n(t)) - m(Z_n(t))] \to 0$ and $n \to \infty$. Hence it follows that $\hat{m}_m(t)$ converges (pointwise) in probability to $m(t)$ as $k_n \to \infty$. This completes the proof of (i) in Theorem 8.2.

(b) Proof of Asymptotic Normality

First, notice that we can write,

$$\sqrt{n}(\hat{m}_m(t) - m(t)) = \sqrt{n}(\hat{m}_m(t) - \hat{m}_e(t)) + \sqrt{n}(\hat{m}_e(t) - m(t)), \tag{8.12}$$

where it is known from previous literature that $\sqrt{n}(\hat{m}_e(t) - m(t)) \sim GP(0, \sigma(\cdot,\cdot))$ and expression of the covariance function $\sigma(\cdot,\cdot)$ are as given in the statement of Theorem 8.2. Thus, it is sufficient to establish that first term in Eq. 8.12 converges in probability to zero as $n \rightarrow$ by choosing a suitable growth rate of the k_n sequence as a function of n.

Using the scale mixture formulation it follows that $\sqrt{n}(\hat{m}_m(t) - \hat{m}_e(t)) = \sqrt{n}E[\frac{\hat{m}_e(tY_n)}{Y_n} - \hat{m}_e(t)]$ where $Y_n \sim Ga(k_n + 1, 1/k_n)$

We use a first order Taylor's expansion around t to write

$$\frac{\hat{m}_e(tY_n)}{Y_n} = \frac{\hat{m}_e(t)}{Y_n} + \frac{(tY_n - t)\hat{m}_e'(t_n^*)}{Y_n},$$

where $t_n^* \xrightarrow{P} t$ as $n \rightarrow \infty$ because $Y_n \xrightarrow{P} 1$. It can be seen from (8.5) that $\hat{m}_e(t)$ is differentiable if $t \in (X_l, X_{l+1}), l = 1, \ldots, n-1$ and $\hat{m}_e(t)$ is not differentiable if $t = X_l, l = 1, \ldots, n-1$. Thus, $\hat{m}_e'(t_n^*)$ exists for $t_n^* \in [0, \infty)\backslash\{X_1, \ldots X_n\}$.

Second, we substitute the Taylor's expansion into $\sqrt{n}E[\frac{\hat{m}_e(tY_n)}{Y_n} - \hat{m}_e(t)]$

$$\begin{aligned}\sqrt{n}(\hat{m}_m(t) - \hat{m}_e(t)) &= \sqrt{n}E[\frac{\hat{m}_e(tY_n)}{Y_n} - \hat{m}_e(t)] \\ &= \sqrt{n}E\left[\frac{\hat{m}_e(t)}{Y_n} - \hat{m}_e(t) + \frac{(tY_n - t)\hat{m}_e\prime(t_n^*)}{Y_n}\right] \\ &= E\left[\sqrt{n}\left(\frac{1}{Y_n} - 1\right)\hat{m}_e(t) - \sqrt{n}\left(\frac{1}{Y_n} - 1\right)t\hat{m}_e\prime(t_n^*)\right]\end{aligned}$$

In order to complete the proof it is now sufficient to show that $\sqrt{n}\left(\frac{1}{Y_n} - 1\right) \xrightarrow{P} 0$ as $n \rightarrow \infty$. However, as $Y_n \sim Ga(k_n + 1, 1/k_n)$, it follows that

$$E\left[\sqrt{n}\left(\frac{1}{Y_n} - 1\right)\right] = \sqrt{n}\left(E\left[\frac{1}{Y_n}\right] - 1\right) = \sqrt{n}\left(\frac{k_n}{k_n + 1 - 1} - 1\right) = 0$$

and

$$Var\left[\sqrt{n}\left(\frac{1}{Y_n} - 1\right)\right] = n\ Var\left[\frac{1}{Y_n}\right] = n\frac{k_n^2}{k_n^2(k_n - 1)} = \frac{n}{k_n - 1}.$$

Thus id we assume that $k_n/n \rightarrow \infty$, i.e., $k_n = cn^{1+\epsilon}$ where $\epsilon > 0$, it can be seen that $var\left[\sqrt{n}\left(\frac{1}{Y_n} - 1\right)\right] \rightarrow 0$ as $n \rightarrow \infty$. Therefore, $\sqrt{n}\left(\frac{1}{Y_n} - 1\right) \xrightarrow{P} 0$ as $n \rightarrow \infty$ and this completes the proof of Theorem 8.2.

Remark 8.1 Notice that the asymptotic properties of $\hat{m}_m(t)$ are the same as those of the estimator of Yang [26] for complete data and the same as those of the estimator of Ghorai et al. [8] for censored data.

References

1. Abdous, B., and A. Berred. 2005. Mean residual life estimation. *Journal of Statistical Planning and Inference* 132: 3–19.
2. Agarwal, S.L., and S.L. Kalla. 1996. A generalized gamma distribution and its application in reliability. *Communications in Statistics—Theory and Methods* 25: 201–210.
3. Bhattacharjee, M.C. 1982. The class of mean residual lives and some consequences. *SIAM Journal of Algebraic Discrete Methods* 3: 56–65.
4. Chaubey, Y.P., and P.K. Sen. 1999. On smooth estimation of mean residual life. *Journal of Statistical Planning and Inference* 75: 223–236.
5. Chaubey, Y.P., and A. Sen. 2008. Smooth estimation of mean residual life under random censoring. In Ims collections—beyond parametrics in interdisciplinary research: Festschrift in honor of professor pranab k. *Sen* 1: 35–49.
6. Elandt-Johnson, R.C., and N.L. Johnson. 1980. *Survival models and data analysis*. New York: Wiley.
7. Feller. 1968. *An introduction to probability theory and its applications*. vol. I, 3rd ed. New York: Wiley.
8. Ghorai, J., A. Susarla., V, Susarla., and Van-Ryzin, J. 1982. Nonparametric Estimation of Mean Residual Life Time with Censored Data. In *Nonparametric statistical inference. vol. I*, Colloquia Mathematica Societatis, 32. North-Holland, Amsterdam-New York, 269-291.
9. Guess, F, and Proschan, F. (1988). Mean residual life theory and applications. In *Handbook of statistics 7, reliability and quality control*, ed. P.R. Krishnaiah., and Rao, C.R. 215–224.
10. Gupta, R.C., and D.M. Bradley. 2003. Representing the mean residual life in terms of the failure rate. *Mathematical and Computer Modelling* 37: 1271–1280.
11. Gupta, R.C., and S. Lvin. 2005. Monotonicity of failure rate and mean residual life function of a gamma-type model. *Applied Mathematics and Computation* 165: 623–633.
12. Hall, W.J., and J.A. Wellner. 1981. Mean residual life. In *Statistics and related topics*, ed. M. Csorgo, D.A. Dawson, J.N.K. Rao, and AKMdE Saleh, 169–184. Amsterdam, North-Holland.
13. Hille, E. (1948). *Functional analysis and semigruops*. American Mathematical Society vol.31.
14. Kalla, S.L., H.G. Al-Saqabi, and H.G. Khajah. 2001. A unified form of gamma-type distributions. *Applied Mathematics and Computation* 118: 175–187.
15. Kaplan, E.L., and P. Meier. 1958. Nonparametric estimation from incomplete observations. *Journal of American Statistical Association* 53: 457–481.
16. Kopperschmidt, K., and U. Potter. 2003. A non-parametric mean residual life estiamtor: An example from market research. *Developmetns in Applied Statistics* 19: 99–113.
17. Kulasekera, K.B. 1991. Smooth Nonparametric Estimation of Mean Residual Life. *Microelectronics Reliability* 31 (1): 97–108.
18. Lai, C.D., L. Zhang, and M. Xie. 2004. Mean residual life and other properties of weibull related bathtub shape failure rate distributions. *International Journal of Reliability, Quality and Safety Engineering* 11: 113–132.
19. Liu, S. (2007). *Modeling mean residual life function using scale mixtures* NC State University Dissertation. http://www.lib.ncsu.edu/resolver/1840.16/3045.
20. McLain, A., and S.K. Ghosh. 2011. Nonparametric estimation of the conditional mean residual life function with censored data. *Lifetime Data Analysis* 17: 514–532.
21. Morrison, D.G. 1978. On linearly increasing mean residual lifetimes. *Journal of Applied Probability* 15: 617–620.

22. Petrone, S., and P. Veronese. 2002. Non parametric mixture priors based on an exponential random scheme. *Statistical Methods and Applications* 11 (1): 1–20.
23. Ruiz, J.M., and A. Guillamon. 1996. nonparametric recursive estimator of residual life and vitality funcitons under mixing dependence condtions. *Communcation in Statistics–Theory and Methods* 4: 1999–2011.
24. Swanepoel, J.W.H., and F.C. Van Graan. 2005. A new kernel distribution function estimator based on a non-parametric transformation of the data. *The Scadinavian Journal of Statistics* 32: 551–562.
25. Tsang, A.H.C., and A.K.S. Jardine. 1993. Estimation of 2-parameter weibull distribution from incomplete data with residual lifetimes. *IEEE Transactions on Reliability* 42: 291–298.
26. Yang, G.L. 1978. Estimation of a biometric function. *Annals of Statistics* 6: 112–116.

Chapter 9
Something Borrowed, Something New: Precise Prediction of Outcomes from Diverse Genomic Profiles

J. Sunil Rao, Jie Fan, Erin Kobetz and Daniel Sussman

Abstract Precise outcome predictions at an individual level from diverse genomic data is a problem of great interest as the focus on precision medicine grows. This typically requires estimation of subgroup-specific models which may differ in their mean and/or variance structure. Thus in order to accurately predict outcomes for new individuals, it's necessary to map them to a subgroup from which the prediction can be derived. The situation becomes more interesting when some predictors are common across subgroups and others are not. We describe a series of statistical methodologies under two different scenarios that can provide this mapping, as well as combine information that can be shared across subgroups, with information that is subgroup-specific. We demonstrate that prediction errors can be markedly reduced as compared to not borrowing strength at all. We then apply the approaches in order to predict colon cancer survival from DNA methylation profiles that vary by age groups, and identify those significant methylation sites that are shared across the age groups and those that are age-specific.

9.1 Introduction

Traditional mixed effect model has long been used by animal geneticists to incorporate population structure and familial relationships [2, 5, 15]. Linear mixed models have been widely used to test for association in genome-wide association studies (GWAS) because of their demonstrated effectiveness in accounting for relatedness among samples and in controlling for population stratification and other confounding factors [14, 17, 25, 26]. Methods like efficient mixed-model association (EMMA, [13]) and genome-wide efficient mixed-model association (GEMMA, [27]) have been developed for exact computation of standard test statistics. As noted in Jiang [10], (Sect. 2.3), there are two types of prediction problems associated with the mixed effects model. The first type, which is encountered more often in practice,

J. Sunil Rao (✉) · J. Fan · E. Kobetz · D. Sussman
Division of Biostatistics, Department of Public Health Sciences,
Miller School of Medicine, University of Miami, Miami, FL 33136, USA
e-mail: jrao@miami.edu

A. Adhikari et al. (eds.), *Mathematical and Statistical Applications in Life Sciences and Engineering*, https://doi.org/10.1007/978-981-10-5370-2_9

is prediction of mixed effects; the second type is prediction of future observation. The prediction of mixed effect has a long history, starting with C.R. Henderson in his early work in the field of animal breeding [4]. The best-known method for this kind of prediction is best linear unbiased prediction, or BLUP. Robinson [19] gave a wide-ranging account of BLUP with examples and applications. In practice, any assumed model is subject to misspecification. Jiang et al. [11] developed the observed best prediction (OBP) method to obtain estimators, which is more robust to model misspecification in terms of the predictive performance. The prediction of future observations has received less attention, although there are plenty of such prediction problems with practical interest [12]. For the prediction of mixed effect, recent work [3, 23] neglects the role of the random effect if the class of the new observation is unknown. This will result in missing an important part if only the estimated fixed effect is used as the estimation of the mixed effect. This is crucial when the variance of the random effect is large. It is important to find a group that the new observation is similar to in order to make precise prediction. Classified mixed-model prediction (CMMP) [9] classifies the new observation to a group in the population and then make predictions for the mixed effect and future observation on top of the classified random effect even though the class of the new observation is unknown.

The hunt for refined sub-typing of disease by techniques like clustering of genomic profiles is based on the premise that mapping individuals to distinct subtypes/subgroups/groups can lead to more precise predictions of outcomes like survival (see for example, [1, 20, 24]). New individuals are mapped to a given subgroup using a distance-type metric based on their genomic profiles to cluster centers, and then a model-based prediction derived using subgroup-specific information only. If all profiles are identical across the subgroups, but the effects of the individual elements might vary, then improved predictions can be estimated using CMMP [9].

Briefly, under an assumed nested error linear mixed model relating the outcome to the predictors, the CMMP procedure optimally classifies a new observation to the subgroup from which it is derived, by minimizing the mean squared error of the (empirical) best predictor (BP) across subgroups. In essence, the subgroup label associated with the new observation is treated as an unknown parameter, and this is estimated in an optimal way. Once the subgroup is identified, its corresponding random effect is assigned to the new fixed effect, and the full outcome prediction generated.This procedure was proven to be consistent in both a mean squared error sense and a point prediction sense. It also demonstrated significantly better empirical performance in terms of lower prediction errors than using methods which ignore classification of the random effect.

To better understand why simply mapping new observations to cluster centroids may not work, consider an extreme example. Take for instance a situation where covariates are all indicators that define different intervention groups. Many observations might be in the same intervention group, however their responses will not be identical. Here the covariate vector of fixed effects does not provide distinct information at the subject level, and hence the predictions will not be accurate. Hence the random effect plays a crucial role of adding additional information at the subject level. Also note that trying to model correlation structure between the random effects may not be useful since it's often assumed that the random effects are uncorrelated, however for prediction, clearly the new observation's random effect is indeed correlated with one of the original random effects.

While the CMMP is certainly a significant step forward, it's not reasonable to assume that each subgroup will be defined by the exact same genomic profiles (with varying effect sizes). Subgroups are likely to contain some common genomic markers as well as some distinct ones. This is precisely the scenario we study in this paper, where our goal is to predict colon cancer survival from diverse DNA methylation profiles. We will detail a series of statistical methodologies which combine the common information across subgroups with subgroup-specific information. One of these strategies is an extension of the CMMP, while the others derive from optimization of a weighted objective function which combines both pieces of information.

The different scenarios correspond to differences in what information is present and what assumptions are made. In all scenarios, we assume the following : the existence of a training data set from the population where both the response and covariates are observed, the existence of an intermediate dataset consisting of responses and covariates from the same subgroup for which a future prediction is desired, and the new observation for which only the covariates are observed. We considered the scenario where the underlying mixed model is assumed to be correctly specified, and another where it is potentially misspecified. Within the second scenario, we do not assume the new observation comes from one of the original subgroups.

9.2 Methods

We consider the following problem: we want to model the relationship between a response y and vector of covariates $\mathbf{x} = (x_1, x_2, \ldots, x_p)$. We assume the population consists of a finite number of diverse subgroups and that the variation in the data can be captured by a linear mixed effects model with subgroup-specific random intercepts only. Typically, we can write the underlying linear mixed model relating y to $\mathbf{x}$ as,

$$y_{ij} = x_{ij1}\beta_1 + \cdots + x_{ijp}\beta_p + \alpha_i + e_{ij}, \; i = 1, \ldots, m, j = 1, \ldots, n_i, \tag{9.1}$$

where m indicates the number of subgroups with a sample of n_i observations for each, the α_i are $N(0, \sigma_\alpha^2)$ subgroup-specific random effects, and the e_{ij} are $N(0, \sigma_e^2)$ random errors. We assume the random effects and errors are independent. Note that not all of the β_v; $v = 1, \ldots, p$ may be non-zero.

However, our paradigm is a slight variation on this. We assume that we have a training dataset of size $N = \sum_{i=1}^m n_i$ with the response and observed values on only a subset of the covariates $\mathbf{x}^{(1)} = (x_1, \ldots, x_{p_1})$. We also have an additional set of data (what we call *intermediate data*) consisting of n_n observations from one of the subgroups with observed values of the response, $\mathbf{x}^{(1)} = (x_1, \ldots, x_{p_1})$ and an additional set of predictors $\mathbf{x}^{(2)} = (x_{p_1+1}, \ldots, x_p)$. However, we do not always know which subgroup this additional data derives from. Our goal is to then make a prediction for y at a completely newly observed full set of predictors that is independent from each of the two sets of data described above. There is a hint that we are given, however that the new observation comes from the same subgroup as the intermediate data. If we had observed values from all of the subgroups for all of the covariates in the training data, we could fit a random coefficients model and then worry only about classifying the new observation to the right subgroup. However, our training data does not have information on these subgroup-specific covariates.

One may naturally ask when such a situation might present itself in practice. Consider the following example: risk factors for an outcome are determined in a study using patients coming from different subgroups (i.e. the training data). A linear mixed model can be fit to relate the risk factors to the outcome. When making predictions for a new patient though, it's recognized that additional risk factors that were not collected as part of the training data are also potentially at play. These might be thought of as additional co-morbidities. It's important to note that the subgroup label for the new observation is also unknown. So to improve predictions, the intermediate dataset is also collected. This intermediate data can be thought of as a baseline set of information for the new patient for which the prediction at some future point is desired. The question then becomes, can predictions be built using both sets of data that are more accurate than those using the intermediate data only?

We label the parameter vector for the common covariates as b_1, and the parameter vectors for the unique covariates as b_2. We assume no overall intercept in the model and also that the random intercepts α_i are assumed to have a Normal distribution with mean 0, and variance σ_α^2, the errors e_{ij} are i.i.d. random variables from Normal distribution with mean 0, and variance σ_e^2 and that the α_i's and e_i's are independent.

We will examine two different Scenarios for such predictions which differ on whether assuming model (9.1) with only $\mathbf{x}^{(1)}$ for the training data is correct or not.

9.2.1 *Scenario 1*

Suppose we mistakenly assume the training data denoted as $(X^{(1)}, \mathbf{y})$, where $X^{(1)} = (x_{ij1}, \ldots, x_{ijp_1})_{i=1,\ldots,m}^{j=1,\ldots,n_i}$, has all of the relevant covariate information in it. For the intermediate data, we are not sure whether b_2 equals 0 or not. The intermediate data is denoted as $(X_{itm}^{(1)}, X_{itm}^{(2)}, y_{itm})$ (itm indicating intermediate data), with common covariates $X_{itm}^{(1)} = (x_{k1}, \ldots, x_{kp_1})_{k=1,\ldots,n_n}$, group-specific covariates $X_{itm}^{(2)} = (x_{k(p_1+1)}, \ldots, x_{kp})_{k=1,\ldots,n_n}$, and response $y_{itm} = (y_k)'_{k=1,\ldots,n_n}$.

Here are the steps of predicting a new response y_{new} from a corresponding vector $x_{new} = (x_{new}^{(1)}, x_{new}^{(2)})$:

1. Estimate b_1, α under model

$$y_{ij} = x_{ij1}\beta_1 + \cdots + x_{ijp_1}\beta_{p_1} + \alpha_i + e_{ij}, \qquad i = 1, \ldots, m, j = 1, \ldots, n_i \quad (9.2)$$

with training data $(X^{(1)}, y)$, denote the estimators as $\hat{b}_1, \hat{\alpha}$.

2. Estimate the group I that new observation belongs to with CMMP method using $\hat{b}_1, \hat{\alpha}$ and intermediate data $(X_{itm}^{(1)}, y_{itm})$, denote the estimator as $\hat{I}$.

3. Combine the training data and intermediate data as $\begin{pmatrix} X^{(1)} & 0 & y \\ X_{itm}^{(1)} & X_{itm}^{(2)} & y_{itm} \end{pmatrix}$, which is grouped as $g = (1, \ldots, 1, \ldots, m, \ldots, m, \hat{I}, \ldots, \hat{I})'$. Then use this combined data to estimate b_1, b_2, α, and denote the estimators as $\tilde{b}_1, \tilde{b}_2, \tilde{\alpha}$.

4. Estimate I with CMMP method again using $\tilde{b}_1, \tilde{b}_2, \tilde{\alpha}$ and intermediate data $(X_{itm}^{(1)}, X_{itm}^{(2)}, y_{itm})$, and denote the estimator as $\tilde{I}$.

5. The prediction of the new observation is $\tilde{y}_{new} = x_{new}^{(1)}\tilde{b}_1 + x_{new}^{(2)}\tilde{b}_2 + \tilde{\alpha}_{\tilde{I}}$

If we believe the model for the training data is misspecified, we can robustify Scenario 1 by using the best predictive estimator (BPE) which is more robust for model misspecification could be employed instead of the ML estimator and REML estimator in step 1 [8].

9.2.2 *Scenario 2*

In the former situation, we assume the regression coefficients of the group-specific covariates to be 0 for the training data, however, this is not usually the case. In this case, the new observation may or may not be from one of the observed subgroups. We can now frame the problem from a different perspective: as an optimization problem that amounts to minimizing the penalized error sum of squares of training data and intermediate data. Two strategies are adopted as follows: one is no intercept for training data, and the other is a varying intercept by subgroup for the training data.

9.2.2.1 Method 2.1

In Scenario 1, mapping of a new individual to a subgroup is done by optimally assigning a subgroup's associate random effect to the new individual. For Scenario 2, we are more interested in going after the mapping via direct estimation of all the coefficients and random effects when the training and intermediate datasets are combined. We want to borrow strength from the training data to improve the estimation. The objective function formed by combining the two data sources is

$$
\begin{aligned}
Q(b_1, b_2, \alpha_I) = & \sum_{i=1}^{m}\sum_{j=1}^{n_i}(y_{ij} - X_{ij}^{(1)}b_1)^2 \\
& + \sum_{k=1}^{n_n}(y_k - X_k^{(1)}b_1 - X_k^{(2)}b_2 - \alpha_I)^2,
\end{aligned}
\tag{9.3}
$$

subject to $\|b_1\|_1 \le \gamma$, where $\gamma \in [0, \infty)$, $X_{ij}^{(1)} = (x_{ij1}, \ldots, x_{ijp_1})$, $X_k^{(1)} = (x_{k1}, \ldots, x_{kp_1})$, $X_k^{(2)} = (x_{k(p_1+1)}, \ldots, x_{kp})$. We minimize (9.3) over b_1, b_2, and α_I, and get estimators $\tilde{b}_1, \tilde{b}_2, \tilde{\alpha}_I$. Then the prediction of the new observation is $\tilde{y}_{new} = x_{new}^{(1)}\tilde{b}_1 + x_{new}^{(2)}\tilde{b}_2 + \tilde{\alpha}_I$.

The reason for constraining $\|b_1\|_1$ is that we are not sure whether the common covariates are useful in predicting y_{new}. The tuning parameter γ indicates how much confidence we have in the common covariates.

Setting $\gamma = 0$ simply excludes this information from training data. Taking $\gamma = \infty$ leads to including all the common variables in the model. For tuning γ, we use leave-one-out cross validation with $m-1$ groups training data and intermediate data in the cross-validated training set, and the left out cluster in the cross-validated testing set to estimate γ over a grid of values.

Lemma 9.1 *The solution to Method 2.1 is a unique solution as long as* $N = \sum_{i=1}^{m} n_i > p + 1$.

Proof

$$
\begin{aligned}
Q(b_1, b_2, \alpha_I) = & \sum_{i=1}^{m}\sum_{j=1}^{n_i}(y_{ij} - X_{ij}^{(1)}b_1)^2 \\
& + \sum_{k=1}^{n_n}(y_k - X_k^{(1)}b_1 - X_k^{(2)}b_2 - \alpha_I)^2,
\end{aligned}
$$

subject to $\|b_1\|_1 \le \gamma$, where $\gamma \in [0, \infty)$, $X_{ij}^{(1)} = (x_{ij1}, \ldots, x_{ijp_1})$, $X_k^{(1)} = (x_{k1}, \ldots, x_{kp_1})$, $X_k^{(2)} = (x_{k(p_1+1)}, \ldots, x_{kp})$.

Denote $\beta^* = (b_1^{'}, b_2^{'}, \alpha_I)^{'}$, $N = \sum_{i=1}^{m} n_i$. Set $c_1 = \{i, j | i = 1, \ldots, m, j = 1, \ldots, n_i\}$ contains all the observations of the training data; set $c_2 = \{k | k = 1, \ldots, n_n\}$ contains all the observations of the intermediate data.

$$
X^* = \begin{bmatrix} x_{111} & \ldots & x_{11p_1} & 0 & \ldots & 0 \\ \ldots & \ldots & \ldots & \ldots & \ldots & \ldots \\ x_{mn_m1} & \ldots & x_{mn_mp_1} & 0 & \ldots & 0 \end{bmatrix}; \quad X_{itm}^* = \begin{bmatrix} x_{11} & \ldots & x_{1p} & 1 \\ \ldots & \ldots & \ldots & \ldots \\ x_{n_n1} & \ldots & x_{n_np} & 1 \end{bmatrix}
$$

The dimension of X^*, X_{itm}^* is $N \times (p+1)$ and $n_n \times (p+1)$ respectively.
(Or $X^* = (X^{(1)}, O_1, \mathbf{0})$, where O_1 is a matrix of zero with dimension $N \times (p - p_1)$,

$\mathbf{0}$ is a vector of 0 s with length N. $X^*_{itm} = (X^{(1)}_{itm}, X^{(2)}_{itm}, \mathbf{1})$, where $\mathbf{1}$ is a vector of 1 s with length n_n.)

The objective function can be rewritten as

$$\begin{aligned} Q(\beta^*) &= \sum_{i=1}^{m}\sum_{j=1}^{n_i}(y_{ij} - X^{(1)}_{ij} b_1 - 0 \times b_2 - 0 \times \alpha_I)^2 \\ &+ \sum_{k=1}^{n_n}(y_k - X^{(1)}_k b_1 - X^{(2)}_k b_2 - \alpha_I)^2 \\ &= \sum_{i=1}^{m}\sum_{j=1}^{n_i}(y_{ij} - X^*_{ij}\beta^*)^2 + \sum_{k=1}^{n_n}(y_k - X^*_{itm,k}\beta^*)^2 \\ &= \sum_{l\in\{c1,c2\}}(y_l - X^*_l\beta^*)^2 \end{aligned}$$

Thus the solution is a partially constrained LASSO that will have a unique solution due to convexity [22] as long as $N > p + 1$.

9.2.2.2 Method 2.2

It may be more reasonable to include a varying coefficient for the training data in the objective function (9.3). The varying coefficient for each group in the training data corresponds to a random intercept in the mixed effect model. The objective function then becomes:

$$\begin{aligned} Q(b_1, b_2, \alpha, \alpha_I) = &\sum_{i=1}^{m}\sum_{j=1}^{n_i}(y_{ij} - X^{(1)}_{ij} b_1 - \alpha_i)^2 \\ &+ \sum_{k=1}^{n_n}(y_k - X^{(1)}_k b_1 - X^{(2)}_k b_2 - \alpha_I)^2, \end{aligned} \tag{9.4}$$

subject to $\|b_1\|_1 \le \gamma$, i.e. $\sum_{l=1}^{p_1}|\beta_l| \le \gamma$, where $\gamma \in [0, \infty)$.

Similarly by minimizing (9.4), we can get estimators for b_1, b_2, α_I, denoted as $\tilde{b}_1, \tilde{b}_2, \tilde{\alpha}_I$. Then the prediction of the new observation is $\tilde{y}_{new} = x^{(1)}_{new}\tilde{b}_1 + x^{(2)}_{new}\tilde{b}_2 + \tilde{\alpha}_I$. Notice that we do not use the α from the training data in the prediction directly but rather they are at play in the estimation of b_1 and b_2. The choice of the tuning parameter is similar as in Method 2.1. Note that Method 2.2 has m more additional parameters to estimate than Method 2.1.

Lemma 9.2 *The solution to Method 2.2 is a unique solution as long as* $N > p + m + 1$.

Proof

$$Q(b_1, b_2, \alpha, \alpha_I) = \sum_{i=1}^{m} \sum_{j=1}^{n_i} (y_{ij} - X_{ij}^{(1)} b_1 - \alpha_i)^2 + \sum_{k=1}^{n_n} (y_k - X_k^{(1)} b_1 - X_k^{(2)} b_2 - \alpha_I)^2,$$

Denote $\beta^{**} = (b_1^{'}, b_2^{'}, \alpha_1, \ldots, \alpha_m, \alpha_I)^{'}$, $X^{**} = (X^{(1)}, O_1, Z, \mathbf{0})$, where O_1 is a matrix of 0s with dimension $N \times (p - p_1)$, $Z = diag(Z_1, \ldots, Z_m)$, $Z_i = (1, \ldots, 1)^{'}_{n_i,1}$, $\mathbf{0}$ is a vector of 0s with length N. $X_{itm}^{**} = (X_{itm}^{(1)}, X_{itm}^{(2)}, O_2, \mathbf{1})$, where O_2 is a matrix of 0s with dimension $n_n \times m$, $\mathbf{1}$ is a vector of 1s with length n_n. The dimension of X^{**}, X_{itm}^{**} is $N \times (p + m + 1)$ and $n_n \times (p + m + 1)$ respectively.

Similarly as before, objective function can be rewritten as

$$\begin{aligned} Q(\beta^{**}) &= \sum_{i=1}^{m} \sum_{j=1}^{n_i} (y_{ij} - X_{ij}^{(1)} b_1 - \alpha_i)^2 + \sum_{k=1}^{n_n} (y_k - X_k^{(1)} b_1 - X_k^{(2)} b_2 - \alpha_I)^2 \\ &= \sum_{i=1}^{m} \sum_{j=1}^{n_i} (y_{ij} - X_{ij}^{**} \beta^{**})^2 + \sum_{k=1}^{n_n} (y_k - X_{itm,k}^{**} \beta^{**})^2 \\ &= \sum_{l \in \{c1,c2\}} (y_l - X_l^{**} \beta^{**})^2 \end{aligned}$$

Thus the solution is a partially constrained LASSO that will have a unique solution due to convexity [22] as long as $N > (p + m + 1)$.

9.2.2.3 Method 2.3

When the new observation is from one of the m subgroups or from a very similar subgroup, the random effect of the new observation should be very close with the random effect of that group. Therefore we can add another constraint to Eq. (9.4) to force α_I to be close to a certain α_i.

1. Estimate b_1, α under model (9.2) using training data $(X^{(1)}, Y)$ and denote the estimator as $\hat{b}_1, \hat{\alpha}$.
2. Estimate I with CMMP method using $\hat{b}_1, \hat{\alpha}$ and intermediate data $(X_{itm}^{(1)}, Y_{itm})$, and denote the estimator as $\hat{I}$.
3. Minimize equation

$$Q(b_1, b_2, \alpha, \alpha_I) = \sum_{i=1}^{m}\sum_{j=1}^{n_i}(y_{ij} - X_{ij}^{(1)}b_1 - \alpha_i)^2 + \sum_{k=1}^{n_n}(y_k - X_k^{(1)}b_1 - X_k^{(2)}b_2 - \alpha_I)^2 \quad (9.5)$$

subject to $\|b_1\|_1 \leq \gamma$, $\|\alpha_I - \alpha_{\hat{I}}\|_1 \leq \tau$, where $\gamma, \tau \in [0, \infty)$. Denote the estimators as $\tilde{b}_1, \tilde{b}_2, \tilde{\alpha}, \tilde{\alpha}_I$

4. Estimate I with CMMP method using $\tilde{b}_1, \tilde{b}_2, \tilde{\alpha}$ and intermediate data ($X_{itm}^{(1)}, X_{itm}^{(2)}, Y_{itm}$), and denote the estimator as $\tilde{I}$.
5. The prediction of the new observation is $\tilde{y}_{new} = x_{new}^{(1)}\tilde{b}_1 + x_{new}^{(2)}\tilde{b}_2 + \tilde{\alpha}_{\tilde{I}}$

Equation (9.4) is a special case of Eq. (9.5) when $\tau = \infty$. Since the new observation is from one of the m groups (or from a very similar group), we add the second constraint to force the behavior of α_I to be similar to $\alpha_{\hat{I}}$. The value of this tuning parameter can be obtained by cross-validation. However, instead of leave one cluster out cross-validation, we use leave one observation out per group cross-validation to ensure that all the m groups of random effects are estimated. One of the observations in the intermediate data is left in the cross-validated testing set, the rest are in the cross-validated training set. The values of γ, τ are selected optimizing over a grid of values.

9.3 Results

9.3.1 Simulation Studies

We consider a simple example of linear mixed model with two covariates only, where x_1 is the common covariate, and x_2 carries the unique covariate information. We generated the x_{ij1} and x_{ij2} from a Normal distribution with mean 0 and variance 1, the random effects were assumed to be, $\alpha_i \sim N(0, {\sigma_\alpha}^2)$, and the random errors, $e_{ij} \sim N(0, {\sigma_e}^2)$. The true coefficient values were set as $(b_1, b_2) = (2, 3)$. The random effects and errors were uncorrelated. All simulations for the proposed methods are compared against the method that only uses the intermediate data. We call this method the Intermediate Data Model (IDM). This is the most obvious naive estimator to use since we do not know the group the new observation belongs to from the training data. We could instead average predictions across all the groups in the training data. This is usually called the Regression Predictor (RP). However, as shown in [9], the RP can behave quite poorly compared to classified predictions.

9.3.1.1 Scenario 1

For Scenario 1, we set $b_2 = 0$ for the training data, and compare against the IDM method in terms of predicting y_{new}. There are $m = 50$ subgroups in the population with $n_i = 5$ observations for each subgroup. The number of intermediate observations n_n is 5. The intermediate data and new observation are generated from the same group which is a random group of the m groups. The prediction squared error $(\hat{y}_{new} - y_{new})^2$ for the IDM method and prediction squared error $(\tilde{y}_{new} - y_{new})^2$ for Method 1 is calculated. The simulation is repeated for $T = 1000$ times, the prediction mean squared error for the IDM method $PMSE_{IDM} = \sum_{t=1}^{T}(\hat{y}_{t,new} - y_{t,new})^2/T$ is compared to the prediction mean squared error for Method 1 $PMSE_1 = \sum_{t=1}^{T}(\tilde{y}_{t,new} - y_{t,new})^2/T$. The percentage of change $100 * (PMSE_{IDM} - PMSE_1)/PMSE_{IDM}$ is also recorded. Set $\sigma_\alpha^2 = 1$, σ_e^2 changes from 0.1 to 1, 2 and 4. The results are shown in Table 9.1.

From Table 9.1 we can see that Method 1 outperforms the IDM method when the variance of error is large relative to the variance of random effect. When the variance of the error is relatively small, making use of the intermediate data is enough to estimate the coefficients. However, when the variance of the error is relatively large, the IDM estimator is not reliable any more, the proposed Method 1 which borrows strength across all subgroups in the training data in estimating the coefficients shows its benefit.

9.3.1.2 Scenario 2

We now let the coefficient of the unique covariate $b_2 = 3$ for the training data. Everything else remains the same. We compare our three strategies in Scenario 2 (denoted as Method 2.1, Method 2.2, and Method 2.3 respectively) with the IDM method. The value of the tuning parameter γ is set to be 2 and the value of τ is set to be 0.1. The simulation is repeated for $T = 1000$ times, the prediction mean squared error of the IDM method $PMSE_{IDM} = \sum_{t=1}^{T}(\hat{y}_{t,new} - y_{t,new})^2/T$ is compared to the prediction mean squared error of Method 2.1 $PMSE_1 = \sum_{t=1}^{T}(\tilde{y}_{t,new} - y_{t,new})^2/T$, prediction mean squared error of Method 2.2 $PMSE_2 = \sum_{t=1}^{T}(\tilde{y}_{t,new} - y_{t,new})^2/T$ and

Table 9.1 Prediction Mean Squared Error (PMSE) for 1000 realizations of simulation according to Scenario 1. The simulation design used $m = 50$ subgroups for the training data, with 5 observations per subgroup. The number of observations in the intermediate data was also set at 5

$\sigma_e{}^2$	0.1	1	2	4
IDM	0.290	3.698	6.034	14.754
Method 1	0.639	2.006	3.391	6.324
Percentage change	−120.4	45.8	43.8	57.1

Table 9.2 Prediction Mean Squared Error (PMSE) for 1000 realizations of simulation according to Scenario 2. The simulation design used $m = 50$ subgroups for the training data, with 5 observations per subgroup. The number of observations in the intermediate data was also set at 5

${\sigma_e}^2$	0.1	1	2	4
IDM	0.409	3.271	6.275	11.863
Method 2.1	0.229	1.763	3.404	7.283
Percentage change	43.9	46.1	45.8	38.6
Method 2.2	0.359	1.725	3.252	6.791
Percentage change	12.2	47.3	48.2	42.8
Method 2.3	0.616	1.928	3.115	6.575
Percentage change	−50.6	41.1	50.4	44.6

prediction mean squared error of Method 2.3 $PMSE_3 = \sum_{t=1}^{T}(\tilde{y}_{t,new} - y_{t,new})^2/T$. The percentage of change $100 * (PMSE_{IDM} - PMSE_i)/PMSE_{IDM}$, $i = 1, 2, 3$ is also recorded in Table 9.2. Similarly $\sigma_\alpha^2 = 1$, σ_e^2 changes from 0.1 to 1, 2 and 4.

From Table 9.2 we can see that Method 2.1, Method 2.2 and Method 2.3 outperform the IDM method when the variance of error is large relative to the variance of random effect. Moreover, Method 2.1 beats the IDM method even though the variance of error is relatively small (equals 0.1 say). In other words, Method 2.1 outperforms the IDM method in terms of PMSE in all considered situations. When the variance of the error is relatively small, Method 2.3 does not perform as well as Method 2.1 and Method 2.2. But as the variance of the error goes up, the PMSE of Method 2.3 becomes slightly smaller than PMSE of Methods 2.1 and 2.2.

9.3.2 Predicting Colon Cancer Survival from Diverse DNA Methylation Profiles

For this study, we analyze CRC samples from The Cancer Genome Atlas (TCGA) https://tcga-data.nci.nih.gov/tcga. TCGA is a public repository data portal of high-quality pan-cancer tumor samples where clinical information, metadata, histopathology and molecular profiling information is available to researchers. For some cancers, non-tumor samples are also in the repository. It's a data repository that's commonly used to study underlying genomic determinants of cancer.

The total number of patients is 460 with information about 80 variables. There are 295 tumor (with a matched normal) issues. We extracted these 293 observations from the total 460 observations, 2 observations are missing because there are no match for them. The summary of some clinical variables are shown in the following: 134 of the 292 patients are female (46%). 204 of the patients are White (70%), 58 of

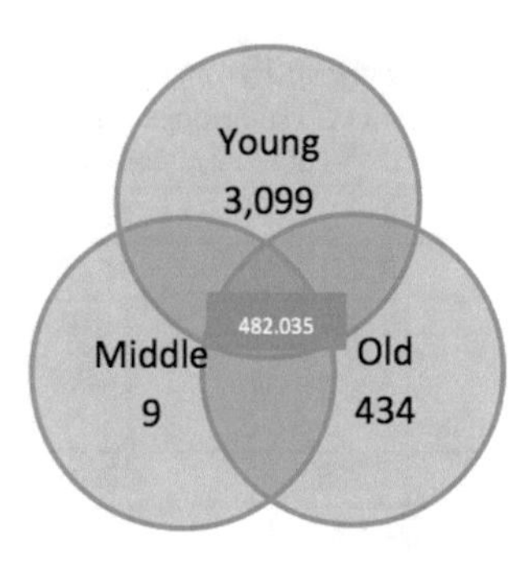

Fig. 9.1 Significantly differential methylation sites (right) for the different age groups

them are Black (20%), 11 of them are Asian (4%), one of them is American Indian, and the race information about the rest is missing (6%). 43 of the patients are dead (14.7%), the rest are censored (85.3%).

Colon cancer samples were assayed using Illumina HumanMethylation 450 K arrays. So-called *M* values were used in the analysis which were available directly on the TCGA website download portal. These values were arrived at after standard preprocessing of raw methylation data (www.bioconductor.org/packages/release/bioc/vignettes/lumi/inst/doc/methylationAnalysis.pdf).

We sample 19 censored from the total 249 censored observations. All the 43 dead observations and these 19 censored observations form a new data set. We grouped the age variable of this data set into three groups: Young, Middle, and Old. There is some growing evidence to suggest that at least some DNA methylation varies by age for colorectal cancer [18], however this has not been examined in a genome-wide manner. The numbers of observations per age grouping is provided in Table 9.3 along with the age ranges within each broad grouping.

To select the significantly differentially methylated sites we used a Bayesian ANOVA analysis [6, 7]. It was done using the Middle age group as a baseline to look for differences between groups in methylation sites with respect to how disease methylation values differ from their matched normal values. Pictorially we can view this analysis in the following Venn diagram Fig. 9.1.

We used the square root of survival time as our response of interest. The squared root of survival time does not differ significantly for different age groups (see Fig. 9.2 and Table 9.4). One thing we notice is that the survival time increases as age increases.

Table 9.3 Summary of age group

	Min	Max	Mean	No. of obv
Old	77	90	81.8	19
Young	34	58	47.3	15
Middle	61	75	69.3	28

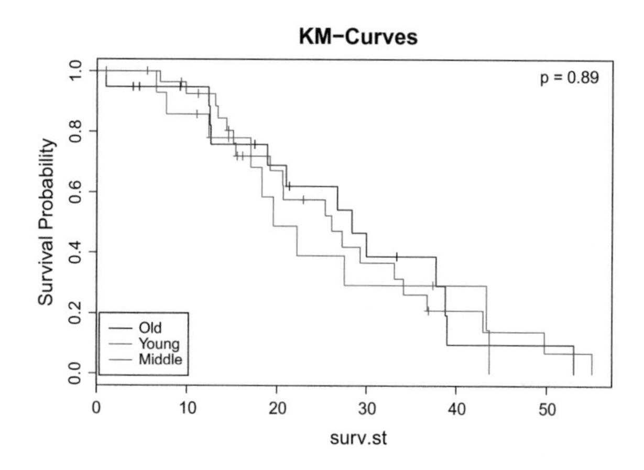

Fig. 9.2 Kaplan-Meier curves for the different age groups

Table 9.4 Summary of surv.st by age group

	Min	Median	Mean	Max	No. of obv
Old	1	21.02	22.22	53.11	19
Young	1	17.03	19.66	43.70	15
Middle	5.57	19.89	22.87	55.15	28

Table 9.5 Summary of stage by age group

	NA	Stage I	Stage II	Stage III	Stage IV	No. of obv
Old	1(5.3%)	0(0%)	10(52.6%)	5(26.3%)	3(15.7%)	19
Young	1(6.7%)	1(6.7%)	1(6.7%)	7(46.7%)	5(33.3%)	15
Middle	1(3.6%)	2(7.1%)	13(46.4%)	4(14.3%)	8(28.6%)	28

This is because that there is larger percentage of advanced cancer stage patients for the young aged group (Table 9.5).

Use the `superpc.train` function from superpc package in R to calculate the Cox scores of each predictor in the four categories (Young, Middle, Old, and overlap), and pick up top three predictors (admittedly an arbitrary cutoff but still illustrative of the methodology), with the largest value of absolute value of Cox score in each categories and use them for future analysis.

We then illustrate our methodologies making predictions for test data for each age group. Let us take middle aged group patients as example to illustrate how. The training data are the 19 old and 15 young patients. There are 3 common predictors for the population data. Among the 28 middle aged patients, 6 (21%) of them were chosen to be the test data and the rest 22 were the intermediate data. There is information of 3 common predictors and 3 group-specific predictors for the middle aged patients. For our newly proposed methods, we dealt with censoring by using Stute weights [21]. We did comparisons against the following methods:

Table 9.6 Comparison of three groups in terms of empirical MSPE

Control	Young	Middle	Old
IDM(Surv)	196.27	229.83	245.68
	(250.38)	(72.11)	(263.87)
Method 1	136.86	177.92	124.28
	(104.38)	(65.90)	(90.05)
Method 2.1	72.98	143. 41	96.34
	(94.02)	(66.22)	(56.15)
Method 2.2	57.87	143.90	96.69
	(49.94)	(61.26)	(53.98)
Enet.wls(All)	19188.09	25329.78	17695.19
	(33367.87)	(36708.73)	(25107.39)
Control	162.77	168.03	190.57
	(69.48)	(83.68)	(132.65)

IDM(Surv): We use the 22 middle aged patients to build a parametric survival model with the squared root of survival being the response, and use this model to predict the survival of the test data. The distribution of data was chosen to be the one that minimize the MSPE of the test data. The survreg function in R was used to fit these models.

Enet.wls (All): Simple elastic net method is applied to the data weighted by the Kaplan-Meier weights [16]. The elastic net estimates are obtained using glmnet function in R. "All" indicates that all of the 485577 predictors are used in the analysis.

Control: Similar to Method 1, we used the 15 young patients and 19 old patients and 22 middle aged patients as the population data and calculated the mean value of the 9 group-specific predictors ($\bar{x}_j^{(i)}, j=1, \ldots, 9; i = 1, 2, 3$ where j indicates the group-specific predictor, $j = 1, 2, 3$ are corresponding to the young group, $j = 4, 5, 6$ to the middle age group, $j = 7, 8, 9$ to the old age group; i indicates the age group, $i = 1, 2, 3$ corresponding to young, middle, and old respectively. The 6 middle aged patients are the test data and we pretend we do not know the group information on them. For the kth test observation, we calculate the distance between the age-specific predictors of the test observation and the mean of the predictors for each group. We then group the test observation by minimizing this distance and assign the mean survival time for the group as the predicted survival time for the test observation.

All scenarios were repeated 10 times using a different seed to determine which observations per group were in the test, intermediate (if the case) and training data while keeping the respective dataset totals fixed throughout. The results of the analyses are presented in Table 9.6. Mean MSPE values (and standard deviations) are shown in Table 9.6. Method 2.1 performs the best with respect to survival predictions for the Middle and Old age groups while Method 2.2 does the best for the Young age group. None of the competing methods examined do better than the newly proposed methods and using the intermediate data alone (ignoring any kind of borrowing strength across groups) was also shown to be suboptimal.

9.4 Discussion

These models begin to explain the contribution of epigenomic markers to observed variability in disease outcomes experienced by different age groups with CRC. Interestingly, the paradigms show that it is not only important to focus on what is unique about a given subpopulation, but also shared variation with methylation of CRCs. In these models, the methylation sites in common served as the common covariates, while methylation sites unique to each group were the only age-specific covariates considered. The findings demonstrate not only the predictive capability of methylation with respect to survival, but also the value of considering the sub-populations from which patients derive when making these predictions of overall survival.

Confidence in our equations comes in part from superiority of their behavior in predicting survival when compared to the IDM only and elastic net, the latter being a technique intended to minimize error in prediction.

Interestingly, only a few methylation sites in total (unique and common) were required to demonstrate marked improvements survival predictions using the new methods.

The identification of methylated sites unique to each group is biologically plausible. Given the known plasticity of methylation events, environmental and cultural differences specific to a particular population subgroup may logically contribute to disparate mortality. Our findings underline the importance of continuing to elucidate the shared and varied molecular markers among these population groups. Our work supports looking for interventions to target not only the shared but unique methylation sites to impact disparate survival.

Funding and Acknowledgements J.S.R. was partially funded by NIH grants R01-CA160593A1, R01-GM085205 and NSF grant DMS 1513266. E.K. was partially funded by NIH grant (put in details here). E.K. and D.S. were partially funded by Bankhead-Coley Team Science grant 2BT02 and ACS Institutional Research Grant 98-277-10. J.S.R., E.K. and D.S. were partially funded by NIH grant UL1-TR000460. The authors declare that they have no competing financial interests.

References

1. Alizadeh, A.A., M.B. Eisen, and R.E. Davis. 2000. Distinct types of diffuse large B-cell lymphoma identified by gene expression profiling. *Nature* 403: 503–511.
2. George, A.W., P.M. Visscher, and C.S. Haley. 2000. Mapping quantitative trait loci in complex pedigrees: a two-step variance component approach. *Genetics* 156: 2081–2092.
3. Gilmour, A., B. Cullis, S. Welham, B. Gogel, and R. Thompson. 2004. An efficient computing strategy for prediction in mixed linear models. *Computational Statistics & Data Analysis* 44 (4): 571–586.

4. Henderson, C.R. 1948. *Estimation of general, specific and maternal combining abilities in crosses among inbred lines of swine*. Ph. D. Thesis, Iowa State University, Ames, Iowa.
5. Henderson, C.R. 1984. *Application of linear models in animal breeding*. Technical Report, (University of Guelph, Ontario).
6. Ishwaran, H., and J.S. Rao. 2003. Detecting differentially expressed genes in microarrays using Bayesian model selection. *Journal of the American Statistical Association* 98: 438–455.
7. Ishwaran, H., and J.S. Rao. 2005. Spike and slab gene selection for multigroup microarray data. *Journal of the American Statistical Association* 100: 764–780.
8. Jiang, J., T. Nguyen, and J.S. Rao. 2011. Best predictive small area estimation. *Journal of the American Statistical Association* 106: 732–745.
9. Jiang, J., J.S., Rao, Fan, J., and Ngyuen, T. 2015. Classified mixed prediction. *Technical Report*, University of Miami, Division of Biostatisics.
10. Jiang, J. 2007. *Linear and generalized linear mixed models and their applications*. New York: Springer.
11. Jiang, J., T. Nguyen, and J.S. Rao. 2011. Best predictive small area estimation. *Journal of American Statistics Association* 106: 732–745.
12. Jiang, J., and W. Zhang. 2002. Distributional-free prediction intervals in mixed linear models. *Statistica Sinica* 12: 537–553.
13. Kang, H.M., et al. 2008. Efficient control of population structure in model organism association mapping. *Genetics* 178: 1709–1723.
14. Kang, H.M., et al. 2010. Variance component model to account for sample structure in genome-wide association studies. *Nature Genetics* 42: 348–354.
15. Kennedy, B.W., M. Quinton, and J.A.M. van Arendonk. 1992. Estimation of effects of single genes on quantitative trait. *Journal of Animal Science* 70: 2000–2012.
16. Khan, M.H.R., and J.E.H. Shaw. 2016. Variable selection for survival data with a class of adaptive elastic net techniques. *Statistics and Computing* 26: 725–741.
17. Listgarten, J., C. Kadie, E.E. Schadt, and D. Heckerman. 2010. Correction for hidden confounders in the genetic analysis of gene expression. *Proceedings of the National Academy of Sciences of the United States of America* 107: 16465–16470.
18. Rao, J.S., Kobetz, E. and Coppede, F. 2016. *PRISM regression models: The anatomical and genetic to gender and age-related changes of DNA methylation in colorectal cancer (submitted)*.
19. Robinson, G.K. 1991. That BLUP is a good thing: The estimation of random effects (with discussion). *Statistical Science* 6: 15–51.
20. Schnitt, S.J. 2010. Classification and prognosis of invasive breast cancer: from morphology to molecular taxonomy. *Modern Pathology* 23: S60–S64.
21. Stute, W. 1993. Consistent estimation under random censorship when covariates are available. *Journal of Multivariate Analysis* 45: 89–103.
22. Tibshirani, R.J. 2013. The lasso problem and uniqueness. *Electronic Journal of Statistics* 7: 1456–1490.
23. Welham, S., B. Cullis, B. Gogel, A. Gilmour, and R. Thompson. 2004. Prediction in linear mixed models. *Australian & New Zealand Journal of Statistics* 46 (3): 325–347.
24. West, L., S.J. Vidwans, N.P. Campbell, J. Shrager, G.R. Simon, R. Bueno, P.A. Dennis, G.A. Otterson, and R. Salgia. 2012. A novel classification of lung cancer into molecular subtypes. *PLoS ONE* 7: e31906. https://doi.org/10.1371/journal.pone.0031906.
25. Yu, J., G. Pressoir, W.H. Briggs, I. Vroh Bi, M. Yamasaki, J.F. Doebley, and E.S. Buckler. 2005. A unified mixed-model method for association mapping that accounts for multiple levels of relatedness. *Nature Genetics* 38 (2): 203–208.
26. Zhang, Z., E. Ersoz, C. Lai, R.J. Todhunter, H.K. Tiwari, M.A. Gore, and E.S. Buckler. 2010. Mixed linear model approach adapted for genome-wide association studies. *Nature Genetics* 42 (4): 355–360.
27. Zhou, X., and M. Stephens. 2012. Genome-wide efficient mixed model analysis for association studies. *Nature Genetics* 44 (7): 821–824.

Chapter 10
Bivariate Frailty Model and Association Measure

Ramesh C. Gupta

Abstract In this paper, we present a bivariate frailty model and the association measure. The relationship between the conditional and the unconditional hazard gradients are derived and some examples are provided. A correlated frailty model is presented and its application in the competing risk theory is given. Some applications to real data sets are also pointed out.

Keywords Hazard gradient · Bivariate proportional hazard model
Bivariate additive model · Association measure · Correlated frailty model
Competing risk

10.1 Introduction

Frailty models are random effect models, where the randomness is introduced as an unobserved frailty. The proportional hazard frailty model is a classical frailty model due to Vaupel et al. [32] in which the baseline failure rate is multiplied by the unknown frailty variable and is given by,

$$\lambda(t|v) = v\lambda_0(t), t > 0, \tag{10.1.1}$$

where $\lambda_0(t)$ is the baseline hazard independent of v.

In addition to the above classical frailty model, various other models, including the additive frailty model and the accelerated failure time frailty model, have also been studied; see [5, 11, 26].

In modeling survival data by frailty models, the choice of the frailty distribution has been of interest. It has been observed that the choice of frailty distribution strongly affects the estimate of the baseline hazard as well as the conditional probabilities, see [1, 15–19]. In the shared frailty models, the assumptions about the frailty distributions play an important role in the model's interpretation since the frailty distribution links

R. C. Gupta (✉)
University of Maine, Orono, ME, USA
e-mail: rcgupta@maine.edu

A. Adhikari et al. (eds.), *Mathematical and Statistical Applications in Life Sciences and Engineering*, https://doi.org/10.1007/978-981-10-5370-2_10

the two processes of interest. For more discussion see [27] and [28]. In order to compare different frailties, in the univariate case, Gupta and Kirmani [10] investigated as to how the well-known stochastic orderings between distributions of two frailties translate into orderings between the corresponding survival functions. More recently, Gupta and Gupta [7, 8] studied a similar problem for a general frailty model which includes the classical frailty model (10.1.1) as well as the additive frailty model.

For some applications of the model (10.1.1) and related models, the reader is referred to Price and Manatunga [31] and Kersey et al. [20], who applied cure models, frailty models and frailty mixture models to analyze survival data.

Xue and Ding [36] applied the bivariate frailty model to inpatients mental health data. Hens et al. [12] applied the bivariate correlated gamma frailty model for type I interval censored data. Wienke et al. [33] applied the correlated gamma frailty model to fit bivariate time to event (occurence of breast cancer) data. Wienke et al. [34] used three correlated frailty models to analyze bivariate survival data by assuming gamma, log normal and compound Poisson distributed frailty. For more applications, the reader is referred to the bibliography in these papers and the books on frailty models.

In this paper, we shall study the bivariate model, whose survival function is given by

$$S(t_1, t_2|v) = e^{-v\psi(t_1,t_2)}, \tag{10.1.2}$$

where $\psi(t_1, t_2)$ is a differentiable function in both arguments such that $S(t_1, t_2|v)$ is a conditional survival function.

The hazard gradient of the above model will be investigated and their properties will be studied in relation to the baseline hazard functions. In particular, the bivariate proportional hazard model, incorporating the frailty effect, will be studied and some examples will be provided. The dependence structure between the two variables will be studied by deriving the local dependence function proposed by Clayton [2] and further studied by Oakes [29].

The organization of the paper is as follows: In Sect. 10.2, we present the definitions of the hazard functions and the association measure. Section 10.3 contains the bivariate frailty model along with some examples. An application in the competing risk theory is also provided. In Sect. 10.4, we present the association measure. Specific examples are provided in the case of proportional hazard frailty model. A correlated frailty model is presented in Sect. 10.5. Finally, in Sect. 10.6, some conclusions and comments are provided.

10.2 Hazard Functions

Let $T_1, T_2, \ldots, T_k$ be independent random variables having absolutely continuous multivariate survival function

$$S(t_1, t_2, \ldots, t_k) = P(T_1 > t_1, T_2 > t_2, \ldots, T_k > t_k).$$

Then, the hazard rates defined below are often used in demography, survival analysis, and biostatistics when analyzing multivariate survival data. These are given by

$$\lambda^{(i)}(t_1, t_2, \ldots, t_k) = \lim it_{\Lambda(t)\to 0} \frac{1}{\Lambda(t_i)} P(t_i \le T_i \le t_i + \Lambda t_i | T_i > t_i, T_j > t_j) \quad (10.2.1)$$
$$= -\frac{\partial}{\partial t_i} \ln S(t_1, t_2, \ldots, t_k), i, j = 1, 2, \ldots, k, i \ne j$$

Clearly (10.2.1) is the hazard rate of T_i given $T_j > t_j (i \ne j)$.

The vector $(\lambda_1(t_1, t_2, \ldots, t_k), \lambda_2(t_1, t_2, \ldots, t_k), \ldots, \lambda_k(t_1, t_2, \ldots, t_k))$ is called the hazard gradient.

Using the result

$$P(T_1 > t_1, T_2 > t_2, \ldots, T_k > t_k) \quad (10.2.2)$$
$$= P(T_1 > t_1)P(T_2 > t_2|T_1 > t_1) \ldots P(T_k > t_k|T_1 > t_1, \ldots T_{k-1} > t_{k-1})$$

It can be seen that $S(t_1, t_2, \ldots, t_k)$ can be recovered from $\lambda^{(i)}(t_1, t_2, \ldots, t_k), i = 1, 2, \ldots, k$ by

$$S(t_1, t_2, \ldots, t_k) = \int_0^{t_1} \lambda^{(1)}(u_1, 0, 0, \ldots, 0)du_1 \quad (10.2.3)$$
$$+ \int_0^{t_2} \lambda^{(2)}(t_1, u_2, 0, \ldots, 0)du_2$$
$$+ \ldots \int_0^{t_k} \lambda^{(k)}(t_1, t_2, \ldots, t_{k-1}, u_k)du_k.$$

In addition to the hazard rates given by (10.2.1), the hazard rates

$$\overline{\lambda^{(i)}}(t_1, t_2, \ldots, t_k) = \lim it_{\Lambda(t)\to 0} \frac{1}{\Lambda(t_i)} P(t_i \le T_i \le t_i + \Lambda t_i | T_i > t_i, T_j = t_j) \quad (10.2.4)$$
$$= -\frac{\partial}{\partial t_i} \ln[-\frac{\partial}{\partial t_j} S(t_1, t_2, \ldots, t_k)], i, j = 1, 2, \ldots, k, i \ne j$$

also play an important role in understanding the dependence structure between the variables.

Clearly , $\lambda^{(i)}(t_1, t_2, \ldots, t_k)$ describes the chances of failure of the ith unit at t_i, given that the jth$(i \ne j)$ unit is surviving at t_j. On the other hand $\overline{\lambda^{(i)}}(t_1, t_2, \ldots, t_k)$ describes the chances of failure of the ith unit at age t_i given that the jth $(i \ne j)$ unit fails at t_j. The deviation of the ratio of these two measures from unity describes the dependence between the life times. From this point of view, Clayton [2] defined

$$\theta_i(t_1, t_2, \ldots, t_k) = \frac{\overline{\lambda^{(i)}}(t_1, t_2, \ldots, t_k)}{\lambda^{(i)}(t_1, t_2, \ldots, t_k)}. \quad (10.2.5)$$

Confining our attention to the bivariate case ($k = 2$), $\theta(t_1, t_2)$ is defined by the ratio

$$\theta(t_1, t_2) = \frac{\overline{\lambda}(t_1, t_2)}{\lambda(t_1, t_2)} = \frac{\overline{\lambda^{(1)}}(t_1, t_2)}{\lambda^{(1)}(t_1, t_2)} = \frac{\overline{\lambda^{(2)}}(t_1, t_2)}{\lambda^{(2)}(t_1, t_2)} \qquad (10.2.6)$$

Clayton [2] proposed this measure by assuming that the association arises because the two members of a pair share some common influence and not because one event influences the other. Thus $\theta(t_1, t_2)$ explains the association between two nonnegative survival times with continuous joint distribution by their common dependence on an unobserved variable. This unobserved random variable is commonly known as frailty or environmental effect, see [29] and [25] for more details on the frailty models.

10.3 Bivariate Frailty Model

We shall confine our discussion for the bivariate case, although the results are similar for the general case.

The model (10.1.2) is given by

$$S(t_1, t_2|v) = e^{-v\psi(t_1,t_2)}, \qquad (10.3.1)$$

where $\psi(t_1, t_2)$ is a differentiable function in both arguments such that $S(t_1, t_2|v)$ is a conditional survival function.

Then

$$\lambda^{(i)}(t_1, t_2|v) = v\frac{\partial}{\partial t_i}\psi(t_1, t_2), i = 1, 2.$$

This gives (for $i = 1, 2$)

$$\begin{aligned} \lambda^{(i)}(t_1, t_2) &= E_{v|T_1>t_1,T_2>t_2}[\lambda^{(i)}(t_1, t_2|v)] \\ &= \int_0^\infty v\frac{\partial}{\partial t_i}\psi(t_1, t_2)h(v|T_1 > t_1, T_2 > t_2)dv, \end{aligned}$$

where $h(v|T_1 > t_1, T_2 > t_2)$ is the *pdf* of V given $T_1 > t_1, T_2 > t_2$. This is given by

$$h(v|T_1 > t_1, T_2 > t_2) = \frac{S(t_1, t_2|v)}{S(t_1, t_2)}$$

The hazard components are given by

$$\lambda^{(i)}(t_1, t_2) = \frac{\partial}{\partial t_i}\psi(t_1, t_2)E(V|T_1 > t_1, T_2 > t_2) \tag{10.3.2}$$
$$= \lambda_0^{(i)}(t_1, t_2)E(V|T_1 > t_1, T_2 > t_2),$$

where $\lambda_0^{(i)}(t_1, t_2)(i = 1, 2)$ is the ith component of the hazard gradient without incorporating the frailty effect. Thus,

$$\frac{\lambda^{(i)}(t_1, t_2)}{\lambda_0^{(i)}(t_1, t_2)} = E(V|T_1 > t_1, T_2 > t_2).$$

It can be verified that

$$\frac{\partial}{\partial t_i}E(V|T_1 > t_1, T_2 > t_2) = -\lambda_0^{(i)}(t_1, t_2)Var(V|T_1 > t_1, T_2 > t_2). \tag{10.3.3}$$

This means that $\lambda^{(i)}(t_1, t_2)/\lambda_0^{(i)}(t_1, t_2)$ is a decreasing function of $t_i (i = 1, 2)$.

Special Case

If T_1 and T_2 are conditionally independent given the frailty, then $\psi(t_1, t_2) = H_1(t_1) + H_2(t_2)$, $\lambda_0^{(1)}(t_1, t_2) = H_1'(t_1)$ and $\lambda_0^{(2)}(t_1, t_2) = H_2'(t_2)$.

The conditional survival function given $V = v$ is given by

$$S(t_1, t_2|v) = \exp[-v(H_1(t_1) + H_2(t_2))].$$

The unconditional survival function is given by

$$S(t_1, t_2) = L_V[(H_1(t_1) + H_2(t_2))],$$

where $L_V(.)$ is the Laplace transform of V.

Thus, the conditional density of V given $T_1 > t_1, T_2 > t_2$ is given by

$$h(v|T_1 > t_1, T_2 > t_2) = \frac{\exp\{-v(H_1(t_1) + H_2(t_2)\}}{L_V(H_1(t_1) + H_2(t_2)}h(v).$$

The hazard components are given by

$$\lambda^{(i)}(t_1, t_2) = -\frac{L_V'[(H_1(t_1) + H_2(t_2))]}{L_V[(H_1(t_1) + H_2(t_2))]}H_i'(t_i), i = 1, 2. \tag{10.3.4}$$

Also

$$E[V|T_1 > t_1, T_2 > t_2] = \frac{L_V'(H_1(t_1) + H_2(t_2))}{L_V(H_1(t_1) + H_2(t_2))}, \tag{10.3.5}$$

and

$$E(V^2|T_1 > t_1, T_2 > t_2] = \frac{L_V''(H_1(t_1) + H_2(t_2))}{L_V(H_1(t_1) + H_2(t_2))}.$$

Hence

$$Var[V|T_1 > t_1, T_2 > t_2] = [\frac{L_V''(H_1(t_1) + H_2(t_2)}{L_V(H_1(t_1) + H_2(t_2)}] - (\frac{L_V'(H_1(t_1) + H_2(t_2))}{L_V(H_1(t_1) + H_2(t_2))})^2 \tag{10.3.6}$$

In the following examples, we assume that T_1 and T_2 are independent given the frailty variable.

Specific Examples

Example 10.3.1 Suppose V has a Gamma distribution with *pdf*

$$h(v) = \frac{1}{\beta^\alpha \Gamma(\alpha)} v^{\alpha-1} e^{-v/\beta}, v > 0, \alpha > 0, \beta > 0.$$

and Laplace transform of V is given by

$$L_V(t) = \frac{1}{(1+\beta t)^\alpha}$$

So

$$S(t_1, t_2) = L_V[H_1(t_1) + H_2(t_2)] = [1 + \beta H_1(t_1) + \beta H_2(t_2)]^{-\alpha}.$$

The hazard components are given by

$$\lambda^{(i)}(t_1, t_2) = -\frac{\partial}{\partial t_i} \ln S(t_1, t_2) = \frac{\alpha\beta H_i'(t_i)}{1 + \beta H_1(t_1) + \beta H_2(t_2)}, i = 1, 2.$$

Also

$$E(V|T_1 > t_1, T_2 > t_2) = \frac{\alpha\beta}{1 + \beta H_1(t_1) + \beta H_2(t_2)}$$

and

$$Var(V|T_1 > t_1, T_2 > t_2) = \frac{\alpha\beta^2}{[1 + \beta H_1(t_1) + \beta H_2(t_2)]^2}.$$

The above expressions yield the square of the coefficient of variation of V given $T_1 > t_1, T_2 > t_2$ as $1/\alpha$. It can be verified that a constant value of the coefficient of variation occurs only in the case of gamma frailty.

Example 10.3.2 Suppose V has an inverse Gaussian distribution with *pdf*

$$h(v) = (2\pi a v^3)^{-1/2} \exp[-(bv-1)^2/2av\}, v > 0, a > 0, b > 0.$$

The Laplace transform of V is given by

$$L_V(t) = \exp[\frac{b}{a}(1-(1+\frac{2a}{b^2}t)^{1/2})].$$

This gives

$$S(t_1, t_2) = \exp[\frac{b}{a}(1-(1-\frac{2a}{b^2}(H_1(t_1)+H_2(t_2)))^{-1/2}].$$

The hazard component is given by

$$\lambda^{(i)}(t_1, t_2) = \frac{H_i(t_i)}{[b^2 + 2a(H_1(t_1)+H_2(t_2))]^{1/2}}, i = 1, 2.$$

Also

$$E(V|T_1 > t_1, T_2 > t_2) = \frac{1}{[b^2 + 2a(H_1(t_1)+H_2(t_2))]^{1/2}},$$

$$Var(V|T_1 > t_1, T_2 > t_2) = \frac{a}{[b^2 + 2a(H_1(t_1)+H_2(t_2))]^{3/2}}.$$

and

$$(CV)^2(V|T_1 > t_1, T_2 > t_2) = \frac{a}{(b^2 + 2a(H_1(t_1 + H_2(t_2))^{1/2}}.$$

Remark 10.3.1 For more general model with covariates, see [37]

10.3.1 An Application in Competing Risk Theory

Let an individual have a common frailty V of both dying of a disease (say, cancer) and other causes (competing causes). Then

$$\lambda(t|V) = V[h_1(t) + h_2(t)],$$

$h_1(t)$ is the failure rate due to cancer and $h_2(t)$ is the failure rate due to other causes.

Inverse Gaussian Shared Frailty Model
The unconditional failure rate is given by

$$\lambda^*(t) = \frac{(h_1(t) + h_2(t))}{(b^2 + 2a(H_1(t + H_2(t))^{1/2}}.$$

In this case, $E(V) = 1/b$ and $Var(V) = a = \sigma^2$.
Assume $E(V) = 1$ so that $b = 1$

$$\lambda^*(t) = \frac{(h_1(t) + h_2(t))}{A(t)}.$$

where

$$A(t) = (1 + 2\sigma^2(H_1(t + H_2(t))^{1/2}.$$

If we consider the two causes separately, we have

$$\lambda_1^*(t) = \frac{h_1(t)}{(1 + 2\sigma^2 H_1(t))^{1/2}}$$

and

$$\lambda_2^*(t) = \frac{h_2(t)}{(1 + 2\sigma^2 H_2(t))^{1/2}}.$$

Then

$$\lambda^*(t) = \lambda_1^*(t) + \lambda_2^*(t) - [(\lambda_1^*(t) - \frac{h_1(t)}{A(t)}) + (\lambda_2^*(t) - \frac{h_2(t)}{A(t)})].$$

It can be shown that

$$\lambda_i^*(t) - \frac{h_i(t)}{A(t)} > 0, i = 1, 2$$

Thus

$$\lambda^*(t) < \lambda_1^*(t) + \lambda_2^*(t).$$

This means that the failure intensity of the shared frailty model does not exceed the sum of the failure intensities obtained by applying the frailties separately.

10.4 The Association Measure

The association measure is given by

$$\theta(t_1, t_2) = \frac{\overline{\lambda}(t_1, t_2)}{\lambda(t_1, t_2)}$$

It can be verified that

$$\theta(t_1, t_2) = 1 - \frac{\frac{\partial}{\partial t_2}\lambda^{(1)}(t_1, t_2)}{\lambda^{(1)}(t_1, t_2)\lambda^{(2)}(t_1, t_2)}, \tag{10.4.1}$$

see [9].

As has already been seen

$$\lambda^{(i)}(t_1, t_2) = \frac{\partial}{\partial t_i}\psi(t_1, t_2)E(V|T_1 > t_1, T_2 > t_2), i = 1, 2 \tag{10.4.2}$$

and

$$\frac{\partial}{\partial t_i}E(V|T_1 > t_1, T_2 > t_2) = -\frac{\partial}{\partial t_i}\psi(t_1, t_2)Var(V|T_1 > t_1, T_2 > t_2) \cdot i = 1, 2, \tag{10.4.3}$$

see Eqs. (10.3.2) and (10.3.3).
Using the above results, it can be verified that

$$\theta(t_1, t_2) = \frac{E(V^2|T_1 > t_1, T_2 > t_2)}{[E(V|T_1 > t_1, T_2 > t_2)]^2} - \frac{\psi_{12}(t_1, t_2)}{\psi_1(t_1, t_2)\psi_2(t_1, t_2)E(V|T_1 > t_1, T_2 > t_2)}, \tag{10.4.4}$$

where $\psi_i(t_1, t_2) = \frac{\partial}{\partial t_i}\psi(t_1, t_2), i = 1, 2$ and $\psi_{12}(t_1, t_2) = \frac{\partial^2}{\partial t_1 \partial t_2}\psi(t_1, t_2)$.
We now present some examples

Example 10.4.1 $\psi(t_1, t_2) = (H_1(t_1) + H_2(t_2) + A(t_1, t_2)$
In this case,

$$\theta(t_1, t_2) = \frac{E(V^2|T_1 > t_1, T_2 > t_2)}{[E(V|T_1 > t_1, T_2 > t_2)]^2} - \frac{A_{12}(t_1, t_2)}{[h_1(t_1) + A_1(t_1, t_2)][h_2(t_2) + A_2(t_1, t_2)]E(V|T_1 > t_1, T_2 > t_2)}, \tag{10.4.5}$$

where $h_i(t_1, t_2) = \frac{\partial}{\partial t_i}H_i(t_1, t_2)$, $A_i(t_1, t_2) = \frac{\partial}{\partial t_i}A_i(t_1, t_2), i = 1, 2$ and $A_{12}(t_1, t_2) = \frac{\partial^2}{\partial t_1 \partial t_2}A(t_1, t_2)$.

Special Case (Proportional Hazard Frailty Model)
In this case,

$$\psi(t_1, t_2) = H_1(t_1) + H_2(t_2)$$

and

$$\theta(t_1, t_2) = \frac{E(V^2|T_1 > t_1, T_2 > t_2)}{[E(V|T_1 > t_1, T_2 > t_2)]^2} = 1 + [c \cdot v \cdot (V|T_1 > t_1, T_2 > t_2)]^2, \tag{10.4.6}$$

where $c \cdot v \cdot (V|T_1 > t_1, T_2 > t_2)$ is the coefficient of variation of V given $T_1 > t_1, T_2 > t_2$.

We now consider some examples of the proportional hazard frailty model.

Example 10.4.2 V has a Gamma distribution with probability density function (*pdf*)

$$h(v) = \frac{1}{\beta^\alpha \Gamma(\alpha)} e^{-v/\beta} v^{\alpha-1}, v > 0, \alpha > 0, \beta > 0. \tag{10.4.7}$$

Using the results in Sect. 10.3, it can be verified that

$$\theta(t_1, t_2) = 1 + \frac{1}{\alpha}. \tag{10.4.8}$$

Note that, in this case, $\theta(t_1, t_2)$ is independent of (t_1, t_2); see Hanagal ([13], p. 83) and Wienke [35].

Example 10.4.3 V has an inverse Gaussian distribution with *pdf*

$$g(v) = (\frac{1}{2\pi a z^3})^{1/2} \exp[-(bv - 1)^2/2av], v, a, b > 0. \tag{10.4.9}$$

Using the results of Sect. 10.3, it can be verified that, in this case

$$\theta(t_1, t_2) = 1 + \frac{a}{[b^2 + 2a(H_1(t_1) + H_2(t_2))]^{1/2}}. \tag{10.4.10}$$

Example 10.4.4 V has a positive stable distribution with *pdf*

$$h(v) = -\frac{1}{\pi v} \sum_{k=1}^{\infty} \frac{\Gamma(k\alpha + 1)}{k!} (-v^{-\alpha})^k \sin(\alpha k \pi), v > 0, 0 < \alpha < 1, \tag{10.4.11}$$

see [4] for more explanation and justification of this distribution as frailty distribution. Note that this density has infinite mean. Therefore, the variance is undetermined.

The Laplace transform of V is given by

$$L_V(t) = e^{-t^\alpha}, 0 < \alpha < 1.$$

whose derivatives are given by

$$L'_V(t) = -\alpha t^{\alpha-1} L_V(t),$$

and

$$L''_V(t) = L_V(t)[\alpha^2 t^{2\alpha-2} - \alpha(\alpha-1)t^{\alpha-2}].$$

It can be verified that

$$\theta(t_1, t_2) = 1 + \frac{(1-\alpha)}{\alpha[H_1(t_1 + H_2(t_2)]^\alpha}. \tag{10.4.12}$$

10.5 Correlated Frailty Model

Suppose $Y_{0,} Y_1$ and Y_2 are independent. Let

$$V_1 = Y_0 + Y_1,\ V_2 = Y_0 + Y_2.$$

This means that V_1 and V_2 are correlated.
The conditional survival function

$$S(t_1, t_2 | V_1, V_2) = \exp\{-(H_1(t_1)V_1 + H_2(t_2)V_2)\}.$$

This means that given V_1 and V_2, the life spans T_1 and T_2 are independent unconditional survival function.

$$\begin{aligned} S(t_1, t_2) = & \int\int\int \exp\{-(y_0 + y_1)H_1(t_1) - (y_0 + y_2)H_2(t_2)\} \\ & h_0(y_0)h_1(y_1)h_b(y_2)dy_0dy_1dy_2 \\ = & L_{Y_0}[(H_1(t_1) + H_2(t_2)]L_{Y_1}(H_1(t_1))L_{Y_2}(H_2(t_2)). \end{aligned}$$

Some Assumptions
Suppose
$Y_0 \sim$ Gamma $(\alpha_{0,}\beta_0)$, $Y_1 \sim$ Gamma $(\alpha_{1,}\beta_1)$, $Y_2 \sim$ Gamma $(\alpha_{2,}\beta_2)$
Assume $\beta_0 = \beta_1 = \beta_2 = \beta$ (say) so that V_1 and V_2 have Gamma distributions.
$E(V_1) = (\alpha_0 + \alpha_1)\beta$ and $Var(V_1) = (\alpha_0 + \alpha_1)\beta^2$
$E(V_2) = (\alpha_0 + \alpha_2)\beta$ and $Var(V_2) = (\alpha_0 + \alpha_2)\beta^2$
Also, assume $\alpha_1 = \alpha_2 = \alpha(say)$. So that V_1 and V_2 have the same Gamma distribution.

Correlation coefficient between V_1 and V_2

$$\rho_{V_1,V_2} = \frac{Var(Y_0)}{\sqrt{Var(V_1)Var(V_2)}} = \frac{\alpha_0}{\alpha_0 + \alpha}$$

This gives

$$\alpha_0 = \frac{\alpha \rho_{V_1,V_2}}{1 - \rho_{V_1,V_2}}$$

Standard assumption
E(Frailty) = 1,
$Var(V_1) = Var(V_2) = \beta = \sigma_V^2$,
This implies that

$$\alpha_0 = \frac{\rho_{V_1,V_2}}{\sigma_V^2}.$$

This class is still wide enough to include individual frailty models and shared frailty models with Gamma frailty and some particular cases.

Note that

$$L_{Y_0}(t) = \frac{1}{(1 + \beta t)^{\alpha_0}}$$

and

$$L_{Y_1}(t) = L_{Y_2}(t) = \frac{1}{(1 + \beta t)^{\alpha}}.$$

These give

$$S(t_1, t_2) = [1 + \sigma_V^2 (H_1(t_1) + H_2(t_2))]^{-\rho_V/\sigma_V^2} \times [(1 + \sigma_V^2 \cdot H_1(t_1))(1 + \sigma_V^2 \cdot H_2(t_2))]^{-(1-\rho_V)/\sigma_V^2}$$

10.5.1 Competing Risk Revisited (Different Frailties)

In this case,

$$S(t|V_1, V_2) = \exp\{-H_1(t)v_1 - H_2(t)v_2\}$$

and

$$S(t) = L_{Y_0}[(H_1(t) + H_2(t))]L_{Y_1}[(H_1(t) + H_2(t))]$$

Unconditional Failure Rate

$$\lambda^*(t) = [h_1(t) + h_2(t)]\frac{L'_{Y_0}[H_1(t) + H_2(t)]}{L_{Y_0}[H_1(t) + H_2(t)]} + \frac{L'_{Y_1}(H_1(t))h_1(t)}{L_{Y_1}(t)} + \frac{L'_{Y_2}(H_2(t))h_2(t)}{L_{Y_2}(t)}.$$

For the case of Gamma distribution of V_1 and V_2

$$\lambda^*(t) = \rho_V \frac{[h_1(t) + h_2(t)]}{1 + \sigma_V^2(H_1(t) + H_2(t))} + (1 - \rho_V)[\frac{h_1(t)}{1 + \sigma_V^2 H_1(t)} + \frac{h_2(t)}{1 + \sigma_V^2 H_2(t)}].$$

Particular Cases

Shared Frailty Model ($\rho_V = 1$)

$$\lambda^*(t) = \frac{[h_1(t) + h_2(t)]}{1 + \sigma_V^2(H_1(t) + H_2(t))}.$$

Remark 10.5.1 Recently Hanagal and Dabade [14] have considered four shared frailty models. These models have been illustrated with real-life bivariate survival data related to a kidney infection.

Independent Case ($\rho_V = 0$)

$$\lambda^*(t) = \frac{h_1(t)}{1 + \sigma_V^2 H_1(t)} + \frac{h_2(t)}{1 + \sigma_V^2 H_2(t)}.$$

10.6 Conclusion and Comments

In this paper, we have presented a general bivariate frailty model. Frailty models are introduced in the proportional hazard model to take into account positive correlations among multivariate failure times, see [3]. Note that the frailty V effects multiplicatively on the baseline hazard function. It may be pointed out that in addition to the proportional hazard frailty model presented in this paper, various other forms of frailty model are available in the literature. For example, the additive frailty model and the accelerated failure time frailty model, see [11, 21–23, 30] and the references therein. We hope that the bivariate frailty model presented in this paper will be useful to researchers who are interested in studying this area of research further [6, 24].

Acknowledgements The author is thankful to the referee for some useful suggestions which enhanced the presentation.

References

1. Agresti, A., B. Caffo, and P. Ohman-Strickland. 2004. Examples in which misspecification of a random effects distribution reduces efficiency and possible remedies. *Compuatational Statistics and Data Analysis* 47: 639–653.
2. Clayton, D.G. 1978. A model for association in bivariate life tables and its application in epidemiological studies of family tendancy in chronic disease incidence. *Biometrika* 65: 141–151.
3. Clayton, D.G., and J. Cuzick. 1985. Multivariate generalization of the proprtional hazard model. *Journal of the Royal Statistical Society, Sereis A* 148: 82–117.
4. Duchateau, L., and P. Janssen. 2008. *The Frailty Model*. NY: Springer.
5. Finkelstein, M.S., and V. Esaulova. 2006. Asymptotic behaviour of a general class of mixture failure rates. *Advances in Applied Probability* 38 (1): 244–262.
6. Gupta, P.L., and R.C. Gupta. 1996. Ageing charaterstics of the Weibull mixtures. *Probability in the Engineering and Informational Sciences* 10: 591–600.
7. Gupta, R.C., and R.D. Gupta. 2009. General frailty model and stochastic orderings. *Journal of Statistical Planning and Inference* 139: 3277–3287.
8. Gupta, R.C., and R.D. Gupta. 2010. Random effect survival models and stochastic comparisons. *Journal of Applied Probability* 47: 426–440.
9. Gupta, R.C. 2010. Reliability functions of bivariate distributions in modeling marked point processes. *Stochastic Models* 26 (2): 195–211.
10. Gupta, R.C., and S.N. Kirmani. 2006. Stochastic comparisons in frailty models. *Journal of Statistical Planning and Inference* 136: 3647–3658.
11. Gupta, R.C. 2016. Properties of additive frailty model in survival analysis. *Metrika* 79: 1–17.
12. Hens, N., A. Wienke, M. Aerts, and G. Molenberghs. 2009. The correlated and shared gamma frailty model for bivariate current status data: an illustration for cross-sectional serological data. *Statistics in Medicine* 28: 2785–2800.
13. Hanagal, D.D. 2011. *Modeling Survival Data Using Frailty Models*. Boca Raton, FL: Chapman and Hall.
14. Hanagal, D.D., and A.D. Dabade. 2015. Comparison of shared frailty models for kidney infection data under exponential power baseline distribution. *Communications in Statistics, Theory and Methods* 44: 5091–5108.
15. Heckman, J.J., and B. Singer. 1984. The identifibility of the proportional hazard model. *Review Economic Studies* 231–241.
16. Hougaard, P. 1984. Lifetable methods for heterogeneous populations: distributions describing the heterogeneity. *Biometrika* 71: 75–83.
17. Hougaard, P. 1991. Modeling hetereogeneity in survival data. *Journal of Applied Probability* 28: 695–701.
18. Hougaard, P. 1995. Frailty models for survival data. *Lifetime Data Analysis* 1: 255–273.
19. Hougaard, P. 2000. *Analysis of Multivariate Survival Data*. New York: Springer.
20. Kersey, H., D. Weisdorf, M.E. Nesbit, T.W. Lebien, P.B. McGlave, T. Kim, D.A. Vellera, A.I. Goldman, B. Bostrom, D. Hurd, and N.K.C. Ramsay. 1987. Comparison of autologous and allogenic bone merrow transplantation for treatment of high-risk refractory acute lymphoblastic leukemia. *New England Journal of Medicine* 317: 461–467.

21. Keiding, N., and P.K. Andersen. 1997. The role of frailty models and accelerated failure time models in describing heterogeneity due to omitted covariates. *Statistics in Medicine* 16: 215–224.
22. Korsgaard, I.R., and A.H. Anderson. 1998. The additive genetic gamma frailty model. *Scandinavian Journal of Statistics* 25: 255–269.
23. Lambert, P., D. Collett, A. Kimber, and R. Johnson. 2004. Parametric accelerated failure time models with random effects and an application to kidney transplant survival. *Statistics in Medicine* 23: 3177–3192.
24. Liang, K.Y., S.G. Self, K.J. Bandeen-Roche, and S. Zeger. 1995. Some recent developments for regression analysis of multivariate failure time data. *Lifetime Data Analysis* 1: 403–406.
25. Manatunga, A.K., and D. Oakes. 1996. A measure of association for bivariate frailty ditributions. *Journal of Multivariate Analysis* 56: 60–74.
26. Missov, T.I., and M.S. Finkelstein. 2011. Admissible mixing distributions for a general class of mixture survival models with known asymptotics. *Theoretical Population Biology* 80 (1): 64–70.
27. Rizopoulos, D., G. Verbke, and G. Molenberghs. 2008. Shared parameter models under random effect misspecification. *Biometrika* 95 (1): 63–74.
28. Sargent, D.J. 1998. A general framework for random effects survival analysis in the Cox proportional hazards setting. *Biometrics* 54: 1486–1497.
29. Oakes, D. 1989. Bivariate survival models induced by frailties. *Journal of the American Statistical Association* 84: 497–493.
30. Pan, W. 2001. Using frailties in the accelarated failure time model (2001). *Lifetime Data Analysis* 7: 55–64.
31. Price, D.L., and A.K. Manatunga. 2001. Modelling survival data with a cure fraction using frailty models. *Statistics in Medicine* 20: 1515–1527.
32. Vaupel, J.W., K.G. Manton, and E. Sttalard. 1979. The impact of heterogeneity in individual frailty on the dynamics of mortality. *Demography* 16 (3): 439–454.
33. Wienke, A., P. Lichtenstein, and A.I. Yashin. 2003. A bivariate frailty model with a cure fraction for modelling familial correlations in diseases. *Biometrics* 59: 1178–1183.
34. Wienke, A., I. Licantelli, and A.I. Yashin. 2006. the modeling of a cure fraction in bivariate time to event data. *Austrian Journal of Statistics* 35 (1): 67–76.
35. Wienke, A. 2010. *Frailty Models in Survival Analysis*. Boca Raton: Chapman & Hall/CRC.
36. Xue, X., and A.Y. Ding. 1999. Assesing heterogeneity and correlation of paired failure times with the bivariate frailty model. *Statistics in Medicine* 18: 907–918.
37. Yin, G., and J.G. Ibrahim. 2005. A class of Bayesian shared gamma frailty models with multivariate failure time data. *Biometrics* 61: 208–216.

Chapter 11
On Bayesian Inference of $R = P(Y < X)$ for Weibull Distribution

Debasis Kundu

Abstract In this paper, we consider the Bayesian inference on the stress-strength parameter $R = P(Y < X)$, when X and Y follow independent Weibull distributions. We have considered different cases. It is assumed that the random variables X and Y have different scale parameters and (a) a common shape parameter or (b) different shape parameters. Moreover, both stress and strength may depend on some known covariates also. When the two distributions have a common shape parameter, Bayesian inference on R is obtained based on the assumption that the shape parameter has a log-concave prior, and given the shape parameter, the scale parameters have Dirichlet-Gamma prior. The Bayes estimate cannot be obtained in closed form, and we propose to use Gibbs sampling method to compute the Bayes estimate and also to compute the associated highest posterior density (HPD) credible interval. The results have been extended when the covariates are also present. We further consider the case when the two shape parameters are different. Simulation experiments have been performed to see the effectiveness of the proposed methods. One data set has been analyzed for illustrative purposes and finally, we conclude the paper.

11.1 Introduction

The problem of estimating the stress-strength parameter $R = P(Y < X)$ and its associated inference, when X and Y are two independent random variables, have received considerable attention since the pioneering work of Birnbaum [1]. In spite of its apparent simplicity, extensive work has been done since then both from the parametric and nonparametric points of view. The estimation of R occurs quite naturally in the statistical reliability literature. For example, in a reliability study, if X is the strength of a system, which is subject to stress Y, then R is the measure of system performance and arises quite frequently in the mechanical reliability of a system. Alternatively, in survival analysis, the area under the receiving operating

D. Kundu (✉)
Department of Mathematics and Statistics, Indian Institute of Technology Kanpur,
Kanpur 208016, India
e-mail: kundu@iitk.ac.in

A. Adhikari et al. (eds.), *Mathematical and Statistical Applications in Life Sciences and Engineering*, https://doi.org/10.1007/978-981-10-5370-2_11

characteristic (ROC) curve, which is a plot of the sensitivity versus, 1—specificity, at different cut-off points of the range of possible test values, is equal to R. A book-length treatment on estimation of R, and its associated inference can be obtained in Kotz et al. [2]. See also Zhou [3], Kundu and Raqab [4], Ventura and Racugno [5], Kizilaslan and Nadar [6] and the references cited therein, for recent developments.

Although extensive work has been done on this particular problem under different assumptions on X and Y, not much attention has been paid when both X and Y depend on some covariates. Guttman et al. [7] and Weerahandi and Johnson [8] considered the estimation of R, and also obtained the associated confidence interval of R, when both stress and strength depend on some known covariates. It has been assumed in both the papers that both X and Y are normally distributed, and their respective means depend on the covariates, but their variances do not depend on the covariates. Guttman and Papandonatos [9] also considered the same model from the Bayesian point of view. They proposed different approximate Bayes estimates under non-informative priors. Interestingly, although it has been mentioned by Guttman et al. [7] that it is important to develop a statistical inferential procedure for the stress-strength parameter in case of covariates for non-normal distributions mainly for small sample sizes, nothing has been developed along that line till date. This is an attempt towards that direction.

The aim of this paper is to consider the inference on R, when both X and Y are independent Weibull random variables. They may or may not have the same shape parameters. It is assumed that both stress and strength distributions may depend on some known covariates. Here, we are proposing the covariates modeling in the following manner. It is assumed that for both X and Y, the scale parameter depends on some known covariates. Since the lifetime distributions are always nonnegative, it is more natural to use Weibull, gamma, log-normal, etc. rather than normal distribution for this purpose. Moreover, using the covariates through the scale parameter also ensures that both the mean and variance of the lifetime of an item/ individual depend on the covariates. In case of normal distribution, the covariates are modeled through mean only, see for example Guttman et al. [7], Weerahandi and Johnson [8] or Guttman and Papandonatos [9], which may not be very reasonable.

Another important point should be mentioned that the statistical inference on $R = P(Y < X)$, when X and Y have independent Weibull random variables have been considered by many authors, see for example Kotz et al. [2], Kundu and Gupta [10], Kundu and Raqab [4], and see the references cited therein. But in all these cases it has been assumed that X and Y have a common shape parameter. It has been assumed mainly due to analytical reason, although it may not be reasonable in many situation. In this paper, we have also considered the case when X and Y may not have the same shape parameters, that is also another significant contribution of this paper.

Our approach in this paper is fully Bayesian. For the Bayesian inference, we need to assume some priors on the unknown parameters. First, it is assumed that X and Y have a common shape parameter and it is known. Assumptions of known shape parameter in case of a Weibull distribution is not very unreasonable, see for example Murthy et al. [11]. In many reliability experiments the experimenter has a prior knowledge about the shape parameter of the corresponding Weibull model. If the shape parameter is known, and there are no covariates, then the most convenient but quite general conjugate prior on the scale parameters is a Dirichlet-gamma prior, as suggested by Peña and Gupta [12]. The Bayes estimate cannot be obtained in explicit form, but it is quite convenient to generate samples from the posterior distribution of R. Hence, we use Gibbs sampling procedure to compute the Bayes estimate and the associated highest posterior density (HPD) credible interval of R.

When the covariates are also present, it is assumed that the covariate parameters have independent normal priors. In case of unknown common shape parameter, the conjugate prior on the shape parameter does not exist. In this case following the approach of Berger and Sun [13], it is assumed that the prior on the shape parameter has the support on $(0, \infty)$, and it has a log-concave density function. Based on the above prior distributions, we obtain the joint posterior distribution function of the unknown parameters. The Bayes estimate of R cannot be obtained in explicit form and we have proposed an effective importance sampling procedure to compute the Bayes estimate and the associated HPD credible interval of the stress-strength parameter.

We further consider the case when the two shape parameters of the Weibull distributions are different and unknown. In this case the stress-strength parameter cannot be obtained in explicit form, and it can be obtained only in an integration form. In this case, the priors on the scale parameters are same as before, and for the shape parameters it is assumed that the two prior distributions are independent, both of them have support on $(0, \infty)$ and they have log-concave density functions. We have used importance sampling technique to compute the Bayes estimate and the associated HPD credible interval of R. We perform some simulation experiments to see the effectiveness of the proposed methods. One small data set has been analyzed for illustrative purposes and to show how the proposed methods work for small sample sizes.

Rest of the paper is organized as follows. In Sect. 11.2, we provide the model description, and the prior assumptions. In Sect. 11.3, we provide the posterior analysis when there is no covariate. In Sect. 11.4, we consider the case when the covariates are present. Simulation results are provided in Sect. 11.5. The analysis of one data set is presented in Sect. 11.6. Finally, in Sect. 11.7 we conclude the paper.

11.2 Model Formulation and Prior Assumptions

11.2.1 Model Formulation and Available Data

A Weibull distribution with the shape parameter $\alpha > 0$ and scale parameter $\lambda > 0$, has the probability density function (PDF)

$$f_{WE}(x; \alpha, \lambda) = \alpha \lambda x^{\alpha-1} e^{-\lambda x^{\alpha}}; \quad x > 0, \tag{11.1}$$

and it will be denoted by WE(α, λ).

Two Shape Parameters are Same: It is assumed that X follows $(\sim)$ WE(α, λ_1) and $Y \sim$ WE(α, λ_2), and they are independently distributed. The choice of a common α can be justified as follows. The logarithm of a Weibull random variable has an

extreme value distribution, which belongs to a location scale family. The parameter α is the reciprocal of the scale parameter. In an analogy to the two-sample normal case, where it is customary to assume a common variance, we assume a common shape parameter α here.
In this case,

$$R = P(Y < X) = \int_0^{\infty} \alpha \lambda_2 y^{\alpha-1} e^{-(\lambda_1+\lambda_2)y^{\alpha}} dy = \frac{\lambda_2}{\lambda_1 + \lambda_2}.$$

If both X and Y depend on some covariates, $u = (u_1, \ldots, u_p)^T$ and $v = (v_1, \ldots, v_q)^T$, respectively, as follows;

$$\lambda_1 - \theta_1 e^{\beta_1^T u} \quad \text{and} \quad \lambda_2 = \theta_2 e^{\beta_2^T v},$$

where $\beta_1 = (\beta_{11}, \ldots, \beta_{1p})^T$ and $\beta_2 = (\beta_{21}, \ldots, \beta_{2q})^T$ are p and q dimensional regression parameters, (p may not be equal to q), then

$$R(u, v) = P(Y < X|u, v) = \frac{\theta_2 e^{\beta_2^T v}}{\theta_1 e^{\beta_1^T u} + \theta_2 e^{\beta_2^T v}}. \tag{11.2}$$

From now on we use R instead of $R(u, v)$ for brevity. But if it is needed we shall make it explicit.
Two Shape Parameters are Different: Now we discuss the case when the two shape parameters are different. In this case, it is assumed that $X \sim \text{WE}(\alpha_1, \lambda_1)$ and $Y \sim \text{WE}(\alpha_2, \lambda_2)$, and they are independently distributed. In this case, R cannot be obtained in explicit form. It can be obtained only in the integration form as follows:

$$R = P(Y < X) = \alpha_2 \lambda_2 \int_0^{\infty} y^{\alpha_2 - 1} e^{-(\lambda_1 y^{\alpha_1} + \lambda_2 y^{\alpha_2})} dy. \tag{11.3}$$

Moreover, when X and Y depend on some covariates as before, then

$$R(u, v) = P(Y < X|u, v) = \alpha_2 \theta_2 \int_0^{\infty} e^{\beta_2^T v} y^{\alpha_2 - 1} e^{-(\theta_1 e^{\beta_1^T u} y^{\alpha_1} + \theta_2 e^{\beta_2^T v} y^{\alpha_2})} dy. \tag{11.4}$$

It is assumed that we have the following stress-strength data as $\{x_i, u_{i1}, \ldots, u_{ip}\}$, for $i = 1, \ldots, m$, and $\{y_j, v_{j1}, \ldots, v_{jq}\}$, for $j = 1, \ldots, n$, respectively, and all the observations are independently distributed.

11.2.2 Prior Assumptions

We use the following notation. A random variable is said to have a gamma distribution with the shape parameter $\alpha > 0$ and scale parameter $\lambda > 0$, if it has the PDF

$$f_{GA}(x; \alpha, \lambda) = \frac{\lambda^{\alpha}}{\Gamma(\alpha)} x^{\alpha-1} e^{-\lambda x}; \quad x > 0. \tag{11.5}$$

From now on it will be denoted by GA(α, λ). A random variable is said to have a Beta distribution with parameters $a > 0$ and $b > 0$, if it has the PDF

$$f_{BE}(x; a, b) = \frac{\Gamma(a+b)}{\Gamma(a)\Gamma(b)} x^{a-1}(1-x)^{b-1}; \quad 0 < x < 1, \tag{11.6}$$

and it will be denoted by Beat(a, b). A p-variate normal random vector, with mean vector a and dispersion matrix B, will be denoted by $N_p(a, B)$.

We make the following prior assumptions on the different parameters as follows. Let us assume $\theta = \theta_1 + \theta_2$, then similarly as in Peña and Gupta [12], it is assumed that $\theta \sim$ GA(a_0, b_0), with $a_0 > 0$, $b_0 > 0$, and $\theta_1/(\theta_1 + \theta_2) \sim$ Beta(a_1, a_2), with $a_1 > 0$, $a_2 > 0$, and they are independently distributed. After simplification, it can be easily seen that the joint PDF of θ_1 and θ_2 takes the following form;

$$\begin{aligned}\pi_{BG}(\theta_1, \theta_2 | a_0, b_0, a_1, a_2) = & \frac{\Gamma(a_1 + a_2)}{\Gamma(a_0)} (b_0\theta)^{a_0 - a_1 - a_2} \times \frac{b_0^{a_1}}{\Gamma(a_1)} \theta_1^{a_1 - 1} e^{-b_0\theta_1} \times \\ & \frac{b_0^{a_2}}{\Gamma(a_2)} \theta_2^{a_2-1} e^{-b_0\theta_2}.\end{aligned} \tag{11.7}$$

The joint PDF (11.7) is known as the PDF of a Beta-Gamma distribution, and it will be denoted by BG(b_0, a_0, a_1, a_2). The above Beta-Gamma prior is a very flexible prior. If $a_0 = a_1 + a_2$, then θ_1 and θ_2 become independent. If $a_0 > a_1 + a_2$, then θ_1 and θ_2 are positively correlated, and for $a_0 < a_1 + a_2$, they are negatively correlated. The following result will be useful for posterior analysis.

Result If $(\theta_1, \theta_2) \sim$ BG(b_0, a_0, a_1, a_2), then for $i = 1, 2$,

$$E(\theta_i) = \frac{a_0 a_i}{b_0(a_1 + a_2)} \quad \text{and} \quad V(\theta_i) = \frac{a_0 a_i}{b_0^2(a_1 + a_2)} \times \left\{ \frac{(a_i + 1)(a_0 + 1)}{a_1 + a_2 + 1} - \frac{a_0 a_i}{a_1 + a_2} \right\}. \tag{11.8}$$

Moreover, Kundu and Pradhan [14] suggested a very simple method to generate samples from a Beta-Gamma distribution, and that will be useful to generate samples from the posterior distribution. When the common shape parameter is unknown, it is assumed that the prior on α, $\pi_2(\alpha)$, is absolute continuous, and it has log-concave PDF.

In presence of covariates, we make the following prior assumptions on the unknown parameters:

$$\begin{aligned}(\theta_1, \theta_2) &\sim \pi_1(\theta_1, \theta_2) = \text{BG}(b_0, a_0, a_1, a_2) \\ \alpha &\sim \pi_2(\alpha) \\ \beta_1 &\sim \pi_3(\beta_1) = N_p(0, \Sigma_1) \\ \beta_2 &\sim \pi_4(\beta_2) = N_q(0, \Sigma_2),\end{aligned}$$

and they are all independently distributed. It is further assumed that $\pi_2(\alpha)$ is absolute continuous and has a log-concave probability density function. If the two shape parameters, α_1 and α_2, are different, then for (θ_1, θ_2), β_1, β_2, we assume the same prior as before, and for α_1 and α_2, it is assumed that

$$\alpha_1 \sim \pi_{21}(\alpha_1) \quad \text{and} \quad \alpha_2 \sim \pi_{22}(\alpha_2), \tag{11.9}$$

and they are independently distributed. Here, $\pi_{21}(\alpha_1)$ and $\pi_{22}(\alpha_2)$ are both absolute continuous and having log-concave probability density functions.

11.3 Posterior Analysis: No Covariates

In this section, we provide the Bayesian inference of the unknown stress-strength parameter based on the prior assumptions provided in Sect. 11.2, and when covariates are absent. We consider the case in the presence of covariates in the next section. In developing the Bayes estimate, it is assumed that the error is squared error, although any other loss function can be easily incorporated. In this section, we consider two cases separately, namely when (i) common shape parameter is known and (ii) common shape parameter is unknown.

11.3.1 Two Shape Parameter are Same: Known

Based on the observations, and the prior assumptions as provided in Sect. 11.2, we obtain the likelihood function as

$$l(data|\alpha, \lambda_1, \lambda_2) = \alpha^{m+n} \lambda_1^m \lambda_2^n \prod_{i=1}^{m} x_i^{\alpha-1} \prod_{j=1}^{n} y_j^{\alpha-1} e^{-\lambda_1 \sum_{i=1}^{m} x_i^{\alpha} - \lambda_2 \sum_{j=1}^{n} y_j^{\alpha}}. \tag{11.10}$$

Therefore, for known α, the posterior distribution of λ_1 and λ_2 becomes

$$\pi(\lambda_1, \lambda_2|\alpha, data) \propto \lambda_1^{m+a_1-1} \lambda_2^{n+a_2-1} (\lambda_1 + \lambda_2)^{a_0-a_1-a_2} e^{-\lambda_1 T_1(\alpha) - \lambda_2 T_2(\alpha)}, \tag{11.11}$$

where

$$T_1(\alpha) = b_0 + \sum_{i=1}^{m} x_i^{\alpha} \quad \text{and} \quad T_2(\alpha) = b_0 + \sum_{j=1}^{n} y_j^{\alpha}.$$

Now observe that for a given α, if $a_0 > 0$, $a_1 > 0$, $a_2 > 0$ and $b_0 > 0$

$$\int_0^\infty \int_0^\infty \lambda_1^{m+a_1-1} \lambda_2^{n+a_2-1} (\lambda_1 + \lambda_2)^{a_0-a_1-a_2} e^{-\lambda_1 T_1(\alpha) - \lambda_2 T_2(\alpha)} d\lambda_1 d\lambda_2 \le$$
$$\int_0^\infty \int_0^\infty \lambda_1^{m+a_1-1} \lambda_2^{n+a_2-1} (\lambda_1 + \lambda_2)^{a_0-a_1-a_2} e^{-(\lambda_1+\lambda_2)\min\{T_1(\alpha), T_2(\alpha)\}} d\lambda_1 d\lambda_2 < \infty.$$

Hence, if the prior is proper, the corresponding posterior is also proper. Note that in this case even if $a_0 = a_1 = a_2 = b_0 = 0$, then also the posterior PDF becomes the product of two independent gamma PDFs, hence it is proper. The following result will be useful for further development.

Theorem 1 *The posterior distribution of* $R = \dfrac{\lambda_1}{\lambda_1 + \lambda_2}$ *given* α *is given by*

$$\pi(R|data, \alpha) \propto \frac{R^{m+a_1-1}(1-R)^{n+a_2-1}}{(RT_1(\alpha) + (1-R)T_2(\alpha))^{m+n+a_1+a_2}}; \quad 0 < R < 1.$$

Proof Let us make the following transformation:

$$R = \frac{\lambda_1}{\lambda_1 + \lambda_2} \quad \text{and} \quad \lambda = \lambda_1 + \lambda_2.$$

Therefore, the joint posterior distribution of R and λ becomes

$$\pi(R, \lambda|data, \alpha) \propto R^{m+a_1-1}(1-R)^{n+a_2-1} \lambda^{m+n+a_1+a_2-1} e^{-\lambda(RT_1(\alpha)+(1-R)T_2(\alpha))}. \tag{11.12}$$

Now integrating out λ from 0 to ∞, the result follows. □

Therefore, the Bayes estimate of R with respect to the squared error loss function becomes

$$\widehat{R}_{Bayes} = E(R|data, \alpha) = K \int_0^1 \frac{R^{m+a_1}(1-R)^{n+a_2-1}}{(RT_1(\alpha) + (1-R)T_2(\alpha))^{m+n+a_1+a_2}} dR. \tag{11.13}$$

Here K is the normalizing constant, *i.e.*

$$K^{-1} = \int_0^1 \frac{R^{m+a_1-1}(1-R)^{n+a_2-1}}{(RT_1(\alpha) + (1-R)T_2(\alpha))^{m+n+a_1+a_2}} dR.$$

Clearly, $\widehat{R}_{Bayes}$ cannot be obtained in explicit forms. It is possible to use Lindley's approximation or Laplace's approximation to compute an approximate Bayes estimate of R. But it may not be possible to construct the highest posterior density (HPD) credible interval of R in that way. Observe that

$$\pi(R|data, \alpha) \leq K \frac{R^{m+a_1-1}(1-R)^{n+a_2-1}}{(\min\{T_1(\alpha), T_2(\alpha)\})^{m+n+a_1+a_2}}, \tag{11.14}$$

therefore, acceptance-rejection method can be easily used to generate samples directly from the posterior distribution of R, and the generated samples can be used to compute Bayes estimate and also to construct HPD credible interval of R.

11.3.2 Common Shape Parameter Unknown

In this case, the joint posterior density function of α, λ_1 and λ_2 can be written as

$$\pi(\lambda_1, \lambda_2, \alpha|data) \propto \lambda_1^{m+a_1-1}\lambda_2^{n+a_2-1}(\lambda_1+\lambda_2)^{a_0-a_1-a_2}e^{-\lambda_1 T_1(\alpha)-\lambda_2 T_2(\alpha)}\alpha^{m+n} S^{\alpha-1}\pi_2(\alpha), \tag{11.15}$$

where $S = \prod_{i=1}^{m} x_i \prod_{j=1}^{n} y_j$. Therefore, we have the similar result as Theorem 1, and whose proof also can be obtained along the same line. Hence it is avoided.

Theorem 2 *The joint posterior distribution of* $R = \dfrac{\lambda_1}{\lambda_1+\lambda_2}$ *and* α *for* $0 < R < 1$ *and* $0 < \alpha < \infty$*, is given by*

$$\pi(R, \alpha|data) \propto \frac{R^{m+a_1-1}(1-R)^{n+a_2-1}}{(RT_1(\alpha)+(1-R)T_2(\alpha))^{m+n+a_1+a_2}} \times \alpha^{m+n} S^{\alpha-1}\pi_2(\alpha).$$

Therefore, in this case, the Bayes estimate of R with respect to the squared error loss function becomes

$$\widehat{R}_{Bayes} = K_1 \int_0^1 \int_0^\infty \frac{R^{m+a_1}(1-R)^{n+a_2-1}}{(RT_1(\alpha)+(1-R)T_2(\alpha))^{m+n+a_1+a_2}} \times \alpha^{m+n} S^{\alpha-1}\pi_2(\alpha)\; d\alpha\, dR, \tag{11.16}$$

here K_1 is the proportionality constant, and it can be obtained as

$$K_1^{-1} = \int_0^1 \int_0^\infty \frac{R^{m+a_1-1}(1-R)^{n+a_2-1}}{(RT_1(\alpha)+(1-R)T_2(\alpha))^{m+n+a_1+a_2}} \times \alpha^{m+n} S^{\alpha-1}\pi_2(\alpha)\; d\alpha\, dR.$$

Clearly, the Bayes estimate of R with respect to the squared error loss function cannot be obtained in closed form. Again, in this case also the Laplace's or Lindley's approximation may be used to approximate the Bayes estimate of R, but the associated credible interval cannot be obtained. We propose to use the importance sampling procedure to compute Bayes estimate and also the associated credible interval as follows. Let us rewrite the joint posterior density of R and α as follows:

$$\pi(R, \alpha|data) = K_1 \times \text{Beta}(R; m + a_1, n + a_2) \times g_1(\alpha|data) \times h(\alpha, R)$$

Here $g_1(\alpha|data)$ is a proper density function, such that

$$g_1(\alpha|data) \propto \alpha^{m+n} S^{\alpha-1} \pi_2(\alpha) \tag{11.17}$$

and

$$h(\alpha, R) = \frac{1}{(RT_1(\alpha) + (1 - R)T_2(\alpha))^{m+n+a_1+a_2}}.$$

Note that $g_1(\alpha|data)$ is log-concave, hence using the method of Devroye [15], it is very easy to generate a sample from $g_1(\alpha|data)$. The following algorithm can be used to compute Bayes estimate of R, and also to construct associated credible interval.

Algorithm 1:

- Step 1: Generate $\alpha_1 \sim g_1(\alpha|data)$ and $R_1 \sim \text{Beta}(m + a_1, n + a_2)$.
- Step 2: Repeat Step 1, and obtain $(\alpha_1, R_1), \ldots, (\alpha_N, R_N)$.
- Step 3: A simulation consistent Bayes estimate of R can be obtained as

$$\widehat{R}_{Bayes} = \frac{\sum_{i=1}^{N} R_i h(\alpha_i, R_i)}{\sum_{j=1}^{N} h(\alpha_j, R_j)}.$$

- Step 4: Now to construct a $100(1 - \gamma)\%$ HPD credible intervals, we propose the following method, see also Chen and Shao [16] in this respect. let us denote

$$w_i = \frac{h(\alpha_i, R_i)}{\sum_{j=1}^{N} h(\alpha_j, R_j)}; \quad \text{for } i = 1, \ldots, N.$$

Rearrange, $\{(\alpha_1, R_1), \ldots, (\alpha_N, R_N)\}$, as follows $\{(R_{(1)}, w_{[1]}), \ldots, (R_{(N)}, w_{[N]})\}$, where $R_{(1)} < R_{(2)} < \cdots < R_{(N)}$. In this case, $w_{[i]}$'s are not ordered, they are just associated with $R_{(i)}$. Let N_p be the integer satisfying

$$\sum_{i=1}^{N_p} w_{[i]} \leq p < \sum_{i=1}^{N_p+1} w_{[i]},$$

for $0 < p < 1$. A $100(1-\gamma)\%$ credible interval of R can be obtained as $(R_{(N_\delta)}, R_{(N_{\delta+1-\gamma})})$, for $\delta = w_{[1]}, w_{[1]} + w_{[2]}, \ldots, \sum_{i=1}^{N_{1-\gamma}} w_{[i]}$. Therefore, a $100(1-\gamma)\%$ HPD credible interval of R becomes $(R_{(N_{\delta^*})}, R_{(N_{\delta^*+1-\gamma})})$, where

$$R_{(N_{\delta^*+1-\gamma})} - R_{(N_{\delta^*})} \leq R_{(N_{\delta+1-\gamma})} - R_{(N_\delta)} \quad \text{for all } \delta.$$

11.4 Inference on *R*: Presence of Covariates

11.4.1 Two Shape Parameters are Same

In this section, we consider the Bayesian inference of R in presence of covariates (u, v), based on the observations and prior assumptions provided in Sect. 11.2. In this section, we will make it explicit that $R = R(u, v) = P(Y < X|u, v)$. Let us use the following notations:

$$T_1(\alpha, \beta_1, U) = \sum_{i=1}^{m} x_i^{\alpha} e^{\beta_1^T u_i} \quad \text{and} \quad T_2(\alpha, \beta_2, V) = \sum_{j=1}^{n} y_j^{\alpha} e^{\beta_2^T v_j}.$$

Here, U and V are covariate vectors of orders $m \times p$ and $n \times q$, respectively, as follows

$$U = \begin{bmatrix} u_{11} & \ldots & u_{1p} \\ \vdots & \ddots & \vdots \\ u_{m1} & \ldots & u_{mp} \end{bmatrix} = \begin{bmatrix} u_1 \\ \vdots \\ u_m \end{bmatrix} \quad \text{and} \quad V = \begin{bmatrix} v_{11} & \ldots & v_{1q} \\ \vdots & \ddots & \vdots \\ v_{n1} & \ldots & v_{nq} \end{bmatrix} = \begin{bmatrix} v_1 \\ \vdots \\ v_n \end{bmatrix}.$$

Therefore, based on the model assumptions, and the posterior distribution, the posterior distribution function of $\theta_1, \theta_2, \alpha, \beta_1$, and β_2 can be written as

$$\begin{aligned} &\pi(\theta_1, \theta_2, \alpha, \beta_1, \beta_2|data) \propto \\ &\quad \theta_1^{m+a_1-1} \exp\{-\theta_1(b_0 + T_1(\alpha, \beta_1))\} \times \theta_2^{n+a_2-1} \exp\{-\theta_1(b_0 + T_2(\alpha, \beta_2))\} \\ &\quad \times (\theta_1 + \theta_2)^{a_0 - a_1 - a_2} \times \pi(\alpha)\alpha^{m+n} s^{\alpha} \times \exp\left\{\sum_{i=1}^{m} \beta_1^T u_i\right\} \prod_{k=1}^{p} \frac{1}{\sqrt{2\pi}\sigma_{1k}} \exp\left(-\frac{\beta_{1k}^2}{2\sigma_{1k}^2}\right) \\ &\quad \times \exp\left\{\sum_{j=1}^{n} \beta_2^T v_j\right\} \prod_{k=1}^{q} \frac{1}{\sqrt{2\pi}\sigma_{2k}} \exp\left(-\frac{\beta_{2k}^2}{2\sigma_{2k}^2}\right). \end{aligned} \tag{11.18}$$

Therefore, for a given u and v, with respect to squared error loss function, the Bayes estimate of R becomes

$$\widehat{R}_B(u, v) = \int_0^\infty \int_0^\infty \int_0^\infty \int_{\mathbb{R}^p} \int_{\mathbb{R}^q} \frac{\theta_2 e^{\beta_2^T v}}{\theta_1 e^{\beta_1^T u} + \theta_2 e^{\beta_2^T v}} \pi(\theta_1, \theta_2, \alpha, \beta_1, \beta_2 | data) \, d\beta_1 d\beta_2 \, d\theta_1 \, d\theta_2 \, d\alpha. \quad (11.19)$$

Clearly, the Bayes estimate of R cannot be obtained in closed form. For a given (u, v), we use the following importance sampling technique to compute the Bayes estimate of R , and the associated HPD credible interval of R. Note that (11.18) can be written as

$$\pi(\theta_1, \theta_2, \alpha, \beta_1, \beta_2 | data) = K \, h(\theta_1, \theta_2) \pi_1(\theta_1 | \alpha, \beta_1, data) \pi_2(\theta_2 | \alpha, \beta_2, data) \times \pi_3(\alpha | \beta_1, \beta_2, data) \pi_4(\beta_1 | data) \pi_5(\beta_2 | data). \quad (11.20)$$

Here, K is the normalizing constant, $\pi_1(\cdot|\alpha, \beta_1, data)$, $\pi_2(\cdot|\alpha, \beta_2, data)$, $\pi_3(\cdot|\beta_1, \beta_2, data)$, $\pi_4(\cdot|data)$ and $\pi_5(\cdot|data)$ are proper density functions, and they are as follows:

$$\pi_1(\theta_1|\alpha, \beta_1, data) \sim \text{Gamma}(\theta_1 | m + a_1, (b_0 + T_1(\alpha, \beta_1))) \quad (11.21)$$

$$\pi_2(\theta_2|\alpha, \beta_2, data) \sim \text{Gamma}(\theta_2 | n + a_2, (b_0 + T_2(\alpha, \beta_2))) \quad (11.22)$$

$$\pi_3(\alpha|\beta_1, \beta_2, data) \propto \frac{\pi(\alpha)\alpha^{m+n} S^\alpha}{(b_0 + T_1(\alpha, \beta_1))^{m+a_1} \times (b_0 + T_2(\alpha, \beta_2))^{n+a_2}} \quad (11.23)$$

$$\pi_4(\beta_1|data) = \prod_{k=1}^{p} N(c_k \sigma_{1k}, \sigma_{1k}^2)$$

$$\pi_5(\beta_2|data) = \prod_{k=1}^{q} N(d_k \sigma_{2k}, \sigma_{2k}^2),$$

where $c_k = \sum_{i=1}^{m} u_{ik}$ for $k = 1, \ldots, p$, and $d_k = \sum_{j=1}^{n} v_{jk}$, for $k = 1, \ldots, q$, and

$$h(\theta_1, \theta_2) = (\theta_1 + \theta_2)^{a_0 - a_1 - a_2}.$$

The following result will be useful for further development.

Theorem 3 *$\pi_3(\alpha|\beta_1, \beta_2, data)$ is log-concave.*

Proof See in the Appendix.

Note that it is quite standard to generate random samples from $\pi_1(\theta_1|\alpha, \beta_1, data)$, $\pi_2(\theta_2|\alpha, \beta_2, data)$, $\pi_4(\beta_1|data)$, $\pi_5(\beta_2|data)$, and using the method of Devroye [15] or Kundu [17], random samples from $\pi_3(\alpha|\beta_1, \beta_2, data)$ also can be obtained quite conveniently.

The following Algorithm 2 can be used to compute a simulation consistent estimate of (11.19) and the associated HPD credible interval.

Algorithm 2:

- Step 1: Generate β_1 and β_2 from $\pi_4(\beta_1|data)$ and $\pi_5(\beta_2|data)$, respectively.
- Step 2: For a given β_1 and β_2, generate α from $\pi_3(\alpha|\beta_1, \beta_2, data)$, using the method suggested by Devroye [15] or Kundu [17].
- Step 3: Now for a given α, β_1 and β_2, generate θ_1 and θ_2, from $\pi_1(\theta_1|\alpha, \beta_1, data)$ and $\pi_2(\theta_2|\alpha, \beta_2, data)$, respectively.
- Step 4: Repeat Step 1 to Step 4, N times and obtain

$$\{(\alpha_i, \beta_{1i}, \beta_{2i}, \theta_{1i}, \theta_{2i}), i = 1, \ldots, N\},$$

and also compute for $i = 1, \ldots, N$,

$$R_i(u, v) = \frac{\theta_{2i} e^{\beta_{2i}^T v}}{\theta_{1i} e^{\beta_{1i}^T u} + \theta_{2i} e^{\beta_{2i}^T v}}.$$

- Step 5: A simulation consistent Bayes estimate of $R(u, v)$ can be obtained as

$$\widehat{R}_B(u, v) = \frac{\sum_{i=1}^{N} R_i(u, v) h(\theta_{1i}, \theta_{2i})}{\sum_{j=1}^{N} h(\theta_{1j}, \theta_{2j})}.$$

- Step 6: Now to construct a $100(1-\gamma)\%$ HPD credible interval of $R(u, v)$, first let us denote

$$R_i = R_i(u, v) \quad \text{and} \quad w_i = \frac{h(\theta_{1i}, \theta_{2i})}{\sum_{j=1}^{N} h(\theta_{1j}, \theta_{2j})}; \quad \text{for } i = 1, \ldots, N.$$

Rearrange, $\{(R_1, w_1), \ldots, (R_N, w_N)\}$ as $\{(R_{(1)}, w_{[1]}), \ldots, (R_{(N)}, w_{[N]})\}$, where $R_{(1)} < \ldots, R_{(N)}$, and $w_{[i]}$'s are not ordered as before, and they are just associated with $R_{(i)}$. Let N_p be the integer satisfying

$$\sum_{i=1}^{N_p} w_{[i]} \leq p < \sum_{i=1}^{N_p+1} w_{[i]},$$

for $0 < p < 1$. A $100(1-\gamma)\%$ credible interval of R can be obtained as $(R_{(N_\delta)}, R_{(N_{\delta+1-\gamma})})$, for $\delta = w_{[1]}, w_{[1]} + w_{[2]}, \ldots, \sum_{i=1}^{N_{1-\gamma}} w_{[i]}$. Therefore, a $100(1-\gamma)\%$ HPD credible interval of $R(u, v)$ becomes $(R_{(N_{\delta^*})}, R_{(N_{\delta^*+1-\gamma})})$, where

$$R_{(N_{\delta^*+1-\gamma})} - R_{(N_{\delta^*})} \leq R_{(N_{\delta+1-\gamma})} - R_{(N_\delta)} \quad \text{for all } \delta.$$

11.4.2 Two Shape Parameters are Different

In this section, we consider the case when the two shape parameters are not same. In this case, it is assumed that $X \sim \text{WE}(\alpha_1, \lambda_1)$, $Y \sim \text{WE}(\alpha_2, \lambda_2)$, λ_1 and λ_2 follow similar relations as in Sect. 11.2. We make the following prior assumptions on the unknown parameters.

$$\begin{aligned}(\theta_1, \theta_2) &\sim \pi_1(\theta_1, \theta_2) = \text{DG}(b_0, a_0, a_1, a_2)\\ \alpha_1 &\sim \pi_{21}(\alpha_1), \quad \alpha_2 \sim \pi_{22}(\alpha_2)\\ \beta_1 &\sim \pi_3(\beta_1) = N_p(0, \Sigma_1)\\ \beta_2 &\sim \pi_4(\beta_2) = N_q(0, \Sigma_2).\end{aligned}$$

Here π_{21} and π_{22} have absolute continuous PDFs, and both the PDFs are log-concave, and all are independently distributed.

Therefore, based on the above prior assumptions, and using the same notations as in Sect. 11.4.1, the posterior distribution function of $\theta_1, \theta_2, \alpha_1, \alpha_2, \beta_1$ and β_2 can be written as

$$\begin{aligned}&\pi(\beta_1, \beta_2, \theta_1, \theta_2, \alpha_1, \alpha_2 | data) \propto\\ &\quad \theta_1^{m+a_1-1} \exp\{-\theta_1(b_0 + T_1(\alpha_1, \beta_1))\} \times \theta_2^{n+a_2-1} \exp\{-\theta_2(b_0 + T_2(\alpha_2, \beta_2))\}\\ &\quad \times (\theta_1 + \theta_2)^{a_0-a_1-a_2} \times \pi_{21}(\alpha_1)\alpha_1^m S_1^{\alpha_1} \times \pi_{22}(\alpha_2)\alpha_2^n S_2^{\alpha_2}\\ &\quad \times \exp\left\{\sum_{i=1}^{m} \beta_1^T u_i\right\} \prod_{i=1}^{p} \frac{1}{\sqrt{2\pi}\sigma_{1i}} \exp\left(-\frac{\beta_{1i}^2}{2\sigma_{1i}^2}\right)\\ &\quad \times \exp\left\{\sum_{j=1}^{n} \beta_2^T v_j\right\} \prod_{j=1}^{q} \frac{1}{\sqrt{2\pi}\sigma_{2j}} \exp\left(-\frac{\beta_{2j}^2}{2\sigma_{2j}^2}\right).\end{aligned} \tag{11.24}$$

Here $S_1 = \prod_{i=1}^{m} x_i$ and $S_2 = \prod_{j=1}^{n} y_j$. Therefore, for a given u and v, with respect to squared error loss function, the Bayes estimate of R becomes

$$\widehat{R}_B(u, v) = \int_0^\infty \int_0^\infty \int_0^\infty \int_{\mathbb{R}^p} \int_{\mathbb{R}^q} \int_0^\infty g(\Gamma, y|u, v) \times \pi(\Gamma|data)\, dy d\Gamma, \tag{11.25}$$

where $\Gamma = (\beta_1, \beta_2, \theta_1, \theta_2, \alpha_1, \alpha_2)$, $d\Gamma = (d\beta_1, d\beta_2, d\theta_1, d\theta_2, d\alpha_1, d\alpha_2)$ and

$$g(\Gamma, y|u, v) = \alpha_2\theta_2 e^{\beta_2^T v} y^{\alpha_2-1} e^{-(\theta_1 e^{\beta_1^T u} y^{\alpha_1} + \theta_2 e^{\beta_2^T v} y^{\alpha_2})}.$$

Clearly, (11.25) cannot be obtained in explicit form. We proceed as follows. Let us rewrite

$$\widehat{R}_B(u, v) = E(g(Y, \Theta_1, \alpha_1, \Theta_2, \alpha_2, \beta_1, \beta_2; u, v)|data), \tag{11.26}$$

here

$$g(y, \theta_1, \alpha_1, \theta_2, \alpha_2, \beta_1, \beta_2; u, v) = e^{-\theta_1 e^{\beta_1^T u} y^{\alpha_1} - \theta_2 e^{\beta_2^T v} y^{\alpha_2} + \beta_2^T v + \theta_2 y^{\alpha_2}},$$

and the joint PDF of Δ given the *data*, where $\Delta = (Y, \Theta_1, \alpha_1, \Theta_2, \alpha_2, \beta_1, \beta_2)$ can be written as

$$\begin{aligned}\pi(\Delta|data) = K &\times \pi_0(y|\alpha_2, \theta_2, data) \times \pi_1(\theta_1|\alpha_1, \beta_1, data) \times \pi_2(\theta_2|\alpha_2, \beta_2, data) \times \\ &\pi_3(\alpha_1|\beta_1, data) \times \pi_4(\alpha_2|\beta_2, data) \times \pi_5(\beta_1|data) \times \pi_6(\beta_2|data) \times \\ &h(\theta_1, \theta_2),\end{aligned}$$

and

$$\begin{aligned}\pi_0(y|\alpha_2, \theta_2, data) &\sim \text{WE}(\alpha_2, \theta_2) \\ \pi_1(\theta_1|\alpha_1, \beta_1, data) &\sim \text{Gamma}(\theta_1|m + a_1, (b_0 + T_1(\alpha_1, \beta_1))) \\ \pi_2(\theta_2|\alpha_2, \beta_2, data) &\sim \text{Gamma}(\theta_2|n + a_2, (b_0 + T_2(\alpha_2, \beta_2))) \\ \pi_3(\alpha_1|\beta_1, data) &\propto \frac{\pi_{21}(\alpha_1)\alpha_1^m S_1^{\alpha_1}}{(b_0 + T_1(\alpha_1, \beta_1))^{m+a_1}} \\ \pi_4(\alpha_2|\beta_2, data) &\propto \frac{\pi_{22}(\alpha_2)\alpha_2^n S_2^{\alpha_2}}{(b_0 + T_2(\alpha_2, \beta_2))^{n+a_2}}\end{aligned}$$

$$\begin{aligned}\pi_5(\beta_1|data) &= \prod_{k=1}^{p} N(c_k\sigma_{1k}, \sigma_{1k}^2) \\ \pi_6(\beta_2|data) &= \prod_{k=1}^{q} N(d_k\sigma_{2k}, \sigma_{2k}^2),\end{aligned}$$

where $c_k = \sum_{i=1}^{m} u_{ik}$ for $k = 1, \ldots, p$, and $d_k = \sum_{j=1}^{n} v_{jk}$, for $k = 1, \ldots, q$, and

$$h(\theta_1, \theta_2) = (\theta_1 + \theta_2)^{a_0 - a_1 - a_2}.$$

Following Theorem 3, it can be easily shown that $\pi_3(\alpha_1|\beta_1, data)$ and $\pi_4(\alpha_2|\beta_2, data)$ both are log-concave. An exactly similar algorithm like Algorithm 2, with an extra generation of $Y \sim \text{WE}(\alpha_2, \theta_2)$, can be used to compute a simulation consistent estimate of $\widehat{R}_B(u, v)$ and the associated HPD credible interval. The explicit details are not provided to avoid repetition.

11.5 Simulation Experiments

In this section, we perform some simulation experiments mainly to compare the nonparametric estimates of R with the MLE and the Bayes estimates of R. We would also like to see whether the parametric estimates are robust or not with respect to the distributional assumptions. We have taken four different cases namely (i) $X \sim$ GA(2,1), $Y \sim$ GA(3,2), (ii) $X \sim$ GA(2,1), $Y \sim$ GA(4,2), (iii) $X \sim$ WE(2,1), $Y \sim$ WE(3,2), (iv) $X \sim$ WE(2,1), $Y \sim$ WE(4,2), and different sample sizes namely $m = n$ = 20, 40, 60, 80 and 100. In each case we estimate R nonparametrically (NPE) and also obtain the MLE and the Bayes estimate of R based on the assumption that X and Y follow Weibull distributions with different shape and scale parameters. To compute the Bayes estimate of R we have taken the following prior distributions of the unknown parameters:

$$\alpha_1 \sim \text{GA}(0.0001, 0.0001), \quad \lambda_1 \sim \text{GA}(0.0001, 0.0001),$$
$$\alpha_2 \sim \text{GA}(0.0001, 0.0001), \quad \lambda_2 \sim \text{GA}(0.0001, 0.0001).$$

We replicate the process 1000 times in each case and obtain the average estimates and the mean squared errors (MSEs). The results are reported in Table 11.1 and Table 11.2. In each box, the first figure represents the average estimate and the corresponding MSE is reported within bracket below.

Some of the points are quite clear from this simulation experiments. The performances of the MLEs and the Bayes estimates based on the non-informative priors are very similar both in terms of biases and MSEs. It is observed that as the sample size increases in all the cases for the nonparametric estimates the biases and the MSEs decrease. It shows the consistency property of the nonparametric estimates. In case of MLEs and Bayes estimates, the MSEs decrease but when the model assumptions are not correct the biases increase. Therefore, it is clear that if we know the distributions of X and Y, it is better to use the parametric estimate otherwise it is better to use the nonparametric estimate, which is more robust with respect to the model assumptions, as expected.

11.6 Data Analysis

In this section, we present the analysis of a real data set to illustrate different methods suggested in this paper. The data set represents the measurements of shear strength of spot welds for two different gauges of steel. In this case, the weld diameter (in units of 0.001 in.) is the explanatory variable for both the cases. Let X and Y denote the weld strengths for 0.040–0.040—in and 0.060–0.060—in steel, respectively. The data are presented in Table 11.3 for convenience. The main interest here is on $R = P(Y < X|u, v)$.

Table 11.1 Comparison of the parametric and nonparametric estimates

$\|n\|$	$X \sim$ GA(2,1), $Y \sim$ GA(3,2)			$X \sim$ WE(2,1), $Y \sim$ WE(3,2)		
	$R = 0.4074$			$R = 0.3953$		
	NPE	MLE	Bayes	NPE	MLE	Bayes
20	0.4056	0.4081	0.4079	0.3948	0.3919	0.3923
	(0.0116)	(0.0020)	(0.0018)	(0.0116)	(0.0015)	(0.0016)
40	0.4065	0.4119	0.4117	0.3961	0.3934	0.3929
	(0.0062)	(0.0013)	(0.0014)	(0.0057)	(0.0011)	(0.0013)
60	0.4047	0.4130	0.4128	0.3979	0.3943	0.3939
	(0.0042)	(0.0009)	(0.0010)	(0.0040)	(0.0007)	(0.0009)
80	0.4045	0.4138	0.4136	0.3979	0.3949	0.3948
	(0.0029)	(0.0007)	(0.0008)	(0.0031)	(0.0006)	(0.0007)
100	0.4066	0.4138	0.4139	0.3981	0.3951	0.3952
	(0.0025)	(0.0006)	(0.0006)	(0.0025)	(0.0005)	(0.0005)

Table 11.2 Comparison of the parametric and nonparametric estimates

$\|n\|$	$X \sim$ GA(2,1), $Y \sim$ GA(4,2)			$X \sim$ WE(2,1), $Y \sim$ WE(4,2)		
	$R = 0.5391$			$R = 0.4381$		
	NPE	MLE	Bayes	NPE	MLE	Bayes
20	0.5354	0.4031	0.4025	0.4348	0.4316	0.4321
	(0.0118)	(0.0201)	(0.0198)	(0.0135)	(0.0042)	(0.0039)
40	0.5396	0.4052	0.4055	0.4361	0.4334	0.4337
	(0.0065)	(0.0194)	(0.0190)	(0.0076)	(0.0032)	(0.0034)
60	0.5385	0.4105	0.4101	0.4361	0.4343	0.4351
	(0.0040)	(0.0186)	(0.0181)	(0.0056)	(0.0028)	(0.0029)
80	0.5360	0.4129	0.4127	0.4375	0.4351	0.4358
	(0.0031)	(0.0175)	(0.0173)	(0.0047)	(0.0016)	(0.0018)
100	0.5383	0.4156	0.4151	0.4381	0.4381	0.4382
	(0.0024)	(0.0145)	(0.0144)	(0.0040)	(0.0009)	(0.0009)

Before progressing further, first we have made some preliminary analysis of the data. We look at the scaled TTT for both X and Y. It is well known that it provides some indication of the shape of the empirical hazard function, see for example Aarset [18]. The scaled TTT plots for X and Y are provided in Fig. 11.1. From the scaled TTT plots it is clear that both X and Y variables have increasing hazard functions, hence Weibull distribution can be used to fit these data sets.

We have fitted WE(α_1, λ_1) to X and WE(α_2, λ_2) to Y. The maximum likelihood estimators (MLEs), the maximized log-likelihood value (MLL), the Kolmogorov-Smirnov (KS) distance between the fitted and empirical distribution function and the associated p value are presented in Table 11.4.

Table 11.3 Shear strength data of welds for two gauges of steel

Obs. no.	X	u	Y	v
1.	350	380	680	190
2.	380	155	800	200
3.	385	160	780	209
4.	450	165	885	215
5.	465	175	975	215
6.	185	165	1025	215
7.	535	195	1100	230
8.	555	185	1030	250
9.	590	195	1175	265
10.	605	210	1300	250

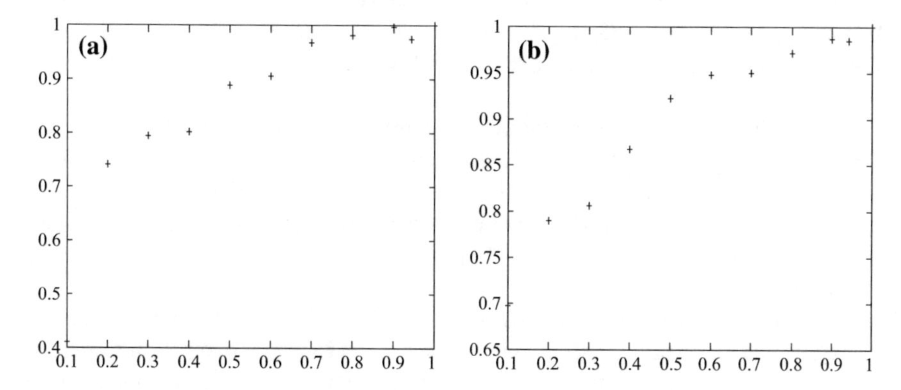

Fig. 11.1 Scaled TTT plot for **a** X and **b** Y

Table 11.4 The MLEs, KS distances and the associated p values for different cases

Data	$\widehat{\alpha}$	$\widehat{\lambda}$	MLL	KS	p
X	4.4439	22.8226	7.0302	0.1574	0.9653
Y	5.9647	0.7434	2.7520	0.1216	0.9984

From the KS distances and the associated p values, it is clear that the Weibull distribution fits both X and Y quite well. We would like to test the following hypothesis:

$$H_0 : \alpha_1 = \alpha_2 \quad \text{vs.} \quad H_1 : \alpha_1 \neq \alpha_2.$$

Under H_0, we obtain the MLEs of $\alpha, \lambda_1, \lambda_2$ and MLL as $\widehat{\alpha} = 5.1335, \widehat{\lambda}_1 = 34.8707, \widehat{\lambda}_2 = 0.8189$, MLL = 9.4476, respectively. Based on the likelihood ratio test (test statistic

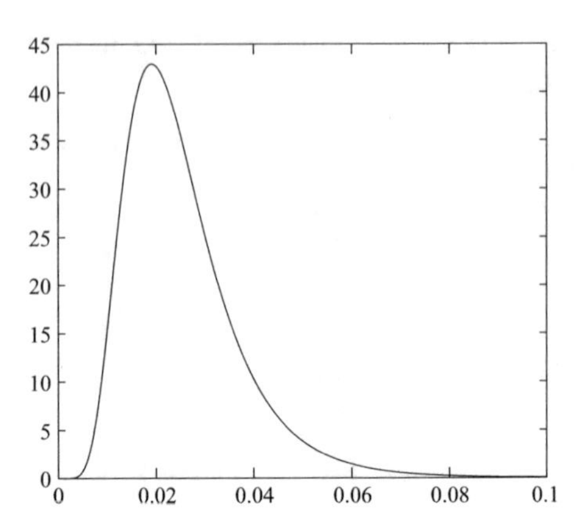

Fig. 11.2 Posterior PDF of R for known α

value becomes $2(7.0302 + 2.7520 - 9.4476) = 0.6692$), we cannot reject the null hypothesis as $p > 0.41$. Hence for this data set, it is assumed that $\alpha_1 = \alpha_2 = \alpha$. Based on this assumption, the MLE of $R = P(Y < X)$ without the covariates becomes 0.0229.

At the beginning we consider the Bayesian inference of R ignoring the covariates. For illustrative purposes, first let us assume that the common shape parameter α is known, and we would like to obtain the Bayes estimate of R and the associated HPD credible interval. Since we do not have any prior knowledge, it is assumed throughout $a_0 = b_0 = a_1 = a_2 \approx 0$. We provide the posterior distribution of R with known α in Fig. 11.2.

Now we generate samples directly from $\pi(R|data, \alpha)$ using acceptance-rejection principle, and based on 10000 samples we obtain the Bayes estimate with respect to the squared error loss function (posterior mean) as 0.0254, and the associated 95% HPD credible interval becomes (0.0123, 0.0502).

Now we would look at the case when the common shape parameter α is not assumed to be known. To compute the Bayes estimate of R we need to assume some specific form of $\pi_2(\alpha)$, and it is assumed that $\pi_2(\alpha) \sim \text{Gamma}(a, b)$. Since we do not have any prior knowledge about the hyper parameters, in this case also it is assumed that $a = b \approx 0$. Based on the above prior distribution, we obtain the posterior distribution of α, $g_1(\alpha|data)$, as in (11.17). The PDF of the posterior distribution of α is provided in Fig. 11.3.

We use Algorithm 1, and based on 10000, we obtain the Bayes estimate of R as 0.0238, and the associated 95% HPD credible intervals as (0.0115, 0.0518).

Now we want to estimate $R(u, v) = P(Y < X|u, v)$, when $u = 180$ and $v = 215$. These are the median values of the covariates of the respective groups, namely for X and Y. Here we have only one covariate each for both the groups. We obtain the MLEs of the unknown parameters, and they are as follows: $\widehat{\alpha} = 5.4318$, $\widehat{\theta_1} = 3.9597$, $\widehat{\theta_2} = 0.0406$, $\widehat{\beta_1} = -0.0518$, $\widehat{\beta_2} = -0.0372$. Hence we obtain the MLE of $R(u, v)$ as 0.0326. To compute the Bayes estimate of $R(u, v) = P(Y < X|u, v)$, we have further assumed $\beta_1 \sim \text{N}(0,0.01)$ and $\beta_2 \sim \text{N}(0,0.01)$. Based on the above assumption, using

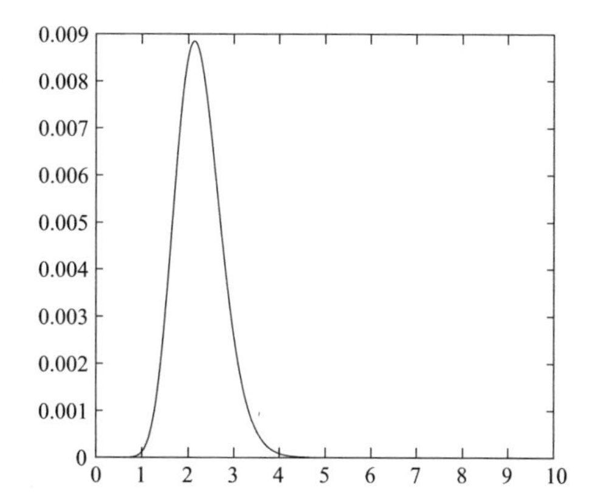

Fig. 11.3 Posterior PDF of α when the two shape parameters are equal

Algorithm 2, we obtain the Bayes estimate of $R(u, v) = P(Y < X|u, v)$ as 0.0298 and the associated 95% HPD credible interval as (0.0118, 0.0594).

For illustrative purposes, we obtain the Bayes estimates of R and $R(u, v)$ without the assumption $\alpha_1 = \alpha_2$ of the same data set. We have already observed that without the covariates, the MLEs of the unknown parameters are as follows: $\widehat{\alpha}_1 = 4.4439$, $\widehat{\lambda}_1 = 22.8226$, $\widehat{\alpha}_2 = 5.9646$ and $\widehat{\lambda}_2 = 0.7434$. Hence, the MLE of R based on (11.3) can be obtained as 0.0131. In presence of the covariates, the MLEs of the unknown parameters are as follows: $\widehat{\alpha}_1 = 4.4724$, $\widehat{\theta}_1 = 3.3638$, $\widehat{\beta}_1 = -0.0453$, $\widehat{\alpha}_2 = 5.9982$, $\widehat{\theta}_2 = 0.0286$, $\widehat{\beta}_2 = -0.0449$. The MLE of $R(u, v)$ becomes 0.0234. To compute the Bayes estimate of $R(u, v)$, it is assumed that $\pi_{21}(\alpha_1) \sim \text{Gamma}((a_{21}, b_{21}), \pi_{22}(\alpha_2) \sim \text{Gamma}((a_{22}, b_{22})$ and $a_{21} = b_{21} = a_{22} = b_{22} \approx 0$. The other prior distributions have taken same as before. Using the algorithm similar to Algorithm 2, based on 10000 samples, we obtain the Bayes estimate of $R(u, v)$, for $u = 180$, $v = 250$ as 0.0289, and the associated 95% HPD credible interval as (0.0078, 0.0634).

11.7 Conclusions

In this paper, we have considered the Bayesian inference of the stress-strength parameter $R = P(Y < X)$, when both X and Y have Weibull distribution. We have considered different cases namely when the two shape parameters are equal and when they are different. We have also addressed the issue when both X and Y may have some covariates also. We have assumed fairly general priors on the shape and scale parameters. In most of the cases, the Bayes estimate and the corresponding HPD credible interval cannot be obtained in explicit form and we propose to use Gibbs sampling and importance sampling methods to compute simulation consistent Bayes estimate and the associate HPD credible interval. We have demonstrated different methods using one data set, and it is observed that the proposed methods work well in practice.

Acknowledgements The author would like to thank one unknown referee for his/her many constructive suggestions which have helped to improve the paper significantly.

Appendix

Proof of Theorem 3: Note that

$$\ln \pi_3(\alpha|\beta_1, \beta_2, data) = const. + \ln \phi(\alpha) + (m+n)\ln \alpha + \alpha \ln S - (m+a_1)\ln(b_0 + \sum_{i=1}^{m} x_i^{\alpha} e^{\beta_1{}^T u_i}) - (n+a_2)\ln(b_0 + \sum_{j=1}^{n} y_j^{\alpha} e^{\beta_2{}^T v_j}).$$

It has been shown in the proof of Theorem 2 of Kundu [17], that

$$\frac{d^2}{d\alpha^2}\ln(b_0 + \sum_{i=1}^{m} x_i^{\alpha} e^{\beta_1{}^T u_i}) \geq 0 \text{ and } \frac{d^2}{d\alpha^2}\ln(b_0 + \sum_{j=1}^{n} y_j^{\alpha} e^{\beta_2{}^T v_j}) \geq 0.$$

Since $\pi(\alpha)$ is log-concave, it immediately follows that

$$\frac{d^2}{d\alpha^2}\ln \pi_3(\alpha|\beta_1, \beta_2, data) \leq 0.$$

References

1. Birnbaum, Z.W. 1956. On a use if Mann-Whitney statistics. In *Proceedings of third berkeley symposium in mathematical statistics and probability*, vol. 1, 13–17. Berkeley, CA: University of California Press.
2. Kotz, S., Y. Lumelskii, and M. Pensky. 2003. *The stress-strength model and its generalizations*. Singapore: World Scientific Press.
3. Zhou, W. 2008. Statistical inference for $P(X<Y)$. *Statistics in Medicine* 27: 257–279.
4. Kundu, D., and M.Z. Raqab. 2009. Estimation of $R = P(Y<X)$ for three parameter Weibull distribution. *Statistics and Probability Letters* 79: 1839–1846.
5. Ventura, L., and W. Racugno. 2011. Recent advances on Bayesian inference for $P(X<Y)$. *Bayesian Analysis* 6: 1–18.
6. Kizilaslan, F., and M. Nadar. 2016. Estimation of reliability in a multicomponent stress-strength model based on a bivariate Kumaraswamy distribution. *Statistical Papers, to appear*. https://doi.org/10.1007/s00362-016-0765-8.
7. Guttman, I., R.A. Johnson, G.K. Bhattacharya, and B. Reiser. 1988. Confidence limits for stress-strength models with explanatory variables. *Technometrics* 30: 161–168.
8. Weerahandi, S., and R.A. Johnson. 1992. Testing reliability in a stress-strength model when X and Y are normally distributed. *Technometrics* 34: 83–91.
9. Guttman, I., and G.D. Papandonatos. 1997. A Bayesian approach to a reliability problem; theory, analysis and interesting numerics. *Canadian Journal of Statistics* 25: 143–158.
10. Kundu, D., and R.D. Gupta. 2006. Estimation of $P(Y<X)$ for Weibull distribution. *IEEE Transactions on Reliability Theory* 55: 270–280.

11. Murthy, D.N.P., M. Xie, and R. Jiang. 2004. *Weibull Models*. New York: Wiley.
12. Peña, E.A., and A.K. Gupta. 1990. Bayes estimation for the Marshall-Olkin exponential distribution. *Journal of the Royal Statistical Society Series B* 52: 379–389.
13. Berger, J.O., and D. Sun. 1993. Bayesian analysis for the Poly-Weibull distribution. *Journal of the American Statistical Association* 88: 1412–1418.
14. Kundu, D., and B. Pradhan. 2011. Bayesian analysis of progressively censored competing risks data. *Sankhyā Series B* 73: 276–296.
15. Devroye, L. 1984. A simple algorithm for generating random variables using log-concave density function. *Computing* 33: 247–257.
16. Chen, M.H., and Q.M. Shao. 1999. Monte carlo estimation of bayesian credible and hpd intervals. *Journal of Computational and Graphical Statistics* 8: 69–92.
17. Kundu, D. 2008. Bayesian inference and life testing plan for the Weibull distribution in presence of progressive censoring. *Technometrics* 50: 144–154.
18. Aarset, M.V. 1987. How to identify a bathtub failure rate? *IEEE Transactions on Reliability* 36: 106–108.

Chapter 12
Air Pollution Effects on Clinic Visits in Small Areas of Taiwan: A Review of Bayesian Spatio-Temporal Analysis

Atanu Biswas and Jean-Francois Angers

Abstract The complete daily clinic visit records and environmental monitoring data at 50 townships and city districts of Taiwan for the year 1998 is considered. This data set has been analyzed in different directions by Hwang and Chan (Am J Epidemiol 155:1–16 (2002) [1]), Angers et al. (Commun Stat Simul Comput 38:1535–1550 (2009) [2]), Angers et al. (Commun Stat Simul Comput (2016) [3]), Biswas et al. (Environ Ecol Stat 22:17–32 (2015) [4]) over the years. The earlier analyses, all Bayesian, are based on the two-stage modelling (first-order autoregressive and Bayesian hierarchical modelling), Bayesian analysis using regression spline model and a Bayesian analysis using Daubechies wavelet. In the present paper, we revisit the dataset once again. We find that NO_2, SO_2, O_3, PM_{10} and temperature are the important pollutants in different areas following some spatial pattern. In this present article, some averages of the dew points temperature, and revisit the data with the wavelet-based modelling of Angers et al. (Commun Stat Simul Comput (2016) [3]). Although the results vary a little bit across different approaches, the basic features are almost same in all the studies.

Keywords Bayesian hierarchical modelling · Bayesian model averaging
Daily clinic visit rate · Daubechies wavelet · Regression spline

12.1 Taiwan Air Pollution Data

Hwang and Chan [1] described the Taiwan air pollution health effect study and the resultant data obtained in the year 1998, covering 50 townships and city districts of Taiwan, where ambient air monitoring stations of Taiwan Air Quality

---

A. Biswas (✉)
Applied Statistics Unit, Indian Statistical Institute, 203 B.T. Road,
Kolkata 700108, India
e-mail: atanu@isical.ac.in

J.-F. Angers
University of Montreal, Montreal, QC, Canada
e-mail: angers@dms.umontreal.ca

A. Adhikari et al. (eds.), *Mathematical and Statistical Applications in Life Sciences and Engineering*, https://doi.org/10.1007/978-981-10-5370-2_12

Monitoring Network (TAQMN) are situated. Quite naturally a large number of monitoring stations cluster in and around the three major cities of the island, namely Taipei, Kaohsiung and Taichung.

Several possible pollutants were measured and these are available in the dataset. The population at risk were estimated using sensible approach by Hwang and Chan [1]. The approach of Hwang and Chan [1] is similar to the popular *species estimation* problem of ecological studies; see Chao et al. [5] and Efron and Thisted [6] in this context.

The following variables are considered in different studies so far. The daily clinic visit rate for the 50 stations (areas) are the data points from the dependent variable. The associated covariates include the indicators of special holidays, indicators of Mondays, indicators of Saturdays, indicators of Sundays, indicators of different months, the daily averages of NO_2, SO_2, O_3 and CO measured in ppb for different areas, the daily average of PM_{10} measured in $\mu g/m^3$ for different areas, the daily average temperature for different areas, the daily average dew point for different areas, indicators of the value of the maximum temperature if it equals or exceeds 32 °C, indicator of the value of the maximum temperature if it is less than 32 °C, and the level of pollutants for different areas.

In Sect. 12.2, we indicate the nature of modelling and results in the earlier studies. Then, we present a new analysis of the data in Sect. 12.3. Section 12.4 presents conclusions.

12.2 Earlier Analyses

In the seminal work of Hwang and Chan [1], the monthly clinic visit rates for respiratory illness for each area in Taiwan in 1998 are modelled using some covariates. Under the assumption of normality of log rate, the modelling, computation and inference are relatively easy and follow standard theory.

Hwang and Chan [1] carried out a different but convenient approach. In fact, they used two phase modelling. They observed that the daily clinic visit rates were associated with current-day concentrations of nitrogen dioxide, carbon monoxide, sulphur dioxide and PM_{10}. Also, the elderly population (of age 65+) were the most susceptible.

Hwang et al. [7] carried out some subsequent analysis of the dataset. But, we are not going to describe that in this present review. Interested readers can go through Hwang et al. [7].

Angers et al. [2] considered this data once again. They considered a regression spline model (with reference to He and Shi [8]), and assuming a conjugate prior they obtained the Bayesian predictive values of the clinic visit rates. Angers et al. [2] implemented the popular Occam's Razor principle (cf. Madigan and Raftery [9]) to find out the appropriate model using Bayesian model averaging. In their study, Angers et al. [2] considered the third group of individuals only (i.e. the elderly population having age 65+) for their analysis. They ignored some of the covariates such as the density of the population in the area, the number of doctors per 10,000 persons, the number of doctors per km^2, and the relative distance of the area from a base point, as these are constant for any given area.

For model selection, once again they used the Occam's Razor principle Madigan and Raftery [9]. The argument of using Occam's Razor principle was that the standard criteria like the BIC and AIC are too conservative, and they often lead choosing to model with only one covariate.

The main conclusion of Angers et al. [2] was that the month of the year is a good predictor for the log of the monthly clinic visit rate for elderly patients. Then the principal component called 'Temperature', which is obtained from the standardized average monthly temperature and the standardized average monthly dew point, came out as the second best predictor [10–12].

Biswas et al. [4] again considered the Bayesian regression spline. However, they tried to improve upon the results of Angers et al. [2] in many aspects. The most important improvement in this modified analysis of TAQMN data set is that the daily clinic visit rates were considered instead of monthly averages.

In Angers et al. [2], a principal component analysis was carried out for covariate reduction. However, it is well known that principal component has the conceptual problem of interpretation. Keeping that in mind Biswas et al. [4] considered all the seven covariates for all the 50 monitoring stations. Hence, the approach of Biswas et al. [4] is much more complete and concrete.

Biswas et al. [4] concluded that NO_2, SO_2, O_3, PM_{10} and temperature are important pollutants in different areas. However, they exhibited some spatial pattern. Interestingly, temperature is believed to be a very influential risk factor for the respiratory illness in several parts of northern Taiwan. The analysis of Biswas et al. [4] successfully identified this factor. Similarly, they identified ozone as a serious risk factor in different parts of southern Taiwan.

Angers et al. [3] considered the Taiwan air pollution data set once again and provided a regression model based on the Daubechies wavelet. Their wavelet model was very much appropriate in term of fitting the data. The temperature, dew point and the oxides (NO_2 and CO) of the current day and the day before were identified as the pollutants in different areas following some spatial pattern.

Note that temperature emerged as a very important factor in all of the above-mentioned analyses. It is known that the cold current often hit northern Taiwan and had a big influence in the health of the inhabitants of the whole region.

12.3 The Data Revisited

In this section, we analyze the same air pollution data set of Taiwan using the same model as Angers et al. [3]. However, in addition to the one-day lagged version of the pollutants, five more variables have been added (see [1]) and these variables Z_{cjt} were not transformed by principal components transformations. These new variables are :

$$Z_{c8t} := \text{average dew point temperature 2 days priors;}$$
$$Z_{c9t} := \text{average dew point temperature 3 days priors;}$$
$$Z_{c10t} := \text{wind speed, coded from 1 to 7;}$$

and indicator functions for the winter and summer seasons. The number of pollutants/ neighbouring stations in the model averaging used to predict the log og daily clinic visit rate values are given in Table 12.1.

The histogram of the correlation between V_j and $\widehat{V}_j$ is given in Fig. 12.1. The mean (median) and standard deviation (interquartile distance) of these correlation values are respectively 0.890 (0.895) and 0.034 (0.045). The minimum and maximum correlation values are 0.771 and 0.946, respectively. The plots of V_j and $\widehat{V}_j$ for stations with thc smallest and largest correlation values are given in Figs. 12.2 and 12.3, respectively. The pollutants cntering into the model averaging for each station and its neighbour are given in Fig. 12.4. In this figure, the black circle indicates that the value of the pollutant for a given day at the station is used, while the red '+' sign means that the value is either a lag of one day or from a neighbouring station. The

Table 12.1 Number of pollutants/neighbouring stations entering in the models averaging

Number of models	1 to 5	6 to 10	11 to 15	16 to 20	21 to 25	26 to 30	≥ 31
Frequency	11	18	7	3	5	4	3

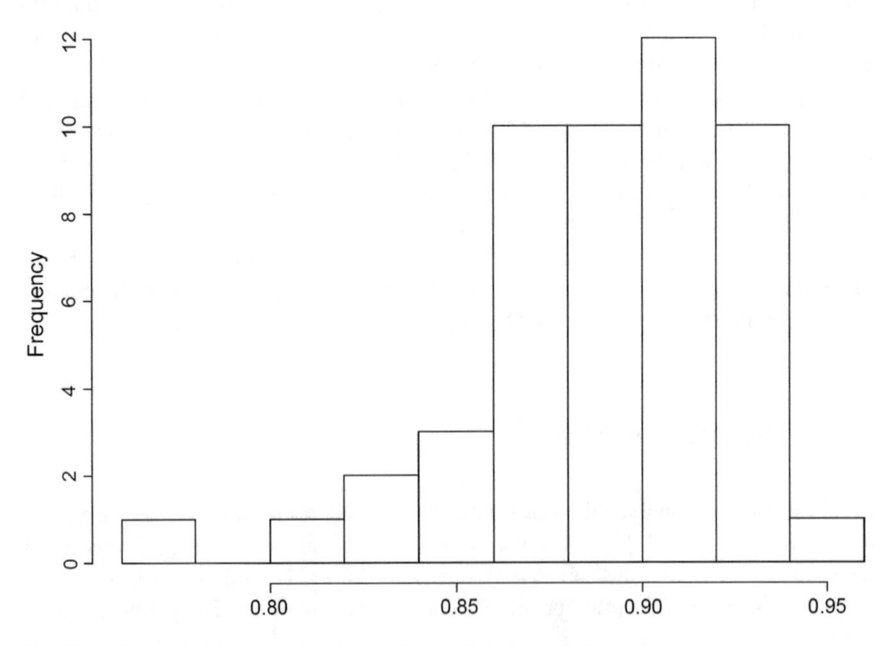

Fig. 12.1 Correlation between the observations and their predictions

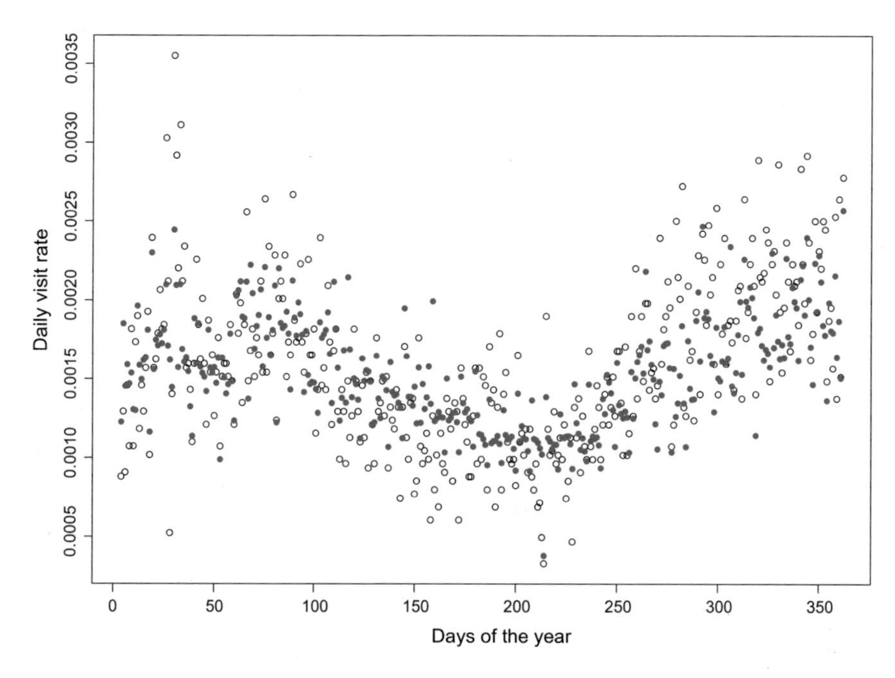

Fig. 12.2 Observed (black circle) and fitted values (red points) for the station with the smallest correlation (station 44)

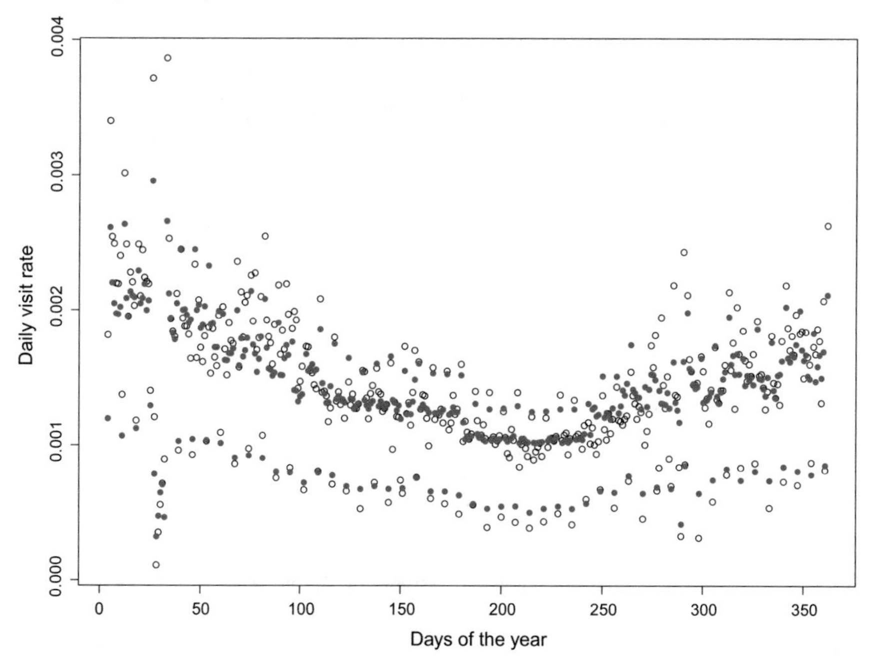

Fig. 12.3 Observed (black circle) and fitted values (red points) for the station with the largest correlation (station 8)

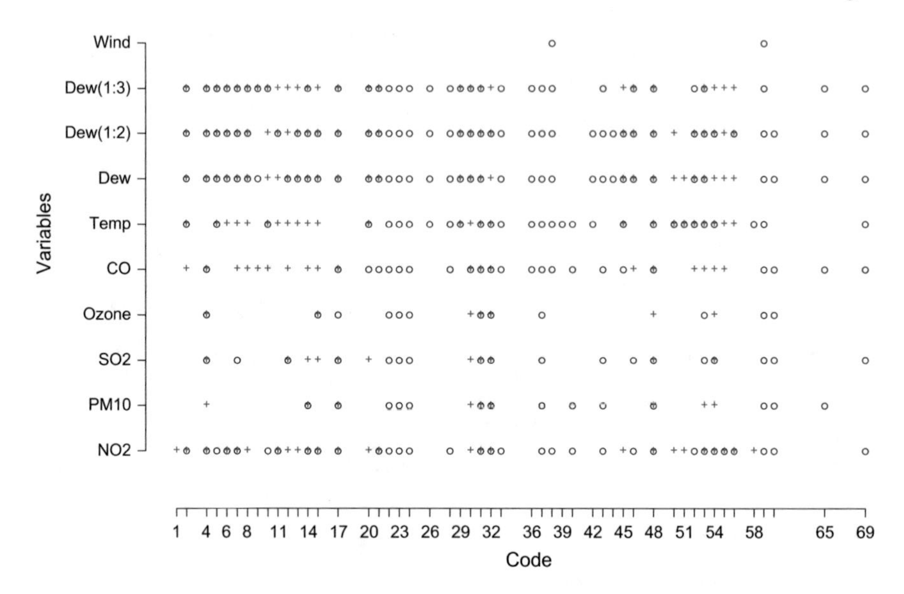

Fig. 12.4 Pollutants used to explain the daily clinic rates

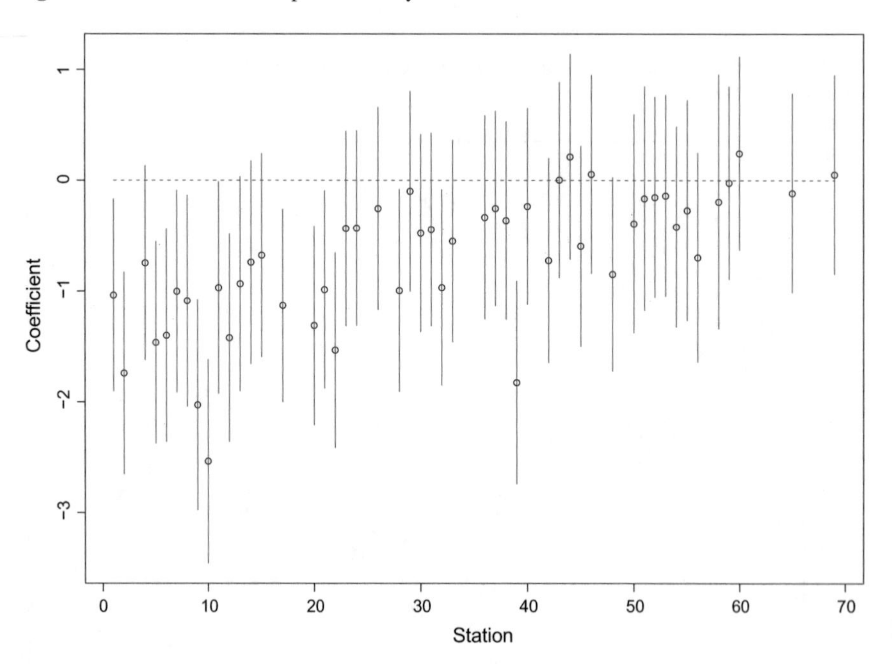

Fig. 12.5 Coefficient (±2 posterior standard deviations) of 'Special holiday' for each station

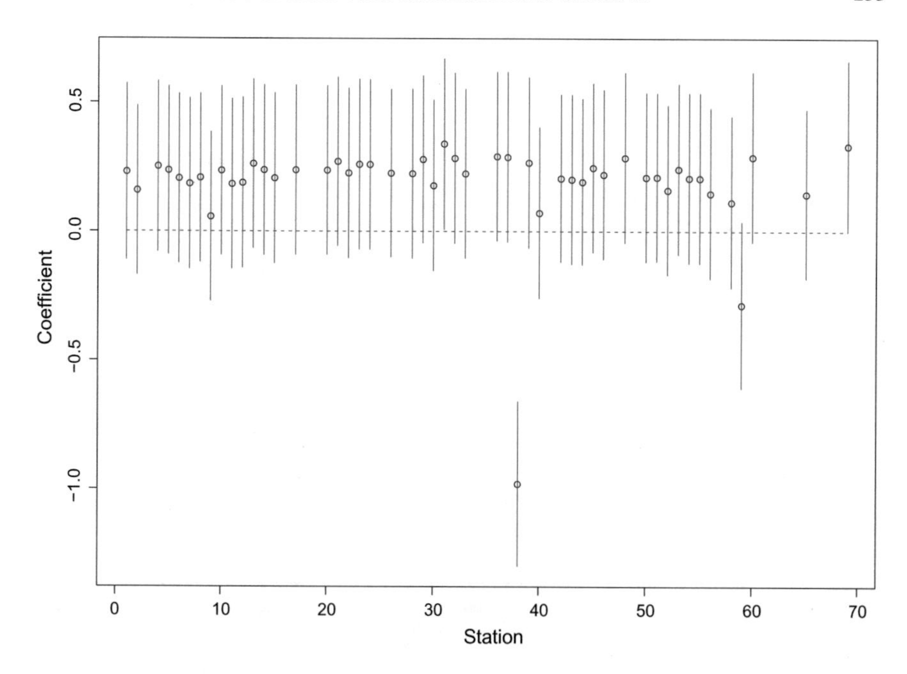

Fig. 12.6 Coefficient (±2 posterior standard deviations) of 'Monday' for each station

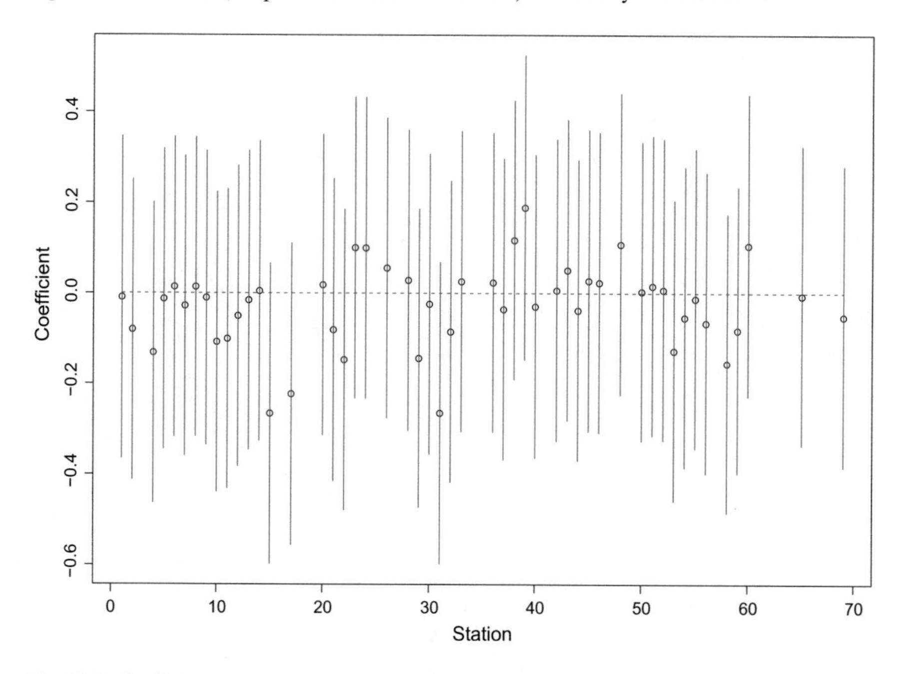

Fig. 12.7 Coefficient (±2 posterior standard deviations) of 'Saturday' for each station

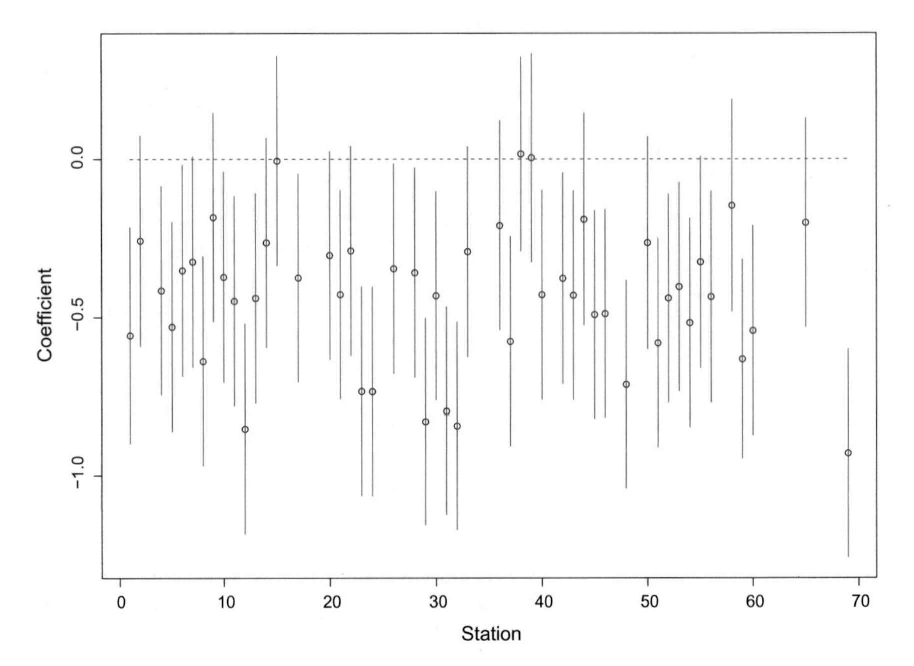

Fig. 12.8 Coefficient (±2 posterior standard deviations) of 'Sunday' for each station

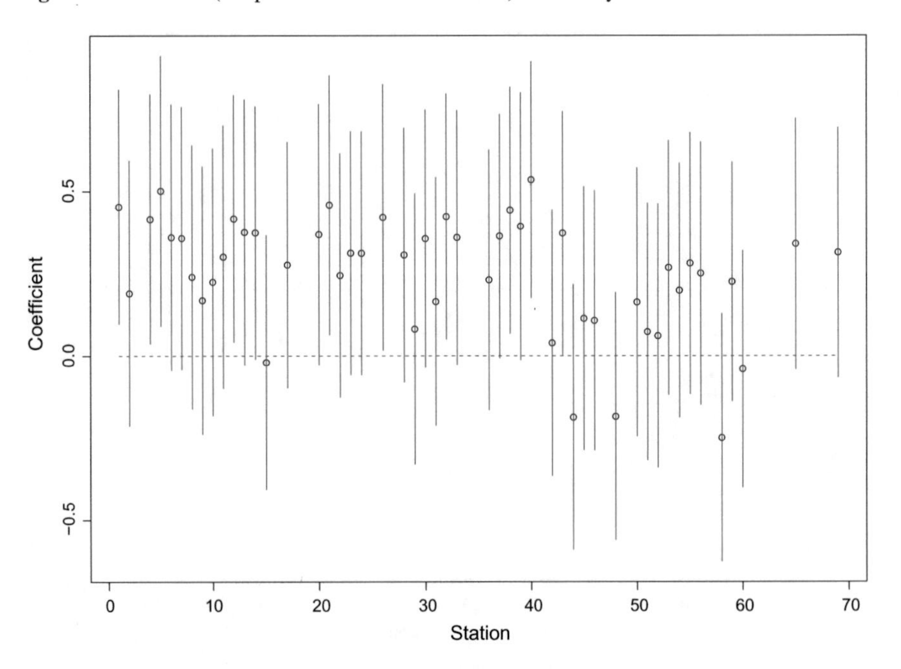

Fig. 12.9 Coefficient (±2 posterior standard deviations) of 'Winter' for each station

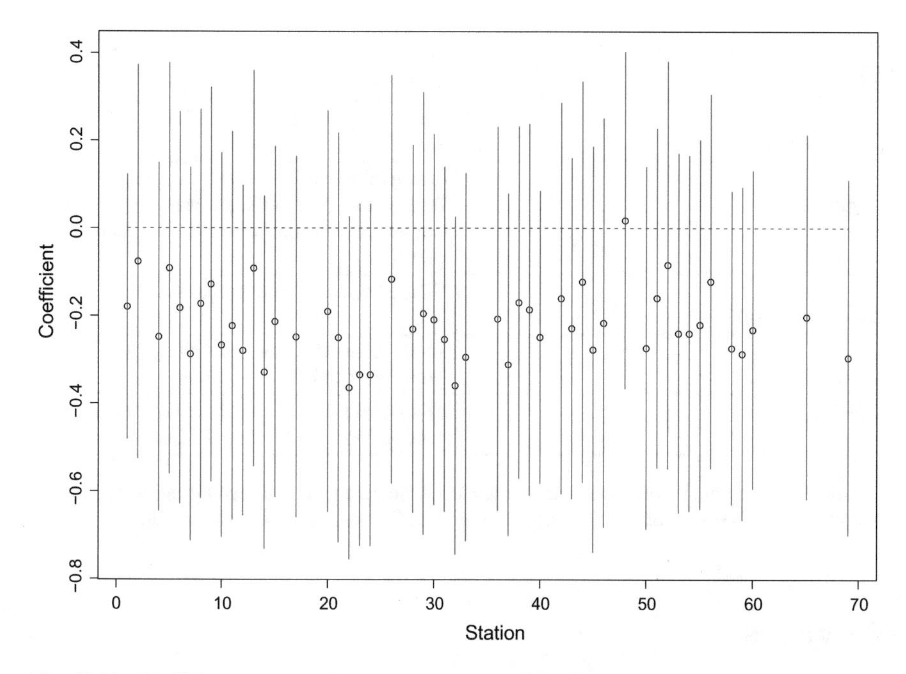

Fig. 12.10 Coefficient (±2 posterior standard deviations) of 'Summer' for each station

importance of the factors (special holiday, Monday, Saturday, Sunday, Winter and Summer) are given in Figs. 12.5, 12.6, 12.7, 12.8, 12.9 and 12.10. The values of the coefficients are plotted along with ±2 posterior standard deviations. Except for the variables 'Monday' and 'Winter', most of these variables reduce the daily visit rates.

12.4 Concluding Remarks

In this present article, we review four published works on the analyses of one real data set. All the analyses are Bayesian, however, their methodologies differ considerably—they vary from cyclic ARMA modelling to spline to wavelet. We also revisit the data set using wavelet modelling, but increased the number of covariates. But, the nature of finding is more or less similar. The objective of this present discussion is to provide different possible solutions for such type of data to the practitioners. In Table 12.2 we present the findings of different methods in tabular form.

One important point to mention is that wind direction is an important covariate in many such modelling of health hazard data on environmental pollutants. However, this important covariate is grossly omitted due to lack of technology to model this type of circular data.

Table 12.2 Findings (important risk factors) from different methods

Method	Important risk factors
Hwang and Chan [1]	Current-day concentrations of NO_2, CO, SO_2, PM_{10}
Angers et al. [2]	Month of the year, principal component Temperature (standardized average monthly temperature, standardized average monthly dew point)
Biswas et al. [4]	NO_2, SO_2, O_3, PM_{10}, temperature
Angers et al. [3]	Temperature, dew point and NO_2, CO of the current day and the day before
Present	Additional factors: special holiday, Saturday, Sunday, Monday, Winter, and Summer

Acknowledgements The authors wish to thank the reviewer for careful reading and one important suggestion which led to some improvement over an earlier version of the manuscript.

References

1. Hwang, J.S., and C.C. Chan. 2002. Effects of air pollution on daily clinic visits for lower respiratory tract illness. *American Journal of Epidemiology* 155: 1–16.
2. Angers, J.-F., A. Biswas, and J.-S. Hwang. 2009. Bayesian nonlinear regression for the air pollution effects on daily clinic visits in small areas of Taiwan. *Communications in Statistics—Simulation and Computation* 38: 1535–1550.
3. Angers, J.-F., A. Biswas, and J.-S. Hwang. 2016. Wavelet-based Bayesian nonlinear regressin for the air pollution effects on clinic in small areas of Taiwan. *Communications in Statistics—Simulation and Computation*. https://doi.org/10.1080/03610918.2016.1165839.
4. Biswas, A., J.-S. Hwang, and J.-F. Angers. 2015. Air pollution effects on clinic visits in small areas of Taiwan revisited. *Environmental and Ecological Statistics* 22: 17–32.
5. Chao, A., P. Yip, and H.S. Lin. 1996. Estimating the number of species via a martingale estimating function. *Statistica Sinica* 6: 403–418.
6. Efron, B., and R. Thisted. 1976. Estimating the number of unseen species: How many words did Shakespeare know? *Biometrika* 63: 433–447.
7. Hwang, J.S., T.H. Hu, and C.C. Chan. 2004. Air pollution mix and emergency room visits for respiratory and cardiac diseases in Taipei. *Journal of Data Science* 2: 311–327.
8. He, X., and P. Shi. 1998. Monotone B-spline smoothing. *Journal of the American Statistical Association* 93: 643–650.
9. Madigan, D., and A.E. Raftery. 1994. Model selection and accounting for model uncertainty in graphical models using Occam's window. *Journal of the American Statistical Association* 89: 1535–1546.
10. Burnett, R.T., R.E. Dales, M.R. Raizenne, D. Krewski, P.W. Summers, G.R. Roberts, M. RaadYoung, T. Dann, and J. Brook. 1994. Effects of low ambient levels of ozone and sulphates on the frequency of respiratory admissions to Ontario hospitals. *Environmental Research* 65: 172–194.
11. Chattopadhyay, A.K., S. Mondal, and A. Biswas. 2015. Independent Component Analysis and clustering for pollution data. *Environmental and Ecological Statistics* 22: 33–43.
12. Dominici, F., J.M. Samet, and S.L. Zeger. 2000. Combining evidence on air pollution and daily mortality from the 20 largest US cities: A hierarchical modelling strategy (with discussion). *Journal of the Royal Statistical Society Series B* 163: 263–302.

Chapter 13
On Competing Risks with Masked Failures

Isha Dewan and Uttara Naik-Nimbalkar

Abstract Competing risks data arise when the study units are exposed to several risks at the same time but it is assumed that the eventual failure of a unit is due to only one of these risks, which is called the "cause of failure". Statistical inference procedures when the time to failure and the cause of failure are observed for each unit are well documented. In some applications, it is possible that the cause of failure is either missing or masked for some units. In this article, we review some statistical inference procedures used when the cause of failure is missing or masked for some units.

13.1 Introduction

In a competing risks setup, a subject or a unit fails due to one of the many causes. Statistical inference for competing risks when the data consist of the failure time and the cause of failure is well documented (see [9, 10]). However, in many situations, the subject or unit is known to fail, but the cause of failure cannot be determined. In some situations, it is possible that the cause of failure is not known exactly but can be narrowed down to a subset of the possible types of failures containing the true type. This phenomenon is known as masking. Masking generally occurs due to constraints of time and the expense of failure analysis. This article gives an overview of the analysis of competing risks when the causes of failure are missing or are masked for some units.

A series system with k components can be considered as a unit exposed to k risks, and the cause of failure can be considered as the (label of) component which

I. Dewan (✉)
Theoretical Statistics and Mathematics Unit, Indian Statistical Institute,
7, S. J. S. Sansanwal Marg, New Delhi 110016, India
e-mail: isha@isid.ac.in

U. Naik-Nimbalkar
Department of Mathematics, Indian Institute of Science Education
and Research (IISER), Dr. Homi Bhabha Road, Pashan, Pune 411008, India
e-mail: uvnaik@gmail.com

A. Adhikari et al. (eds.), *Mathematical and Statistical Applications in Life Sciences and Engineering*, https://doi.org/10.1007/978-981-10-5370-2_13

failed and led to the system failure. To assess the effect of a treatment for a particular disease in a clinical trial or an epidemiological study, it is not uncommon to have missing information on the cause of death. We use the words system/subject/unit interchangeably in the following. Throughout it is assumed that the failure of each subject/unit/system is caused by only one of the competing causes/risks.

An example from animal bioanalysis where all causes were not available is considered in [29]. In [31], it is observed that 40% of the death certificates of people who had died in motor accidents had no information on the cause. Some other examples of masked survival data available in the literature are the survival data of heart transplant patients [25] and the longitudinal study of breast cancer patients [11].

We first set up the notation. Let T be the random variable denoting the failure time (or the time of occurrence of the event), and let δ denote the cause/risk of failure. Suppose there are k causes of failures. The joint distribution of (T, δ) can be expressed in terms of the sub-distribution function $F(j,t)$ or the sub-survival function $S(j,t)$ of the risk j, which are defined, respectively, as

$$F(j,t) = P[T \le t, \delta = j] \text{ and } S(j,t) = P[T > t, \delta = j], \; j = 1, \ldots, k.$$

Let $F(t)$ and $S(t)$, respectively, denote the distribution function and the survivor function of the failure time T. Let $f(j,t)$ denote the sub-density function corresponding to risk j and $f(t)$ the density function of T. We have

$$F(t) = \sum_{j=1}^{k} F(j,t), \quad S(t) = \sum_{j=1}^{k} S(j,t), \quad f(t) = \sum_{j=1}^{k} f(j,t).$$

The cause-specific hazard rates for $j = 1, \ldots, k$ are defined as

$$\lambda(j,t) = f(j,t)/S(t) = \lim_{h \downarrow 0} \frac{P[t < T \le t+h, \delta = j | T \ge t]}{h}.$$

We now consider the latent variables approach. Let U_j denote the failure time of the unit due to the j-th risk, $j = 1, \ldots, k$. That is, the series system fails due to the failure of the j-th component. Then the failure time T of the unit/system is

$$T = min(U_1, \ldots, U_k).$$

Define $\delta = j$ if $T = U_j$. As before, the actual observation is the pair (T, δ). The variables U_j, $j = 1, \ldots, k$ are called "latent" random variables. Let $F_j(t)$, $S_j(t)$, and $f_j(t)$, respectively, denote the distribution function, the survival function, and the density function of the latent random variable U_j, $j = 1, \ldots, k$. We note that, under the assumption of independent risks,

$$S(t) = \prod_{j=1}^{k} S_j(t) \text{ and } f(t) = \sum_{j=1}^{k} \left(f_j(t) \prod_{\substack{l=1 \\ l \neq j}}^{k} S_l(t) \right).$$

In some situations, the values of δ_i's are missing for some units under study. Let O_i be an indicator variable which takes value one if δ_i is observed and zero if δ_i is missing. The indicator variables $O_1, \cdots O_n$ are observed. Further, assume that the failure times can be right censored. Let C denote the censoring time and ξ the censoring indicator, that is, $\xi_i = 1$, if the failure time T_i is observed for the unit i and $\xi_i = 0$, otherwise. Also, the future cause of failure is not known if $C(\leq T)$ is observed instead of T. Let $X = min(T, C)$. Thus for unit i, we have observations $(X_i, O_i\xi_i\delta_i, \xi_i)$.

The types of "missingness" considered in the literature are as follows:

1. Missing completely at random (MCAR): In this setup, it is assumed that the missing mechanism is independent of everything else, that is.

   $$P[O = 1|T, \delta, C, \xi = 1] = P[O = 1|\xi = 1],$$

   and

   $$P[O = 0|T, \delta, C, \xi = 0] = 1.$$

2. Under the missing at random (MAR) assumption (see [40]), the missing mechanism can depend on the time but not on the cause of failure when conditioning on observed data, that is,

   $$P[O = 1|X, \delta, \xi = 1] = P[O = 1|X, \xi = 1].$$

3. Informative missingness I: $P[O = 1 \mid X, \delta, \xi = 1] = P[O = 1 \mid \delta, \xi = 1]$. In this case, whether the cause is observed or not depends on the true value of δ and hence, the missingness carries the information about the unobserved cause.
4. Informative missingness II: In this case, the missingness depends on both, the cause of failure and the fully observed failure time.
5. The missingness is said to be missing not at random (MNAR) if the missing mechanism depends on the missing variables also.
6. Suppose one does not observe the exact cause of failure but knows that the cause of failure belongs to some proper subset $\mathcal{G}$ of $\{1, 2, \ldots, k\}$, the set of all causes of failure. We have observations on $(X, \xi, \mathcal{G})$ for each unit under study. In this situation, the failure type is said to be masked in the set $\mathcal{G}$.

The article [18] is among the first to consider the estimation of survival due to different failure types when the information on failure type was either completely available or not available at all. In [37], MLEs and MVUEs of the parameters of exponential distributions for a two-component series system are obtained when the cause of failure for some systems is missing; and approximate and asymptotic properties of these estimators and confidence intervals are discussed in [30]. Results of [37] were extended in [47] to a three-component series system, under the same constant failure rates assumption but with masked failure data. The results were further extended to series systems with larger number of components in [26, 41, 42]. The likelihood is written in terms of densities of the component failure times with masked failure data under the MAR assumption. An iterative maximum likelihood procedure in the case of two-component series system under the assumption that components have Weibull failure time distributions and under the MAR assumption is given in [48].

In some articles (see [7, 8, 20, 21]), it is considered that for some units with masked failure at the first stage, the cause of failure is identified at the second stage by further failure analysis like autopsy. In [20], maximum likelihood estimation under a model with proportional (crude) hazard functions for the competing risks is discussed and in [21], a model with parametric densities is considered. A semiparametric model with piecewise constant cause-specific hazard functions and with the missing mechanism or the masking probabilities depending on the cause of failure and the failure time (informative missingness II) is considered in [7]. Complete parametric modeling with the masking probabilities depending on the true cause of failure (informative missingness I) is considered in [8].

Use of multiple imputation methods in the parametric setup is proposed in [32, 34, 46]. A semiparametric Bayesian approach for analyzing competing risks survival data with masked cause of death is proposed in [43]. The article does not assume independence among the causes.

The regression problems for missing failure types using partial likelihood for two types of failures under the assumption of proportional cause-specific hazards for the two failure types are considered in [15, 24, 35] under the MAR assumption. Semi-parametric inference of competing risks data with additive cause-specific hazards and missing cause of failure under MCAR and MAR assumptions are considered in [5, 36].

Nonparametric estimators of the survival function in the missing failure cause setup are mostly obtained under either the MAR or the MCAR assumptions. The first article to consider a nonparametric maximum likelihood estimator (NPMLE) in this setup with right-censored failure times is [18]. The EM algorithm is used to obtain an NPMLE. In [33], it is shown that there are infinitely many NPMLEs and some of them are inconsistent but an estimator which is consistent and asymptotically normal is proposed. In [49], a NPMLE of the survival function is proposed and is shown to be efficient. Two nonparametric procedures for masked failure cause are proposed in [16]. One approach is under the MAR assumption and the other assumes that certain information on the conditional probability of the true type given a set of possible failure types is available from the experimentalists. We describe these procedures in the next section. The article [22] considers the nonparametric estimation of the survival function and estimation in the Cox regression model and establishes the asymptotic properties of the proposed estimators. In [19], a nonparametric estimator of the sub-distribution function $F(j, t|z)$ (also known as the cumulative incidence function) is obtained in the presence of a continuous covariate vector z under the

MCAR assumption of missingness. The asymptotic normality of the normalized estimator is established.

A modified log-rank test for the equality of two competing risks with missing failure type is considered in [23] and is extended in [15]. A nonparametric weighted log-rank (WLR)-type test for testing equality of conditional survival functions, for the missing failure cause setup, is proposed in [3]. In [4], a test for the equality of the survival functions corresponding to two competing risks, based on the weighted Kaplan–Meier-type statistic is proposed and its asymptotic normality under the null hypothesis is established.

For some recent work on competing risks with missing data, see [12, 17, 27, 38, 45, 50, 51].

In the next section, we consider estimation procedures when for some units the cause of failure is either masked or missing. We first review the parametric setup when the likelihood is based on the distributions of the latent random variables and also when the likelihood is written in terms of the cause-specific hazard rates. We then consider two nonparametric procedures. The tests for equality of two risks are reviewed in Sect. 13.3. We consider Locally Most Powerful (LMP) tests, Locally Most Powerful Rank (LMPR) tests, tests based on U-statistics, and tests based on counting processes. A small numerical study is also done. Areas of future work are indicated in Sect. 13.4.

13.2 Estimation

We first consider the parametric setup with the likelihood based on the densities of the latent variables. We follow it up with the likelihood based on the cause-specific hazard rates and then discuss two nonparametric procedures. Unless mentioned otherwise, the risks and hence the latent variables are assumed to be independent. The failure times of the units are also assumed to be independent.

13.2.1 Parametric Inference

Consider n identical series systems each with k components. Let U_{ij} denote the failure time of component j in system i (that is, the latent variable corresponding to risk j for unit i); $j = 1, \cdots, k$, $i = 1, \ldots, n$. The failure time T_i of system i is

$$T_i = min\{U_{i1}, U_{i2}, \ldots, U_{ik}\}.$$

Below, we discuss the likelihood function given in [26]. Let $f_j(t)$ and $S_j(t)$ denote the probability density and survival functions of the random variable U_{ij}. The values T_i are observed for $i = 1, \ldots, n$. Let $\mathcal{G}_i$ denote the set of components (labels) that may cause the system i to fail. The data are (t_i, g_i); observed values of $(T_i, \mathcal{G}_i)$,

$i = 1, \ldots, n$. Assuming no censoring, the contribution of (t_i, g_i) to the likelihood is

$$L_i = \sum_{j \in g_i} \left(f_j(t_i) \prod_{\substack{l=1 \\ l \neq j}}^{k} S_l(t_i) \right) P(\mathcal{G}_i = g_i | T_i = t_i, \delta_i = j).$$

Assuming the MAR condition, we have for j and $j' \in g_i$ and $j \neq j'$

$$P(\mathcal{G}_i = g_i | T_i = t_i, \delta_i = j) = P(\mathcal{G}_i = g_i | T_i = t_i, \delta_i = j'). \tag{13.1}$$

The term $P(\mathcal{G}_i = g_i | T_i = t_i, \delta_i = j)$ then can be factored outside the sum over j and

$$L_i = P\left(\mathcal{G}_i = g_i | T_i = t_i, \delta_i = j' \right) \sum_{j \in g_i} \left(f_j(t_i) \prod_{\substack{l=1 \\ l \neq j}}^{k} S_l(t_i) \right).$$

The full likelihood is

$$L = \prod_{i=1}^{n} L_i.$$

A parametric model is assumed for the component failure times. It is assumed that the masking probabilities $P_{g_i|j}(t) = P(\mathcal{G}_i = g_i | T_i = t_i, \delta_i = j)$ do not depend on the parameters of the failure time distributions. Under this assumption, to obtain MLEs of the parameters of the failure time distributions, the partial likelihood

$$L_R = \prod_{i=1}^{n} \left\{ \sum_{j \in g_i} \left(f_j(t_i) \prod_{\substack{l=1 \\ l \neq j}}^{k} S_l(t_i) \right) \right\}$$

is maximized.

The case, where the exact cause of failure for some systems (or subjects), say for m systems, is known and for the remaining $n - m$ systems only the failure time is known, is covered by the above likelihood. If the cause of failure of system i is type j, then $g_i = \{j\}$ and for a system i, if only the failure time is known, then $g_i = \{1, \ldots, k\}$.

Censored failure time data

For unit i, let C_i denote the censoring variable and ξ_i the indicator $I[T_i \leq C_i]$. Let $H_i(t)$, $\bar{H}_i(t)$ and $h_i(t)$, respectively, denote the distribution function, the survival function, and the density of C_i. Let $X_i = min(T_i, C_i)$. The data are observations on $(X_i, \mathcal{G}_i, \xi_i)$, $i = 1, \ldots, n$. If $\xi_i = 0$ then $\mathcal{G}_i = \{1, \ldots, k\}$. Further assume that T_i and C_i are independent and that $H_i(t)$ does not depend on the parameters of the failure time distributions. Under the MAR assumption and the assumption that the masking probabilities do not depend on the parameters of the failure time distributions, the partial likelihood for obtaining the MLEs of the parameters of the failure time distributions is

$$L_c = \prod_{i=1}^{n} \left\{ (\sum_{j \in g_i} (f_j(t_i) \prod_{\substack{l=1 \\ l \neq j}}^{k} S_l(t_i))) \bar{H}_i(t_i) \right\}^{\xi_i} \left\{ h_i(t_i) \prod_{l=1}^{k} S_l(t_i) \right\}^{1-\xi_i}.$$

Since the H_i's do not depend on the failure time parameters, the reduced likelihood is

$$L_R = \prod_{i=1}^{n} \left\{ \left(\sum_{j \in g_i} \left(f_j(t_i) \prod_{\substack{l=1 \\ l \neq j}}^{k} S_l(t_i) \right) \right) \right\}^{\xi_i} \left\{ \prod_{l=1}^{k} S_l(t_i) \right\}^{1-\xi_i}.$$

In [20, 21], a two-stage procedure is considered, where if for a unit the failure is masked in stage-I, then a further failure analysis, such as an autopsy, is done to determine the exact cause of failure. They assume informative type-I missingness, that is, the missingness depends on the cause of failure. They split the likelihood in the following manner. First, we set up the notation:
n_j denotes the number of failures due to cause j and let $t_i^{(j)}$, $i = 1, \ldots, n_j$ denote the corresponding failure times.
n_g is the number of failures having masking group g and with failure times $t_i^{(g)}$, $i = 1, \ldots, n_g$.
n_c denotes the number of censored systems. The corresponding censoring (survival) times are $t_i^{(c)}$, $i = 1, \ldots, n_c$.
$n_{g,j}$ is the number of system failures with masking group g in stage-I and identified due to cause j in stage-II.
$n_g^+ = \sum_{j=1}^{k} n_{g,j}$ is the total number of failed units with masking group g in stage-I with the failure cause identified in stage-II.
$\tilde{n}_g$ is the number of failed units with masking group g in stage-I that are not considered in stage-II for identification.
$n_j^* = n_j + \sum_{i \in g} n_{i,g}$ is the total number of failed units due to cause j identified either in stage-I or stage-II

Let $\bar{t}_i$ denote the i-th event time that corresponds either to a failure or a censoring time; $i = 1, \ldots, n$.
$\tilde{t}_i^{(g)}$ is the i-th failure time among all unresolved failure times with masking group g.
$\tilde{t}_i^{(g,j)}$ is the i-th failure time among all failure times of units restricted to masking group g in stage-I and identified with cause j in stage-II.
P_j is the probability that a system failure due to cause j is correctly identified in stage-I.
$P_{g|j}$ (the masking probability) is the probability that system failure due to cause j is restricted to the masking group g in stage-I.
It is assumed that P_i and $P_{g|j}$ do not depend on the time and the competing causes act independently of each other.

Let θ_j be the parameter(s) and let $f_j(t; \theta_j)$ and $S_j(t : \theta_j)$, respectively, denote the probability density and the survival functions associated with the failure time distribution of cause j. Let $\theta = (\theta_1, \ldots, \theta_k)$ and $f(t; \theta)$ and $S(t; \theta)$, respectively, denote the probability density and the survival functions associated with the system.

The likelihood function using both stage-I and stage-II data is as follows:

$$L = \prod_{i=1}^{n_c} S\left(t_i^{(c)}; \theta\right) \prod_{j=1}^{k} \prod_{i=1}^{n_j} \left\{ P_j f_j \left(t_i^{(j)}; \theta_j\right) \prod_{\substack{l=1 \\ l \neq j}}^{k} S_l \left(t_i^{(j)}; \theta_l\right) \right\}$$

$$\times \prod_{g} \prod_{i=1}^{\tilde{n}_g} \left[\sum_{r \in g} P_{g|r} f_r \left(\tilde{t}_i^{(g)}; \theta_r\right) \prod_{\substack{l=1 \\ l \neq r}}^{k} S_l \left(\tilde{t}_i^{(g)}; \theta_l\right) \right]$$

$$\times \prod_{j=1}^{k} \prod_{g \in \mathcal{G}_j^*} \prod_{i=1}^{n_{g,j}} \left[P_{g|j} f_j \left(t_i^{(g,j)}; \theta_j\right) \prod_{\substack{l=1 \\ l \neq j}}^{k} S_l \left(t_i^{(g,j)}; \theta_l\right) \right], \quad (13.2)$$

where $\mathcal{G}_j^*$ denotes the set of proper groups containing cause $\{j\}$ (with the exception of group $\{j\}$).

The first line of (13.2) corresponds to the censored failure times and the failure times identified in stage-I; the second line corresponds to the failure causes masked and not resolved; and the third line to the failure causes resolved in stage-II. If no unit is taken to stage-II, then the likelihood would consist of the first two lines of (13.2). Assuming Weibull distributions for the competing failure times, [21] suggest an iterative procedure for obtaining maximum likelihood estimates (MLE) of $\bar{\theta}$, P_j, $j =, \ldots k$, and of $P_{g|j}$ for all possible values of j and g.

Let $\pi_{j|g}(t)$ denote the probability that a failure at time t restricted to a masking group g is due to cause j. Then by the Bayes theorem,

$$\pi_{j|g}(t) = \frac{P_{g|j} f_j(t; \theta_j)}{\sum_{r \in g} P_{g|r} f_r(t; \theta_r)}.$$

The diagnostic probabilities $\pi_{j|g}(t)$ can be estimated by plugging in the estimates of θ and the $P_{g|j}$'s.

In [20], it is shown that under the assumption of proportional hazards for the competing risks the resulting likelihood function is over-parametrized and the model parameters are unidentifiable.

Dependent Competing Risks

Estimation of the cause-specific hazard rates and sub-distribution functions for dependent competing risks when failure type is masked is considered in [8]. A two-stage observation scheme as in [21] is considered. It is supposed that n systems are observed for a period of time length τ. Suppose there are G proper masking groups (that is, they contain more than one cause), and let $M = G + k$. The observation on each unit i is $(x_i, \gamma_{ig_1}, \ldots, \gamma_{ig_M}; \delta_{i1}, \ldots, \delta_{ik})$, where x_i is either the failure time or the censoring time; γ_{ig} is the indicator that unit i's masking group is g at the first stage (if the failure cause is known to be j at stage-I, then the unit is said to be masked to $g = \{j\}$); and δ_{ij} is the indicator that unit i's failure cause j is observed. If a unit is masked in stage-I and not taken to stage-II, then all the δ_{ij}'s are unknown. If unit i is right censored, then all the indicators $\delta_{ij},\ j = 1, \ldots, k$, take value 0, the γ_{ig}'s are unknown.

Piecewise constant cause-specific hazard rates are assumed for each cause j. For each cause j, the interval $(0, \tau]$ is divided into M_j subintervals $(a_{j(m-1)}, a_{jm}]$, $m = 1, \ldots, M_j$, $(0 = a_{j0} < a_{j1} < \ldots < a_{jM_j})$; and

$$\lambda(j, t) = \sum_{m=1}^{M_j} \lambda_{jm} I_{jm}(t),$$

where $I_{jm}(t)$ is the indicator that $t \in (a_{j(m-1)}, a_{jm}]$. Let θ denote the vector of parameters to be estimated; $\theta = (\lambda_{11}, \ldots, \lambda_{kM_k}, P_{g_1|1}, \ldots, P_{g_G|k})$. Let $\mathcal{G}_j^*$ denote the set of proper groups containing cause $\{j\}$ (with the exception of group $\{j\}$.)

Conditional on j being the cause of failure of masked unit i, the random vector $\{\gamma_{ig} : g \in \{g_1, \ldots, g_{G+k}\}, j \in g\}$ has a multinomial distribution with total 1. Moreover $P_{g|j} = P(\gamma_{ig} = 1|j)$. Using $S(t) = exp(-\int_0^t \sum_{j=1}^k \lambda(j, u)du)$ and assuming that all the δ_{ij}'s are observed, the conditional log-likelihood function given in [8] is

$$l_C(\theta) = \sum_{i=1}^{n}\sum_{j=1}^{k}\Bigg\{\Bigg[\delta_{ij} ln \sum_{m=1}^{M_j} \lambda_{jm} I_{jm}(x_i) - \sum_{m=1}^{M_j} \lambda_{jm} \int_0^{x_i} I_{jm}(u)du\Bigg] + \delta_{ij}\Bigg[\Bigg(1 - \sum_{g\in\mathcal{G}_j^*} \gamma_{ig}\Bigg) ln \Bigg(1 - \sum_{g\in\mathcal{G}_j^*} P_{g|j}\Bigg) + \sum_{g\in\mathcal{G}_j^*} \gamma_{ig} ln P_{g|j}\Bigg]\Bigg\}.$$

In [8], an estimator of the vector θ is obtained using the EM algorithm by conditioning on the observed data; and estimator of the sub-distribution functions are obtained using the relation

$$F(j, t) = \int_0^t \lambda(j, u) exp\Bigg(-\int_0^u \sum_{l=1}^{k} \lambda(l, v)dv\Bigg)du.$$

13.2.2 Nonparametric Estimation

Nonparametric estimation of the different cause-specific hazards, based on data with the above-mentioned general missing pattern in failure types and censored failure times is considered in [16]. The MAR condition (13.1) is assumed. We describe this approach below.

Let A_i denote the set of labels for the individuals failed or censored at time x_i, and D_i the set of labels for the individuals failed at time x_i.

The likelihood in terms of the cause-specific hazard rates is proportional to

$$L = \prod_{=1}^{n} \Big[\prod_{l \in A_i} \Big\{ \Big(\sum_{j \in g_l} \lambda(j, x_i) \Big)^{\xi_l} S(x_i) \Big\} \Big].$$

Since the nonparametric maximum likelihood estimates of cause-specific hazard rates have mass at most at the observed failure times, $s_1 < s_2 < \cdots < s_m$, say. Let λ_{ji} denote the discrete cause-specific hazard of type j at time s_i, the above likelihood reduces to

$$L_R = \prod_{i=1}^{m} \Big[\Big\{ \prod_{l \in D_i} \Big(\sum_{j \in g_l} \lambda_{ji} \Big) \Big\} \Big(1 - \sum_{j=1}^{k} \lambda_{ji} \Big)^{n_i - d_i} \Big],$$

where d_i denotes the number of failures at s_i (number of labels in D_i) and $n_i =$ number of individuals at risk just prior to time s_i. Using the EM algorithm, a method is proposed for obtaining the estimates of the λ_{ji}'s.

In [16], a Nelson–Aalen-type estimator is also proposed for situations when certain information on the conditional probability of the true type given a set of possible failure types is available from the experimentalists. We consider this estimator below.

As introduced earlier, $P_{g|j}(t) = P[\mathcal{G} = g | T = t, \delta = j, \xi = 1]$; if g does not contain j, then $P_{g|j}(t) = 0$. For a fixed j, $\sum_g P_{g|j}(t) = 1$. It is assumed that the missing mechanism is independent of the censoring mechanism. The hazard rate for failure due to cause j at time t and with g (containing j) observed as the set of possible causes is $P_{g|j}(t)\lambda(j, t))$. Hence, the hazard rate for failure at time t with g observed as the set of possible causes is

$$\lambda^*(g, t) = \sum_{j \in g} P_{g|j}(t) \lambda(j, t). \tag{13.3}$$

To obtain the Nelson–Aalen-type estimators, it is assumed that $P_{g|j}(t) = P_{g|j}$ is independent of time t but may depend on g and j, that is, the informative missingness I setup is assumed. Let $N_g(t)$ denote the number of failures up to time t, with g as the observed set of possible causes. A multiplicative intensity model is assumed for counting process $\{N_g(t), t \geq 0\}$, that is,

$$dN_g(t) = \lambda^*(g, t) Y(t) dt + dM_g(t),$$

where $Y(t)$ denotes the number of individuals at risk just prior to time t and $\{M_g(t)\}$ is a local square integrable martingale, for each nonempty subset g. The Nelson–Aalen estimator of $\Lambda^*(g, t) = \int_0^t \lambda^*(g, u) du$ is given by [1]

$$\hat{\Lambda}^*(g,t) = \int_0^t \frac{I\{Y(s) > 0\}}{Y(s)} dN_g(s), \tag{13.4}$$

which converges in distribution to a Gaussian process with mean $\Lambda^*(g,t)$ and a variance function which can be consistently estimated by

$$\hat{V}_g(t) = \int_0^t \frac{I\{Y(s) > 0\}}{Y^2(s)} dN_g(s). \tag{13.5}$$

Let $\underline{\Lambda}^*(t)$ denote the $(2^k - 1) \times 1$ vector of $\Lambda^*(g,t)$'s and $\underline{\Lambda}(t)$ be the $k \times 1$ of the cumulative cause-specific hazards $\Lambda(j,t)$'s, then from (13.3)

$$\underline{\Lambda}^*(t) = \mathbf{P}\underline{\Lambda}(t), \tag{13.6}$$

where $\mathbf{P}$ is the $(2^k - 1) \times m$ matrix of the $P_{g|j}$'s. From (13.4) and (13.6),

$$\hat{\underline{\Lambda}}^*(t) = \mathbf{P}\underline{\Lambda}(t) + \underline{\epsilon}(t), \tag{13.7}$$

where $\hat{\underline{\Lambda}}^*(t)$ is the vector of $\hat{\Lambda}^*(g,t)$'s and $\underline{\epsilon}(t)$ is a vector process converging to a vector of Gaussian martingales whose variance function is consistently estimated by the matrix $diag(\hat{V}_g(t))$. The expression (13.7) can be considered as a linear model with the "design" matrix P, which can be estimated as given below. Let $\hat{P}$ denote a consistent estimator of P. Then, using the principle of weighted least squares and the consistent estimator (13.5), a consistent estimator of $\underline{\Lambda}(t)$ is

$$\hat{\underline{\Lambda}}(t) = (\hat{P}^T W(t) \hat{P})^{-1} \hat{P}^T W(t) \hat{\underline{\Lambda}}^*(t),$$

where $W(t) = diag(1/\hat{V}_g(t))$.
For g containing j,

$$P_{g|j} = P(\mathcal{G} = g|\delta = j) = \frac{P(\delta = j|\mathcal{G} = g)P(\mathcal{G} = g)}{\sum_{g' \in \mathcal{G}_j^*} P(\delta = j|\mathcal{G} = g')P(\mathcal{G} = g')}.$$

The fraction of failures with $\mathcal{G}$ observed as g can be taken as an estimator of $P(\mathcal{G} = g)$ and information from the experimenter can be used to estimate $P(\delta = j|\mathcal{G} = g)$, which lead to an estimate of the $P_{g|j}$. In [16], an estimator of the cause-specific hazard is obtained by using kernel smoothing suggested by [39]. Also, a simulation study is reported, which shows that for sufficiently large number of observations, the bias may be small, even for high proportion of missing data but the estimates seem to be sensitive to misspecification of the conditional probabilities of the true types when the missing proportion is high.

13.3 Testing

In this section, we restrict ourselves to the case when there are two causes of failure, that is $k = 2$. And information on some causes of failure is missing. The following testing problems have been considered in literature by [6]:

$$\begin{aligned}
&H_0 : F(1,t) = F(2,t) \text{ for all t against } H_1 : F(1,t) \leq F(2,t) \text{with strict inequality for some t,}\\
&H_0 : S(1,t) = S(2,t) \text{ for all t against } H_2 : S(1,t) \leq S(2,t) \text{ with strict inequality for some t,}\\
&H_0 : \lambda(1,t) = \lambda(2,t) \text{ for all t against } H_3 : \lambda(1,t) \leq \lambda(2,t) \text{ with strict inequality for some t.}
\end{aligned} \tag{13.8}$$

Under each of the three alternatives risk 2 is more "effective" than risk 1 stochastically. The three hypotheses mentioned above are not equivalent, but H_3 implies both H_1 and H_2. Sometimes, the sub-distribution functions may cross but the sub-survival functions could be ordered or vice versa.

In what follows we consider the LMP and LMPR tests for testing H_0 against H_1. We also propose U-statistics for this testing problem. Then, we look at tests based on counting process for testing H_0 against H_3 [14]. A small numerical study is also done.

13.3.1 *Locally Most Powerful Tests*

We want to test the hypothesis H_0 versus the alternative H_1 that the sub-distribution functions are ordered when information on causes of failure for some individuals is missing. We have information on failure times and causes of failure for n individuals. For the remaining $N - n$ individuals, only the cause of failure is known.

The likelihood function based on $(T_i, \delta_i), i = 1, 2, \ldots, n$ and $T_i, i = n + 1, n + 2, \ldots, N$ is given by

$$L(\underline{t}, \underline{\delta}) = \prod_{i=1}^{n} \left\{ f(1, t_i) \right\}^{I(\delta_i = 1)} \left\{ f(2, t_i) \right\}^{I(\delta_i = 2)} \prod_{i=n+1}^{N} f(t_i). \tag{13.9}$$

Here n is random. Suppose T and δ are independent. Then

$$F(1,t) = \theta F(t), \;\; F(2,t) = (1-\theta) F(t),$$

where $\theta = P[\delta = 1]$.

The likelihood reduces to

$$L(\theta, \underline{t}, \underline{\delta}) = \theta^{\sum_{i=1}^{n} I(\delta_i=1)} (1-\theta)^{I(\delta_i=2)} \prod_{i=1}^{N} f(t_i). \tag{13.10}$$

Testing, $F(1,t) = F(2,t)$ is same as testing $\theta = 1/2$. The optimal statistic is

$$U_1 = \sum_{i=1}^{n} I(\delta_i = 1). \tag{13.11}$$

U_1 is the generalization of the sign test to the case when some causes of failure are missing. Unlike the sign statistic in the complete sample case, this is the sum of random number of indicator functions. Note that n has $B(N, p)$ distribution, where $p = P(\delta$ is observed). For fixed n, nU_1 has $B(n, \theta)$ distribution.

We assume that n is independent of $\delta_i^{\prime}s$. The exact distribution of U_1 is discussed below.

$$\begin{aligned}
&P(U_1 = u) \\
&= \sum_{k=0}^{N} P(U_1 = u | n = k) P(n = k) \\
&= \sum_{k=0}^{N} B(u, k, \theta) B(k, N, p) \\
&= \sum_{k=0}^{N} \binom{k}{u} \theta^u (1-\theta)^{k-u} \binom{N}{k} p^k (1-p)^{N-k} \\
&= \sum_{k=0}^{N} \frac{N!}{u!(k-u)!(N-k)!} (\theta p)^u ((1-\theta)p)^{k-u} (1-p)^{N-k} \\
&= \sum_{j=0}^{N} \frac{N!}{u!j!(N-j-u)!} (\theta p)^u ((1-\theta)p)^{N-j-u} (1-p)^j.
\end{aligned} \tag{13.12}$$

Hence,

$$P(U_1 \le u) = \sum_{i=0}^{u} \sum_{j=0}^{N} \frac{N!}{i!j!\ell!} (\theta p)^i ((1-\theta)p)^{\ell} (1-p)^j. \tag{13.13}$$

13.3.2 Locally Most Powerful Rank Tests

Let

$$f(1,t) = f(t,\theta), \ f(2,t) = f(t) - f(t,\theta)$$

where $f(t)$ and $f(t,\theta)$ are known density and sub-density functions such that

$$f(t,\theta_0) = \frac{1}{2} f(t).$$

Let $T_{(1)} < T_{(2)} < \ldots < T_{(n)}$ be the ordered failure times. Let

$$W_i = \begin{cases} 1 \text{ if } T_{(i)} \text{ corresponds to first risk} \\ 0 \quad \text{otherwise.} \end{cases} \tag{13.14}$$

Note that $W_i's$ are known only for n individuals and are missing for the remaining.

If all $W_i's$ were known, the likelihood of ranks would be

$$\int \cdots \int_{0<t_1<\ldots<t_N<\infty} \prod_{i=1}^{N} \Big[f(t_i,\theta) \Big]^{w_i} \Big[f(t_i) - f(t_i,\theta) \Big]^{1-w_i} dt_i. \tag{13.15}$$

However, now it is given by (we sum over possible values of $W_i's$ that are missing)

$$P(\underline{R}, \underline{W}, \theta) = \int \cdots \int_{0<t_1<\ldots<t_N<\infty} \prod_{i=1}^{n} \Big[f(t_i,\theta) \Big]^{w_i} \Big[f(t_i) - f(t_i,\theta) \Big]^{1-w_i} \prod_{i=n+1}^{N} f(t_i) \prod_{i=1}^{N} dt_i. \tag{13.16}$$

Let

$$A = \prod_{i=1}^{n} \Big[f(t_i,\theta) \Big]^{w_i} \Big[f(t_i) - f(t_i,\theta) \Big]^{1-w_i} \prod_{i=n+1}^{N} f(t_i).$$

When $\theta = \theta_0$, $A = \frac{1}{2^n} \prod_{i=1}^{N} f(t_i)$. Note that n is random.

Differentiating A with respect to θ and putting $\theta = \theta_0$, we get

$$\sum_{i=1}^{n} \left[w_i \frac{f'(t_i,\theta_0)}{f(t_i,\theta_0)} - (1-w_i) \frac{f'(t_i,\theta_0)}{f(t_i,\theta_0)} \right] A. \tag{13.17}$$

Hence, we have the following result.

Theorem 1 *If $f'(t,\theta)$ is the derivative of $f(t,\theta)$ with respect to θ, then the locally most powerful rank test for $H_0 : \theta = \theta_0$ against $H_1 : \theta > \theta_0$ is given by the following: Reject H_0 for large values of $L_c = \sum_{i=1}^{n} w_i a_i$, where*

$$a_i = \frac{1}{2^n} \int \cdots \int_{0<t_1<\ldots<t_N<\infty} \frac{f'(t_i,\theta_0)}{f(t_i,\theta_0)} \prod_{i=1}^{N} \Big[f(t_i,\theta_0) dt_i \Big]. \tag{13.18}$$

Some special choices of the scores a_i are listed below :

(i) If T and δ are independent, then $a_i = \frac{1}{2^n}$.
(ii) In case of Lehmann-type alternative defined by

$$F(1,t) = \left[\frac{H(t)}{2}\right]^{\theta}, \quad F(2,t) = H(t) - \left[\frac{H(t)}{2}\right]^{\theta},$$

LMPR test is based on scores $a_i = \frac{1}{2^n} E(E_{(j)})$ where $E_{(j)}$ is the j-th-order statistic from a random sample of size n from standard exponential distribution.
(iii) If $f(1,t) = \frac{1}{2} g(t,0)$ and $f(2,t) = \frac{1}{2} g(t,\theta), \theta > 0$ and $g(t,\theta)$ is the logistic density function $g(t,\theta) = \frac{e^{(x-\theta)}}{[1+e^{(x-\theta)}]^2}$, then the LMPR test is based on the statistic

$$W^+ = \sum_{i=1}^{n} \frac{1}{2^n} W_i R_i,$$

which is the analogue of the Wilcoxon signed rank statistic for competing risks data.

For most other distributions, the scores are complicated and need to be solved using numerical integration techniques.

The scores are similar to those for the case of complete competing risks data. However, the statistic is a sum of random number of components (n instead of N in the complete case). Besides, there is a factor $\frac{1}{2^n}$, which is random. For the case when all causes of failure are known, that is, $N = n$, $\frac{1}{2^N}$ is a fixed number.

13.3.3 U-Statistics

In this section, we propose tests based on U-statistics for testing

$$H_0 : F(1,t) = F(2,t) = F(t)/2, \quad \text{for all t}$$

against the alternative

$$H_1 : F(1,t) < F(2,t), \quad \text{for some t.}$$

A measure of deviation from the null hypothesis is $F(2,t) - F(1,t)$, which is non-negative under the alternative H_1. Consider

$$\int_0^{\infty} [F(2,t) - F(1,t)] dF(t) = 2\int_0^{\infty} F(2,t) dF(t) - \frac{1}{2} = 2P[T_1 \leq T_2, \delta_1 = 2] - \frac{1}{2}. \quad (13.19)$$

When (T_i, δ_i), $i = 1, \ldots, N$ are available, a U-statistic (U_F) for testing H_0 against H_1 is based on the kernel, which is an estimator of the above measure (13.19) without the constant term, defined as follows:

$$\begin{aligned}\phi_F(T_i, \delta_i, T_j, \delta_j) &= 1 \text{ if } T_i < T_j, \delta_i = 2 \text{ or, } T_j < T_i, \delta_j = 2,\\ &= 0 \text{ otherwise.}\end{aligned}$$

Let U_F be the U-statistic corresponding to the kernel $\phi_F(.)$

$$U_F = \frac{1}{\binom{N}{2}} \sum_{1 \le i < j \le N} \phi_F(T_i, \delta_i, T_j, \delta_j). \tag{13.20}$$

Then, the expected value of U_F, is

$$E(U_F) = 2 \int_0^\infty F(2, t) dF(t). \tag{13.21}$$

Recall that $E(U_F \mid H_0) = 1/2$, $E(U_F \mid H_1) > 1/2$, and $var(U_F \mid H_0) = 1/3$ (see [13, 28]).

If δ_i are missing for some i, then the above kernel cannot be defined for each pair (i, j). Following table shows the situations when the kernel cannot be defined (m indicates missing δ and ? indicates that the kernel cannot be defined).

(δ_i, δ_j)	(1,1)	(1,2)	(1,m)	(2,1)	(2,2)	(2,m)	(m,1)	(m,2)	(m,m)
$T_i > T_j$	0	1	?	0	1	?	0	1	?
$T_i \le T_j$	0	0	0	1	1	1	?	?	?

Note that the kernel is defined in four cases even if one of the δ is missing. This is because the order of the failure times also gives information about ϕ_F, and hence ignoring $T_i's$ for which δ_i is missing will result in loss of information. Out of 18 combinations of a pair of observations, the kernel cannot be defined for six combinations when either δ_i or δ_j or both are missing. In these cases, the observations neither support nor negate the null hypothesis but the information on the ordering of failure times is fully available. Hence, in order to retrieve the best possible information, we assign weight $1/2$ for these six combinations. Now, we redefine the kernel as follows:

$$\begin{aligned}\phi_{FM}(T_i, \delta_i, O_i, T_j, \delta_j, O_j) &= 1 \text{ if } T_i < T_j, \delta_i = 2, O_i = 1 \text{ or, } T_j < T_i, \delta_j = 2, O_j = 1,\\ &= 1/2 \text{ if } T_i < T_j, O_i = 0 \text{ or, } T_j < T_i, O_j = 0,\\ &= 0 \text{ otherwise.}\end{aligned}$$

Now, the U-statistic which can be used to test the hypothesis is

$$U_{FM} = \frac{1}{\binom{N}{2}} \sum_{1 \le i < j \le N} \phi_{FM}(T_i, \delta_i, O_i, T_j, \delta_j, O_j). \quad (13.22)$$

$$E(U_{FM}) = 2p \int_0^\infty F(2,t)dF(t) + (1-p)/2 = pE(U_F) + (1-p)/2, \quad (13.23)$$

where $p = pr(O_i = 1)$ is the probability that δ is observed.

$E(U_{FM} \mid H_0) = 1/2$ and $E(U_{FM} \mid H_1) > 1/2$.

$$\lim_{n \to \infty} var(\sqrt{N}U_{FM} \mid H_0) = 4[(p+3)/12 - 1/4] = p/3.$$

If $p = 1$, that is, there are no missing causes, then the variance is equal to $1/3$ which is the asymptotic variance of $\sqrt{N}U_F$. As p decreases, variance of $\sqrt{N}U_{FM}$ linearly decreases and is 0 if causes are missing for all units. In practice, p is generally unknown and hence, the variance need to be estimated by replacing p by its empirical estimator, $\hat{p} = n/N$.

Using the results from [44], it follows that under H_0 $\sqrt{N}(U_{FM} - 1/2)$ converges in distribution to normal random variable with mean zero and variance $p/3$ as $N \to \infty$. Hence, we reject H_0 if $\sqrt{3N}(U_{FM} - 1/2)/\sqrt{\hat{p}} > Z_\alpha$ where Z_α is the upper α point of the null distribution of standard normal distribution.

13.3.4 Exact Null Distribution of the Statistic U_{FM}

Let R_i be the rank of T_i among $T_1, T_2, \ldots, T_N$. Then

$$\begin{aligned}\binom{N}{2}U_{FM} &= 1/2\sum_{i=1}^{N}\Big[N - R_i\Big]\Big(1 - O_i\Big) + \sum_{i=1}^{N}\Big[N - R_i\Big]O_i I(\delta_i = 2) \quad (13.24)\\ &= 1/2\sum_{i=1}^{N}\Big[N - i + 1\Big]\Big(1 - O_{(i)}\Big) + \sum_{i=1}^{N}\Big[N - i + 1\Big]O_{(i)} I(\delta_{(i)} = 2),\end{aligned}$$

where $O_{(i)}$ and $\delta_{(i)}$ denote the observations corresponding to $T_{(i)}$, i^{th} ordered T. If all causes of failure are observed, then

$$\binom{N}{2}U_{FM} = \sum_{i=1}^{N}\Big[N - R_i\Big]I(\delta_i = 2).$$

The joint distribution of O_i and δ_i is specified by

$$pr(O_i = 0, \delta_i = 1) = (1-p)\theta, \;\; pr(O_i = 0, \delta_i = 2) = (1-p)(1-\theta),$$
$$pr(O_i = 1, \delta_i = 1) = p\theta, \;\; pr(O_i = 1, \delta_i = 2) = p(1-\theta),$$

where $\theta = pr(\delta_i = 1) = 1 - pr(\delta_i = 2)$.

It is easy to see that under H_0,

$$pr(O_i = r, \delta_i = s) = pr(O_{(i)} = r, \delta_{(i)} = s), \;\; r = 0, 1; s = 1, 2. \qquad (13.25)$$

The moment-generating function of $\binom{N}{2} U_{FM}$ under H_0 is

$$\begin{aligned}
M(t) &= E\left(\exp\left\{t\binom{N}{2}U_{FM}\right\}\right)\\
&= E\left(\exp\left\{t\sum_{i=1}^{N}\left[N-i+1\right]\left[(1-O_{(i)})/2 + O_{(i)}I(\delta_{(i)}=2)\right]\right\}\right)\\
&= \prod_{i=1}^{N} E\left(\exp\{t(N-i+1)[(1-O_{(i)})/2 + O_{(i)}I(\delta_{(i)}=2)]\}\right)\\
&= \prod_{i=1}^{N}\left[p\theta + p(1-\theta)\exp\{t(N-i+1)\} + (1-p)\exp\{t(N-i+1)/2\}\right].
\end{aligned}$$

Under H_0, $\theta = 1/2$ the moment-generating function depends on the unknown p. Hence, the statistic is not distribution-free even under the null hypothesis. However, the exact null distribution can be worked out by replacing the unknown p by its consistent estimator. Note that p is a nuisance parameter in the sense that it is extraneous to the joint distribution of (T, δ).

13.3.5 Simulation Studies

We carry out a small simulation study to consider the performance of the statistic U_{FM}.

Example 1 Block and Basu's bivariate exponential distribution

Consider a bivariate density function

$$\begin{aligned}
f(x, y) &= \lambda\lambda_1\frac{\lambda_3+\lambda_2}{\lambda_1+\lambda_2}\exp\left\{-\lambda_1 x - (\lambda_3+\lambda_2)y\right\} \;\; x < y\\
&= \lambda\lambda_2\frac{\lambda_3+\lambda_1}{\lambda_1+\lambda_2}\exp\left\{-(\lambda_3+\lambda_1)x - \lambda_2 y\right\} \;\; y \le x,
\end{aligned}$$

where $\lambda = \lambda_1 + \lambda_2 + \lambda_3$. Let $T = min(X, Y)$ and $\delta = I(T = X)$, where (X, Y) has the above-mentioned joint survival function $S(x, y)$. The cause-specific hazards are $\lambda(j, t) = \lambda_j \lambda/(\lambda_1 + \lambda_2)$, $j = 1, 2$. If $\lambda_3 = 0$, then X and Y are independent. Since cause-specific hazard $\lambda(j, t)$ is constant in t, T and δ are independent for all choices of $\lambda_1, \lambda_2, \lambda_3$.

We simulated random samples by varying N, p, and $(\lambda_1, \lambda_2, \lambda_3)$ from the above distribution. Empirical levels of significance and power were calculated by using 1000 replications for each combination of N, p and $(\lambda_1, \lambda_2, \lambda_3)$. Table 13.1 gives the empirical level of significance and Table 13.2 gives the empirical power of tests based on U_{FM}.

The test based on U_{FM} attains its level even for sample sizes as small as 25 and p as small as 0.5 (about 50% of the causes missing). The tests are able to detect even small departures from null hypothesis. The power increases as the sample size increases and as the parameter λ_2 moves further away from λ_1. The empirical power was computed for various choices of λ_3 and in all cases, the tests showed good power. For the sake of illustration, we have reported results for $\lambda_3 = 0.5$ only.

Example 2 Farlie–Gumbel–Morgenstern bivariate exponential family

Consider a bivariate exponential distribution with survival function

Table 13.1 Empirical level of significance of U_{FM} for Block and Basu's bivariate exponential distribution $(\lambda_1, \lambda_2, \lambda_3) = (1, 1, 0.5)$

p	$N = 25$	$N = 50$	$N = 100$
1	0.049	0.048	0.051
0.9	0.054	0.054	0.051
0.8	0.056	0.051	0.059
0.5	0.046	0.055	0.052

Table 13.2 Empirical power of U_{FM} for Block and Basu's bivariate exponential distribution

$(\lambda_1, \lambda_2, \lambda_3)$	p	$N = 25$	$N = 50$	$N = 100$
(1, 1.5, 0.5)	1	0.215	0.328	0.537
(1, 1.5, 0.5)	0.9	0.198	0.318	0.508
(1, 1.5, 0.5)	0.8	0.200	0.309	0.469
(1, 2, 0.5)	1	0.437	0.667	0.897
(1, 2, 0.5)	0.9	0.412	0.613	0.880
(1, 2, 0.5)	0.8	0.376	0.593	0.824
(1, 3, 0.5)	1	0.742	0.947	0.997
(1, 3, 0.5)	0.9	0.720	0.907	0.998
(1, 3, 0.5)	0.8	0.627	0.883	0.989
(1, 3, 0.5)	0.5	0.461	0.723	0.935

Table 13.3 Empirical level of significance of U_{FM} for Farlie–Gumbel–Morgenstern bivariate exponential distribution $(\alpha, \lambda_1, \lambda_2) = (0.1, 1, 1)$

p	$N = 50$	$N = 100$
1	0.038	0.030
0.9	0.032	0.025
0.8	0.038	0.030

Table 13.4 Empirical power of U_{FM} for Farlie–Gumbel–Morgenstern bivariate exponential distribution

$(\lambda_1, \lambda_2, \lambda_3)$	p	$N = 50$	$N = 100$
(0.1, 1, 1.5)	1	0.288	0.427
(0.1, 1, 1.5)	0.9	0.249	0.395
(0.1, 1, 1.5)	0.8	0.254	0.407
(0.1, 1, 2)	1	0.654	0.864
(0.1, 1, 2)	0.9	0.558	0.809
(0.1, 1, 2)	0.8	0.539	0.800
(0.1, 1, 3)	1	0.930	0.996
(0.1, 1, 3)	0.9	0.890	0.995
(0.1, 1, 3)	0.8	0.876	0.992
(0.1, 1, 3)	0.5	0.876	0.918

$$S(x, y) = \exp\{-\lambda_1 x\}\exp\{-\lambda_2 y\}[1 + \alpha(1 - \exp\{-\lambda_1 x\})(1 - \exp\{-\lambda_2 y\})],$$

where $x, y > 0$, $\lambda_1, \lambda_2 > 0$, $-1 \leq \alpha \leq 1$. When $\alpha = 0$, X and Y are independent and so are T and δ. The cause-specific hazard rates are

$$\lambda(1, t) = \lambda_1 \frac{1 + \alpha(1 - exp(-2\lambda_1 t)(1 - exp(-\lambda_2 t))}{1 + \alpha \prod_{j=1}^{2}(1 - exp(-\lambda_j t))},$$

$$\lambda(2, t) = \lambda_2 \frac{1 + \alpha(1 - exp(-2\lambda_2 t)(1 - exp(-\lambda_1 t))}{1 + \alpha \prod_{j=1}^{2}(1 - exp(-\lambda_j t))}.$$

For $\lambda_1 < \lambda_2$, $\lambda(1, t) < \lambda(2, t)$, for all $t > 0$.

In this case the level attained is less than 0.05, the test is conservative (see Table 13.3). However, given the level, the power attained is good. It increases with increase in sample size and with departure from null hypothesis (Table 13.4).

13.3.6 Tests for H_0 Against H_3 - Counting Process

In this section, we review the tests discussed in [14] for testing H_0 against the alternative that the cause-specific hazard rates are ordered. We base the test on the following counting processes:

$$N_1^{(n)}(t) = \sum_{i=0}^{n} I\Big[T_i \leq t, \delta_i = 1, O_i = 1\Big],\ N_2^{(n)}(t) = \sum_{i=0}^{n} I\Big[T_i \leq t, \delta_i = 2, O_i = 1\Big],$$

$$N_3^{(n)}(t) = \sum_{i=0}^{n} I\Big[T_i \leq t, \delta_i = 1, O_i = 0\Big],\ N_4^{(n)}(t) = \sum_{i=0}^{n} I\Big[T_i \leq t, \delta_i = 2, O_i = 0\Big].$$

The corresponding intensity functions are $\alpha(j;t)Y^{(n)}(t)$, $i = 1, 2, 3, 4$, where

$$Y^{(n)}(t) = \sum_{i=1}^{n} I\big[T_i > t\big]$$

and $\alpha(j;t)$ are the cause-specific hazard functions. Let $A_1(t)$, $A_2(t)$, $A_{1,3}(t)$, $A_{2,4}(t)$, and $A_{3,4}(t)$ denote the cumulative hazard functions corresponding to the counting processes $N_1^{(n)}$, $N_2^{(n)}$, $N_{1,3}^{(n)} = N_1^{(n)} + N_3^{(n)}$, $N_{2,4}^{(n)} = N_2^{(n)} + N_4^{(n)}$ and $N_{3,4}^{(n)} = N_3^{(n)} + N_4^{(n)}$. The processes $N_3^{(n)}$ and $N_4^{(n)}$ are not observable but their sum $N_{3,4}^{(n)}$ is.

Further suppose that $\beta(t) = P[\delta = 1|O = 0, T = t]$ is a known function. Our interest is in comparing $\lambda(1;t)$ and $\lambda(2;t)$, which are the cause-specific hazard functions corresponding, respectively, to the processes $N_{1,3}^{(n)}$ and $N_{2,4}^{(n)}$. Then

$$\lambda(1;t) = \alpha(1;t) + \alpha(3;t), \text{ and } \lambda(2;t) = \alpha(2;t) + \alpha(4;t).$$

Suppose $\alpha_{3,4}(t)Y^{(n)}(t)$ denotes the intensity function of the process $N_{3,4}^{(n)}(t)$, then we have

$$\alpha(3;t) = \beta(t)\alpha_{3,4}(t) \text{ and } \alpha(4;t) = (1 - \beta(t))\alpha_{3,4}(t).$$

Then the Nelson–Aalen estimators of $A_{1,3}(t)$ and $A_{2,4}(t)$ are, respectively,

$$\hat{A}_{1,3}(t) = \int_0^t \frac{1}{Y^n(s)} dN_1^n(s) + \int_0^t \frac{\beta(s)}{Y^n(s)} dN_{3,4}^n(s),$$

$$\hat{A}_{2,4}(t) = \int_0^t \frac{1}{Y^n(s)} dN_2^n(s) + \int_0^t \frac{1-\beta(s)}{Y^n(s)} dN_{3,4}^n(s).$$

A test for the hypothesis $H_0 : \lambda(1;t) = \lambda(2;t)$ for all t against H_3, is based on the statistics

$$S_{2n}(\tau) = \hat{A}_{2,4}(\tau) - \hat{A}_{1,3}(\tau),$$

where τ is some fixed time point. Under the null, $S_{2n}(\tau)$ has zero mean. Large positive values of S_{2n} show evidence against H_0.

Using the Doob–Meyer decompositions of the counting processes and the Rebelledo martingale central limit theorem ([2] p. 83), we obtain the following theorem.

Theorem 2 *Suppose the sub-distribution functions are absolutely continuous. As* $n \to \infty$ *and under* $H_0 : \lambda(1,t) = \lambda(2,t)$, *the process* $\{\sqrt{n}S_{2n}(t),\ 0 \le t \le \tau\}$ *converges weakly to a process* $U = \{U(t),\ 0 \le t \le \tau\}$ *in* $D[0,\tau]$ *with the Skorohod topology, where* $\{U(t), 0 \le t \le \tau\}$ *Is a continuous zero-mean martingale and* $cov(U(s), U(t)) = \sigma^2 min(t,s)$ *with*

$$\sigma^2(t) = \int_0^t \frac{\alpha(1,s) + \alpha(2,s) + (1 - 2\,\beta(s))^2\,\alpha_{3,4}(s)}{S(t)} ds.$$

Here, $D[0,\tau]$ *denotes the space of real valued functions on* $[0,\tau]$ *that are continuous from the right and have limits from the left everywhere. A consistent estimator for* $\sigma^2(t)$ *is given by*

$$\sigma_n^2(t) = \int_0^t \frac{dN_1^n(s)}{Y^n(s)^2} + \int_0^t \frac{dN_2^n(s)}{Y^n(s)^2} + \int_0^t \left(1 - 2\,\beta(s)\right)^2 \frac{dN_{3,4}^n(s)}{Y^n(s)^2}.$$

From the above results, we have that

$$\frac{\sqrt{n}S_{2n}(\tau)}{\sigma_n(\tau)} \to N(0,1), \quad as\ n \to \infty.$$

Thus, a value of $\frac{\sqrt{n}S_{2n}(\tau)}{\sigma_n(\tau)}$ *larger than 1.64 shows evidence in favor of* H_3 *against* H_0 *at 5% level of significance.*

13.4 Discussion and Future Work

This is an expository article to consider the estimation and testing issues involved in the study of competing risks when some of the causes of failure are missing. Limiting distributions of U_1 and U_{FM} need to be studied carefully as n; the number of observations for which both failure time and cause of failure are observable is a random variable. In [14], tests based on counting processes for testing H_0 versus H_3 are studied. The tests can be extended to the case when k, the number of causes involved, is greater than 2. In case some failure times are censored, then one can carry out the testing problem by considering censoring as another risk. An extensive simulation study to compare the performance of the proposed steps is worth considering.

One can extend the tests based on counting processes to compare a given risk in two populations.

Most of the articles in the literature assume either the MCAR or MAR condition, and some exceptions are [7, 8, 16]. Methods to handle the informative missingness I, informative missingness II, and the MNAR condition need to be developed.

Some of the problems mentioned are under consideration.

Acknowledgements We thank Prof. J. V. Deshpande and Prof. Sangita Kulathinal for several fruitful discussions.

References

1. Andersen, P.K., and O. Borgan. 1985. Counting process models for life history data: A review. *Scandinavian Journal of Statistics* 12: 97–158.
2. Anderson, P.K., O. Borgan, R.D. Gill, and N. Keiding. 1993. *Statistical models based on counting processes*. New York: Springer.
3. Bandyopadhyay, D., and S. Datta. 2008. Testing equality of survival distributions when the population marks are missing. *Journal of Statistical Planning and Inference* 138 (6): 1722–1732.
4. Bandyopadhyaya, D., and M.A. Jácomeb. 2016. Comparing conditional survival functions with missing population marks in a competing risks models. *Computational Statistics and Data Analysis* 95: 150–160.
5. Bordes, L., J.Y. Dauxois, and P. Joly. 2014. Semiparametric inference of competing risks data with additive hazards and missing cause of failure under MCAR or MAR assumptions. *Electronic Journal of Statistics* 8: 41–95.
6. Carriere, K.C., and S.C. Kochar. 2000. Comparing sub-survival functions in a competing risks model. *Lifetime Data Analysis* 6: 85–97.
7. Craiu, R.V., and T. Duchesne. 2004. Inference based on the EM algorithm for the competing risks model with masked causes of failure. *Biometrika* 91: 543–558.
8. Craiu, R.V., and B. Reiser. 2006. Inference for the dependent competing risks model with masked causes of failure. *Lifetime Data Analysis* 12: 21–33.
9. Crowder, M.J. 2001. *Classical competing risks*. London: Chapman and Hall/CRC.
10. Crowder, M.J. 2012. *Multivariate survival analysis and competing risks*. Boca Raton: CRC Press.
11. Cummings, F.J., R. Gray, T.E. Davis, D.C. Tormey, J.E. Harris, G.G. Falkson, and J. Arseneau. 1986. Tamoxifen versus placebo : Double blind adjuvant trial in elderly woman with stage II breast cancer. *National Cancer Institute Monographs* 1: 119–123.
12. Datta, S., D. Bandyopadhyay, and G.A. Satten. 2010. Inverse probability of censoring (2008). weighted U-statistics for right-censored data with an application to testing hypotheses. *Scandinavian Journal of Statistics* 37: 680–700.
13. Dewan, I., and J.V. Deshpande. 2005. Tests for some statistical hypotheses for dependent competing risks - A review. In *Modern statistical methods in reliability*, ed. A. Wilson, et al., 137–152. New Jersey: World Scientific.
14. Dewan, I., and Naik-Nimbalkar, U.V. 2013. Statistical analysis of competing risks with missing causes of failure. In *Proceedings 59th ISI World Statistics Congress*, 1223–1228.
15. Dewnaji, A. 1992. A note on a test for competing risks with missing failure type. *Biometrika* 79: 855–857.
16. Dewnaji, A., and D. Sengupta. 2003. Estimation of competing risks with general missing pattern in failure types. *Biometrics* 59: 1063–1070.
17. Dewnaji, A., P.G. Sankaran, D. Sengupta, and B. Karmakar. 2016. Regression analysis of competing risks data with general missing pattern in failure types. *Statistical Methodology* 29: 18–31.

18. Dinse, G.E. 1982. Nonparametric estimation for partially complete time and type of failure data. *Biometrics* 38: 417–431.
19. Effraimidis, G., and C.M. Dahl. 2014. Nonparametric estimation of cumulative incidence functions for competing risks data with missing cause of failure. *Statistics and Probability Letters* 89: 1–7.
20. Flehinger, B.J., B. Reiser, and E. Yashchin. 1998. Survival with competing risks and masked causes of failures. *Biometrika* 85: 151–164.
21. Flehinger, B.J., R. Reiser, and E. Yashchin. 2002. Parametric modeling for survival with competing risks and masked failure causes. *Lifetime Data Analysis* 8: 177–203.
22. Gijbels, I., D.Y. Lin, and Z. Ying. 2007. Non- and semi-parametric analysis of failure time data with missing failure indicators. IMS lecture notes-monograph series complex datasets and inverse problems (2008). *Tomography, Networks and Beyond* 54: 203–223.
23. Goetghebeur, E., and L. Ryan. 1990. A modified log rank test for competing risks with missing failure type. *Biometrika* 77: 207–211.
24. Goetghebeur, E., and L. Ryan. 1995. Analysis of competing risks survival data when some failure types are missing. *Biometrika* 82: 821–833.
25. Greenhouse, J.B., and R.A. Wolfe. 1984. A competing risks derivation of a mixture model for the analysis of survival data. *Communications in Statistics - Theory and Methods* 13: 3133–3154.
26. Guess, F.M., J.S. Usher, and T.J. Hodgson. 1991. Estimating system and component reliabilities under partial information on the cause of failure. *Journal of Statistical Planning and Inference* 29: 75–85.
27. Hyun, S., J. Lee, and Y. Sun. 2012. Proportional hazards model for competing risks data with missing cause of failure. *Journal of Statistical Planning and Inference* 142: 1767–1779.
28. Kochar S.C. 1995. A review of some distribution-free tests for the equality of cause specific hazard rates. In *Analysis of Censored Data*, Eds. Koul H.L, Deshpande J.V, IMS, Hayward, 147–162.
29. Kodell, R.L., and J.J. Chen. 1987. Handling cause of death in equivocal cases using the EM algorithm (with rejoinder). *Communications in Statistics - Theory and Methods* 16: 2565–2585.
30. Kundu, D., and S. Basu. 2000. Analysis of incomplete data in presence of competing risks. *Journal of Statistical Planning and Inference* 87: 221–239.
31. Lapidus, G., M. Braddock, R. Schwartz, L. Banco, and L. Jacobs. 1994. Accuracy of fatal motorcycle injury reporting on death certificates. *Accident Analysis and Prevention* 26: 535–542.
32. Lee, M., K.A. Cronin, M.H. Gail, J.J. Dignam, and E.J. Feuer. 2011. Multiple imputation methods for inference on cumulative incidence with missing cause of failure. *Biometrical Journal* 53: 974–993.
33. Lo, S.H. 1991. Estimating a survival function with incomplete cause-of-death data. *Journal of Multivariate Analysis* 39: 217–235.
34. Lu, K., and A.A. Tsiatis. 2001. Multiple imputation methods for estimating regression coefficients in the competing risks model with missing cause of failure. *Biometrics* 57: 1191–1197.
35. Lu, K., and A.A. Tsiatis. 2005. Comparison between two partial likelihood approaches for the competing risks model with missing cause of failure. *Lifetime Data Analysis* 11: 29–40.
36. Lu, W., and Y. Liang. 2008. Analysis of competing risks data with missing cause of failure under additive hazards model. *Statistica Sinica* 18: 219–234.
37. Miyakawa, M. 1984. Analysis of incomplete data in competing risks model. *IEEE Transactions in Reliability* 33: 293–296.
38. Moreno-Betancur, M., G. Rey, and A. Latouche. 2015. Direct likelihood inference and sensitivity analysis for competing risks regression with missing causes of failure. *Biometrics* 71: 498–507.
39. Ramlau-Hansen, H. 1983. Smoothing counting process intensities by means of kernel functions. *Annals of Statistics* 11: 453–466.
40. Rubin, D.B. 1976. Inference and missing data. *Biometrika* 63: 581–592.

41. Sarhan, A.M. 2001. Reliability estimations of components from masked system life data. *Reliability Engineering and System Safety* 74: 107–113.
42. Sarhan, A.M. 2003. Estimation of system components reliabilities using masked data. *Applied Mathematics and Computation* 136: 79–92.
43. Sen, A., M. Banerjee, Y. Li, and A.M. Noone. 2010. A Bayesian approach to competing risks analysis with masked cause of death. *Statistics in Medicine* 29: 1681–1695.
44. Serfling, R.J. 1980. *Approximation theorems of mathematical statistics*. New York: Wiley.
45. Sun, Y., H. Wang, and P.B. Gilbert. 2012. Quantile regression for competing risks data with missing cause of failure. *Statistica Sinica* 22: 703–728.
46. Tsiatis, A.A., M. Davidian, and B. McNeney. 2002. Multiple imputation methods for testing different treatment differences in survival distributions with missing cause of failure. *Biometrika* 89: 238–244.
47. Usher, J.S., and T.J. Hodgson. 1988. Maximum likelihood estimation of component reliability using masked system life test data. *IEEE Transactions on Reliability* 37: 550–555.
48. Usher, J.S. 1996. Weibull component reliability - prediction in the presence of masked data. *IEEE Transactions on Reliability* 45: 229–232.
49. Van der Laan, M.J., and I.W. McKeague. 1998. Efficient estimation from right-censored data when failure indicators are missing at random. *Annals of Statistics* 26: 164–182.
50. Wang, J., and Q. Yu. 2012. Consistency of the generalized MLE with interval-censored and masked competing risks data. *Communications in Statistics - Theory and Methods* 41: 4360–4377.
51. Yu, Q., and J. Li. 2012. The NPMLE of the joint distribution function with right-censored and masked competing risks data. *Journal of Nonparametric Statistics* 24: 753–764.

Chapter 14
Environmental Applications Based on Birnbaum–Saunders Models

Víctor Leiva and Helton Saulo

Abstract We discuss some environmental applications of methodologies based on the Birnbaum–Saunders model, which is an asymmetrical statistical distribution that is being widely considered to describe data collected in earth sciences. We present a formal justification, by means of the proportionate effect law, to use the Birnbaum–Saunders model as a useful distribution for environmental and regional variables. The methodologies discussed in this work include exceedance probabilities, X-bar control charts, np control charts, and spatial models. Applications with real-world environmental data sets are carried out for each discussed methodology.

14.1 Introduction

Statistical distributions have been widely considered to describe variables studied in earth and environmental sciences. The use of these distributions may be beneficial to determine, for example, the effect of atmospheric contaminants on human health or the spatial variability of fertilizer concentrations in the soil for agricultural management; see Marchant et al. [1] and Garcia-Papani et al. [2]. In epidemiological monitoring, average atmospheric pollutant concentrations are employed to indicate levels that induce adverse human effects, as for example, myocardial infarction and chronic bronchitis; see McConnell et al. [3] and Nuvolone et al. [4]. In agricultural management, in order to evaluate the effects of agriculture on environmental quality, agricultural systems are exposed to natural actions and human activities, where defi-

The original version of this chapter was revised: Incorrect affiliations have been corrected. The erratum to this chapter is available at https://doi.org/10.1007/978-981-10-5370-2_17

V. Leiva (✉)
School of Industrial Engineering, Pontificia Universidad católica de Valparaíso,
Avenida Brasil 2241,Valparaíso 2362807, Chile
e-mail: victorleivasanchez@gmail.com

H. Saulo
Department of Statistics, University of Brasilia, Brasilia 70910-900, Brazil
e-mail: heltonsaulo@gmail.com

A. Adhikari et al. (eds.), *Mathematical and Statistical Applications in Life Sciences and Engineering*, https://doi.org/10.1007/978-981-10-5370-2_14

ciency and imbalance of nutrients in the soil are the main problems; see De Bastiani et al. [5].

Due to the inherent variation of environmental and regional variables, fertilizer and pollutant concentrations are considered as random variables (RVs), which are nonnegative. These RVs can be modeled by statistical distributions and are often positively skewed (asymmetry to the right). The interested reader is referred to Marchant et al. [1] for a complete study about different statistical distributions used to model environmental data. Thus, the Gaussian (or normal) distribution, which is symmetrical, should not be used to model this type of RVs. In order to avoid problems when data transformations are carried to reach normality, one can model the data directly with a suitable asymmetrical distribution; see Leiva et al. [6].

Several statistical distributions have been often considered to describe asymmetrical data. For example, the Birnbaum–Saunders (BS), exponential, gamma, inverse Gaussian (IG), log-normal, and Weibull distributions can be mentioned; see Johnson et al. [7, 8], Leiva and Saunders [9] and Leiva [10]. The BS distribution is being widely studied and applied in different fields, including earth and environmental sciences; see Leiva et al. [11–18], Podlaski [19], Balakrishnan [20], Kotz et al. [21], Vilca et al. [22, 23], Ferreira et al. [24], Marchant et al. [1], and Saulo et al. [25, 26]. In contrast to its original derivation in material fatigue problems, Leiva et al. [14] formalized the BS distribution as an adequate model to describe environmental data using the proportionate effect law. This is because the contaminants are diluted or concentrated in a volume varying according to environmental factors that move these contaminants from their original place, but retaining their original amount.

The objective of this work is to discuss some environmental applications of methodologies based on the BS distribution. We present a mathematical derivation, employing the proportionate effect law, which formalizes the use of the BS model as an appropriate distribution for describing environmental and regional variables. We discuss methodologies that include exceedance probabilities, X-bar control charts, np control charts, and spatial models. We illustrate these methodologies with several real-world data sets.

The rest of the work proceeds as follows. In Sect. 14.2, we introduce the BS distribution and provide expressions for the distribution of the sum of RVs following the BS model, which we name the BSsum distribution; see Raaijmakers [27, 28], Fox et al. [29], Leiva et al. [30], and Saulo et al. [25]. In Sect. 14.3, we present a justification for using the BS model as a concentration distribution. This model is useful to describe data of environmental pollutant concentrations and fertilizer concentrations in the soil for agricultural management. Based on this motivation, we discuss BS exceedance probabilities in Sect. 14.4, as well as X-bar and np control charts for the BS distribution in Sects. 14.5 and 14.6, respectively. In Sect. 14.7, we provide a formulation of the BS spatial log-linear model. Some conclusions are presented in Sect. 14.8.

14.2 The BS and BSsum Distributions

In this section, we introduce some features and shapes of the BS and BSsum distributions.

14.2.1 The BS Distribution

If an RV X is BS distributed, with shape $\alpha > 0$ and scale $\beta > 0$ parameters, which is denoted by $X \sim \text{BS}(\alpha, \beta)$, we have the following probabilistic features:

(F1) The cumulative distribution function (CDF) of X at x is given by

$$F_X(x; \alpha, \beta) = \Phi\left(\frac{1}{\alpha}\xi\left(\frac{x}{\beta}\right)\right), x > 0, \tag{14.1}$$

where Φ is the CDF of the standard normal distribution, denoted by N(0, 1), and $\xi(a) = a^{1/2} - a^{-1/2} = 2\sinh(\log(a^{1/2}))$, for $a > 0$.

(F2) The probability density function (PDF) of X is read to be

$$f_X(x; \alpha, \beta) = \frac{1}{\sqrt{2\pi}}\exp\left(-\frac{1}{2\alpha^2}\left(\frac{x}{\beta} + \frac{\beta}{x} - 2\right)\right)\frac{x^{-3/2}(x+\beta)}{2\alpha\sqrt{\beta}}, x > 0. \tag{14.2}$$

(F3) The quantile function (QF) of X is given by

$$x(q; \alpha, \beta) = F_X^{-1}(q; \alpha, \beta) = \beta\left(\alpha\, z(q)/2 + \left((\alpha\, z(q)/2)^2 + 1\right)^{1/2}\right)^2, 0 < q < 1,$$

where $z(q)$ denotes the N(0, 1) QF (or $q \times 100$th quantile) and F_X^{-1} is the inverse function of F_X given in (14.1). From the BS FQ, note that if $q = 0.5$, then β is the BS median. The BS QF can be used to generate random numbers from the BS distribution; see Leiva et al. [31].

(F4) The survival function (SF) and hazard rate (HR) of X are given, respectively, as

$$S_X(x; \alpha, \beta) = \Phi\left(-\frac{1}{\alpha}\xi\left(\frac{x}{\beta}\right)\right), x > 0,$$

$$h_X(x; \alpha, \beta) = \frac{\phi(\xi(x/\beta)/\alpha)(x^{-3/2}(x+\beta))/(2\alpha\sqrt{\beta})}{\Phi(-(\xi(x/\beta)/\alpha)))}, x > 0,$$

where ϕ is the N(0, 1) PDF and ξ is defined in (F1). An HR is defined in general by $h_X(x) = f_X(x)/S_X(x)$, where f_X is the PDF of X and $S_X(x) = 1 - F_X(x)$ is the corresponding SF, with F_X being the associated CDF. The BS HR $h_X(x; \alpha, \beta)$ given in (F4) has the following characteristics: (a) it is

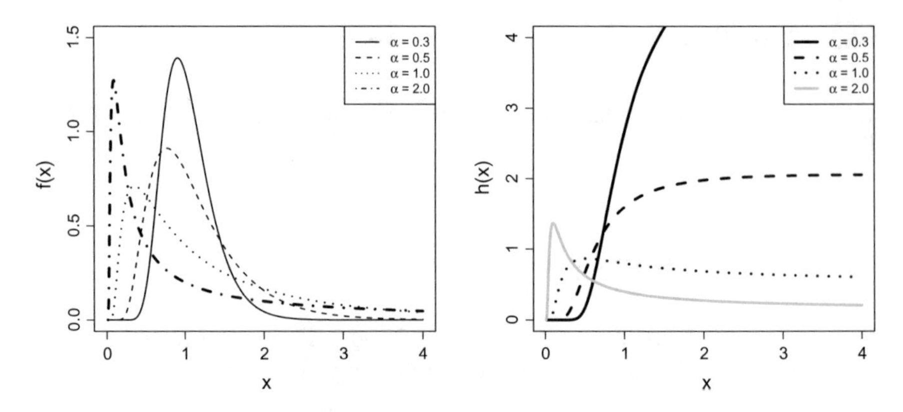

Fig. 14.1 Plots of the BS PDF (left) and BS HR (right) for the indicated value of α with $\beta = 1$

unimodal for any α, increasing for $x < x_c$, and decreasing for $x > x_c$, where x_c denotes its change-point; (b) it goes to $1/(2\alpha^2\beta)$ as $x \to \infty$; (c) it tends to be decreasing for $\alpha > 2$, as $\alpha \to \infty$; and (d) it tends to be increasing as $\alpha \to 0$; see Kundu et al. [32].

Figure 14.1 (left) shows graphs of the BS PDF given in (F2) for different values of α and $\beta = 1$, without loss of generality because β is a scale parameter. Note that the BS distribution is continuous, unimodal and positively skewed (asymmetry to the right). Also, note that, as α goes to zero, the BS distribution tends to be symmetrical around β (the median of the distribution) and its variability reduces. Furthermore, as α increases, the distribution has heavier tails. Thus, α not only changes its shape, but also its skewness and its kurtosis. Figure 14.1 (right) shows graphs of the BS HR for different values of α and $\beta = 1$. Theoretical considerations mentioned in (F4) are confirmed by this graphical shape analysis.

Let $X \sim \text{BS}(\alpha, \beta)$. Then, the following properties of the BS distribution hold:

(P1) For $Z \sim \text{N}(0, 1)$,

$$X = \beta\left(\frac{\alpha Z}{2} + \left(\left(\frac{\alpha Z}{2}\right)^2 + 1\right)^{1/2}\right)^2 \sim \text{BS}(\alpha, \beta).$$

(P2) By using the transformation in (P1) and its monotonicity, it follows that

$$Z = \frac{1}{\alpha}\xi\left(\frac{X}{\beta}\right) \sim \text{N}(0, 1).$$

(P3) From (P2), the RV

$$K = Z^2 = \frac{1}{\alpha^2}\xi^2\left(\frac{X}{\beta}\right) \sim \chi^2(1),$$

that is, K is chi-squared distributed with one degree of freedom.

(P4) Its proportionality (scaling) property is $c\,X \sim \mathrm{BS}(\alpha, c\,\beta)$, with $c > 0$.

(P5) Its reciprocation (inversion) property is $1/X \sim \mathrm{BS}(\alpha, 1/\beta)$.

(P6) The mean and variance of X are given, respectively, by

$$\mathrm{E}(X) = \beta\left(1 + \frac{\alpha^2}{2}\right), \quad \mathrm{Var}(X) = \beta^2\alpha^2\left(1 + \frac{5\alpha^2}{4}\right).$$

(P7) The coefficients of variation (CV), skewness or asymmetry (CS), and kurtosis (CK) of X are expressed, respectively, by

$$\mathrm{CV}(X) = \frac{\alpha\left(5\alpha^2+4\right)^{1/2}}{(2+\alpha^2)}, \mathrm{CS}(X) = \frac{4\alpha(11\alpha^2+6)}{(5\alpha^2+4)^{3/2}}, \mathrm{CK}(X) = 3 + \frac{6\alpha^2(40+93\alpha^2)}{(4+5\alpha^2)^2}.$$

The estimation of the BS model parameters can be performed by the maximum likelihood (ML) and modified moment (MM) methods by using the random sample $X_1, \ldots, X_n$ collected from the population $X \sim \mathrm{BS}(\alpha, \beta)$, where $x_1, \ldots, x_n$ are their observed values. The ML estimate of β, denoted by $\widehat{\beta}$, is obtained maximizing the corresponding likelihood function, which conducts to solving numerically the nonlinear equation

$$\beta^2 - \beta\,(2r + K(\beta)) + r\,(s + K(\beta)) = 0,$$

where

$$K(u) = \left(\frac{1}{n}\sum_{i=1}^{n}\frac{1}{u + x_i}\right)^{-1}, u > 0,$$

and

$$s = \frac{1}{n}\sum_{i=1}^{n} x_i, \quad r = \left(\frac{1}{n}\sum_{i=1}^{n}\frac{1}{x_i}\right)^{-1}$$

denote the sample arithmetic and harmonic means, respectively. The ML estimate of α, denoted by $\widehat{\alpha}$, is also obtained maximizing the corresponding likelihood function conducting to

$$\widehat{\alpha} = \left(\frac{s}{\widehat{\beta}} + \frac{\widehat{\beta}}{r} - 2\right)^{1/2}.$$

The asymptotic joint distribution of the ML estimators $(\widehat{\alpha}, \widehat{\beta})$ is used to obtain

$$\sqrt{n}\begin{pmatrix}\widehat{\alpha} - \alpha \\ \widehat{\beta} - \beta\end{pmatrix} \sim \mathrm{N}\left(\begin{pmatrix}0 \\ 0\end{pmatrix}, \begin{pmatrix}\frac{\alpha^2}{2} & 0 \\ 0 & \frac{\beta^2}{(0.25+\alpha^{-2}+I(\alpha))}\end{pmatrix}\right),$$

where

$$I(\alpha) = 2\int_0^\infty \left(\frac{1}{1 + 1 + (\alpha u)^2/2 + \alpha u(1 + (\alpha u)^2/4)^{1/2}} - \frac{1}{2}\right)^2 \mathrm{d}\Phi(u).$$

The MM estimates of α and β, denoted by $\widetilde{\alpha}$ and $\widetilde{\beta}$, are obtained equating the expressions $\mathrm{E}(X) = \beta(1 + \alpha^2/2)$ and $\mathrm{E}(1/X) = (1/\beta)(1 + \alpha^2/2)$, generated from (P5) and (P6), to their corresponding sample values, which solution conducts to

$$\widetilde{\alpha} = \left(2\left(\left(\frac{s}{r}\right)^{1/2} - 1\right)\right)^{1/2}, \quad \widetilde{\beta} = \sqrt{s\,r}.$$

The corresponding asymptotic joint distribution of $(\widetilde{\alpha}, \widetilde{\beta})$ is used to obtain

$$\sqrt{n}\begin{pmatrix}\widetilde{\alpha} - \alpha \\ \widetilde{\beta} - \beta\end{pmatrix} \sim \mathrm{N}\left(\begin{pmatrix}0 \\ 0\end{pmatrix}, \begin{pmatrix}\frac{\alpha^2}{2} & 0 \\ 0 & (\alpha\beta)^2\left(\frac{1+3/4\alpha^2}{(1+1/2\alpha^2)^2}\right)\end{pmatrix}\right).$$

For details about the estimation results presented above, see Birnbaum and Saunders [33], Engelhardt et al. [34], Ng et al. [35], and Leiva [10].

14.2.2 The BSsum Distribution

Raaijmakers [27, 28] proposed an approximate expression for the PDF of the sum of BS RVs; see also Leiva et al. [30] and Saulo et al. [25]. In order to obtain the distribution of the sum of BS RVs, we can approximate it by using the Laplace transform to the BS PDF given in (14.2). The Laplace transform of real argument v of a function f is given by

$$Lf(v) = Q(v) = \int_0^\infty \exp(-vx) f(x)\mathrm{d}x.$$

Thus, the PDF and CDF of the sum of k BS RVs, $S = \sum_{i=1}^{k} X_i$ say, at s are given, respectively, by

$$f_S(s; \alpha, \beta = 1, k) = \frac{a}{2^k}\exp(2ka(1 - s))\sum_{i=0}^{k}\binom{k}{i}(2ka)^{i-2}\varsigma_i\left(\frac{s}{4k^2 a}\right), s > 0,$$

$$F_S(s; \alpha, \beta = 1, k) = \frac{1}{2^k}\exp(2ka(1 - s))\sum_{i=2}^{k}\frac{l_i\,\varsigma_i(s/(4k^2 a))}{(2ka)^{2-i}} + \Phi\left(\frac{\varphi(s; k)}{\alpha}\right),$$

where $s > 0$, $\alpha > 0$, $\beta > 0$, $k = 1, 2, \ldots, a = 1/(2\alpha^2)$, $l_i = l_{i+2} - \binom{k}{i}$, with $l_{k+2} = l_{k+1} = 0$, for $i = 2, \ldots, k$, and $\varphi(s; k) = \sqrt{s} - k/\sqrt{s}$. Note that $L\varsigma_i(s) = \exp(-\sqrt{s})/s^{i/2}$ is the Laplace transform of the function ς_i. If an RV S is BSsum distributed, then the notation $S \sim \text{BSsum}(\alpha, \beta, k)$ is used and its QF is given by

$$Q_S(q; \alpha, \beta, k) = F_S^{-1}(q; \alpha, \beta, k), 0 < q < 1. \tag{14.3}$$

Note that (14.3) does not have an analytical solution and must be obtained numerically.

Fox et al. [29] proposed an exact expression for the PDF of the sum of BS RVs assuming the following. Consider X_i as the ith inter-occurrence time (the time between events $i - 1$ and i), which is a nonnegative continuous RV. We suppose inter-occurrence times are independent and identically distributed RVs, but this supposition is relaxed later. Assuming that the first inter-occurrence is measured with respect to the zero time (see Ross [36]), the CDF of the RV of counting C at n in the time interval $[0, T]$ is given by

$$\Pr(C \leq n) = \Pr\left(\sum_{i=1}^{n+1} X_i > T\right) = 1 - \Pr\left(\sum_{i=1}^{n+1} X_i \leq T\right). \tag{14.4}$$

Consider the inter-occurrence distribution has mean μ and standard deviation σ. Despite the counting distribution is known to be asymptotically normal $\text{N}(T/\mu, T_2/\mu_3)$ as T approaches infinity (see Theorem 3.3.5 of Ross [36]), this result does not allow us to obtain a distribution when T is finite.

By using (14.4) and the standard central limit theorem, the probability of $C \leq n$ is read to be

$$\Pr(C \leq n) = \Phi\left(\frac{T/(n+1) - \mu}{\sigma/\sqrt{n+1}}\right).$$

Approximating the discrete RV C by the continuous RV $X > 0$, the PDF of X is given by

$$f_X(x; T, \mu, \sigma) = \frac{1}{2\sigma\sqrt{2\pi}} \exp\left(-\frac{1}{2}\left(\frac{T - (x+1)\mu}{\sigma\sqrt{x+1}}\right)^2\right) \frac{(T + (x+1)\mu)}{(x+1)^{3/2}}, x > 0. \tag{14.5}$$

Note that Birnbaum and Saunders [37] used n instead of $n + 1$ for describing the amount of cycles until failure. This is due to $n = 0$ is not a possibility in their model, but it is possible in (14.5). Then, the corresponding PDF proposed by Birnbaum and Saunders [37] is defined as

$$f_X(x; T, \mu, \sigma) = \frac{1}{2\sigma\sqrt{2\pi}} \exp\left(-\frac{1}{2}\left(\frac{T - x\mu}{\sigma\sqrt{x}}\right)^2\right) \frac{(T + x\mu)}{x^{3/2}}, x > 0. \tag{14.6}$$

In addition, note that Birnbaum and Saunders [37] defined the reparameterization $\alpha = \sigma/\sqrt{\mu T}$, $\beta = T/\mu$ and reformulated their PDF based on the parameters α and β. As μ and σ are observable in the formulation of Fox et al. [29], such as in many applications of counting problems, and to exploit the connection between inter-occurrence time and counting distributions, the parameters μ, σ, and T are retained in the sequel. The moment-generating function (MGF) of the BS distribution with PDF defined in (14.6) is obtained as

$$M_X(u) = \frac{1}{2}\exp\left(\frac{T\mu}{\sigma^2}\left(1-\sqrt{1-\frac{2u\sigma^2}{\mu^2}}\right)^2\right)\left(1+\frac{1}{\sqrt{1+2u\sigma^2/\mu^2}}\right),\ |u| < \frac{\mu^2}{\sigma^2}. \quad (14.7)$$

The probability of $C = n$ considering the PDF given in (14.6) is the area between n and $n-1$, which is not centered at n but at $n-1/2$. This may be corrected by shifting (14.6) to the right by $1/2$ unit. In that case, the PDF of $X > 0$, which keeps the linkage to the lifetime distribution and considers the continuity correction, is given by

$$f_X(x; T, \mu, \sigma) = \frac{1}{2\sigma\sqrt{2\pi}}\exp\left(-\frac{1}{2}\left(\frac{T-(x+0.5)\mu}{\sigma\sqrt{(x+0.5)}}\right)^2\right)\frac{(T+(x+0.5)\mu)}{(x+0.5)^{3/2}},\ x > 0. \quad (14.8)$$

The distribution associated with the PDF expressed in (14.8), which is unimodal, with its mode being less than its median and it being less than its mean, is named here as time–BS distribution; see Fox et al. [29]. The correction added in (14.8) is particularly important in problems of counting. The interested reader is refer to Fox et al. [29] for more details about a shape analysis of the PDF given in (14.8).

Let the mean and standard deviation of the (stationary) inter-occurrence time distribution be μ and σ, respectively. Then, for the associated counting distribution, we have

(i) $\mathrm{E}(C) = \frac{T}{\mu} - 0.5 + \frac{\sigma^2}{2\mu^2}$.
(ii) $\mathrm{E}((C-\mathrm{E}(C))^2) = \frac{5\sigma^2}{4\mu^2} + \frac{T}{\mu}\frac{\sigma^2}{\mu^2}$.
(iii) $\mathrm{E}((C-\mathrm{E}(C))^3) = \frac{11\sigma^6}{2\mu^6} + \frac{T}{\mu}\frac{\sigma^4}{\mu^4}$.

Note that result (i) is $1/2$ unit less than the corresponding result given in Fox et al. [37], whereas result (ii) is identical. Result (iii) may be reached from Johnson et al. [8] after a simple algebra. Observe that results (i)–(iii) can be obtained and corroborated from the MGF presented in (14.7). Notice that the moment formulas given above are all functions of two quantities: the CV of the inter-occurrence time distribution, that is, of σ/μ, and the ratio T/μ. Furthermore, these moments are all increasing functions of both quantities. Moreover, the third moment about the mean is always positive and then the counting distribution is always positively skewed.

The probability that the RV C equals n may be computed exactly. Thus, a comparison between the time–BS distribution and any other known counting distribution is possible. The inter-occurrence time distribution must hold that (a) it has nonnegative support and (b) the distribution for the sum may be determined conveniently. The interested reader is referred to Fox et al. [29] for comparisons between distributions of sums based on gamma and uniform models. In many applications, summing RVs of counting is needed, for example, in business and economics. Specifically, the demand distribution may vary over time and so demand in a fixed period may be represented as the sum of demands through disjoint subintervals. Furthermore, in inventory problems, it is necessary to establish the distribution of demands summed over a lag or lead-time interval.

The distribution of the sum of BS RVs can be obtained by the MGF of the BS distribution. Here, the classical BS PDF defined in (14.6) is used due to its most prevalent form found in the literature on the topic. It simplifies comparisons with some previous results. The MGF of the time–BS distribution, which considers a 1/2 unit shift by comparison to the classical BS, introduces the multiplicative factor $\exp(t^2)$. Thus, obtaining identical results for the time–BS distribution is quite simple.

Note that the BS distribution is the discrete mixture of two distributions in equal proportion: an IG distribution with parameters $\omega = T/\mu$ and $\lambda = T^2/\sigma^2$, and a sum of an IG distribution (with the same parameters) and an independent gamma distribution with shape parameter $k = 1/2$ and scale parameter $\theta = 2\sigma^2/\mu^2$. Note that this derivation of the BS distribution proposed by Fox et al. [29] is different from that provided by Desmond [38]; see also Balakrishnan et al. [20]. In addition, the BS MGF given in (14.7) has been determined in a closed-form expression for the first time also by Fox et al. [29] using the new mixture interpretation mentioned above. This is done by recognizing that the BS MGF may be expressed as a sum of the MGF of an IG distribution and the derivative of the same MGF. Furthermore, the mixture interpretation provided by Fox et al. [29] permits one to analyze sums of independent BS RVs having different parameters T_i, μ_i, and σ_i, which Desmond's interpretation does not permit. Moreover, this mixture result implies that the reciprocal IG distribution is equivalent to the sum of RVs with IG and gamma distributions, respectively; see details in Fox et al. [29].

Summing RVs following the BS distribution needs the usage of confluent hypergeometric functions, which provide a solution to the differential equation $z\mathrm{d}\omega/\mathrm{d}z^2 + (b-z)\mathrm{d}\omega/\mathrm{d}z - a\omega = 0$. Such a solution is the confluent hypergeometric function of the first kind (also known as the Kummer function of the first kind), whose infinite series is given by

$$K_1(a, b, z) = 1 + \frac{a}{b}z + \frac{a(a+1)}{b(b+1)}\frac{z^2}{2!} + \frac{a(a+1)(a+2)}{b(b+1)(b+2)}\frac{z^3}{3!} + \cdots .$$

A second independent solution to the above differential equation is given by the confluent hypergeometric function of the second kind (the Kummer function of the second kind) given by

$$K_2(a, b, z) = \frac{\pi}{\sin(\pi b)}\left(\frac{K_1(a, b, z)}{\Gamma(1+a-b)\Gamma(b)} - \frac{z^{1-b}\,K_1(1+a-b, 2-b, z)}{\Gamma(a)\Gamma(2-b)}\right),$$

where Γ is the usual gamma function. For more details about Bessel functions, Hermite polynomials, Laguerre polynomials, and the error function, all which are special cases of confluent hypergeometric functions, the reader interested is referred to Abramowit and Stegun [39] (Chap. 13).

In order to obtain closed-form expressions for the BSsum distribution, assume the following. Consider an RV X_1 with IG distribution of parameters $\omega = T/\mu$ and $\lambda = T^2/\sigma^2$, whose PDF is given by

$$f_{X_1}(x; T, \mu, \sigma) = \left(\frac{\lambda}{2\pi x^3}\right)^{1/2} \exp\left(\left(\frac{-\lambda(x-\omega)^2}{2x\omega^2}\right)^2\right), x > 0. \qquad (14.9)$$

In addition, consider a second RV X_2 with gamma distribution of shape parameter k ($k = 0.5, 1, 1.5, 2, \ldots$) and scale parameter $\theta = 2\sigma^2/\mu^2$. Then, based on the PDF given in (14.9), the RV $S = X_1 + X_2$ has a PDF given by

$$f_S(s; T, \mu, \sigma, k) = \frac{T\mu^{2k}}{\sqrt{2\pi}\sigma(2\sigma^2)^k} \exp\left(-\frac{1}{2}\left(\frac{T - s\mu}{\sqrt{s}\sigma}\right)^2\right) s^{k-3/2} K_2\left(k, \frac{3}{2}, \frac{T^2}{2s\sigma^2}\right), s > 0. \qquad (14.10)$$

Note that, from the PDF given in (14.10), it is possible to deduce that the sum of an RV with IG distribution of parameters $\omega = T/\mu$ and $\lambda = T^2/\sigma^2$, and other RV with gamma distribution of shape parameter $k = 1/2$ and scale parameter $\theta = 2\sigma^2/\mu^2$, both of them independent, has a reciprocal IG distribution.

Now, consider an RV X_i following a BS distribution with parameters T_i, μ_i, and σ_i, whose X_is are independent. As indicated by Raaijmakers [27, 28], $S = \sum_{i=1}^n X_i$ does not follow the BS distribution. However, it is possible to find the PDF of this sum by assuming that a positive constant v exists, such that $\sigma_i/\mu_i = v$, for all i. This existence permits the mean and standard deviation of the inter-occurrence distribution to vary over time; see details in Fox et al. [29]. Therefore, the RV $S = \sum_{i=1}^n X_i$ corresponds to a mixture distribution whose PDF is given by

$$f_S(s; T, \mu, \sigma, n) = \frac{1}{2^n} f_0(s) + \sum_{j=1}^{n} \frac{1}{2^n}\binom{n}{j} f_j(s), \ s > 0, \qquad (14.11)$$

where

$$f_j(s) = \frac{T\mu^j}{\sqrt{2\pi}2^{j/2}\sigma^{j+1}} \exp\left(-\frac{1}{2}\left(\frac{T - s\mu}{\sqrt{s}\sigma}\right)^2\right) s^{j/2-3/2} K_2\left(\frac{j}{2}, \frac{3}{2}, \frac{T^2}{2s\sigma^2}\right), s > 0,$$

with

$$\mu = \sqrt{\sum_{i=1}^{n} \mu_i}, \quad \sigma = \sqrt{\sum_{i=1}^{n} \sigma_i}, \quad T = \mu \sum_{i=1}^{n} \frac{T_i}{\mu_i}.$$

In (14.11), note that, for $j = 0$, $K_2(0, 3/2, T^2/(2s\sigma^2)) = 1$, and, for $j = 1$, $K_2(1/2, 3/2, T^2/(2s\sigma^2)) = \sqrt{2s}\sigma/T$. For more details about these results and a shape analysis for the PDF given in (14.11), see Fox et al. [29]. Other probabilistic functions of the BSsum distribution, as well as its parameter estimation aspects, can be obtained such as in Sect. 14.2.1 and directly from there.

14.3 The BS Model as a Contaminant Distribution

The usage of the BS model like an atmospheric contaminant distribution may be justified relating the studies by Ott [40] and Desmond [41] (see Leiva et al. [14]). Based on the proportionate effect model, Ott [40] proposed a physical explanation of the log-normal model as a concentration distribution (see Aitchison and Brown [42], p. 22). However, Desmond [41] indicated the unsuitability in the use of Cramer's [43] biological model, which is linked to the proportionate effect model, to justify the employment of the log-normal model as a life distribution. Desmond [41] showed that the Cramér [43] model corresponds to a BS distribution; see Cramér [43], p. 219.

Consider Cramér [43]'s biological (or proportionate effect) model as follows. Suppose that n effects $H_1, \ldots, H_n$ are acting in the order of their indices. These effects are assumed to be independent RVs. Let W_j be the size of an organ produced by $H_1, \ldots, H_j$. In addition, assume that the organ increase provoked by H_{j+1} is proportional to itself and to a function g of the organ size in that instant given by

$$W_{j+1} = W_j + H_{j+1}\, g(W_j),\ j = 0, 1, \ldots \tag{14.12}$$

From (14.12), observe that the log-normal distribution is obtained when $g(W) = W$, whereas the BS distribution is obtained when $g(W) = 1$; see Desmond [41]. By applying the standard central limit theorem in (14.12) and considering a small enough increment $\Delta W_j = W_{j+1} - W_j$, so that summation can be changed by integration, we get

$$\sum_{j=1}^{n} H_j = \sum_{j=1}^{n} \frac{\Delta W_j}{g(W_j)} \approx \int_{W_0}^{W_n} \frac{\mathrm{d}w}{g(w)} \to I(W_t) = \int_{W_0}^{W_x} \frac{1}{g(w)}\,\mathrm{d}w \sim \mathrm{N}(x\eta, x\rho^2), \tag{14.13}$$

where W_0 is the initial organ size, W_t is the organ size at time x, and η and ρ^2 are the mean and variance of H_j, respectively. Assume that $W_c > W_0$ is the critical organ size at which the event of interest occurs and that W_c, W_0 are nonrandom. Then, the time until this event is given by $X = \inf\{x\colon W_x > W_c\}$. From (14.13) and the equivalent events $\{X \leq x\}$ and $\{W_x > W_c\}$, the CDF of X at x is given by

$$F_X(x) = \Phi\left(\frac{x\eta - I(W_c)}{\sqrt{x}\rho}\right).$$

Note that the model in (14.12) leads to life distributions in the BS family regardless of the form of $g(W)$. The dependence of the rate of organ extension on previous organ size is determined by the choice of the function $g(W)$. Here, a power function $g(W) = W^\delta$ is reasonable, for $\delta \geq 0$ and $\delta \neq 1$; see Desmond [41]. Thus,

$$I(W_x) = \int_{W_0}^{W_x} \frac{\mathrm{d}w}{g(w)} = \frac{1}{\delta - 1}\left(\frac{1}{W_0^{\delta-1}} - \frac{1}{W_x^{\delta-1}}\right) = \frac{W_0^{1-\delta} - W_x^{1-\delta}}{\delta - 1} \sim \mathrm{N}(x\eta, x\rho^2). \tag{14.14}$$

From (14.14), note that $W_x^{1-\delta} \sim \mathrm{N}(W_0^{1-\delta} + (1-\delta)x\eta, (1-\delta)^2 x\rho^2)$. Then, the CDF of X at x is given by

$$F_X(x) = \begin{cases} \Phi\left(\frac{W_c^{1-\delta} - W_0^{1-\delta} + (\delta-1)x\eta}{(\delta-1)\sqrt{x}\rho}\right), & \text{if } \delta > 1; \\ \Phi\left(\frac{W_0^{1-\delta} - W_c^{1-\delta} + (1-\delta)x\eta}{(1-\delta)\sqrt{x}\rho}\right), & \text{if } \delta < 1. \end{cases} \tag{14.15}$$

The BS distribution is obtained from (14.15) when $\delta = 0$. Nevertheless, the case $\delta = 1$, which corresponds to the log-normal distribution when $g(W) = W$ in the proportionate effect model given in (14.12), cannot be obtained from (14.15). Therefore, the CDF expressed in (14.15) corresponds to a BS type and not to a log-normal type.

The correspondence between Cramér's [43] biological model and Desmond's [41] fatigue model can be associated with contamination by making a parallel between the proportionate effect and pollutant concentration models. In a contamination context, suppose that an environment has a pollutant concentration W_0 and an air mass V_0 at an initial time instant equal to zero. Let $q_0 = W_0\, V_0$ be the total quantity of pollutant in the environment. Also, let V_1 be the volume of the mixture after first dilution and W_1 be the pollutant concentration in that diluted mixture. Then, $q_0 = W_0\, V_0 = W_1\, V_1$. If D_j stands for the corresponding factor for the jth dilution, the concentration W_2 in the second dilution is given by $W_2 = D_2\, W_1 = D_2\, D_1\, W_0$. For n successive dilutions, we have

$$W_n = W_0 \prod_{j=1}^{n} D_j. \tag{14.16}$$

In logarithmic terms, (14.16) becomes

$$\sum_{j=1}^{n} \log(D_j) = \log(W_n) - \log(W_0) = \int_{W_0}^{W_n} \frac{\mathrm{d}w}{w}. \tag{14.17}$$

Such in (14.13), one could assume a more general expression for (14.17) as

$$\sum_{j=1}^{n} H_j \approx \int_{W_0}^{W_n} \frac{\mathrm{d}w}{g(w)},$$

which should conduct to a BS distribution under certain conditions. This result permits the modeling of concentration data by a statistical distribution, which is positively skewed; see Ott [40]. Note that a similar principle can be used to justify the use of the BS distribution for describing fertilizer concentrations in the soil for agricultural management.

14.4 BS Exceedance Probabilities

The justification of the BS model as an environmental contaminant distribution described in Sect. 14.3 supports its use as an air pollutant concentration distribution. Usually, official environmental guidelines employ a contaminant concentration distribution to compute exceedance probabilities, which are important to establish regulatory environmental alerts.

The particulate matter (PM) is a type of air pollutant frequently monitored by environmental agencies because of its high risks to human health. A PM with a diameter below 10 μm (PM10) can cause an increment of respiratory diseases; see Box [44], Clyde [45] and Marchant et al. [1]. According to Chilean/American and European guidelines, the maximum permitted PM10 concentrations are 150 and 100 μg/normalized cubic meters (μg/m^{3}N) over a 24 h period, respectively.

Let $X \sim \mathrm{BS}(\alpha, \beta)$ be an atmospheric contaminant concentration as PM10. Then, the exceedance probability or of detecting levels of PM10 greater than x is given by

$$\mathrm{P}(X > x) = 1 - F_X(x; \alpha, \beta) = \Phi\left(-\frac{1}{\alpha}\left(\sqrt{x/\beta} - \sqrt{\beta/x}\right)\right), x > 0, \quad (14.18)$$

where Φ, α, and β are as in (14.1).

Example 14.4.1 (Marchant et al. [1]) We here illustrate the use of BS exceedance probabilities given in (14.18) as a tool to declare environmental alerts. We consider PM10 concentrations collected in 2003 at two following monitoring stations in Santiago, Chile: Las Condes (LS) and El Bosque (ES). We compute the probability for detecting PM10 levels greater than 150 μg/m^{3}N, which is the maximum allowed level according to Chilean air quality guidelines. The BS distribution can reasonably be assumed to describe the PM10 concentration data; see Marchant et al. [1]. By using the ML estimates of α and β, denoted by $\widehat{\alpha}$ and $\widehat{\beta}$, and plugging them into (14.18), we obtain

$$\mathrm{P}(X > 150) = 1 - F_X(150; \widehat{\alpha}, \widehat{\beta}) = \Phi\left(-\frac{1}{\widehat{\alpha}}\left(\sqrt{150/\widehat{\beta}} - \sqrt{\widehat{\beta}/150}\right)\right). \quad (14.19)$$

Based on (14.19), the exceedance probabilities are 0.0908 and 0.2063 for LS and for ES, respectively. These results suggest a lower capability of detecting higher pollution levels for LS, whereas a different situation is encountered at ES, as expected. The interested reader is referred to Marchant et al. [1], for details about this example.

14.5 BS X-Bar Control Charts

The BSsum distribution discussed in Sect. 14.2 is useful for developing X-bar control charts in order to detect environmental risk, when the contaminant concentration data follow a BS distribution; see Saulo et al. [25]. The lower (LCL) and (UCL) control limits for the mean concentration are computed by using the BSsum QF presented in (14.3). In Algorithm 1, we list the steps introduced in Saulo et al. [25] to construct X-bar control charts based on the BS and BSsum distributions.

Algorithm 1 X-bar control chart based on the BS and BSsum distributions

1: Collect $x_1, \ldots, x_k$ at k sampling points and compute their sample arithmetic mean $\bar{x} = \sum_{i=1}^{k} x_i/k$.
2: Based on the observed values from the random sample, calculate $s_i = \sum_{j=k(i-1)+1}^{ik} x_j$, for $i = 1, \ldots, n$, and obtain the estimates of α and β of the BSsum distribution.
3: Choose a value for γ, which is the out-of-control probability when the process is actually under control.
4: Based on estimates of Step 2 and the $(\gamma/2) \times 100$th and $(1 - \gamma/2) \times 100$th quantiles of the BSsum distribution divided by k, generate the LCL and UCL of the BS X-bar control chart. Add a central line (CL) by using the median of the data.
5: If $\bar{x} \geq$ UCL or $\bar{x} \leq$ LCL, declare the process as out of control, otherwise it is under control.
6: Repeat Steps 1 to 5 m times, where m denotes the number of groups to be evaluated.

Example 14.5.1 (Saulo et al. [25]) By means of an example, we illustrate the applicability of X-bar control charts based on the BS and BSsum models. We analyze the pH concentration level of five rivers from the South Island of New Zealand; (see Manly [46], pp. 135–138). These data range from January 1989 to December 1997. A correlation analysis indicates the absence of serial correlation. Moreover, the Kolmogorov–Smirnov test result (p-value $= 0.078$) favors the assumption that the data do follow a BS distribution. Figure 14.2 depicts a X-bar control chart, constructed according to Algorithm 1, to monitor the mean pH levels. This X-bar control chart is used to search for changes in the average value of pH levels over time. From Fig. 14.2, note that no points outside the control limits are detected, suggesting that the contamination levels are under control. The interested reader is referred to Saulo et al. [25], for details about this example.

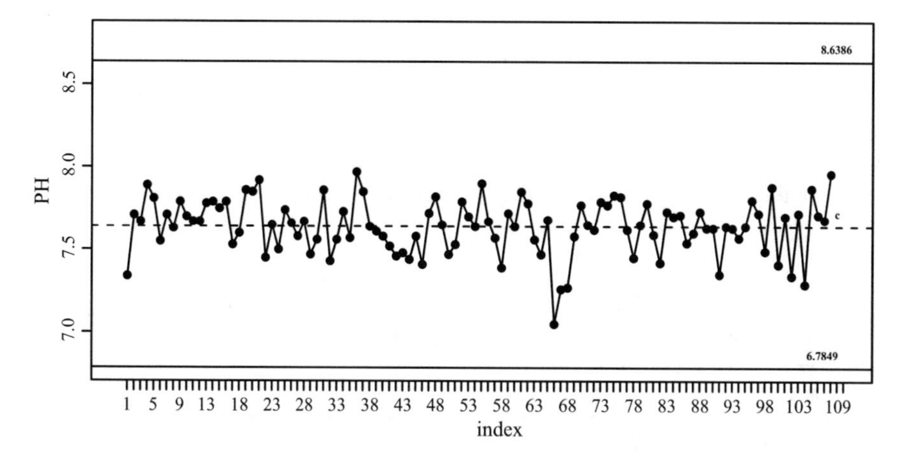

Fig. 14.2 BS X-bar control chart for the mean with pH data

14.6 BS np Control Charts

The np control chart can be thought as a modified version of the control chart for non-conforming fraction (p), when samples of equal size (n) are taken from the process. Consider an RV corresponding to the number (D) of times that the concentration of an atmospheric contaminant (X) exceeds a predetermined value (x). This value is considered by some environmental law and/or regulation and allows us to compute an exceedance probability $p = \mathrm{P}(X > x) = 1 - F_X(x)$. Note that D has a binomial distribution with parameters n and p, that is,

$$\mathrm{P}(D = d) = \binom{n}{d} p^d (1 - p)^{n-d}, d = 0, 1, \ldots, n,$$

with $\mathrm{E}(D) = np$ and $\mathrm{Var}(D) = np(1 - p)$. Leiva et al. [14] proposed an np control chart when X follows a BS distribution, where the LCL, CL, and UCL are given by

$$\begin{aligned} \mathrm{LCL} &= \max\left\{0, np_0 - k\sqrt{np_0(1 - p_0)}\right\}, \\ \mathrm{CL} &= np_0, \\ \mathrm{UCL} &= np_0 + k\sqrt{np_0(1 - p_0)}. \end{aligned} \tag{14.20}$$

In (14.20), k stands for a control coefficient ($k = 2$ is a warning level and $k = 3$ a dangerous level), p_0 is the non-conforming fraction corresponding to a target mean μ_0 under control, and n is the size of the subgroup. Note that p_0 is the probability that the atmospheric contaminant exceeds a dangerous concentration x_0, that is, $\mathrm{P}(X > x_0) = F_X(x_0)$. By using a reparameterized version of the BS distribution, namely, $X \sim \mathrm{BS}(\alpha, \mu)$, with $\mu = \beta(2 + \alpha^2)/2$, we obtain

$$p_0 = 1 - F_X(x_0; a, \alpha) = \Phi\left(-\frac{1}{\alpha}\xi\left(a(1+\alpha^2/2)\right)\right), \tag{14.21}$$

where ξ is defined in (F1). Here, $x_0 = a\mu_0$, where a is a proportionality constant. Official air quality guidelines can be used to provide the values of the target mean μ_0 and then the dangerous concentration x_0. Algorithm 2 is presented in Leiva et al. [14] as a criterion for environmental assessment in cases when the atmospheric contaminant follows a BS distribution.

Algorithm 2 np control chart based on the BS distribution

1: Obtain N subgroups of size n.
2: Collect data $x_1, \ldots, x_n$ for each subgroup.
3: Remove (if detected) any seasonal and/or serial dependence in the data.
4: Set values for the constants μ_0, a and k.
5: Compute in each subgroup of n data the number d of times that x_i exceeds $x_0 = a\mu_0$, for $i = 1, \ldots, n$.
6: Calculate LCL $= \max\{0, n\widehat{p}_0 - k\sqrt{n\widehat{p}_0(1-\widehat{p}_0)}\}$ and UCL $= n\widehat{p}_0 + k\sqrt{n\widehat{p}_0(1-\widehat{p}_0)}$, where $\widehat{p}_0 = \Phi(-(1/\widetilde{\alpha})\xi(a(1+\widetilde{\alpha}^2/2)))$ is as in (14.21) and $\widetilde{\alpha} = \sqrt{2(\sqrt{s/r}-1)}$ is the MM estimate of α, with $s = (1/n)\sum_{i=1}^n x_i$ and $r = \left((1/n)\sum_{i=1}^n (1/x_i)\right)^{-1}$.
7: If $d \geq$ UCL or $d \leq$ LCL, declare the process as out of control, otherwise it is under control.

Example 14.6.1 (Leiva et al. [14]) We illustrate the results established above by constructing a BS np charts for assessing environmental risk in Santiago, Chile, which has serious atmospheric contamination problems. We focus on PM10 (see Sect. 14.4) concentration data, which are obtained as 1h (hourly) average values. These data are based on the month of May 2008 and refer to the Independencia (IN) monitoring station. As mentioned previously, 150 and 100 μg/m^{3}N are the maximum permitted PM10 concentrations by Chilean/American and European guidelines,respectively. The BS distribution can reasonably be assumed to describe these PM10 concentration data; see Leiva et al. [14]. We apply Algorithm 2 and obtain a BS np control chart for the PM10 data; see Fig. 14.3. This plot evidences the coherence with the alerts provided by the Chilean Ministry of Health during the days May 12–16, 2008 and pre-emergence for the May 30, 2008; see www.seremisaludrm.cl/sitio/pag/aire/indexjs3airee001.asp. The interested reader is referred to Leiva et al. [14], for details about this example.

14.7 BS Spatial Models

Consider a stochastic process $\{X(\boldsymbol{s}), \boldsymbol{s} \in D\}$ with $D \subset \mathbb{R}^2$. Consider also n measurements $\boldsymbol{X} = (X_1, \ldots, X_n)^\top$, where $X_i = X(\boldsymbol{s}_i)$, for $i = 1, \ldots, n$, taken from the set of known spatial locations $\{\boldsymbol{s}_1, \ldots, \boldsymbol{s}_n\}$. A spatial model based on the BS distribution can be written as

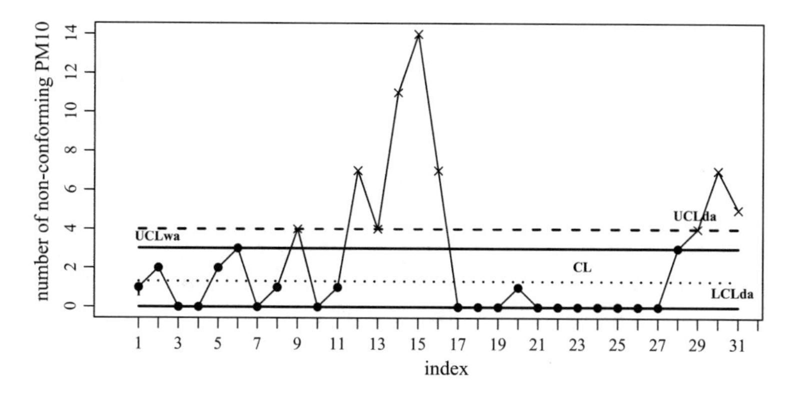

Fig. 14.3 BS np chart with $x_0 = 150$, where subindex "wa" indicates warning ($k = 2$, solid line) and subindex "da" dangerous ($k = 3$, dashed line) situations, for PM10 data in IN station

$$X_i = \exp(\mu_i)\,\eta_i, i = 1, \ldots, n. \tag{14.22}$$

By assuming stationarity, $\mu_i = \mu(\boldsymbol{s}_i) = \mu$ holds, and $\eta_i = \eta(\boldsymbol{s}_i) \sim \text{BS}(\alpha, 1)$, for $i = 1, \ldots, n$. Note that $\exp(\mu)$ is the median of the model. By applying logarithm in (14.22), we obtain

$$Y_i = \mu + \varepsilon_i, i = 1, \ldots, n, \tag{14.23}$$

where $Y_i = \log(X_i)$, whereas ε_i follows a log-BS distribution with shape parameter α and location parameter $\mu = 0$, denoted by $\varepsilon_i = \log(\eta_i) \sim \text{log-BS}(\alpha, 0)$, for $i = 1, \ldots, n$; see Garcia-Papani et al. [2]. Note that Y_i in (14.23) follows the log-BS distribution denoted by $Y_i \sim \text{log-BS}(\alpha, \mu)$. Then, $Y_1 = \log(X_1), \ldots, Y_n = \log(X_n)$ can be considered as a sample from $Y \sim \text{log-BS}(\alpha, \mu)$ with CDF of Y at y and PDF given, respectively, by

$$F_Y(y; \alpha, \mu) = \Phi\left(\frac{2}{\alpha}\sinh\left(\frac{y_i - \mu}{2}\right)\right), y \in \mathbb{R}, \mu \in \mathbb{R}, \alpha > 0,$$

$$f_Y(y; \alpha, \mu) = \frac{1}{\alpha\sqrt{2\pi}} \cosh\left(\frac{y - \mu}{2}\right) \exp\left(-\frac{2}{\alpha^2}\sinh^2\left(\frac{y - \mu}{2}\right)\right).$$

By written (14.23) in matrix form, we obtain

$$\boldsymbol{Y} = \mu\mathbf{1} + \varepsilon, \tag{14.24}$$

with $\boldsymbol{Y} = (Y_1, \ldots, Y_n)^\top$, $\mathbf{1} = (1, \ldots, 1)^\top$ and $\varepsilon = (\boldsymbol{\varepsilon_1, \ldots, \varepsilon_n})^\top$ being $n \times 1$ vectors. Note that ε is a stationary process with $\text{E}(\varepsilon) = \mathbf{0}$.

The structure of spatial dependence is modeled as follows. For the $n \times n$ positive definite (non-singular) scale and dependence matrix $\boldsymbol{\Sigma}$, we have the parametric form

$$\boldsymbol{\Sigma} = \varphi_1 \boldsymbol{I}_n + \varphi_2 \boldsymbol{R}, \tag{14.25}$$

where $\boldsymbol{I}_n$ is the $n \times n$ identity matrix and $\boldsymbol{R} = (r_{ij})$ is an $n \times n$ symmetric matrix with diagonal elements $r_{ii} = 1$ given in the family of Matérn models by

$$r_{ij} = \begin{cases} 1, i = j; \\ \frac{1}{2^{\delta-1}\Gamma(\delta)}\left(\frac{h_{ij}}{\varphi_3}\right)^{\delta} K_\delta\left(\frac{h_{ij}}{\varphi_3}\right), i \neq j; \end{cases} \tag{14.26}$$

with δ being a shape parameter, Γ being the usual gamma function, and K_δ being the modified Bessel function of third kind of order δ. We obtain from (14.26) that the elements σ_{ij} of $\boldsymbol{\Sigma}$ defined in (14.25) are given as

$$\sigma_{ij} = \begin{cases} \varphi_1 + \varphi_2, i = j; \\ \frac{\varphi_2}{2^{\delta-1}\Gamma(\delta)}\left(\frac{h_{ij}}{\varphi_3}\right)^{\delta} K_\delta\left(\frac{h_{ij}}{\varphi_3}\right), i \neq j. \end{cases}$$

Note that $\varphi_1 \geq 0$ and $\varphi_2 \geq 0$ are parameters known as nugget effect and partial sill, respectively, whereas $\varphi_3 \geq 0$ is a parameter related to the effective range or spatial dependence radius $a = g(\varphi_3)$. The vector of unknown parameters $\boldsymbol{\theta} = (\alpha, \mu, \varphi_1, \varphi_2, \varphi_3)^\top$ of the spatial model defined in (14.24) can be estimated by the ML method. Then, the corresponding log-likelihood function for $\boldsymbol{\theta}$, based on the observations $\boldsymbol{y} = (y_1, \ldots, y_n)^\top$ of $\boldsymbol{Y}$ defined in (14.24), is given by

$$\begin{aligned} \ell(\boldsymbol{\theta}) = & -\frac{n}{2}\log(2\pi) - \frac{1}{2}\log(|\boldsymbol{\Sigma}|) \\ & -n\log(\alpha) - \frac{2}{\alpha^2}\boldsymbol{V}^\top\boldsymbol{\Sigma}^{-1}\boldsymbol{V} + \sum_{i=1}^{n}\log\left(\cosh\left(\frac{y_i - \mu}{2}\right)\right), \end{aligned}$$

where $\boldsymbol{V} = (V_1, \ldots, V_n)^\top$ is an $n \times 1$ vector with elements $V_i = \sinh((y_i - \mu)/2)$, for $i = 1, \ldots, n$. The ML estimate $\widehat{\boldsymbol{\theta}}$ of $\boldsymbol{\theta}$ is obtained by maximizing $\ell(\boldsymbol{\theta})$ as $\widehat{\boldsymbol{\theta}} = \arg\max_{\boldsymbol{\theta}} \ell(\boldsymbol{\theta})$.

Example 14.7.1 (Garcia-Papani et al. [2]) We present an illustrative example concerning the soil phosphorus concentration which has a positive effect on plant growth and nutrition. The experimental study refers to the 2012–2013 crop year in a 167.35 ha commercial area of grain production in Cascavel, Paraná, Brazil. A total of $n = 102$ locations are geo-referenced and considered in this study. The sample CV, CS, and CK for these data are CV = 0.41 (41%), CS = 1.787, and CK = 5.104, respectively. Figure 14.4 shows the box plot and model map of the phosphorus concentration data. Note that the box plot suggests that cases #32, #53, #57, and #59 are potential influential observations. Note also that these points are identified (circled) in the model map and they are located in the lower part of the studied region. The BS distribution can reasonably be assumed to describe the phosphorus concentration data; see Garcia-Papani et al. [2]. The ML estimates (with estimated asymptotic standard errors in parenthesis) of the BS spatial model (assuming $\delta = 2.5$) in (14.24) are $\widehat{\alpha} = 0.997(3.521)$, $\widehat{\mu} = 2.807(0.082)$, $\widehat{\varphi}_1 = 0.134(0.946)$, $\widehat{\varphi}_2 = 0.020(0.142)$,

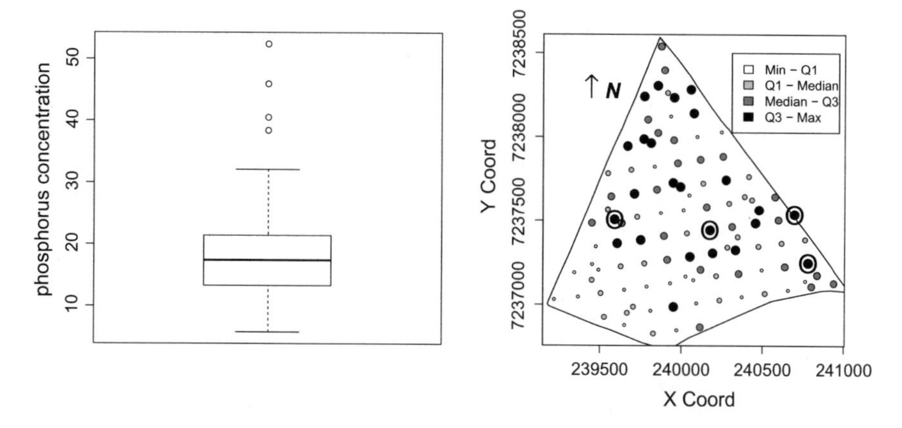

Fig. 14.4 Box plot (left) and model map (right) for phosphorus data

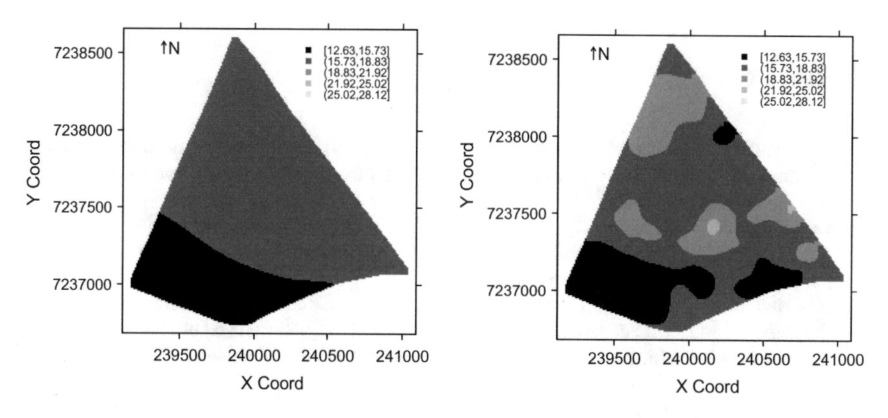

Fig. 14.5 Shaded contour plots with complete data (left) and removed cases (right) for phosphorus data

$\widehat{\varphi}_3 = 177.940(0.0000014)$, and $\widehat{a} = 1.053(0.0000083)$. By using influence diagnostic tools, it is found that cases #2, #48, and #94 are identified as influential, which are all of them different from the points detected by the box plot. Figure 14.5 shows contour maps of the soil phosphorus concentration based on the BS spatial model and ordinary Kriging interpolation; see Krige [47]. In the left part of this figure, the complete data set (reference map) is considered, whereas in the right part the influential cases #2, #48, and #94 are removed. Note that both maps are different, which shows the importance of a diagnostic analysis in all process of construction of maps when using spatial models. The interested reader is referred to Garcia-Papani et al. [2], for details about this example.

14.8 Concluding Remarks

In this work, we have presented some environmental applications of the Birnbaum–Saunders distribution. We have described a justification which indicates why this distribution can be a good contaminant model. We have also shown Birnbaum–Saunders exceedance probabilities which are used to declare environmental alerts. Moreover, we have discussed X-bar and np control charts based on the Birnbaum–Saunders distribution proposed to monitor environmental risk. Furthermore, we have presented a Birnbaum–Saunders spatial log-linear model. The presented methodologies have been illustrated by means of applications to different real-world data sets.

Acknowledgements The authors thank the editors and reviewers for their constructive comments on an earlier version of this manuscript. This work was partially supported by FONDECYT 1160868 grant from the Chilean government.

References

1. Marchant, C., V. Leiva, M. Cavieres, and A. Sanhueza. 2013. Air contaminant statistical distributions with application to PM10 in Santiago, Chile. *Reviews of Environmental Contamination and Toxicology* 223: 1–31.
2. Garcia-Papani, F., M. Uribe-Opazo, V. Leiva, and R. Aykroyd. 2016. Birnbaum-Saunders spatial modelling and diagnostics applied to agricultural engineering data. *Stochastic Environmental Research and Risk Assessment* 31: 105–124.
3. McConnell, R., K. Berhane, F. Gilliland, J. Molitor, D. Thomas, F. Lurmann, E. Avol, W.J. Gauderman, and J.M. Peters. 2003. Prospective study of air pollution and bronchitic symptoms in children with asthma. *American Journal of Respiratory and Critical Care Medicine* 168: 790–797.
4. Nuvolone, D., D. Balzi, M. Chini, D. Scala, F. Giovannini, and A. Barchielli. 2011. Short-term association between ambient air pollution and risk of hospitalization for acute myocardial infarction: results of the cardiovascular risk and air pollution in tuscany (RISCAT) study. *American Journal of Epidemiology* 174: 63–71.
5. De Bastiani, F., A. Cysneiros, M. Uribe-Opazo, and M. Galea. 2015. Influence diagnostics in elliptical spatial linear models. *TEST* 24: 322–340.
6. Leiva, V., A. Sanhueza, S. Kelmansky, and E. Martínez. 2009. On the glog-normal distribution and its association with the gene expression problem. *Computational Statistics and Data Analysis* 53: 1613–1621.
7. Johnson, N., S. Kotz, and N. Balakrishnan. 1994. *Continuous Univariate Distributions*, vol. 1. New York, US: Wiley.
8. Johnson, N., S. Kotz, and N. Balakrishnan. 1995. *Continuous Univariate Distributions*, vol. 2. New York, US: Wiley.
9. Leiva, V. and S.C. Saunders. 2015. Cumulative damage models. *Wiley StatsRef: Statistics Reference Online (available at* http://onlinelibrary.wiley.com/doi/10.1002/9781118445112.stat02136.pub2/abstract) 1–10.
10. Leiva, V. 2016. *The Birnbaum-Saunders Distribution*. New York, US: Academic Press.
11. Leiva, V., E. Athayde, C. Azevedo, and C. Marchant. 2011. Modeling wind energy flux by a Birnbaum-Saunders distribution with unknown shift parameter. *Journal of Applied Statistics* 38: 2819–2838.
12. Leiva, V., M. Barros, G. Paula, and A. Sanhueza. 2008. Generalized Birnbaum-Saunders distribution applied to air pollutant concentration. *Environmetrics* 19: 235–249.

13. Leiva, V., M. Ferreira, M.I. Gomes, and C. Lillo. 2016. Extreme value Birnbaum-Saunders regression models applied to environmental data. *Stochastic Environmental Research and Risk Assessment* 30: 1045–1058.
14. Leiva, V., C. Marchant, F. Ruggeri, and H. Saulo. 2015. A criterion for environmental assessment using Birnbaum-Saunders attribute control charts. *Environmetrics* 26: 463–476.
15. Leiva, V., M. Ponce, C. Marchant, and O. Bustos. 2012. Fatigue statistical distributions useful for modeling diameter and mortality of trees. *Revista Colombiana de Estadística* 35: 349–367.
16. Leiva, V., A. Sanhueza, and J.M. Angulo. 2009. A length-biased version of the Birnbaum-Saunders distribution with application in water quality. *Stochastic Environmental Research and Risk Assessment* 23: 299–307.
17. Leiva, V., A. Sanhueza, A. Silva, and M. Galea. 2008. A new three-parameter extension of the inverse Gaussian distribution. *Statistical and Probability Letters* 78: 1266–1273.
18. Leiva, V., F. Vilca, N. Balakrishnan, and A. Sanhueza. 2010. A skewed sinh-normal distribution and its properties and application to air pollution. *Communications in Statistics: Theory and Methods* 39: 426–443.
19. Podlaski, R. 2008. Characterization of diameter distribution data in near-natural forests using the Birnbaum-Saunders distribution. *Canadian Journal of Forest Research* 18: 518–527.
20. Balakrishnan, N., V. Leiva, A. Sanhueza, and E. Cabrera. 2009. Mixture inverse Gaussian distribution and its transformations, moments and applications. *Statistics* 43: 91–104.
21. Kotz, S., V. Leiva, and A. Sanhueza. 2010. Two new mixture models related to the inverse Gaussian distribution. *Methodology and Computing in Applied Probability* 12: 199–212.
22. Vilca, F., A. Sanhueza, V. Leiva, and G. Christakos. 2010. An extended Birnbaum-Saunders model and its application in the study of environmental quality in Santiago, Chile. *Stochastic Environmental Research and Risk Assessment* 24: 771–782.
23. Vilca, F., L. Santana, V. Leiva, and N. Balakrishnan. 2011. Estimation of extreme percentiles in Birnbaum-Saunders distributions. *Computational Statistics and Data Analysis* 55: 1665–1678.
24. Ferreira, M., M.I. Gomes, and V. Leiva. 2012. On an extreme value version of the Birnbaum-Saunders distribution. *Revstat Statistical Journal* 10: 181–210.
25. Saulo, H., V. Leiva, and F. Ruggeri. 2015. Monitoring environmental risk by a methodology based on control charts. In *Theory and Practice of Risk Assessment*, ed. C. Kitsos, T. Oliveira, A. Rigas, and S. Gulati, 177–197. Switzerland: Springer.
26. Saulo, H., V. Leiva, F.A. Ziegelmann, and C. Marchant. 2013. A nonparametric method for estimating asymmetric densities based on skewed Birnbaum-Saunders distributions applied to environmental data. *Stochastic Environmental Research and Risk Assessment* 27: 1479–1491.
27. Raaijmakers, F. 1980. The lifetime of a standby system of units having the Birnbaum-Saunders distribution. *Journal of Applied Probability* 17: 490–497.
28. Raaijmakers, F. 1981. Reliability of standby system for units with the Birnbaum-Saunders distribution. *IEEE Transactions on Reliability* 30: 198–199.
29. Fox, E., B. Gavish, and Semple, J. 2008. A general approximation to the distribution of count data with applications to inventory modeling. Available at https://papers.ssrn.com/sol3/papers.cfm?abstract_id=979826
30. Leiva, V., G. Soto, E. Cabrera, and G. Cabrera. 2011. New control charts based on the Birnbaum-Saunders distribution and their implementation. *Revista Colombiana de Estadística* 34: 147–176.
31. Leiva, V., A. Sanhueza, P. Sen, and G. Paula. 2008. Random number generators for the generalized Birnbaum-Saunders distribution. *Journal of Statistical Computation and Simulation* 78: 1105–1118.
32. Kundu, D., N. Kannan, and N. Balakrishnan. 2008. On the hazard function of Birnbaum-Saunders distribution and associated inference. *Computational Statistics and Data Analysis* 52: 2692–2702.
33. Birnbaum, Z.W., and S.C. Saunders. 1969. Estimation for a family of life distributions with applications to fatigue. *Journal of Applied Probability* 6: 328–347.
34. Engelhardt, M., L. Bain, and F. Wright. 1981. Inferences on the parameters of the Birnbaum-Saunders fatigue life distribution based on maximum likelihood estimation. *Technometrics* 23: 251–256.

35. Ng, H.K.T., D. Kundu, and N. Balakrishnan. 2003. Modified moment estimation for the two-parameter Birnbaum-Saunders distribution. *Computational Statistics and Data Analysis* 43: 283–298.
36. Ross, S. 1983. *Stochastic Processes*. New York, US: Wiley.
37. Birnbaum, Z.W., and S.C. Saunders. 1969. A new family of life distributions. *Journal of Applied Probability* 6: 319–327.
38. Desmond, A. 1986. On the relationship between two fatigue life models. *IEEE Transactions on Reliability* 35: 167–169.
39. Abramowitz, M., and I. Stegun. 1972. *Handbook of Mathematical Functions*. New York, US: Dover Press.
40. Ott, W. 1999. A physical explanation of the lognormality of pollution concentrations. *Journal of the Air and Waste Management Association* 40: 1378–1383.
41. Desmond, A. 1985. Stochastic models of failure in random environments. *Canadian Journal of Statistics* 13: 171–183.
42. Aitchison, J., and J. Brown. 1973. *The Lognormal Distribution*. London, UK: Cambridge University Press.
43. Cramér, H. 1946. *Mathematical Methods of Statistics*. Princeton, US: Princeton University Press.
44. Box, L. 2000. Statistical issues in the study of air pollution involving airborne particulate matter. *Environmetrics* 11: 611–626.
45. Clyde, M. 2000. Model uncertainty and health effect studies for particulate matter. *Environmetrics* 11: 745–763.
46. Manly, B. 2009. *Statistics for Environmental Science and Management*. Boca Raton: Chapman and Hall.
47. Krige, D. 1951. A statistical approach to some basic mine valuation problems on the Witwatersrand. *Journal of the Chemical, Metallurgical and Mining Society of South Africa* 52: 119–139.

Chapter 15
Analysis of Chronic Disease Processes Based on Cohort and Registry Data

Richard J. Cook and Jerald F. Lawless

Abstract In this chapter, we review the types of observation schemes which arise in the analysis of data on chronic conditions from individuals in disease registries. We consider the utility of multistate modeling for such disease processes, and deal with both right-censored data and data arising from intermittent observation of individuals. The assumptions necessary to support standard likelihood or partial likelihood inference are highlighted and adaptations to deal with dependent censoring or dependent inspection are described and examined in simulation studies and through application.

15.1 Introduction

Disease registries offer a valuable opportunity to gain scientific understanding about chronic conditions through the collection and recording of longitudinal data. Often interest lies in characterizing the rates of movement through different stages of a process and learning about fixed and dynamic factors that influence such changes. Life history data is the term used to describe the information collected on the occurrence of events experienced by individuals over the course of observation and life history analysis is based on such data. The techniques employed must be able to deal with incomplete observation and selective sampling schemes.

Often there is a relationship between the observation process and the disease process of interest. Subjects fairing poorly may be predisposed to withdrawing from a registry or cohort study, creating challenges in analyzing the available data due to induced dependent censoring. In other settings, individuals may only be observed intermittently and marker data and their disease status may only be available at periodic assessment times. In such cases care is required when analyzing the available data as it may offer a biased impression of the underlying process. Inverse probability weighting schemes can be employed to correct for these biased observation schemes and we discuss them in this chapter.

R. J. Cook (✉) · J. F. Lawless
Department of Statistics and Actuarial Science, University of Waterloo,
200 University Avenue West, Waterloo, ON N2L 3G1, Canada
e-mail: rjcook@uwaterloo.ca

A. Adhikari et al. (eds.), *Mathematical and Statistical Applications in Life Sciences and Engineering*, https://doi.org/10.1007/978-981-10-5370-2_15

A careful consideration of censoring and intermittent observation processes is important in order to avoid biased inference. We will give a careful discussion of the assumptions necessary for the construction of valid likelihood functions for settings where individuals are under continuous observation over a random period of time, as well as settings where they are under periodic examination. In the former case the life history processes are subject to right censoring, and in the latter, they are under intermittent observation and so yield interval censored event times and other types of incomplete data. Many of the issues we consider can be conveniently discussed within the framework of multistate models, which we describe next.

15.2 Multistate Modeling of Chronic Disease Processes

15.2.1 Intensity Functions

We let $Z(s)$ reflect the state occupied at time $s > 0$ in a K-state multistate process $\{Z(s), 0 < s\}$ with the states labeled $1, \ldots, K$. Figure 15.1 contains an illustrative state space diagram of an illness-death process with state 1 representing the condition of being alive and healthy, state 2 represents the state of alive with disease, and state 3 represents death. Transitions between these states represent the onset of disease (i.e., a $1 \to 2$ transition) or death (i.e., a transition into state 3). This simple model can play a powerful role in modeling and understanding the onset of disease and its consequent impact on risk of death.

To characterize the stochastic features of multistate models we define counting processes such that there is one counting process for each possible type of transition in the multistate model. Let $N_{jk}(t)$ count the number of $j \to k$ transitions realized over the interval $(0, t]$, $\Delta N_{jk}(t) = N_{jk}(t + \Delta t^-) - N_{jk}(t^-)$ count the number of $j \to k$ transitions over $[t, t + \Delta t)$, and let $dN_{jk}(t) = \lim_{\Delta t \downarrow 0} \Delta N_{jk}(t) = 1$ if a $j \to k$ transition occurs at time t. We may then define the vector of counting processes for transitions out of state j as $N_j(t) = (N_{j1}(t), \ldots, N_{jK}(t))'$, let $N(t) = (N'_1(t), \ldots, N'_K(t))'$ denote the vector of all counting processes, and let $dN(t)$ be the vector of indicators of transitions at time t. In many applications there will be one or more absorbing states; if so we omit the corresponding vectors $dN_k(t)$ from $dN(t)$ since these are all zero by definition.

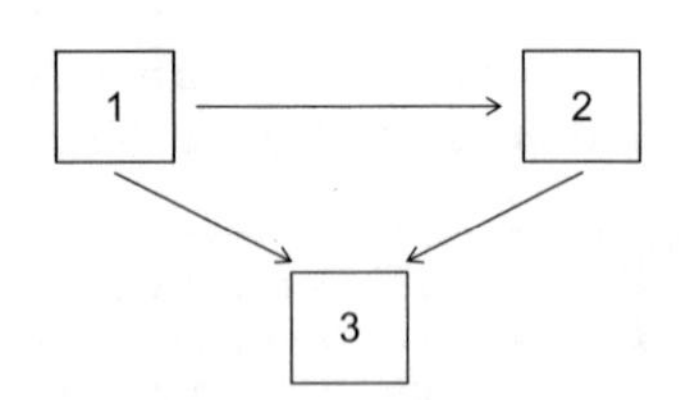

Fig. 15.1 An illness-death process

We let $\{X(s), 0 < s\}$ denote a left-continuous bounded covariate process. The increment of the covariate process over $[t, t + \Delta t)$ is $\Delta X(t) = X(t + \Delta t) - X(t)$ and we let $dX(t) = \lim_{\Delta t \downarrow 0} \Delta X(t)$. The history of the multistate and covariate processes up to time t is denoted by $\mathcal{H}(t) = \{dN(s), dX(s); 0 < s < t\}$. We let

$$\lim_{\Delta t \downarrow 0} \frac{P\left(Z((t + \Delta t)^-) = k | Y_j(t) = 1, \mathcal{H}(t)\right)}{\Delta t} = \lambda_{jk}\left(t | \mathcal{H}(t)\right) , \qquad (15.1)$$

where $Y_j(t) = I(Z(t^-) = j)$ indicates that a subject is at risk of transition out of state j at time t and $\lambda_{jk}(t|\mathcal{H}(t))$ is the intensity of a $j \to k$ transition at t; we assume that two transitions cannot occur at the same time.

Suppose a subject is to be observed continuously over the interval $(0, E]$ where E is the administrative censoring time. Let D denote a possible random dropout time so that $C = \min(D, E)$ is the net censoring time. We let $Y(t) = I(t \le C)$ indicate that the subject is still under observation at time t. We let $\{C(s), 0 < s\}$ denote the counting process for censoring, where $C(t) = I(C \le t)$, $\Delta C(t) = C(t + \Delta t^-) - C(t^-)$, and $dC(t) = \lim_{\Delta t \downarrow 0} \Delta C(t) = 1$ if censoring occurs at time t. We then let $d\bar{N}_{jk}(t) = Y(t)dN_{jk}(t) = 1$ if a $j \to k$ transition *is observed* at time t. Next, we define the vectors $d\bar{N}_j(t) = (d\bar{N}_{j1}(t), \dots, d\bar{N}_{jK}(t))'$ and let $d\bar{N}(t) = (d\bar{N}_1'(t), \dots, d\bar{N}_K'(t))'$ denote the vector of all variables indicating transitions observed at time t; note only one element in $d\bar{N}(t)$ will be 1 at any time for a particular individual and all other elements will be zero. We likewise define $\Delta\bar{X}(t) = Y(t)\Delta X(t)$ and $d\bar{X}(t) = \lim_{\Delta t \downarrow 0} \Delta\bar{X}(t)$. The history of *the observable process* is then $\bar{\mathcal{H}}(t) = \{d\bar{N}(s), d\bar{X}(s), C(s); 0 < s < t\}$. The intensity functions (Andersen et al. [2]) for the observable multistate process are then

$$\lim_{\Delta t \downarrow 0} \frac{P\left(\Delta\bar{N}_{jk}(t) = 1 | \bar{Y}_j(t) = 1, \bar{\mathcal{H}}(t)\right)}{\Delta t} = \bar{\lambda}_{jk}(t|\bar{\mathcal{H}}(t)) , \quad j \ne k \qquad (15.2)$$

where $\bar{Y}_j(t) = Y(t)Y_j(t)$ indicates individual is "under observation and at risk of transition out of state j" at time t. Under conditionally independent censoring $\bar{\lambda}_{jk}(t|\bar{\mathcal{H}}(t)) = Y(t)\lambda_{jk}(t|\mathcal{H}(t))$ (see Lawless [18]).

15.2.2 *Product Integration and the Partial Likelihood*

Inference is often most naturally and efficiently based on the likelihood function which here is proportional to the joint probability of the multistate, covariate, and observation process. To construct this we use product integration (Andersen et al. [2]) and begin by dividing the interval $(0, E]$ into R subintervals with cut-points $0 = u_0 < u_1 < \cdots < u_{R-1} < u_R = E$ and $\Delta u_r = u_r - u_{r-1}$. We let $\Delta\bar{N}_{jk}(u_r) = \bar{N}_{jk}(u_r^-) - \bar{N}_{jk}(u_{r-1}^-)$ and consider the total contributions corresponding to the probabilities of what may be realized over each interval $[u_{r-1}, u_r)$ among those individuals still conveying information. For a generic individual this gives

$$\prod_{r=1}^{R} \Bigg\{ \Bigg[P(\Delta \bar{N}(u_r) | Y(u_r) = 1, \bar{\mathcal{H}}(u_r)) \tag{15.3}$$

$$\times \; P(\Delta \bar{X}(u_r) | \Delta \bar{N}(u_r), Y(u_r) = 1, \bar{\mathcal{H}}(u_r)) \Bigg]^{Y(u_r)} P(\Delta C(u_r) | \bar{\mathcal{H}}(u_r)) \Bigg\}^{Y(u_{r-1})}.$$

When interest lies in the multistate process only we may not wish to model the covariate or censoring processes and so would like to ignore the second and third terms in (15.3). This incurs no loss in efficiency as long as the models for these processes do not contain any parameters of the response process; in this case, we say the covariate and censoring processes are noninformative (Lawless [18]). Retaining the first term in (15.3) we focus on the "partial likelihood" which we write as

$$\prod_{r=1}^{R} P(\Delta \bar{N}(u_r) | Y(u_r) = 1, \bar{\mathcal{H}}(u_r))^{Y(u_r)} \tag{15.4}$$

$$= \prod_{r=1}^{R} \prod_{j=1}^{K} P(\Delta \bar{N}_j(u_r) | \bar{Y}_j(u_r) = 1, \bar{\mathcal{H}}(u_r))^{Y(u_r) Y_j(u_{r-1})}$$

since the only vector which will be nonzero with probability less than one is the one corresponding to the state occupied at t^- (i.e., $\Delta \bar{N}_j(u_r)$ if $\bar{Y}_j(u_{r-1}) = 1$). We then note that $P(\Delta \bar{N}_j(u_r) | \bar{Y}_j(u_r) = 1, \bar{\mathcal{H}}(u_r))$ can be written as

$$\Bigg[\prod_{k \neq j = 1}^{K} P(\Delta \bar{N}_{jk}(u_r) = 1 | \bar{Y}_j(u_r) = 1, \bar{\mathcal{H}}(u_r))^{\Delta \bar{N}_{jk}(u_r)} \Bigg]$$

$$\times \; P(\Delta \bar{N}_{j\cdot}(u_r) = 0 | \bar{Y}_j(u_r) = 1, \bar{\mathcal{H}}(u_r))^{1 \;\; \Delta \bar{N}_{j\cdot}(u_r)}$$

where $\Delta \bar{N}_{j\cdot}(t) = \sum_{k \neq j=1}^{K} \Delta \bar{N}_{jk}(t)$. These probabilities can be expressed in terms of the parameters of the underlying multistate process provided censoring is conditionally independent of the multistate process. Assuming censoring is conditionally independent given the observed history, then

$$P(\Delta \bar{N}_{jk}(t) = 1 | \bar{Y}_j(t) = 1, \bar{\mathcal{H}}(t)) = \bar{Y}_j(t) \; \lambda_{jk}(t | \mathcal{H}(t)) \Delta t + o(\Delta t)$$

and

$$P(\Delta \bar{N}_{j\cdot}(t) = 0 | \bar{Y}_j(t) = 1, \bar{\mathcal{H}}(t)) = \bar{Y}_j(t) \big[1 - \lambda_{j\cdot}(t | \mathcal{H}(t)) \Delta t \big] + o(\Delta t),$$

where $\lambda_{j\cdot}(u_r|\mathcal{H}(u_r)) = \sum_{k=1}^{K} \lambda_{jk}(u_r|\mathcal{H}(u_r))$. Moreover, assuming that at most one transition can occur at any instant, then $P(\Delta \bar{N}_{j\cdot}(t) \geq 2|\bar{\mathcal{H}}(t)) = o(\Delta t)$. The likelihood is obtained by substituting these expressions into (15.4), dividing by $\prod_{r=1}^{R}(\Delta u_r)^{Y(u_r)}$, and taking the limit as $R \to \infty$ to obtain (Andersen et al. [2])

$$L \propto \prod_{j=1}^{K} \prod_{k \neq j=1}^{K} \Bigg[\Bigg(\prod_{t_l \in \mathcal{D}_{jk}} \lambda_{jk}\Big(t_l|\mathcal{H}(t_l)\Big) \Bigg) \times \exp\Bigg(- \int_0^{\infty} \bar{Y}_j(u) \lambda_{jk}\Big(u|\mathcal{H}(u)\Big) \Bigg) du \Bigg] \tag{15.5}$$

where $\mathcal{D}_{jk} = \{t_l$: a $j \to k$ transition was observed at $t_l\}$. This likelihood can be written as $L \propto \prod_{j=1}^{K} \prod_{k \neq j=1}^{K} L_{jk}$ and the log-likelihood can then be written as

$$\ell = \sum_{j=1}^{K} \sum_{k \neq j=1}^{K} \ell_{jk}(\theta_{jk})$$

where θ_{jk} parameterizes the $j \to k$ transition intensity, and

$$\ell_{jk}(\theta_{jk}) = \int_0^{\infty} \bar{Y}_j(u) \ \log \lambda_{jk}(u|\mathcal{H}(u)) \, dN_{jk}(u) - \int_0^{\infty} \bar{Y}_j(u) \ \lambda_{jk}(u|\mathcal{H}(u)) \, du \ . \tag{15.6}$$

If the different transition intensities do not share any parameters then maximization of (15.5) can be carried out by separately maximizing each element in the sum of the log-likelihood.

15.2.3 *Estimation with Markov Models*

In the absence of covariates, Markov models have intensities which depend only on the state currently occupied and the time since the start of the process. They are often suitable when the process "ages" and there is a degenerative aspect to it. Examples include conditions like arthritis, kidney disease, etc. where the time since the origin of the process (i.e., "disease onset") is the natural time scale. In such settings we write $\lambda_{jk}(t|Y_j(t) = 1, \mathcal{H}(t)) = Y_j(t) q_{jk}(t)$ and let $Q_{jk}(t) = \int_0^t q_{jk}(u) du$ denote the cumulative $j \to k$ transition intensity; $q_{jk}(t)$ is often referred to in this case as a transition rate. We may define a matrix of cumulative transition intensities $\mathbb{Q}(t)$ with (j, k) element $Q_{jk}(t)$ and diagonal elements $-\sum_{k \neq j=1}^{K} Q_{jk}(t)$. The transition probability matrix $\mathbb{P}(s, t)$ with (j, k) entry $p_{jk}(s, t) = P(Z(t) = k|Z(s) = j)$ is obtained by product integration as

$$\mathbb{P}(s,t) = \prod_{u\in(s,t]} [\mathbb{I} + d\mathbb{Q}(u)] = \lim_{R\uparrow\infty} \prod_{r=1}^{R} [\mathbb{I} + \Delta\mathbb{Q}(u_r)] \tag{15.7}$$

where $\mathbb{I}$ is a $K \times K$ identity matrix and $\Delta\mathbb{Q}(u) = \mathbb{Q}(u_r^-) - \mathbb{Q}(u_{r-1}^-)$.

Nonparametric estimates of Markov transition intensities and probabilities take a simple form. With a sample of m independent individuals, we introduce a subscript i and write the partial log-likelihood based on (15.6) as

$$\ell = \sum_{i=1}^{m}\sum_{j=1}^{K}\sum_{k\neq j=1}^{K} \int_0^\infty \bar{Y}_{ij}(u)\left[\log dQ_{jk}(u)dN_{ijk}(u) - dQ_{jk}(u)\right] .$$

Then differentiating with respect to $dQ_{jk}(u)$ gives $d\widehat{Q}_{jk}(u) = d\bar{N}_{\cdot jk}(u)/\bar{Y}_{\cdot j}(u)$ where $d\bar{N}_{\cdot jk}(u) = \sum_{i=1}^{m} \bar{Y}_{ij}(u)dN_{ijk}(u)$ and $\bar{Y}_{\cdot j}(u) = \sum_{i=1}^{m} \bar{Y}_{ij}(u)$. The Nelson–Aalen estimate of the cumulative $j \to k$ transition intensity is $\widehat{Q}_{jk}(t) = \int_0^t d\widehat{Q}_{jk}(u)$ (Lawless [18]). The nonparametric estimate of the transition probability matrix is then

$$\widehat{\mathbb{P}}(s,t) = \prod_{u\in(s,t]} \left[\mathbb{I} + d\widehat{\mathbb{Q}}(u)\right]$$

where $d\widehat{\mathbb{Q}}(u)$ is obtained by replacing the unknown quantities by the corresponding estimate (Andersen et al. [2]). This is known as the Aalen–Johansen estimate and is available from R software such as the `etm` package. Aalen et al. [1] and Datta and Satten [8] noted that while this estimator is justified by a Markov model it is consistent more generally provided censoring is independent of the multistate process.

With fixed or time-dependent covariates, modulated Markov models take the form

$$\lambda_{jk}\left(t|Y_j(t), \mathcal{H}(t)\right) = Y_j(t) \cdot q_{jk}(t) \cdot \exp(X'(t)\beta_{jk}) , \tag{15.8}$$

where here we assume for simplicity that the same sets of covariates are of interest for all transition intensities. We use the term "modulated" where the baseline Markov intensity is modified by the effects of fixed or external time-dependent covariates.

With a sample of m independent individuals, after introducing the subscript i to index individuals, substituting (15.8) into (15.6) and summing over individuals we obtain

$$\ell_{jk} = \sum_{i=1}^{m}\left[\int_0^\infty \bar{Y}_{ij}(u)\log dQ_{ijk}(u)dN_{ijk}(u) - \int_0^\infty \bar{Y}_{ij}(u)dQ_{ijk}(u)\right] .$$

which looks like an ordinary likelihood for a survival model (Kalbfleisch and Prentice [16]) except here $dQ_{ijk}(t) = dQ_{jk}(t)\exp(X_i'(t)\beta_{jk})$ is a transition intensity rather than a hazard and $\bar{Y}_{ij}(u)$ accommodates "delayed entry" (Klein and Moeschberger [17]). Differentiating with respect to $dQ_{jk}(u)$ and β_{jk} gives the two sets of estimating equations

$$\sum_{i=1}^{m} \bar{Y}_{ij}(u)[dN_{ijk}(u) - dQ_{ijk}(u)] = 0\ , \quad u > 0 \tag{15.9a}$$

$$\sum_{i=1}^{m} \int_{0}^{\infty} \bar{Y}_{ij}(u) X_{ijk}(u)[dN_{ijk}(u) - dQ_{ijk}(u)] = 0\ . \tag{15.9b}$$

Let

$$S_{jk}^{(0)}(u; \beta_{jk}) = \sum_{i=1}^{m} \bar{Y}_{ij}(u)\ \exp(X'_{ijk}(u)\beta_{jk})$$

and

$$S_{jk}^{(1)}(u; \beta_{jk}) = \sum_{i=1}^{m} \bar{Y}_{ij}(u)\ X_{ijk}(u)\ \exp(X'_{ijk}(u)\beta_{jk}).$$

If $Q_{jk}(t) = \int_0^t q_{jk}(u)du$ is the cumulative baseline transition intensity, we may profile out $dQ_{jk}(u)$ to get $d\widehat{Q}_{jk}(j; \beta_{jk}) = d\bar{N}_{\cdot jk}(u)/S_{jk}^{(0)}(u; \beta_{jk})$, and substitute the result into (15.9b) to obtain the partial score equation for β_{jk},

$$U_{jk}(\beta_{jk}) = \sum_{i=1}^{m} \int_{0}^{\infty} \left[X_{ijk}(u) - \frac{S_{jk}^{(1)}(u; \beta_{jk})}{S_{jk}^{(0)}(u; \beta_{jk})} \right] d\bar{N}_{ijk}(u) = 0\ . \tag{15.10}$$

We let $\widehat{\beta}_{jk}$ denote the solution to $U_{jk}(\beta_{jk}) = 0$. Because (15.10) has the same form as a partial score equation from a Cox regression model, software for fitting the Cox model can be used to obtain $\widehat{\beta}_{jk}$.

15.2.4 Dependent Withdrawal from Cohorts

Suppose the assumption of conditionally independent censoring is not valid and so we cannot write $P(\Delta\bar{N}_{jk}(t) = 1|\bar{Y}_j(t) = 1, \bar{\mathcal{H}}(t)) = \bar{Y}_j(t)\lambda_{jk}(t|\mathcal{H}(t))\Delta t + o(\Delta t)$ as we did following (15.2). Suppose moreover there is an auxiliary covariate $W(t)$ which we do not wish to regress upon, but which satisfies $P(d\bar{N}(u)|\bar{Y}_j(u) = 1, \bar{\mathcal{H}}(u), W(u)) = Y(u)P(dN(u)|\mathcal{H}(u), W(u))$; this means that conditional on $W(t)$ the censoring process is independent of the response process. We again let $\Delta W(t) = W(t + \Delta t) - W(t)$, $\Delta\bar{W}(t) = Y(t)\Delta W(t)$, and $d\bar{W}(t) = \lim_{\Delta t \downarrow 0} \Delta\bar{W}(t)$. We may then modify (15.9a) and (15.9b) by the introduction of inverse probability of censoring weights as

$$\sum_{i=1}^{n} \frac{\bar{Y}_{ij}(u)}{G_i(u)} [dN_{ijk}(u) - dQ_{ijk}(u)] = 0 \tag{15.11a}$$

$$\sum_{i=1}^{n} \int_{0}^{\infty} \frac{\bar{Y}_{ij}(u)}{G_i(u)} X_{ijk}(u) [dN_{ijk}(u) - dQ_{ijk}(u)] = 0 , \tag{15.11b}$$

where $\bar{\mathcal{H}}^\star(t) = \{d\bar{N}(u), d\bar{X}(u), d\bar{W}(u)\, 0 < u < t\}$ and $G_i(u) = P(D_i > u|\bar{\mathcal{H}}_i^\star(u))$ (Datta and Satten [9]). Of course, we do not know $G_i(u)$ in practise, so we typically fit models for the censoring intensity,

$$\lim_{\Delta t \downarrow 0} \frac{P(\Delta C(t) = 1|\bar{\mathcal{H}}^\star(t))}{\Delta t} = Y(t) \cdot \lambda^c(t|\bar{\mathcal{H}}^\star(t)) .$$

For example, multiplicative models of the form $\lambda^c(t|\bar{\mathcal{H}}^\star(t))) = \lambda_0^c(t) \exp(X'(t)\gamma_1 + W'(t)\gamma_2)$ are often used, where $\gamma = (\gamma_1', \gamma_2')'$ are regression coefficients in a multiplicative censoring model and $\Lambda_0^c(t) = \int_0^t \lambda_0^c(u)du$. Once $\widehat{\Lambda}_0^c(t)$ and $\widehat{\gamma}$ are obtained, we can then compute the estimate

$$\widehat{G}_i(u) = \widehat{P}(D_i > u|\bar{\mathcal{H}}_i^\star(u)) = \prod_{s \in (0,u]} \left[1 - d\widehat{\Lambda}_0^c(s)\, \exp(X_i'(s)\widehat{\gamma}_1 + W_i'(s)\widehat{\gamma}_2)\right] .$$

Provided that the multiplicative censoring model is correctly formulated such that $E(dC_i(t)|\bar{\mathcal{H}}_i^*(t), C(t^-) = 0) = \lambda_0^c(t) \exp(X_i'(t)\gamma_1 + W_i'(t)\gamma_2)$ and $(d\widehat{\Lambda}_0^c(\cdot), \widehat{\gamma}')'$ is consistent, then consistent estimates of the parameters of interest are obtained by solving (15.11a) and (15.11b) with $G_i(u)$ replaced by $\widehat{G}_i(u)$ (Cook et al. [7]; Satten, Datta and Robins [22]).

15.2.5 An Illustrative Example

We consider a simple illustration involving a four-state progressive process $\{Z(s), 0 < s\}$ with states labeled 0, 1, 2, and 3, where for $k = 1, 2, 3$, T_k denotes the entry time to state k, and

$$\lim_{\Delta t \downarrow 0} \frac{P(Z((t + \Delta t)^-) = k|Z(t^-) = k - 1, X_1)}{\Delta t} = \lambda_k \cdot \exp(X_1\beta_k) , \tag{15.12}$$

where X_1 is a covariate of interest. We let $X_2 \sim N(0, 1)$ represent another fixed covariate, discussed below, but our objective is to estimate the λ_k and β_k in (15.12).

We denote the planned observation period as $(0, E]$ where $E = 1$, let D denote a random dropout time, and let $C = \min(D, E)$, $Y(s) = I(s \le C)$ and $C(s) = I(C \le s)$. We suppose that for $t < E = 1$

$$\lim_{\Delta t \downarrow 0} \frac{P(\Delta C(t) = 1 | C(t) = 0, X_2)}{\Delta t} = Y(t) \cdot \rho \cdot \exp(X_2 \alpha)$$

so that when $\alpha \neq 0$, the dropout (and hence censoring) time is associated with the covariate X_2.

We want to illustrate the effects of dependent censoring so we will associate X_2 with the multistate process while preserving the proportional intensity form of (15.12) and the Markov property. To do this we use a copula function to induce a dependence between T_3 and X_2 given X_1. We let $F_k(t|X_1) = P(T_k < t|X_1)$ denote the conditional c.d.f. for the entry time to state k, let $G(d|X_2)$ denote the c.d.f. of the time to withdrawal D with $P(D > d|X_2) = G(d|X_2)$, and let $G_2(X_2)$ denote the c.d.f. of X_2 which is assumed to be standard normal. We let $U_1 = F_3(T_3|X_1)$ and $U_2 = G_2(X_2)$ and with $\mathcal{C}(u_1, u_2; \theta)$ the bivariate Clayton copula function (Nelsen [21]) with dependence parameter θ we define

$$P(T_3 \leq t_3, X_2 \leq x_2 | X_1) = \mathcal{C}(F_3(t_3|X_1), G_2(X_2); \theta) \, .$$

Thus $T_3 \perp D|X_1, X_2$, but $T_3 \not\perp D|X_1$ so although model (15.12) holds, a naive multistate analysis conditioning only on X_1 will be subject to dependent censoring if $\alpha \neq 0$ and $\theta \neq 0$. We first consider a one sample problem in which $\beta_k = 0$, $k = 1, 2, 3$ and X_1 is ignored. We set $\lambda_k = 1.1\lambda_{k-1}, k = 2, 3$, representing increased rates of transition and solve for λ_1 such that $P(T_3 < 1) = 0.9$. We then set $\alpha = 1$ and solve for ρ such that the net censoring rate is 60% for T_3. That is

$$P(T_3 < C) = E_{X_2} \left\{ \int_0^E g(u|X_2) \, \mathcal{F}_3(u) \, du + G(E|X_2) \, \mathcal{F}_3(E) \right\} .$$

Figure 15.2 displays the true state entry time distributions for $k = 1$ and $k = 3$ given by $P_{01}(t) + P_{02}(t) + P_{03}(t)$ and $P_{03}(t)$ respectively, along with the corresponding naive Kaplan–Meier estimates for a sample of size $m = 10000$. Also shown are the estimates obtained based on inverse probability of censoring weights, where the better performance is clearly evident.

We also consider the consequences to fitting parametric and semiparametric models to the multistate process under the assumption of independent censoring to explore which parameters are most sensitive to dependent censoring. We let X_1 be binary with $P(X_1 = 1) = 0.5$ and let $\beta_1 = \beta_2 = \beta_3 = \log 0.75$ in (15.12). We fit a parametric Markov model and a semiparametric Markov model as described in Sect. 15.2; note that these would both yield consistent estimates under independent censoring since they are not misspecified for the multistate process. Table 15.1 reports the empirical bias and empirical standard errors for 1000 data sets of size $m = 1000$.

The impact of dependent censoring is complex in the multistate setting and somewhat difficult to anticipate because dependent censoring induces both a selection effect due to dependent withdrawal times from risk sets as well as dependent entry into risk sets for estimating transitions from noninitial states. In broad terms the biases in the estimated regression coefficients are greater the stronger the

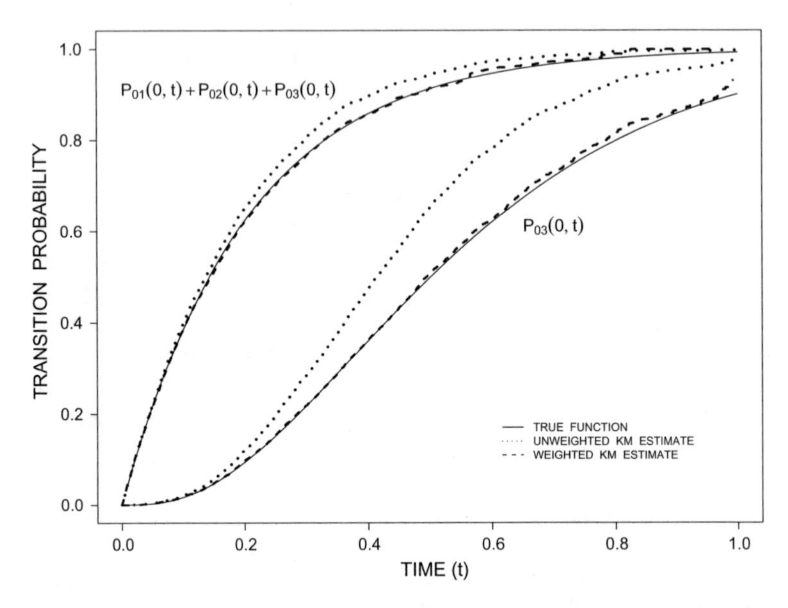

Fig. 15.2 Plots of the true state entry time distributions for states 1 and 3, the unweighted Kaplan–Meier estimate, and an inverse probability of censoring weighted Kaplan–Meier estimate for a sample of size $m = 10000$; $\exp(\alpha) = 2$ for the censoring intensity model and the dependence between X_2 and T_3 is induced by a Clayton copula with Kendall's $\tau = 0.8$; note $\beta_k = 0$ for $k = 1, 2$ and 3 for this one sample setting

association between the censoring times and absorption times for the multistate process for parametric models; for semiparametric models, the empirical biases are smaller and the trends in relation to the strength of the dependent censoring are less apparent.

15.2.6 Application to a Palliative Trial in Metastatic Breast Cancer

We consider the analysis of data from a clinical trial examining the effect of a bisphosphonate, versus placebo treatment, on reducing skeletal complications including bone pain requiring radiotherapy (Hortobagyi et al. [13]). A secondary goal is to estimate the survival distribution for patients in each treatment arm; we focus on patients in the placebo arm. Panel (a) in Fig. 15.3 contains the two-state model for the survival time T_i alone, and panel (b) shows the full model of interest, with the addition of two censoring states. If we conduct a simple survival analysis in this setting we let $N_i^{\dagger}(s) = I(T_i \leq s)$ indicate death by time s. In a one-sample problem, we let $Q(t) = \int_0^t q(s)\, ds$ denote the cumulative hazard for death, where the hazard function is

Table 15.1 Empirical biases and standard errors of estimated regression coefficients under parametric and semiparametric analyses with varying degree of dependent right censoring

		Kendall's $\tau = 0.4$		Kendall's $\tau = 0.8$	
		$\exp(\alpha) = 2$	$\exp(\alpha) = 4$	$\exp(\alpha) = 2$	$\exp(\alpha) = 4$
Parametric analyses					
β_1	Bias	0.012	0.017	0.020	0.028
	ESE	0.075	0.077	0.073	0.073
β_2	Bias	0.021	0.026	0.029	0.033
	ESE	0.089	0.091	0.085	0.086
β_3	Bias	0.027	0.033	0.031	0.034
	ESE	0.099	0.101	0.095	0.092
Semiparametric analyses					
β_1	Bias	0.008	0.011	0.005	−0.003
	ESE	0.077	0.080	0.077	0.080
β_2	Bias	0.018	0.021	0.002	−0.024
	ESE	0.091	0.094	0.090	0.095
β_3	Bias	0.028	0.034	−0.004	−0.050
	ESE	0.101	0.102	0.101	0.105

$$q(s) = \lim_{\Delta s \downarrow 0} \frac{P(s \le T_i < s + \Delta s | s \le T_i)}{\Delta s} . \tag{15.13}$$

If $Y_i^{\dagger}(t) = I(t \le T_i)$, the usual nonparametric estimating function for the hazard at time s is

$$\sum_{i=1}^{m} Y_i(s)\, Y_i^{\dagger}(s) \left\{ dN_i^{\dagger}(s) - dQ(s) \right\} , \tag{15.14}$$

with solution $d\widehat{Q}(s) = d\bar{N}.(s)/\bar{Y}.(s)$ where $d\bar{N}.(s) = \sum_{i=1}^{m} Y_i(s)Y_i^{\dagger}(s)dN_i(s)$ and $\bar{Y}.(s) = \sum_{i=1}^{m} Y_i(s)Y_i^{\dagger}(s)$. The Kaplan–Meier estimate is given by $\widehat{\mathcal{F}}(t) = \prod_{(0,t]} (1 - d\widehat{Q}(s))$.

The five-state model in Fig. 15.3b allows one to consider the joint occurrence of bone pain requiring radiotherapy and death; state 1 corresponds to being alive and radiotherapy-free, state 2 is occupied by individuals who required radiation therapy and are alive, and state 3 is entered upon death. As before we let $\{Z(s), s > 0\}$ denote the three state process, $dN(s) = (dN_{12}(s), dN_{23}(s), dN_{13}(s))'$ indicate the nature of any transitions at time s, $d\bar{N}_{jk}(s) = Y(s)dN_{jk}(s)$, and $d\bar{N}(s) = (d\bar{N}_{12}(s), d\bar{N}_{23}(s), d\bar{N}_{13}(s))'$; the additional states in Fig. 15.3 correspond to the censoring event; we distinguish between the states exited upon censoring and let $\gamma_k(t)$ denote the intensity of censoring from state k and $\Gamma_k(t) = \int_0^t \gamma_k(u)du, k = 1, 2$. Let $\bar{\mathcal{H}}(t) = \{(d\bar{N}^{\dagger}(s), d\bar{N}(s), Y(s)), 0 < s < t\}$,

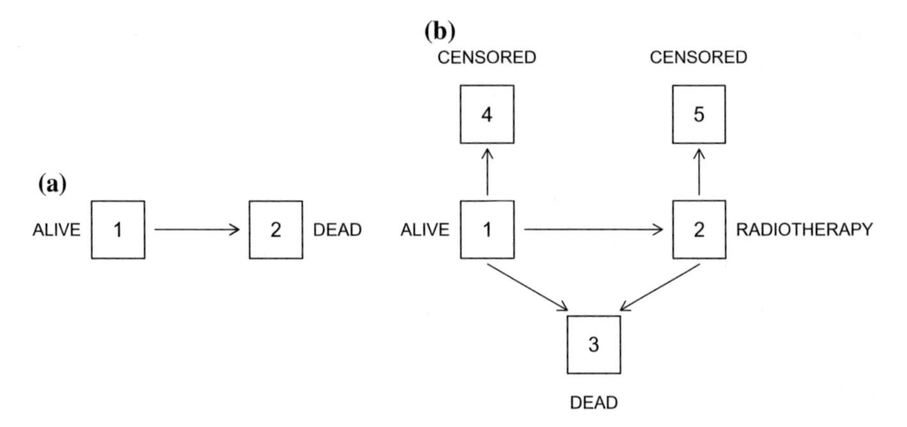

Fig. 15.3 Two-state diagram representing a process for survival time (panel **a**) and a multistate diagram reflecting the joint distribution of the time to radiotherapy, death and censoring (panel **b**)

$$\lim_{\Delta t \downarrow 0} \frac{P(\Delta C(t) = 1 | \bar{\mathcal{H}}(t), Z(t) = k)}{\Delta t} = Y(t)\ \lambda^c(t|\bar{\mathcal{H}}(t)) = Y(t)\ \gamma_k(t)\ . \quad (15.15)$$

We assume the process in panel (b) is Markov. If $\gamma_1(t) = \gamma_2(t)$ then censoring is independent of the event process. If $q_{13}(t) \neq q_{23}(t)$ and $\gamma_1(t) \neq \gamma_2(t)$, then censoring is event (history) dependent and the Kaplan–Meier estimate of the survival distribution will be biased.

The left panel of Fig. 15.4 contains plots of the Nelson–Aalen estimates of the transition intensities $\widehat{Q}_{k\ell}(t) = \int_0^t d\widehat{Q}_{k\ell}(s)$ where $d\widehat{Q}_{k\ell}(s) = \sum_{i=1}^m \bar{Y}_{ik}(s)\, dN_{ik\ell}(s) / \sum_{i=1}^m \bar{Y}_{ik}(s)$. The Nelson–Aalen estimate of the cumulative intensity for censoring out of state k is given by $\widehat{\Gamma}_k(t) = \int_0^t d\widehat{\Gamma}_k(s)$ where $d\widehat{\Gamma}_k(t) = \sum_{i=1}^m \bar{Y}_{ik}(t)\, dC_i(t) / \sum_{i=1}^m \bar{Y}_{ik}(t)$; these estimates are plotted in the right panel of Fig. 15.4. It is apparent that $\gamma_1(t) \neq \gamma_2(t)$ and $q_{13}(t) \neq q_{23}(t)$ and thus $E(Y_i(s)\, dN_i^{\dagger}(s)|T_i \geq s, C_i \geq s) \neq Y_i^{!}(s)\, dQ(s)$, so (15.14) is not unbiased and the resulting estimator is inconsistent.

The inverse probability weighted estimating equation is

$$\sum_{i=1}^{m} \frac{Y_i(s)\ Y_i^{\dagger}(s)}{\widehat{G}_i(s)} \left\{ dN_i^{\dagger}(s) - dQ(s) \right\} \quad (15.16)$$

where $\widehat{G}_i(s) = \widehat{P}(C_i \geq s|\mathcal{H}_i(s))$. Provided $G_i(s)$ is modeled correctly and a consistent estimate of $G_i(s)$ is used, this yields a consistent estimate of the survival distribution. Here we model $d\Lambda^c(s|\mathcal{H}_i(s)) = d\Lambda^c(s|Z_i(s^-) = k) = d\Gamma_k(s)$ and estimate $G_i(t)$ via $\widehat{G}_i(t) = \prod_{s<t}\{1 - d\widehat{\Lambda}^c(s|\mathcal{H}_i(s))\}$. The inverse probability weighted Kaplan–Meier estimate is

$$\widetilde{P}(T \geq t) = \widetilde{\mathcal{F}}(t) = \prod_{(0,t]} \{1 - d\widetilde{Q}(s)\}$$

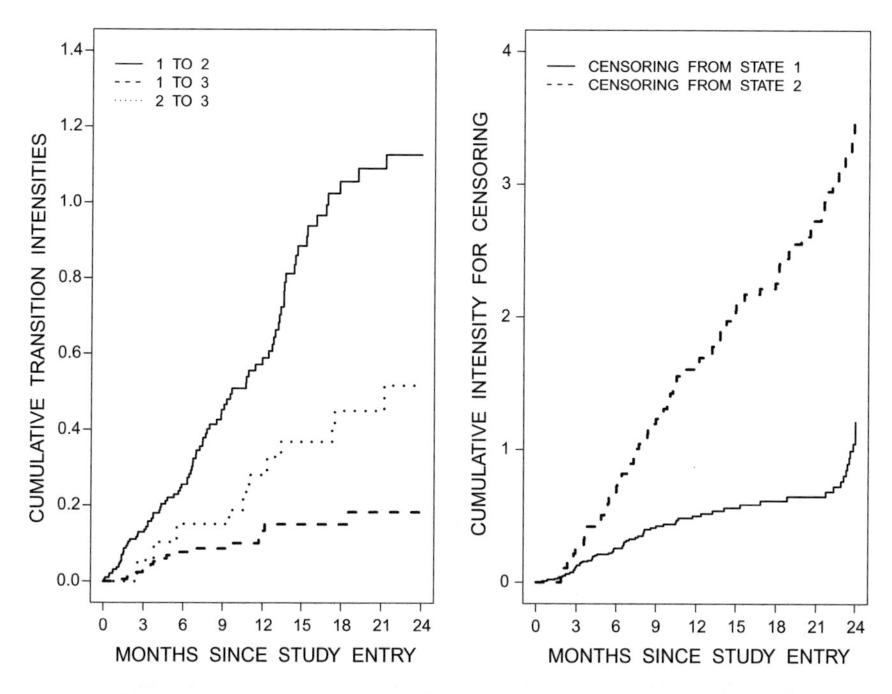

Fig. 15.4 Plots of the Nelson–Aalen estimates of the cumulative intensities for censoring (left panel) and the cumulative intensities for the transition probabilities in the three state process (right panel)

where if $\bar{Y}_i^{\dagger}(t) = Y_i(t)\ Y_i^{\dagger}(t)$, $d\widetilde{Q}(t) = [\sum_{i=1}^{m}\ \bar{Y}_i^{\dagger}(t)\ dN_i^{\dagger}(t)/\widehat{G}_i(t)]/[\sum_{i=1}^{m}\ \bar{Y}_i^{\dagger}(t)\ /\widehat{G}_i(t)]$. The weighted and unweighted estimates are shown in Fig. 15.5. They differ only a little, but the unweighted estimate lying below the weighted one reflects the fact that most individuals enter state 3 from state 2, while at the same time the censoring rate is much higher from state 2.

15.3 Modeling with Data from Intermittent Observations

15.3.1 Likelihood Construction

Here we consider the models and underlying assumptions generating data in clinical disease registries where individuals are under intermittent observation (Kalbfleisch and Lawless [15]). We consider for simplicity an inception cohort in which individuals are recruited and examined at the start of their multistate process, and subsequently, receive treatment for their condition in the clinic maintaining the registry. Let E denote an administrative censoring time and D denote a random time an individual withdraws from the clinic and thereby drops out of the registry. Then

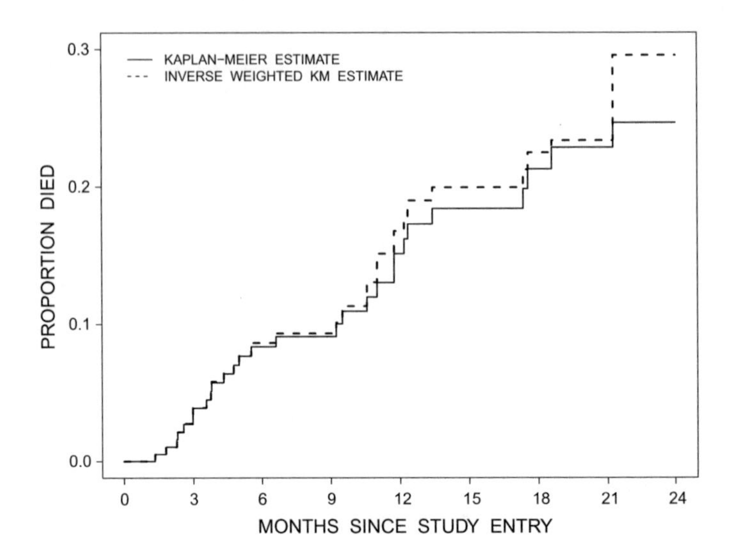

Fig. 15.5 Unweighted Kaplan–Meier and weighted Kaplan–Meier estimates for the cumulative distribution function of the survival time

$C = \min(D, E)$ is the net censoring time with $Y = I(s \leq C)$ indicating that they are on study at time s and $\{C(s), 0 < s\}$ denoting the counting process for censoring such that $C(s) = I(C \leq s)$.

The process by which individuals attend clinics and furnish information on their condition is complex, often influenced by protocol-driven assessments, scheduled follow-up appointments, or unplanned symptom-driven appointments. We consider a general point process models to characterize this aspect of the observation process (Cook and Lawless [6]). Let $A(s)$ be a right-continuous counting process counting the number of assessments over $(0, s]$, $\Delta A(s) = A(s + \Delta s^-) - A(s^-)$, and let $dA(s) = A(s) - A(s^-) = 1$ if an assessment is made at s and $dA(s) = 0$ otherwise. If $0 = v_0 < v_1 < \cdots < v_{A(s)}$ denote assessment times, we observe $Z(v_j)$, $j = 1, \ldots, A(s)$ but not any transition times.

To consider the probability of a sample path and the evolution of information over time, we discretize time and use product integration as in Sect. 15.2. If the intention is to collect information over $(0, E]$, we let $0 = u_0 < u_1 < \cdots < u_R = E$ partition this interval into R subintervals of width $\Delta u_r = \Delta u$, $r = 1, 2, \ldots, R$. Let $\bar{\mathcal{H}}(s) = \{C(u), A(u), Z(u), 0 < u < s\}$ denote the history of the joint processes including the censoring process, the assessment process, and the underlying disease process. The *observed history* at u_r is $\bar{H}(u_r) = \{C(u_s), \Delta\bar{A}(u_s), \Delta\bar{A}(u_s)Z(u_s), s = 1, \ldots, r-1\}$ where $\Delta A(u_s) = A(u_s^-) - A(u_{s-1}^-)$, $\Delta\bar{A}(u_s) = Y(u_s)\Delta A(u_s)$, and $\Delta\bar{A}(u_s)Z(u_s)$ indicates $Z(u_s)$ is observed only if $\Delta\bar{A}(u_s) = 1$. The probability of the observed data over $[0, u_R]$ can be factored as

$$\prod_{r=1}^{R} P(\Delta C(u_r)|\bar{H}(u_r))^{Y(u_{r-1})} \tag{15.17}$$
$$\times \prod_{r=1}^{R} \left\{ P(\Delta A(u_r)|Y(u_r)=1, \bar{H}(u_r))\ P(Z(u_r)|Y(u_r)=1, \Delta A(u_r)=1, \bar{H}(u_r))^{\Delta A(u_r)} \right\}^{Y(u_r)} .$$

Under the assumption that the censoring and inspection processes are noninformative we may ignore the first two terms in (15.17), leaving the partial likelihood

$$\prod_{r=1}^{R} \left\{ P(Z(u_r)|Y(u_r)=1, \Delta A(u_r)=1, \bar{H}(u_r))^{\Delta \bar{A}(u_r)} \right\} . \tag{15.18}$$

Then taking the limit of (15.18) as $R \to \infty$ we obtain

$$L = \prod_{j=1}^{A(C)} P(Z(v_j)|v_j, Y(v_j)=1, dA(v_j)=1, \bar{\mathcal{H}}^{obs}(v_j))$$

where

$$\begin{aligned} \bar{\mathcal{H}}^{obs}(v_j) &= \{Y(s), A(u), 0 < u < s, Z(v_1), \ldots, Z(v_{A(s)})\} \\ &= \{Y(s), v_1, \ldots, v_{A(s)}, Z(v_1), \ldots, Z(v_{A(s)})\}. \end{aligned}$$

This is computable under a MAR assumption because the observed visit times v_j may be treated as a fixed sequence (Gill et al. [11]). To facilitate discussion of visit process models below, we make the plausible assumption of sequential missing at randomness (Gill et al. [11]; Hogan et al. [12]), or SMAR. This stipulates that given $Y(u_r) = 1$ and $\bar{H}(u_r)$, $\Delta A(u_r)$ is independent of $Z(u_s)$, $s = r, \ldots, R$.

Under a Markov model $P(Z(v_j)|\bar{Z}^{obs}(v_j))$ becomes $P(Z(v_j)|Z(v_{j-1}))$ for fixed v_j, v_{j-1} and the score function $\partial \log L/\partial\theta$ become

$$S(\theta) = \sum_{j=1}^{A(C)} \frac{\partial \log P(Z(v_j)|Z(v_{j-1}); \theta)}{\partial\theta} .$$

Kalbfleisch and Lawless [15] develop a Fisher-scoring algorithm which can be used to obtain the maximum likelihood estimates and this is implemented in the `msm` function (Jackson [14]).

15.3.2 Time-Dependent Covariates and Dependent Inspection Processes

With a time-varying covariate $\{X(s), 0 < s\}$ we need to generalize the derivations starting with (15.17). We assume that the covariate values are observed at the same time as the multistate process and let $\bar{\mathcal{H}}(s) = \{C(u), A(u), X(u), Z(u), 0 < u < s\}$ and $\bar{H}(u_r) = \{C(u_s), \Delta\bar{A}(u_s), \Delta\bar{A}(u_s)X(u_s), \Delta\bar{A}(u_s)Z(u_s), s = 1, \ldots, r-1\}$ where if $\Delta\bar{A}(u_s) = 1$ we observe $X(u)$ and $Z(u)$ at u_s, but not if $\Delta\bar{A}(u_s) = 0$.

Given the partition $0 = u_0 < u_1 < \cdots < u_R = E$ we factor the probability of the observed data as

$$\prod_{r=1}^{R} \left\{ P(\Delta C(u_r)|\bar{H}(u_r))\; P(\Delta A(u_r)|Y(u_r) = 1, \bar{H}(u_r))^{Y(u_r)} \right\}^{Y(u_{r-1})}$$
$$\times \prod_{r=1}^{R} \left\{ P(Z(u_r)|\Delta\bar{A}(u_r) = 1, \bar{H}(u_r))\; P(X(u_r)|Z(u_r), \Delta\bar{A}(u_r) = 1, \bar{H}(u_r)) \right\}^{\Delta\bar{A}(u_r)} .$$

Restricting attention to the second row, assuming the covariate process is noninformative, and assuming a SMAR condition, the limit as $R \to \infty$ gives a partial likelihood

$$L \propto \prod_{j=1}^{A(C)} P(Z(v_j)|v_j, \bar{Z}^{obs}(v_j), \bar{X}^{obs}(v_j)) \; .$$

where $\bar{X}^{obs}(v_j) = \{X_k(v_s), 1 \le s \le j\}$ denotes the observed history of the covariate process. Once again, we implicitly condition on the observed assessment times $v_1, \ldots, v_{A(C)}$, which are treated as fixed values. Under a modulated Markov model we can replace $P(Z(v_j)|v_j, \bar{Z}^{obs}(v_j), \bar{X}^{obs}(v_j))$ with $P(Z(v_j)|Z(v_{j-1}), X(v_{j-1}))$ where we leave the conditioning on the observed assessment times as implicit since we are treating them as if they were fixed. Note that the sequentially missing at random assumption is weaker here since we are conditioning on more information.

Suppose however that interest lies in estimating a marginal feature such as $P(Z(t) = k) = P(Z(t) = k|Z(0) = 1)$, where we characterize this as a marginal feature since we do not condition on any intermediate states or time-varying covariates. It may be that $X(s)$ has an effect on both the multistate process and the inspection process and while the SMAR assumption holds given $X(s)$, it does not hold for a model for $\{Z(s), s > 0\}$ in which we do not condition on $\{X(s), s > 0\}$. As an example, $X(s)$ may be comprised of information on markers associated with the disease process of interest and these may be associated with the visit process. In arthritis, for example, inflammatory markers reflecting disease activity (severity of joint pain and inflammation) such as the erythrosedimentation rate (ESR), may be associated with both progression in the disease and the visit process. Physicians of patients with higher values of ESR may naturally schedule future appointments sooner than they would otherwise be scheduled as part of a standard clinic protocol. Interest does not lie, in this scenario, on the effect of ESR on the marginal probability of being in a particular state reflecting the severity of joint damage. The markers of inflammation may, however, naturally be associated with the assessment process $\{A(s), 0 < s\}$.

We let $\bar{X}^{-}(u_r) = \{(u_s, X(u_s)), 1 \le s \le r-1 : \Delta A(u_s) = 1\}$ denote the observed history of the covariate process. If $\bar{H}(u_r) = \{C(u_s), \Delta\bar{A}(u_s), \Delta\bar{A}(u_s)Z(u_s), \Delta\bar{A}(u_s)X(u_s), s = 1, \ldots, r-1\}$, one may specify the marginal model of interest but then $\Delta\bar{A}(u_r)$ is not independent of $Z(u_r)$ unconditionally. We can adjust for this by using inverse intensity of visit weighted log-likelihood contributions. Specifically, if we consider the interval $(u_{r-1}, u_r]$ based on the partition as before, we can let

$$\frac{\Delta\bar{A}(u_r)}{P(\Delta A(u_r)=1|Y(u_r)=1,\bar{H}(u_r),\bar{X}^-(u_r))}\log P(Z(u_r)|Z(0)) ,$$

and taking the limit as $R\to\infty$ leads to the inverse intensity of visit weighted (IIVW) contribution

$$\frac{Y(s)dA(s)}{\lambda^a(s|\bar{H}(s),\bar{X}^-(s))}\log P(Z(s)|Z(0)=1) .$$

for $u_{r-1}<s\le u_r$. For parametric models, this leads to an inverse intensity of visit weighted pseudo-score equation (Lin et al. [20]) of the form

$$\frac{d\bar{A}(t)}{\lambda^a(t|\bar{H}(t),\bar{X}^-(t))}\partial\log P(Z(t)|Z(0))/\partial\theta=0 \tag{15.19}$$

where the probabilities for $Z(v_j)$ are calculated as for a specified set of fixed times. To see that (15.19) has expectation zero we may first note that

$$E_{dA(s)}\left\{\frac{Y(s)dA(s)}{\lambda^a(s|\bar{H}(s),\bar{X}^-(s))}\frac{\partial\log P(Z(s)|Z(0))}{\partial\theta}\middle|Z(s),\bar{H}(s),\bar{X}^-(s)\right\} \tag{15.20}$$

yields $Y(s)\partial\log P(Z(s)|Z(0))/\partial\theta$. Then taking the expectation with respect to $E_{\bar{X}^-(s)}(\cdot|Z(s),\bar{H}(s))$ yields the same expression which, under the assumption of independent dropout, is proportional to the score function for Z(s) and hence is unbiased. We assume that the random withdrawal time is independent of the multistate process; if this is not plausible an additional weight related to the dropout process can be introduced.

15.3.3 Current Status Data and Dependent Inspection: Empirical Studies

Here we present the results of simulation studies involving current status data under a dependent observation scheme. Let T denote a time of interest and $F(t)=P(T\le t)$ denote the cumulative distribution function for T which we wish to estimate. With a current status observation scheme, we simply observe a single inspection time C and the status indicator $Y=I(T<C)$. For a random sample of m independent individuals, we write the data as $\{(C_i,Y_i), i=1,\dots,m\}$.

Let U_i denote a gamma distributed random variable with mean 1 and variance ϕ. We then assume $T_i|U_i=u_i$ is exponentially distributed with hazard $u_i\lambda$ and

$C_i|U_i = u_i$ is exponentially distributed with hazard $u_i\rho$. The marginal survivor functions for T and C are then $\mathcal{F}(t) = P(T_i \geq t) = 1/(1+\phi\lambda t)^{1/\phi}$ and $\mathcal{G}(c) = P(C_i \geq c) = 1/(1+\phi\rho c)^{1/\phi}$ respectively. The joint survival distribution of (T, C) is given by

$$P(T \geq t, C \geq c) = 1/(1+\phi \cdot (\lambda t + \rho c))^{\phi^{-1}} \tag{15.21}$$

and the association as measured by Kendall's τ is $\tau = \phi/(\phi+2)$.

For the simulations, we consider the following parameter settings. Without loss of generality, we let $\lambda = 1$ and solve for ρ such that $P(T_i < C_i) = \lambda/(\lambda+\rho)$ with values of 0.25, 0.50, and 0.75. We let $\phi = 0.1, 0.25$ and 0.50 to reflect mild, moderate and stronger dependencies between T and C. We let $\theta = (\log\ \lambda, \log\ \phi)'$ and write the naive log-likelihood (assuming $T_i \perp C_i$) as

$$\log L(\theta) = \sum_{i=1}^{m} \left[Y_i \cdot \log(1-\mathcal{F}(C_i)) + (1-Y_i) \cdot \log\ \mathcal{F}(C_i)\right] \tag{15.22}$$

We consider nonparametric estimation of $\mathcal{F}(t)$ under the assumption of an independent inspection time (i.e., $T_i \perp C_i$) by maximizing this log-likelihood subject to the monotonicity constraint using the pooled adjacent violators algorithm (PAVA); see Ayer et al. [4] and Barlow et al. [5]. We also consider a weighted log-likelihood of the form

$$\log L^w(\theta) = \sum_{i=1}^{m} \frac{I(C_i = c_i)}{g(c_i|u_i)} \left[Y_i \cdot \log(1-\mathcal{F}(C_i)) + (1-Y_i) \cdot \log\ \mathcal{F}(C_i)\right] \tag{15.23}$$

as suggested by Van Der Laan and Robins [24]; inverse intensity weights could alternatively be used as discussed in Sect. 15.3.2. Here $g(c|u)$ is the conditional density of C given $U = u$, and we suppose that U is observable. Let $c_{(1)} < c_{(2)} < \cdots < c_{(J)}$ denote the J ordered unique inspection times, $m_j = \sum_{i=1}^{n} I(c_i = c_{(j)})/g(c_{(j)}|u_i)$, $r_j = \sum_{i=1}^{n}(I(c_i = c_{(j)})Y_i)/g(c_{(j)}|u_i)$. We apply the isotonic regression of $(r_1/m_1, \ldots, r_J/m_J)'$ with weights $(m_1, \ldots, m_J)'$ to give

$$1 - \widehat{\mathcal{F}}(C_{(j)}) = \max_{u \leq j} \min_{v \geq j} \left(\frac{\sum_{\ell=u}^{v} r_\ell}{\sum_{\ell=u}^{v} m_\ell}\right) \tag{15.24}$$

for $j = 1, \ldots, J$ as a weighted PAVA estimator.

Figure 15.6 displays the results of a simulation study in which a sample of 100,000 individuals was generated and the estimates of $\mathcal{F}(t)$ are plotted; the true value for $\mathcal{F}(t)$ is represented by the black line. We consider the case in which 25% of individuals are expected to have experienced the event at the time of the assessment (i.e., $P(T < C) = 0.25$) and $\phi = 0.10$. Estimates based on unweighted and weighted

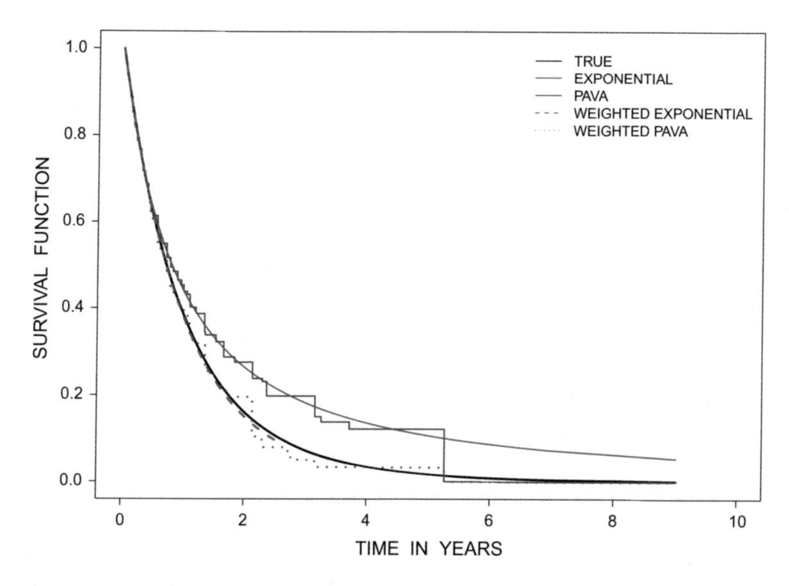

Fig. 15.6 Plots of the true and estimated survivor functions based on unweighted and weighted likelihoods; the nonparametric estimates are based on the PAVA or weighted PAVA given by (15.24) for $P(T < C) = 0.25$ and $\phi = 0.10$

parametric maximum likelihood are given under an exponential model, along with the unweighted and weighted PAVA estimator. It is apparent that the bias in the naive parametric and nonparametric estimators can be appreciable when the inspection time is associated with the event time, and that the weighted estimators correct for this bias quite well.

15.4 Discussion

Large cohort studies are increasingly being used to learn about disease processes. Such processes are often naturally and conveniently characterized by multistate models. Valid analysis of such processes requires an understanding of the assumptions regarding the observation schemes implicit when using standard methods of analysis, as well as methods to generalize these techniques when the standard assumptions are not satisfied. Much work has been done on dealing with dependent right-censoring of disease processes and the use of inverse probability of censoring weights to accommodate dependent censoring.

When processes operate in continuous time but are only observed periodically upon clinic visits, there may be an association between the disease process and the observation or visit process. This can cause standard estimators to be inconsistent but if the observation process is modeled one can derive corrected estimators which are consistent provided the observation model is specified correctly. We discuss inverse intensity-weighted estimating equations for Markov processes under intermittent observation. Often interest lies in descriptive marginal models which examine the effect of fixed covariates on specific features of a disease process such as the probability of being in a particular state. Approaches to analysis include the use of pseudo-observations (Andersen et al. [3]) and direct binomial regression (Scheike and Zhang [23]). Lawless and Nazeri Rad [19] consider applications to the case of intermittent observation schemes. In such settings the assumptions regarding an independent inspection process are even stronger since the history of the response process is not conditioned upon; inverse intensity weighting plays a critical role in such settings.

In some settings involving incomplete data due to dropout, researchers may undertake a more intensive tracing study to track down those individuals lost to follow-up (Farewell et al. [10]). Such studies yield additional data and hence can improve efficiency of estimation, but moreover, can yield insight into the withdrawal process and enable one to fit more comprehensive models to accommodate dependent censoring. An important area of research is the development of design methodology for the selection of individuals for tracing. Such selection models can be based on information on the disease process observed prior to tracing, covariates of interest in the response model, or auxiliary covariates. Use of inverse probability of selection weights may be required to ensure valid inference when integrating the additional data obtained from the tracing study. Moreover in some cases, the data obtained involves surrogate outcome data representing mismeasured responses; knowledge of the misclassification distribution may be required to exploit such information.

References

1. Aalen, O.O., O. Borgan, and H. Fekjaer. 2001. Covariate adjustment of event histories estimated with Markov chains: The additive approach. *Biometrics* 57: 993–1001.
2. Andersen, P.K., O. Borgan, R.D. Gill, and N. Keiding. 1993. *Statistical Models Based on Counting Processes*. New York: Springer.
3. Andersen, P.K., J.P. Klein, and S. Rosthoj. 2003. Generalised linear models for correlated pseudo-observations, with applications to multi-state models. *Biometrika* 90: 15–27.
4. Ayer, M., H.D. Brunk, G.M. Ewing, W.T. Reid, and E. Silverman. 1955. An empirical distribution function for sampling with incomplete observations. *Annals of Mathematical Statistics* 26: 641–647.
5. Barlow, R.E., D.J. Bartholomew, J.M. Bremner, and H.D. Brunk. 1972. *Statistical inference under order restrictions: The theory and application of isotonic regression*. New York: Wiley.
6. Cook, R.J., and J.F. Lawless. 2007. *The statistical analysis of recurrent events*. Berlin: Springer.
7. Cook, R.J., J.F. Lawless, L. Lakhal-Chaieb, and K.-A. Lee. 2009. Robust estimation of mean functions and treatment effects for recurrent events under event-dependent censoring and termination: application to skeletal complications in cancer metastatic to bone. *Journal of the American Statistical Association* 104: 60–75.
8. Datta, S., and G.A. Satten. 2001. Validity of the Aalen–Johansen estimators of stage occupation probabilities and Nelson–Aalen estimators of integrated transition hazards for non-markov models. *Statistics and Probability Letters* 55 (4): 403–411.

9. Datta, S., and G.A. Satten. 2002. Estimation of integrated transition hazards and stage occupation probabilities for non-markov systems under dependent censoring. *Biometrics* 58: 792–802.
10. Farewell, V.T., J.F. Lawless, D.D. Gladman, and M.B. Urowitz. 2003. Tracing studies and analysis of the effect of loss to follow-up on mortality estimation from patient registry data. *Journal of the Royal Statistical Society Series C* 52: 445–456.
11. Gill, R.D., Van der Laan, M.J. and Robins, J.M. 1997. Coarsening at random: characterizations, conjectures, counter-examples. In *Processdings 1st Seattle Sypmposium in Biostatisitcs: Survival Analysis*, eds. Lin D.Y and Fleming T.R, 256–294. New York: Springer.
12. Hogan, J.W., Roy, J. and Korkontzelou, C. 2004. Handling dropouts in longitudinal studies.
13. Hortobagyi, G.N., R.L. Theriault, A. Lipton, L. Porter, D. Blayney, C. Sinoff, H. Wheeler, J.F. Simeone, J.J. Seaman, R.D. Knight, M. Heffernan, K. Mellars, and D.J. Reitsma. 1998. Long-term prevention of skeletal complications of metastatic breast cancer with pamidronate. Protocol 19 Aredia Breast Cancer Study Group. *Journal of Clinical Oncology* 16: 2038–2044.
14. Jackson, C.H. 2011. Multi-state models for panel data: The msm package for R. *Journal Statistical Software* 38: 1–28.
15. Kalbfleisch, J.D., and J.F. Lawless. 1985. The analysis of panel data under a Markov assumption. *Journal of the American Statistical Association* 80: 863–871.
16. Kalbfleisch, J.D., and R.L. Prentice. 2002. *The statistical analysis of failure time data* (2nd ed.). New York: Wiley.
17. Klein, J.P., and M.L. Moeschberger. 2003. *Survival analysis: Techniques for censored and truncated data*, 2nd ed. New York: Springer.
18. Lawless, J.F. 2003. *Statistical models and methods for lifetime data*, 2nd ed. Hoboken: Wiley.
19. Lawless, J.F., and N. Nazeri Rad. 2015. Estimation and assessment of Markov multistate models with intermittent observations on individuals. *Lifetime Data Analysis* 21: 160–179.
20. Lin, H., D.O. Scharfstein, and R.A. Rosenheck. 2004. Analysis of longitudinal data with irregular, outcome-dependent follow-up. *Journal of the Royal Statistical Society: Series B (Statistical Methodology)* 66: 791–813.
21. Nelsen, R.B. 2006. *An introduction to copulas*, 2nd ed. New York: Springer.
22. Satten, G.A., S. Datta, and J. Robins. 2007. Estimating the marginal survival function in the presence of time dependent covariates. *Statistics and Probability Letters* 54: 397–403.
23. Scheike, T.H., and M.J. Zhang. 2007. Direct modelling of regression effects for transition probabilities in multistate models. *Scandinavian Jorunal of Statistics* 34: 17–32.
24. Van Der Laan, M.J., and J.M. Robins. 1998. Locally efficient estimation with current status data and time-dependent covariates. *Journal of the American Statistical Association* 93: 693–701.

Chapter 16
Exact Likelihood-Based Point and Interval Estimation for Lifetime Characteristics of Laplace Distribution Based on a Time-Constrained Life-Testing Experiment

Xiaojun Zhu and N. Balakrishnan

Abstract In this paper, we first derive explicit expressions for the MLEs of the location and scale parameters of the Laplace distribution based on a Type-I right-censored sample arising from a time-constrained life-testing experiment by considering different cases. We derive the conditional joint MGF of these MLEs and use them to derive the bias and MSEs of the MLEs for all the cases. We then derive the exact conditional marginal and joint density functions of the MLEs and utilize them to develop exact conditional CIs for the parameters. We also briefly discuss the MLEs of reliability and cumulative hazard functions and the construction of exact CIs for these functions. Next, a Monte Carlo simulation study is carried out to evaluate the performance of the developed inferential results. Finally, some examples are presented to illustrate the point and interval estimation methods developed here under a time-constrained life-testing experiment.

Acronyms and Abbreviations

CDF	Cumulative density function
CI	Confidence interval
K–M curve	Kaplan–Meier curve
i.i.d.	Independent and identically distributed
MGF	Moment generating function
MLE	Maximum likelihood estimator
MSE	Mean square error
PDF	Probability density function
P–P plot	Probability–probability plot
Q–Q plot	Quantile–quantile plot
SE	Standard error

X. Zhu · N. Balakrishnan (✉)
Department of Mathematics and Statistics, McMaster University Hamilton,
Hamilton, ON L8S 4K1, Canada
e-mail: bala@mcmaster.ca

A. Adhikari et al. (eds.), *Mathematical and Statistical Applications in Life Sciences and Engineering*, https://doi.org/10.1007/978-981-10-5370-2_16

Notation

n	Sample size
r	Number of smallest order statistics observed in the Type-II censored sample
$X_{i:n}$	The i-th-ordered failure time from a sample of size n
L	Likelihood function
$f(t)$	Probability density function
$R(t)$	Reliability or survival function
$F(t)$	Cumulative distribution function
$F_{\Gamma}(t)$	Cumulative distribution function of a gamma variable
$S_{\Gamma}(t)$	Reliability function of a gamma variable
$\Lambda(t)$	Cumulative hazard function
$E(\cdot)$	Expectation
$Var(\cdot)$	Variance
$Cov(\cdot, \cdot)$	Covariance
$E(\sigma)$	Exponential distribution with scale parameter σ
$\Gamma(\alpha, \beta)$	Gamma distribution with shape parameter α and scale parameter β
$\Gamma(t, \cdot, \cdot)$	The CDF of the gamma distribution
$L(\mu, \sigma)$	Laplace distribution with location parameter μ and scale parameter σ
q	Quantile of the standard $L(0, 1)$
Q_{α}	$100\alpha\%$ quantile

16.1 Introduction

The Laplace distribution, also known as the Double Exponential distribution, has its PDF as

$$f(x) = \frac{1}{2\sigma} e^{-\frac{|x-\mu|}{\sigma}}, -\infty < x < \infty, \tag{16.1}$$

where μ and σ are the location and scale parameters, respectively. The CDF corresponding to (16.1) is

$$F(x) = \begin{cases} \frac{1}{2} e^{-\frac{\mu-x}{\sigma}}, & x < \mu, \\ 1 - \frac{1}{2} e^{-\frac{x-\mu}{\sigma}}, & x \geq \mu. \end{cases} \tag{16.2}$$

For Laplace distribution, many inferential results have been developed based on complete and Type-II censored samples; one may refer to Johnson et al. [16] and Kotz et al. [19] for detailed overviews on all these developments. Based on a complete sample, Bain and Engelhardt [3] developed approximate CIs, while Kappenman [17, 18] derived conditional CIs and tolerance intervals. Balakrishnan and Cutler [6] presented the MLEs for general Type-II censored samples in an explicit form. Childs and Balakrishnan [9–11] used these explicit expressions of the MLEs to develop conditional inferential methods for the case of Type-II and progressively Type-II censored samples. Iliopoulos and Balakrishnan [13] developed exact likelihood inferential procedures based on some pivotal quantities, while Iliopoulos and MirMostafaee [14] developed exact prediction intervals based on MLEs for Type-II censored samples. Recently, Balakrishnan and Zhu [8] and Zhu and Balakrishnan [22] developed exact likelihood-based inference for the location and scale parameters as well as some lifetime functions of interest such as the quantile, reliability, and cumulative hazard functions. All these works are based on either Type-II or progressively Type-II censored samples and no work has been developed for the case when the life-testing experiment is time-constrained resulting in a Type-I censored sample. We therefore focus on this situation and derive the MLEs of Laplace parameters based on Type-I censored samples. We then derive conditional marginal and joint distributions of the MLEs, from which we obtain bias, MSEs, and covariance of the estimates. We also develop exact conditional CIs from the exact conditional distributions of the MLEs. Similarly, we develop the MLEs of quantile, reliability, and cumulative hazard functions and use them to develop exact conditional CIs for these functions as well.

The rest of this paper is organized as follows. In Sect. 16.2, we derive closed-form expressions of the MLEs based on Type-I right-censored samples for different censoring cases. In Sect. 16.3, we derive the conditional joint MGF of the MLEs and use it to obtain the mean, variance, and covariance of the MLEs. The exact conditional marginal and joint density functions of the MLEs are derived in Sect. 16.4, which are then used to develop exact conditional CIs for μ and σ. In Sect. 16.5, by using the joint MGF of the MLEs, we obtain the exact distribution of the MLE of quantile, which is then used to develop exact conditional CIs. In Sects. 16.6 and 16.7, we discuss exact conditional CIs for reliability and cumulative hazard functions. A Monte Carlo simulation study is carried out in Sect. 16.8 to evaluate the performance of these point and interval estimates. In Sect. 16.9, we present two examples to illustrate all the methods of inference developed here. Finally, some concluding comments are made in Sect. 16.10. Throughout this paper, we use "$E(\theta)$" to denote a general exponential distribution, by allowing the scale parameter to be any real value. Of course, this would mean that, for example, if $X \sim E(\theta)$ and $\theta < 0$, then $-X \sim E(-\theta)$. Moreover, we use "$NE(\theta)$" and "$N\Gamma(\alpha, \beta)$" with a positive scale parameter to denote the negative exponential and negative gamma distributions, i.e., if $X \sim NE(\theta)$, then $-X \sim E(\theta)$.

16.2 MLEs from a Time-Constrained Life Test

Let $x_{1:n} < x_{2:n} < \cdots < x_{n:n}$ denote the ordered lifetimes of n units under a life test. Suppose the experimenter decides to conduct a life-testing experiment until a pre-fixed time T and terminate the experiment at time T. The data so observed will be $(x_{1:n} < x_{2:n} < \cdots < x_{D:n})$, where D is the random number of units that fail until time T, commonly referred to as a Type-I censored sample. Then, we have the corresponding likelihood function as (see Balakrishnan and Cohen [5] and Arnold et al. [1])

$$L = C_d \prod_{i=1}^{d} f(x_{i:n})[S(T)]^{n-d}, \qquad -\infty < x_{1:n} < x_{2:n} < \cdots < x_{d:n} < T, \tag{16.3}$$

where $C_d = \frac{n!}{(n-d)!}$ and $S(\cdot) = 1 - F(\cdot)$ is the survival function. First of all, it is clear that the MLEs of μ and σ exist only when $D \geq 1$, and so all subsequent results developed here are based on this condition of observing at least one failure.

Result 16.1 *By maximizing the likelihood function in (16.3), the MLEs of μ and σ can be derived as follows:*

$$\hat{\mu} = \begin{cases} [X_{m:n}, X_{m+1:n}], & n = 2m, d \geq m+1, \\ X_{m+1:n}, & n = 2m+1, d \geq m+1, \\ [X_{m:n}, T], & n = 2m, d = m, \\ T + \hat{\sigma}\log(\frac{n}{2d}), & d < \frac{n}{2}; \end{cases} \tag{16.4}$$

$$\hat{\sigma} = \begin{cases} \frac{1}{d}\left[(n-d)T + \sum_{i=m+1}^{d} X_{i:n} - \sum_{i=1}^{m} X_{i:n}\right], & n = 2m, d \geq m, \\ \frac{1}{d}\left[(n-d)T + \sum_{i=m+2}^{d} X_{i:n} - \sum_{i=1}^{m} X_{i:n}\right], & n = 2m+1, d \geq m+1, \\ \frac{1}{d}\sum_{i=1}^{d}(T - X_{i:n}), & d < \frac{n}{2}. \end{cases} \tag{16.5}$$

Proof See Appendix B. We observe that in (16.4), in some cases, $\hat{\mu}$ can be any value in a specific interval with equal likelihood. In these cases, as done usually, we take the mid-points of the intervals to obtain

$$\hat{\mu} = \begin{cases} \frac{1}{2}(X_{m:n} + X_{m+1:n}) & n = 2m, d \geq m+1, \\ X_{m+1:n} & n = 2m+1, d \geq m+1, \\ \frac{1}{2}(X_{m:n} + T) & n = 2m, d = m, \\ T + \hat{\sigma}\log(\frac{n}{2d}) & d < \frac{n}{2}. \end{cases} \tag{16.6}$$

16.3 Exact Conditional MGF of the MLEs

In this section, we derive the exact conditional marginal and joint MGFs of $(\hat{\mu}, \hat{\sigma})$ conditional on observing at least one failure for all the cases presented in the preceding section, and then obtain the bias and MSEs of $\hat{\mu}$ and $\hat{\sigma}$ from these expressions. We describe in detail the procedure for obtaining the conditional marginal MGF of $\hat{\sigma}$ only for the case when $n = 2m$, $d \geq m + 1$, and then just present the final results for all other cases for the sake of brevity since their derivations are similar.

16.3.1 Even Sample Size

Due to the two forms of density function in (16.1), we need to consider the cases of $\mu \geq T$ and $\mu < T$ separately. In the case when $\mu < T$, we will use the conditional approach and let J $(0 \leq J \leq D)$ denote the number of observations in the Type-I censored data that are smaller than μ.

Result 16.2 *The MGF of $\hat{\sigma}$, conditional on observing at least one failure, is as follows:*

$$\begin{aligned} E(e^{t\hat{\sigma}}|D>0) = 1_{\{T>\mu\}} \Bigg\{ & \sum_{d=1}^{m}\sum_{j=0}^{d}\sum_{l=0}^{d-j} p_1 M_{Z_1^{(1)}}(t) + \sum_{d=m+1}^{n}\sum_{j=0}^{m}\sum_{l_1=0}^{m-j}\sum_{l_2=0}^{d-m-1} p_{7\sigma} M_{Z_\sigma^{(7)}}(t) \\ & + \sum_{d=m+1}^{n}\sum_{j=0}^{m}\sum_{l_1=0}^{m-j}\sum_{l_2=0}^{d-m-1} p_{8\sigma} M_{Z_\sigma^{(8)}}(t) \\ & + \sum_{d=m+1}^{n}\sum_{j=m+1}^{d}\sum_{l_1=0}^{j-m-1}\sum_{l_2=0}^{d-j} p_{11} M_{Z_{1,e}^{(11)}}(t) \Bigg\} \\ & + 1_{\{T\leq\mu\}} \Bigg\{ \sum_{d=1}^{m} q_1 M_{Z_1^{(12)}}(t) + \sum_{d=m+1}^{n}\sum_{l=0}^{d-m-1} q_3 M_{Z_{1,e}^{(14)}}(t) \Bigg\}, \end{aligned} \tag{16.7}$$

where the coefficients and variables involved are all as presented in Appendix A.

Proof See Appendix B.

Result 16.3 *The conditional marginal MGF of $\hat{\mu}$ is given by*

$$\begin{aligned} E(e^{s\hat{\mu}}|D>0) = 1_{\{T>\mu\}} \Bigg\{ & \sum_{d=1}^{m-1}\sum_{j=0}^{d}\sum_{l=0}^{d-j} p_1 M_{Z_2^{(1)}}(t) + \sum_{l=0}^{m-1}\left[p_{2\mu} M_{Z_2^{(2)}}(t) + p_{3\mu} M_{Z_2^{(3)}}(t) \right] \\ & + p_4 M_{Z_2^{(4)}}(t) + \sum_{d=m+1}^{n}\sum_{l_1=0}^{m-1}\sum_{l_2=0}^{d-m-1}\Big[p_{5\mu} M_{Z_2^{(5)}}(t) + p_{6\mu} M_{Z_2^{(6)}}(t) \\ & + p_{7\mu,e} M_{Z_{2,e}^{(7)}}(t) + p_{8\mu,e} M_{Z_{2,e}^{(8)}}(t) \Big] + \sum_{d=m+1}^{n}\sum_{l=0}^{d-m-1}\Big[p_9 M_{Z_2^{(9)}}(t) \end{aligned}$$

$$+p_{10}M_{Z_2^{(10)}}(t)\Bigg] + \sum_{d=m+1}^{n}\sum_{l_1=0}^{d-m-1} p_{11\mu}M_{Z_{2,e}^{(11)}}(t)\Bigg\}$$

$$+1_{\{T\le\mu\}}\left\{\sum_{d=1}^{m-1} q_1M_{Z_2^{(12)}}(t) + q_2M_{Z_2^{(13)}}(t) + \sum_{d=m+1}^{n}\sum_{l=0}^{d-m-1} q_3M_{Z_{2,e}^{(14)}}(t)\right\}. \tag{16.8}$$

For obtaining the exact conditional joint distribution of the MLEs from the conditional joint MGF, we first need the following lemma.

Lemma 16.1 *Let $Y_1 \sim \Gamma(\alpha_1, \beta_1)$, $Y_2 \sim N\Gamma(\alpha_2, \beta_2)$, $Z_2 \sim E(1)$, $Z_1 \sim E(1)$, with Y_1, Y_2, Z_1, and Z_2 being independent, and $\beta_1, \beta_2 > 0$. Further, let $W_1 = Y_1 + Y_2 + a_1^*Z_1 + a_2^*Z_2$ and $W_2 = b_1^*Z_1 + b_2^*Z_2$. Then, for any real values a_1^*, a_2^*, b_1^*, and b_2^*, the joint MGF of W_1 and W_2 is given by*

$$E\left(e^{tW_1+sW_2}\right) = (1-t\beta_1)^{-\alpha_1}(1+t\beta_2)^{-\alpha_2}\left(1-a_1^*t-b_1^*s\right)^{-1}\left(1-a_2^*t-b_2^*s\right)^{-1}. \tag{16.9}$$

Proof It is readily obtained from the well-known properties of exponential and gamma distributions; see Johnson et al. [15].

The joint and marginal CDFs of W_1 and W_2 are presented in Appendix B. Balakrishnan and Zhu [8] have presented expressions for the CDF of $Y_1+Y_2+aZ_1$ and so these are not presented here for the sake of conciseness.

By using Lemma 16.1, we readily obtain the following result.

Result 16.4 *The conditional joint MGF of $(\hat\mu, \hat\sigma)$ is as follows:*

$$E(e^{t\hat\sigma+s\hat\mu}|D>0) = 1_{\{T>\mu\}}\left\{\sum_{d=1}^{m-1}\sum_{j=0}^{d}\sum_{l=0}^{d-j} p_1M_{Z_1^{(1)},Z_2^{(1)}}(t,s) + \sum_{j=0}^{m-1}\sum_{l=0}^{m-1-j}\left[p_2M_{Z_1^{(2)},Z_2^{(2)}}(t,s)\right.\right.$$

$$\left.+p_3M_{Z_1^{(3)},Z_2^{(3)}}(t,s)\right] + p_4M_{Z_1^{(4)},Z_2^{(4)}}(t,s) + \sum_{d=m+1}^{n}\sum_{j=0}^{m-1}\sum_{l_1=0}^{m-1-j}\sum_{l_2=0}^{d-m-1}$$

$$\left[p_5M_{Z_1^{(5)},Z_2^{(5)}}(t,s) + p_6M_{Z_1^{(6)},Z_2^{(6)}}(t,s) + p_{7,e}M_{Z_{1,e}^{(7)},Z_{2,e}^{(7)}}(t,s)\right.$$

$$\left.+p_{8,e}M_{Z_{1,e}^{(8)},Z_{2,e}^{(8)}}(t,s)\right] + \sum_{d=m+1}^{n}\sum_{l=0}^{d-m-1}\left[p_9M_{Z_1^{(9)},Z_2^{(9)}}(t,s)\right.$$

$$\left.\left.+p_{10}M_{Z_1^{(10)},Z_2^{(10)}}(t,s)\right] + \sum_{d=m+1}^{n}\sum_{j=m+1}^{d}\sum_{l_1=0}^{j-m-1}\sum_{l_2=0}^{d-j} p_{11}M_{Z_{1,e}^{(11)},Z_{2,e}^{(11)}}(t,s)\right\}$$

$$+1_{\{T\le\mu\}}\left\{\sum_{d=1}^{m-1} q_1M_{Z_1^{(12)},Z_2^{(12)}}(t,s) + q_2M_{Z_1^{(13)},Z_2^{(13)}}(t,s)\right.$$

$$\left.+\sum_{d=m+1}^{n}\sum_{l=0}^{d-m-1} q_3M_{Z_{1,e}^{(14)},Z_{2,e}^{(14)}}(t,s)\right\}. \tag{16.10}$$

16.3.2 Odd Sample Size

Result 16.5 *The conditional joint MGF of* $(\hat{\mu}, \hat{\sigma})$ *is as follows:*

$$
\begin{aligned}
E(e^{t\hat{\sigma}+s\hat{\mu}}|D>0) = 1_{\{T>\mu\}} & \left\{ \sum_{d=1}^{m}\sum_{j=0}^{d}\sum_{l=0}^{d-j} p_1 M_{Z_1^{(1)},Z_2^{(1)}}(t,s) \right. \\
& + \sum_{d=m+1}^{n}\sum_{j=0}^{m}\sum_{l_1=0}^{m-j}\sum_{l_2=0}^{d-m-1}\left[p_{7,o}M_{Z_{1,o}^{(7)},Z_{2,o}^{(7)}}(t,s)+p_{8,o}M_{Z_{1,o}^{(8)},Z_{2,o}^{(8)}}(t,s)\right] \\
& \left. + \sum_{d=m+1}^{n}\sum_{j=m+1}^{d}\sum_{l_1=0}^{j-m-1}\sum_{l_2=0}^{d-j} p_{11}M_{Z_{1,o}^{(11)},Z_{2,o}^{(11)}}(t,s) \right\} \\
& + 1_{\{T\le\mu\}}\left\{\sum_{d=1}^{m} q_1 M_{Z_1^{(12)},Z_2^{(12)}}(t,s) + \sum_{d=m+1}^{n}\sum_{l=0}^{d-m-1} q_3 M_{Z_{1,o}^{(14)},Z_{2,o}^{(14)}}(t,s)\right\}.
\end{aligned}
\tag{16.11}
$$

The conditional marginal MGFs of $\hat{\mu}$ and $\hat{\sigma}$ are deduced from (16.11) by setting $t=0$ and $s=0$, respectively. Also, the MGF of $\hat{\mu}$ can be obtained by setting $t=0$ for $D<m+1$ and utilizing the exact distribution of $X_{m+1:n}$ for $D \geq m+1$. Using this approach, we get the following result for $\hat{\mu}$.

Result 16.6 *The conditional marginal MGF of* $\hat{\mu}$ *is given by*

$$
\begin{aligned}
E(e^{s\hat{\mu}}|D>0) = 1_{\{T>\mu\}} & \left\{ \sum_{d=1}^{m}\sum_{j=0}^{d}\sum_{l=0}^{d-j} p_1 M_{Z_2^{(1)}}(t) + \sum_{d=m+1}^{n}\sum_{l_1=0}^{d-m-1} p_{11\mu}M_{Z_{2,o}^{(11)}}(t) \right. \\
& \left. + \sum_{d=m+1}^{n}\sum_{l_1=0}^{m}\sum_{l_2=0}^{d-m-1}\left[p_{7\mu,o}M_{Z_{2,o}^{(7)}}(t)+p_{8\mu,o}M_{Z_{2,o}^{(8)}}(t)\right]\right\} \\
& + 1_{\{T\le\mu\}}\left\{\sum_{d=1}^{m} q_1 M_{Z_2^{12}}(t) + \sum_{d=m+1}^{n}\sum_{l=0}^{d-m-1} q_3 M_{Z_{2,o}^{(14)}}(t)\right\}.
\end{aligned}
\tag{16.12}
$$

16.4 Exact Conditional Density Functions of MLEs and Exact Conditional Confidence Intervals

From the conditional marginal MGFs of $\hat{\sigma}$ and $\hat{\mu}$ derived in the preceding section, we can readily obtain the conditional density functions of MLEs as presented below.

Result 16.7 *If the sample size is even (i.e.,* $n=2m$*), then the MLEs* $\hat{\sigma}$ *and* $\hat{\mu}$ *are distributed as follows:*

$$\hat{\sigma}|(D>0) \stackrel{d}{=} 1_{\{T>\mu\}}\left\{\sum_{d=1}^{m}\sum_{j=0}^{d}\sum_{l=0}^{d-j} p_1 Z_1^{(1)} + \sum_{d=m+1}^{n}\sum_{j=0}^{m}\sum_{l_1=0}^{m-j}\sum_{l_2=0}^{d-m-1} p_{7\sigma} Z_\sigma^{(7)} \right.$$
$$+ \left.\sum_{d=m+1}^{n}\sum_{j=0}^{m}\sum_{l_1=0}^{m-j}\sum_{l_2=0}^{d-m-1} p_{8\sigma} Z_\sigma^{(8)} + \sum_{d=m+1}^{n}\sum_{j=m+1}^{d}\sum_{l_1=0}^{j-m-1}\sum_{l_2=0}^{d-j} p_{11} Z_{1,e}^{(11)}\right\}$$
$$+ 1_{\{T\le\mu\}}\left\{\sum_{d=1}^{m} q_1 Z_1^{(12)} + \sum_{d=m+1}^{n}\sum_{l=0}^{d-m-1} q_3 Z_{1,e}^{(14)}\right\}, \tag{16.13}$$

$$\hat{\mu}|(D>0) \stackrel{d}{=} 1_{\{T>\mu\}}\left\{\sum_{d=1}^{m-1}\sum_{j=0}^{d}\sum_{l=0}^{d-j} p_1 Z_2^{(1)} + \sum_{l=0}^{m-1}\left[p_{2\mu} Z_2^{(2)} + p_{3\mu} Z_2^{(3)}\right] + p_4 Z_2^{(4)} \right.$$
$$+ \sum_{d=m+1}^{n}\sum_{l_1=0}^{m-1}\sum_{l_2=0}^{d-m-1}\left[p_{5\mu} Z_2^{(5)} + p_{6\mu} Z_2^{(6)} + p_{7\mu,e} Z_{2,e}^{(7)} + p_{8\mu,e} Z_{2,e}^{(8)}\right]$$
$$+ \left.\sum_{d=m+1}^{n}\sum_{l=0}^{d-m-1}\left[p_9 Z_2^{(9)} + p_{10} Z_2^{(10)}\right] + \sum_{d=m+1}^{n}\sum_{l_1=0}^{d-m-1} p_{11\mu} Z_{2,e}^{(11)}\right\}$$
$$+ 1_{\{T\le\mu\}}\left\{\sum_{d=1}^{m-1} q_1 Z_2^{(12)} + q_2 Z_2^{(13)} + \sum_{d=m+1}^{n}\sum_{l=0}^{d-m-1} q_3 Z_{2,e}^{(14)}\right\}, \tag{16.14}$$

where $\sum_{i=1}^{n} P_{X_i} X_i$ *denotes the generalized mixture of distributions of variables* $X_1, \cdots, X_n$ *with probabilities* $P_{X_1}, \cdots, P_{X_n}$, *such that* $\sum_{i=1}^{n} P_{X_i} = 1$ *but* P_{X_i}*'s not necessarily being nonnegative.*

Result 16.8 *If the sample size is odd (i.e., $n = 2m+1$), then the MLEs $\hat{\sigma}$ and $\hat{\mu}$ are distributed as follows:*

$$\hat{\sigma}|(D>0) \stackrel{d}{=} 1_{\{T>\mu\}}\left\{\sum_{d=1}^{m}\sum_{j=0}^{d}\sum_{l=0}^{d-j} p_1 Z_1^{(1)} + \sum_{d=m+1}^{n}\sum_{j=0}^{m}\sum_{l_1=0}^{m-j}\sum_{l_2=0}^{d-m-1}\left[p_{7,o} Z_{1,o}^{(7)} + p_{8,o} Z_{1,o}^{(8)}\right] \right.$$
$$+ \left.\sum_{d=m+1}^{n}\sum_{j=m+1}^{d}\sum_{l_1=0}^{j-m-1}\sum_{l_2=0}^{d-j} p_{11} Z_{1,o}^{(11)}\right\}$$
$$+ 1_{\{T\le\mu\}}\left\{\sum_{d=1}^{m} q_1 Z_1^{(12)} + \sum_{d=m+1}^{n}\sum_{l=0}^{d-m-1} q_3 Z_{1,o}^{(14)}\right\}, \tag{16.15}$$

$$\hat{\mu}|(D>0) \stackrel{d}{=} 1_{\{T>\mu\}}\left\{\sum_{d=1}^{m}\sum_{j=0}^{d}\sum_{l=0}^{d-j} p_1 Z_2^{(1)} + \sum_{d=m+1}^{n}\sum_{l_1=0}^{m}\sum_{l_2=0}^{d-m-1}\left[p_{7\mu,o}Z_{2,o}^{(7)} + p_{8\mu,o}Z_{2,o}^{(8)}\right]\right.$$
$$\left. + \sum_{d=m+1}^{n}\sum_{l_1=0}^{d-m-1} p_{11\mu}Z_{2,o}^{(11)}\right\}$$
$$+ 1_{\{T\le\mu\}}\left\{\sum_{d=1}^{m} q_1 Z_2^{(12)} + \sum_{d=m+1}^{n}\sum_{l=0}^{d-m-1} q_3 Z_{2,o}^{(14)}\right\}. \tag{16.16}$$

From Results 16.7 and 16.8, we readily obtain the conditional moments of $\hat{\mu}$ and $\hat{\sigma}$ as well as the product moment. For example, when the sample size is odd, we have

$$E(\hat{\sigma}|D>0) = 1_{\{T>\mu\}}\left\{\sum_{d=1}^{m}\sum_{j=0}^{d}\sum_{l=0}^{d-j}\frac{p_1}{d}[(T-\mu)(d-l)+(2j-d)\sigma]\right.$$
$$+ \sum_{d=m+1}^{n}\sum_{j=0}^{m}\sum_{l_1=0}^{m-j}\sum_{l_2=0}^{d-m-1}\left[\frac{p_{7,o}}{d}\left((T-\mu)(m-l_2)+(2j+d-n)\sigma\right.\right.$$
$$\left. + \frac{(l_2-l_1)\sigma}{l_1+l_2+1}\right)$$
$$\left. + \frac{p_{8,o}}{d}\left((T-\mu)(m-l_1)+(2j+d-n)\sigma + \frac{(l_2-l_1)\sigma}{l_1+l_2+1}\right)\right]$$
$$+ \sum_{d=m+1}^{n}\sum_{j=m+1}^{d}\sum_{l_1=0}^{j-m-1}\sum_{l_2=0}^{d-j}\frac{p_{11}}{d}\left[(T-\mu)(n-d+l_2)+(d-2j+n)\sigma\right.$$
$$\left.\left. + \frac{(m-l_1)\sigma}{m+l_1+1}\right]\right\}$$
$$+ 1_{\{T\le\mu\}}\sigma\left\{\sum_{d=1}^{m} q_1 + \sum_{d=m+1}^{n}\sum_{l=0}^{d-m-1}\frac{q_3}{d}\left[n-d+\frac{m-l}{l+m+1}\right]\right\}. \tag{16.17}$$

By using Lemma 16.1, we can also obtain the exact marginal and joint conditional CDFs of $\hat{\mu}$ and $\hat{\sigma}$, which can then be utilized to derive the exact marginal and joint conditional CIs.

16.5 Conditional MLE of Quantile and Its Exact Distribution

The MLE of the quantile is given by

$$\hat{Q}_q = q\hat{\sigma} + \hat{\mu}. \tag{16.18}$$

By using the exact conditional MGF of $(\hat{\mu}, \hat{\sigma})$ presented in Results 3 and 4, we readily obtain the exact conditional MGF of $\hat{Q}$ as

$$M(t) = E\left(e^{t\hat{Q}}\right) = E\left(e^{tq\hat{\sigma}+t\hat{\mu}}\right). \tag{16.19}$$

By simplifying the obtained expressions, we obtain the following two results.

Result 16.9 *If the sample size is even (i.e., $n = 2m$), then the MLE of $\hat{Q}$ is distributed as follows:*

$$\begin{aligned}
\hat{Q}_q|D>0 \stackrel{d}{=} 1_{\{T>\mu\}} &\left\{ \sum_{d=1}^{m-1}\sum_{j=0}^{d}\sum_{l=0}^{d-j} p_1 ZQ_1 + \sum_{j=0}^{m-1}\sum_{l=0}^{m-1-j} (p_2 ZQ_2 + p_3 ZQ_3) + p_4 ZQ_4 \right.\\
&+ \sum_{d=m+1}^{n}\sum_{j=0}^{m-1}\sum_{l_1=0}^{m-1-j}\sum_{l_2=0}^{d-m-1} \left(p_5 ZQ_5 + p_6 ZQ_6 + p_{7,e} ZQ_{7,e} + p_{8,e} ZQ_{8,e}\right)\\
&\left. + \sum_{d=m+1}^{n}\sum_{l=0}^{d-m-1} (p_9 Z_9 + p_{10} ZQ_{10}) + \sum_{d=m+1}^{n}\sum_{j=m+1}^{d}\sum_{l_1=0}^{j-m-1}\sum_{l_2=0}^{d-j} p_{11} ZQ_{11,e} \right\}\\
&+ 1_{\{T\le\mu\}} \left\{ T + \sum_{d=1}^{m-1} q_1 ZQ_{12} + q_2 ZQ_{13} + \sum_{d=m+1}^{n}\sum_{l=0}^{d-m-1} q_3 ZQ_{14,e} \right\}.
\end{aligned} \tag{16.20}$$

Result 16.10 *If the sample size is odd (i.e., $n = 2m + 1$), then the MLE of $\hat{Q}$ is distributed as follows:*

$$\begin{aligned}
\hat{Q}_q|D>0 \stackrel{d}{=} 1_{\{T>\mu\}} &\left\{ \sum_{d=1}^{m}\sum_{j=0}^{d}\sum_{l=0}^{d-j} p_1 ZQ_1 + \sum_{d=m+1}^{n}\sum_{j=0}^{m}\sum_{l_1=0}^{m-j}\sum_{l_2=0}^{d-m-1} \left(p_{7,o} ZQ_{7,o} + p_{8,o} ZQ_{8,o}\right) \right.\\
&\left. + \sum_{d=m+1}^{n}\sum_{j=m+1}^{d}\sum_{l_1=0}^{j-m-1}\sum_{l_2=0}^{d-j} p_{11} ZQ_{11,o} \right\}\\
&+ 1_{\{T\le\mu\}} \left\{ T + \sum_{d=1}^{m} q_1 ZQ_{12} + \sum_{d=m+1}^{n}\sum_{l=0}^{d-m-1} q_3 ZQ_{14,o} \right\}.
\end{aligned} \tag{16.21}$$

From Results 16.9 and 16.10, we readily obtain the conditional moments of $\hat{Q}$. For example, when the sample size is odd, we get

$$\begin{aligned}
E(\hat{Q}_q|D>0) = 1_{\{T>\mu\}} &\left\{ \sum_{d=1}^{m}\sum_{j=0}^{d}\sum_{l=0}^{d-j} \frac{p_1}{d}\left[dT + (T-\mu)(d-l)\left(\log\left(\frac{n}{2d}\right)+q\right) + (2j-d)\left(\log\left(\frac{n}{2d}\right)+q\right)\sigma\right] \right.\\
&+ \sum_{d=m+1}^{n}\sum_{j=0}^{m}\sum_{l_1=0}^{m-j}\sum_{l_2=0}^{d-m-1} \left[\frac{p_{7,o}}{d}\left(d\mu + (T-\mu)(m-l_2)q + (2j+d-n)q\sigma + \frac{(l_2-l_1)q+d}{l_1+l_2+1}\sigma\right)\right.\\
&\left. + \frac{p_{8,o}}{d}\left(dT + (T-\mu)(m-l_1)q + (2j+d-n)q\sigma + \frac{(l_2-l_1)q+d}{l_1+l_2+1}\sigma\right)\right]\\
&\left. + \sum_{d=m+1}^{n}\sum_{j=m+1}^{d}\sum_{l_1=0}^{j-m-1}\sum_{l_2=0}^{d-j} \frac{p_{11}}{d}\left[d\mu + (T-\mu)(n-d+l_2)q + (n+d-2j)q\sigma + \frac{(m-l_1)q-d}{m+l_1+1}\sigma\right] \right\}\\
&+ 1_{\{T\le\mu\}} \left\{ T + \sum_{d=1}^{m} q_1\left[q + \log\left(\frac{n}{2d}\right)\right]\sigma + \sum_{d=m+1}^{n}\sum_{l=0}^{d-m-1} \frac{q_3}{d}\left[(n-d)q + \frac{(m-l)q-d}{m+l+1}\right]\sigma \right\}.
\end{aligned} \tag{16.22}$$

By using this exact conditional distribution, we can also develop the conditional CI for any quantile of interest. These CIs can then be used as bounds in the Q–Q plot. The procedure is similar to the one described in Sect. 16.4 and is therefore omitted for the sake of brevity.

16.6 Conditional MLE of Reliability and Its CI

Balakrishnan and Chandramouleeswaran [4] discussed the Best Linear Unbiased Estimator of reliability function. Zhu and Balakrishnan [22] developed the exact CI based on a Type-II censored sample. Here, we consider the MLE of the reliability function based on Type-I censored sample. A natural estimator for the reliability at time t is

$$\hat{S}(t) = \begin{cases} 1 - \frac{1}{2} e^{-\left(\frac{\hat{\mu}-t}{\hat{\sigma}}\right)} & \text{if } t < \hat{\mu}, \\ \frac{1}{2} e^{-\left(\frac{t-\hat{\mu}}{\hat{\sigma}}\right)} & \text{if } t \geq \hat{\mu}. \end{cases} \tag{16.23}$$

The distribution function of $\hat{S}(t)$ can be obtained as

$$P\left(\hat{S}(t) \leq s\right) = \begin{cases} P\left(\hat{\mu} + \log(2(1-s))\hat{\sigma} \leq t\right) & \text{if } t < \hat{\mu}, s < \frac{1}{2}, \\ P\left(\hat{\mu} - \log(2s)\hat{\sigma} \leq t\right) & \text{if } t \geq \hat{\mu}, s \geq \frac{1}{2}. \end{cases} \tag{16.24}$$

Developing an exact equi-tailed $100(1-\alpha)\%$ CI for $S(t)$ is equivalent to finding a s, such that

$$\begin{cases} P\left(\hat{\mu} + \log(2(1-s))\hat{\sigma} \leq t\right) = \frac{\alpha}{2} & \text{if } t < \hat{\mu}, s < \frac{1}{2}, \\ P\left(\hat{\mu} - \log(2s)\hat{\sigma} \leq t\right) = \frac{\alpha}{2} & \text{if } t \geq \hat{\mu}, s \geq \frac{1}{2}. \end{cases} \tag{16.25}$$

and

$$\begin{cases} P\left(\hat{\mu} + \log(2(1-s))\hat{\sigma} \leq t\right) = 1 - \frac{\alpha}{2} & \text{if } t < \hat{\mu}, s < \frac{1}{2}, \\ P\left(\hat{\mu} - \log 2s\hat{\sigma} \leq t\right) = 1 - \frac{\alpha}{2} & \text{if } t \geq \hat{\mu}, s \geq \frac{1}{2}. \end{cases} \tag{16.26}$$

Note that the exact distribution of $\hat{\mu} + \log(2(1-s))\hat{\sigma}$ and $\hat{\mu} - \log(2s)\hat{\sigma}$ can be obtained by setting $q = \log(2(1-s))$ or $q = -\log(2s)$ in (16.13) and (16.14). These CIs can then be used as bounds in the K–M curve or in the P–P plot.

16.7 Conditional MLE of Cumulative Hazard and Its Exact CI

The cumulative hazard function denoted by Λ is defined as

$$\Lambda(t) = -\ln(S(t)). \tag{16.27}$$

So, a natural estimator for the cumulative hazard function at time t is

$$\hat{\Lambda}(t) = -\ln(\hat{S}(t)), \tag{16.28}$$

where $\hat{S}(t)$ is defined as in (16.23). Now, the distribution function of $\hat{\Lambda}(t)$ can be expressed as

$$P(\hat{\Lambda}(t) \leq h) = P(\hat{S}(t) \geq e^{-h}) = 1 - P(\hat{S}(t) < e^{-h}). \tag{16.29}$$

Suppose an exact equi-tailed $100(1-\alpha)\%$ CI for $S(t)$ is (s_l, s_u), then an exact equi-tailed $100(1-\alpha)\%$ CI for $\Lambda(t)$ is simply $(-\log(s_u), -\log(s_l))$.

16.8 Monte Carlo Simulation Study

We carried out a Monte Carlo simulation study for $n = 15, 20$ by taking $\mu = 0$ and $\sigma = 1$, without loss of any generality. The values of T were chosen as $-0.10(0.05)0.10$, and then we computed the first, second, and product moments of $\hat{\mu}$ and $\hat{\sigma}$ through simulations and also by the use of exact formulas derived in the preceding sections. All these results are presented in Table 16.1 from which we observe that in all cases, $\hat{\sigma}$ is negatively biased and that the bias decreases when T increases. Moreover, the second moments of both estimators decrease with increasing T. Finally, it is of interest to observe that the exact values are in close agreement with the corresponding simulated values, thus validating the accuracy of the derived results.

With the values of T chosen as to allow the approximate degree of censoring as 10(10)60%, we also computed the first and second moments of $\hat{Q}$ through Monte Carlo simulations and also by the use of exact formulas derived in the preceding sections. All these results are presented in Table 16.2, from which we once again observe that in all cases the exact values are in close agreement with the corresponding simulated values.

Table 16.1 Simulated values of the first, second, and product moments of $\hat{\mu}$ and $\hat{\sigma}$ when $\mu = 0$, $\sigma = 1$, with the corresponding exact values within parentheses

n	T	$\hat{\mu}$	$\hat{\mu}^2$	$\hat{\sigma}$	$\hat{\sigma}^2$	$\hat{\mu}\hat{\sigma}$
15	−0.10	0.0259(0.0263)	0.1646(0.1593)	0.9830(0.9826)	1.1274(1.1271)	0.0780(0.0771)
	−0.05	0.0169(0.0183)	0.1405(0.1402)	0.9774(0.9773)	1.1056(1.1067)	0.0552(0.0574)
	0.00	0.0088(0.0104)	0.1237(0.1244)	0.9707(0.9707)	1.0831(1.0843)	0.0369(0.0396)
	0.05	0.0022(0.0042)	0.1113(0.1129)	0.9644(0.9648)	1.0623(1.0644)	0.0221(0.0257)
	0.10	−0.0008(0.0008)	0.1051(0.1054)	0.9611(0.9613)	1.0492(1.0505)	0.0141(0.0166)
20	−0.10	0.0144(0.0143)	0.1032(0.1014)	0.9892(0.9891)	1.0959(1.0963)	0.0445(0.0432)
	−0.05	0.0079(0.0077)	0.0904(0.0902)	0.9853(0.9848)	1.0811(1.0810)	0.0299(0.0292)
	0.00	0.0009(0.0012)	0.0803(0.0808)	0.9793(0.9792)	1.0629(1.0634)	0.0165(0.0165)
	0.05	−0.0037(−0.0035)	0.0734(0.0739)	0.9742(0.9743)	1.0469(1.0479)	0.0071(0.0072)
	0.10	−0.0057(−0.0056)	0.0690(0.0695)	0.9715(0.9716)	1.0367(1.0377)	0.0018(0.0017)

16.9 Illustrative Examples

In this section, two known data sets from the reliability literature are used to illustrate the results established in the preceding sections.

Example 16.1 The data presented in Table 16.3, given by Mann and Fertig [20], correspond to lifetimes of 13 aeroplane components with the last 3 lifetimes having been censored. Balakrishnan and Zhu [8] analyzed these data by assuming a Laplace model based on Type-II censored sample and determined the bias-corrected MLEs $\hat{\mu}$ and $\hat{\sigma}$ to be 1.5400 and 1.1711, respectively. Here, we analyze these data by assuming a Laplace distribution and compute the MLEs based on Type-I censored samples with different choices of T. We computed the MSEs and the correlation coefficient of the MLEs based on the exact formulas derived in Sect. 16.3, and these results are presented in Table 16.4. The 95% CIs, constructed from the exact conditional CDFs derived in Sect. 16.4 as well as those obtained by bootstrap, are presented in Table 16.5. The two sets of CIs are seen to be quite close once again. We have presented the Q–Q plot and survival function with $T = 3.00$ in Figs. 16.1 and 16.2. Finally, we carried out formal goodness-of-fit tests based on the correlation coefficient between the theoretical and the empirical quantiles, as well as the Kolmogorov–Smirnov (KS) test. The obtained results are presented in Table 16.6, which do support the Laplace model assumption (Fig. 16.3).

Example 16.2 Davis [12] has given lifetimes in hours of forty-watt incandescent lamps taken from 42 weekly forced-life test samples. The data presented in Table 16.7 are the first 20 observations from this data set. Bain et al. [2] analyzed these data by fitting a logistic distribution. For illustrative purpose, we will analyze these data by assuming a Laplace distribution based on a Type-I censored sample with $T = 1000$. We obtained the MLEs and the MLE of quantiles with bias and SE by using the bootstrap as well as the exact formulas derived earlier. These results are presented in Table 16.8. Finally, we have presented the Q–Q plot and survival functions in

Table 16.2 Simulated and exact (followed by the simulated value) values of the first and second moments (within parentheses) of Q_q when $\mu = 0, \sigma = 1$

n	d.o.c.(T)	$\hat{Q}_{0.10}$		$\hat{Q}_{0.25}$		$\hat{Q}_{0.50}$		$\hat{Q}_{0.75}$		$\hat{Q}_{0.90}$	
15	10%(1.6094)	−1.5619(2.7259)	−1.5612(2.7035)	−0.6731(0.5837)	−0.6724(0.5805)	−0.0006(0.0961)	0.0000(0.0980)	0.6718(0.5844)	0.6724(0.5832)	1.5607(2.7275)	1.5612(2.7098)
	20%(0.9163)	−1.5614(2.7446)	−1.5608(2.7196)	−0.6728(0.5868)	−0.6722(0.5830)	−0.0007(0.0960)	0.0000(0.0978)	0.6715(0.5885)	0.6722(0.5867)	1.5600(2.7484)	1.5608(2.7280)
	30%(0.5108)	−1.5527(2.7444)	−1.5525(2.7276)	−0 6694(0.5861)	−0.6690(0.5827)	−0.0013(0.0951)	−0.0007(0.0955)	0.6668(0.5877)	0.6677(0.5862)	1.5501(2.7481)	1.5512(2.7357)
	40%(0.2231)	−1.5456(2.7537)	−1.5452(2.7503)	−0 6670(0.5858)	−0.6665(0.5839)	−0.0024(0.0969)	−0.0018(0.0960)	0.6622(0.5996)	0.6628(0.5994)	1.5408(2.7857)	1.5415(2.7862)
	50%(0.000)	−1.5521(2.8057)	−1.5519(2.8057)	−0 6630(0.5907)	−0.6625(0.5905)	0.0096(0.1236)	0.0104(0.1244)	0.6821(0.6974)	0.6832(0.7002)	1.5712(3.0534)	1.5726(3.0604)
	60%(−0.2231)	−1.5497(2.8273)	−1.5500(2.8284)	−0 6418(0.6028)	−0.6417(0.6013)	0.0449(0.2258)	0.0453(0.2239)	0.7317(0.9734)	0.7324(0.9724)	1.6396(3.6878)	1.6406(3.6901)
20	10%(1.6094)	−1.5763(2.6926)	−1.5771(2.6972)	−0 6790(0.5527)	−0.6792(0.5541)	−0.0002(0.0660)	0.0000(0.0666)	0.6787(0.5542)	0.6792(0.5556)	1.5760(2.6961)	1.5771(2.7008)
	20%(0.9163)	−1.5772(2.7121)	−1.5777(2.7160)	−0.6794(0.5562)	−0.6795(0.5574)	−0.0003(0.0658)	−0.0001(0.0665)	0.6789(0.5578)	0.6793(0.5592)	1.5767(2.7159)	1.5775(2.7201)
	30%(0.5108)	−1.5734(2.7231)	−1.5724(2.7208)	−0.6787(0.5590)	−0.6780(0.5585)	−0.0018(0.0651)	−0.0015(0.0653)	0.6750(0.5558)	0.6751(0.5560)	1.5697(2.7156)	1.5694(2.7150)
	40%(0.2231)	−1.5687(2.7343)	−1.5676(2.7321)	−0.6789(0.5624)	−0.6783(0.5619)	−0.0058(0.0648)	−0.0055(0.0650)	0.6673(0.5540)	0.6672(0.5540)	1.5571(2.7148)	1.5565(2.7136)
	50%(0.000)	−1.5763(2.7848)	−1.5748(2.7823)	−0.6785(0.5693)	−0.6776(0.5689)	0.0006(0.0803)	0.0012(0.0808)	0.6797(0.6136)	0.6799(0.6147)	1.5775(2.8874)	1.5771(2.8887)
	60%(−0.2231)	−1.5730(2.7946)	−1.5715(2.7923)	−0.6602(0.5661)	−0.6594(0.5658)	0.0302(0.1390)	0.0305(0.1395)	0.7207(0.7959)	0.7205(0.7967)	1.6334(3.3283)	1.6326(3.3284)

Table 16.3 Data from Mann and Fertig [20]

0.22	0.50	0.88	1.00	1.32	1.33	1.54	1.76	2.50	3.00

Table 16.4 MLEs of the parameters based on data in Table 16.3 and their bias, MSEs and correlation coefficient based on the exact formulas

T	$\hat{\mu}$	$bias(\hat{\mu})$	$\hat{\sigma}$	$bias(\hat{\sigma})$	$\widehat{MSE(\hat{\mu})}$	$\widehat{MSE(\hat{\sigma})}$	$\widehat{Cor(\hat{\mu}, \hat{\sigma})}$
1.75	1.5400	−0.0013	0.7500	−0.0368	0.0713	0.0789	0.0727
2.75	1.5400	0.0000	1.1122	−0.0403	0.1511	0.1263	0.0170
3.00	1.5400	0.0000	1.1010	−0.0381	0.1380	0.1094	0.0155

Table 16.5 Exact and bootstrap 95% CIs for μ and σ based on data in Table 16.3

T	Exact results		Bootstrap results	
	μ	σ	μ	σ
1.75	(1.0242, 2.0308)	(0.3113, 1.3089)	(1.0252, 2.0283)	(0.3113, 1.3332)
2.75	(0.7751, 2.3050)	(0.5437, 1.8584)	(0.7766, 2.2997)	(0.5445, 1.8514)
3.00	(0.7828, 2.2973)	(0.5436, 1.8181)	(0.7843, 2.2920)	(0.5442, 1.8144)

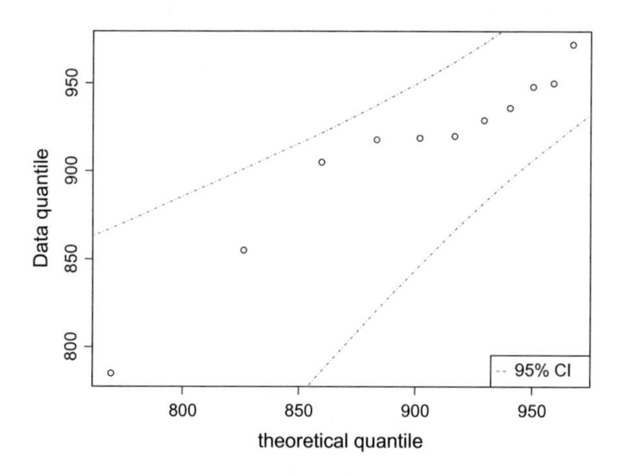

Fig. 16.1 Q–Q plot with 95% confidence bounds based on data in Table 16.3

Figs. 16.3 and 16.4. Here again, we carried out two formal goodness-of-fit tests based on the correlation coefficient and the KS test and the obtained results are presented in Table 16.9, which clearly support the Laplace model assumption.

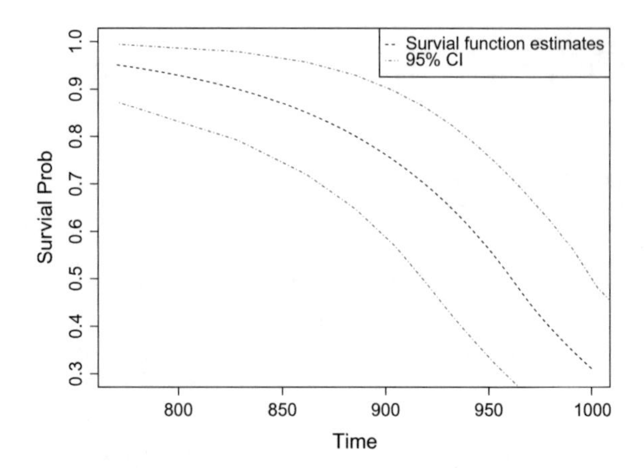

Fig. 16.2 Estimated survival function with 95% confidence bounds based on data in Table 16.3

Table 16.6 Formal goodness-of-fit tests based on data in Table 16.3

	Statistic	P value
Q–Q correlation test	0.9654	0.3988
KS test	0.1535	0.6139

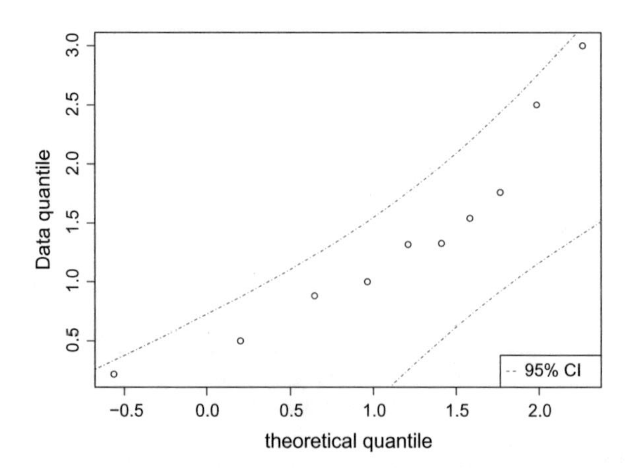

Fig. 16.3 Q–Q plot with 95% confidence bounds based on data in Table 16.7

Table 16.7 Data from Davis [12], where * denotes the unobserved censored data

785	855	905	918	919	920	929	936	948	950
972	1035*	1045*	1067*	1092*	1126*	1156*	1162*	1170*	1196*

Table 16.8 MLEs of quantiles, estimates of their bias, and SEs based on data in Table 16.7

	MLE	$\widehat{bias}$	$\widehat{SE}$
μ	961.0000	−0.1566	20.94
		−0.1499	21.0274
σ	82.4546	−2.0645	22.1333
		−2.0328	22.2117
$Q_{0.10}$	828.2945	3.1661	41.1417
		3.1219	41.3358
$Q_{0.25}$	903.8469	1.2744	25.8362
		1.2592	25.9665
$Q_{0.50}$	961.0000	−0.1566	20.9411
		−0.1499	21.0274
$Q_{0.75}$	1018.1531	−1.5876	26.0821
		−1.5590	26.1556
$Q_{0.90}$	−1093.7055	−3.4793	41.5004
		−3.4216	41.6116

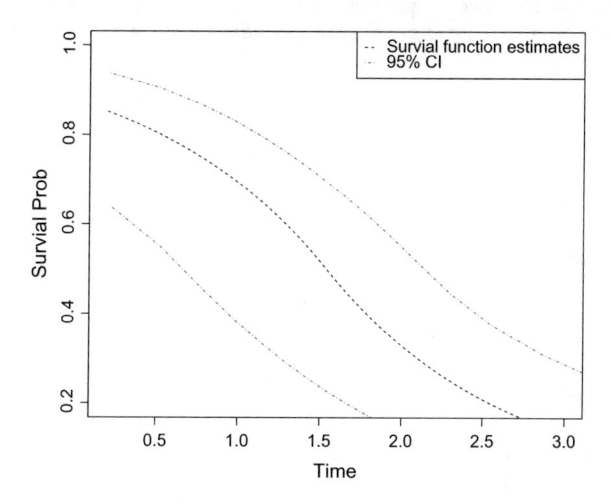

Fig. 16.4 Estimated survival function with 95% confidence bounds based on data in Table 16.7

Table 16.9 Formal goodness-of-fit tests based on data in Table data1

	Statistic	P value
Q–Q correlation test	0.9309	0.2058
KS test	0.1755	0.7430

16.10 Discussion and Concluding Remarks

In this paper, we have derived the MLEs of the location and scale parameters of the Laplace distribution based on a time-constrained life-testing experiment. We have then developed conditional marginal and joint MGFs of the MLEs and exact conditional CIs for both parameters. Moreover, we have derived the exact distributions of the MLEs of quantile, reliability, and cumulative hazard functions. The exact density functions are then used to determine the bias and MSEs of the estimates as well as to derive exact CIs, which are further utilized to develop exact confidence bounds for Q–Q plot and survival function. As a further extension of the work, it will be useful to generalize the present work to a general hybrid-censored sample (see Balakrishnan and Kundu [7]). Puig and Stephens [21] discussed the goodness-of-fit for the Laplace model based on a complete sample. It will naturally be of interest to discuss the goodness-of-fit when the data is Type-I censored. Work is currently under progress on these problems and we hope to report these findings in a future paper.

Acknowledgements The authors express their sincere thanks to the editor and anonymous reviewers for their useful comments and suggestions on an earlier version of this manuscript which led to this improved one.

Appendix

List of notation

$$p_0 = \frac{1}{2^n} e^{-\frac{n(T-\mu)}{\sigma}},$$

$$q_0 = \left(1 - \frac{1}{2} e^{-\frac{\mu-T}{\sigma}}\right)^n,$$

$$p_1 = \frac{(-1)^l n! e^{-\frac{(T-\mu)(n+l-d)}{\sigma}}}{(1-p_0)2^n (n-d)! j! (d-j-l)! l!},$$

$$p_2 = \frac{(-1)^l n! e^{-\frac{(T-\mu)m}{\sigma}}}{2^n j! (l+1)! (m-j-l-1)! (n-m)! (1-p_0)},$$

$$p_3 = -p_2 e^{-\frac{(T-\mu)(l+1)}{\sigma}},$$

$$p_4 = \frac{n! e^{-\frac{(T-\mu)m}{\sigma}}}{2^n m! m! (1-p_0)},$$

$$p_5 = \frac{(-1)^{l_1+d-m-1-l_2} n! e^{-\frac{(T-\mu)(m-1-l_2)}{\sigma}}}{2^n j! (m-1-j-l_1)! (d-m-1-l_2)! (l_2+1)! (n-d)! (l_1+1)! (1-p_0)},$$

$$p_6 = -p_5 e^{-\frac{(T-\mu)(l_2+1)}{\sigma}},$$
$$p_{7,e} = -\frac{p_5}{l_1+l_2+2},$$
$$p_{7,o} = \frac{(-1)^{l_1+d-m-1-l_2} n! e^{-\frac{(T-\mu)(m-l_2)}{\sigma}}}{(1-p_0)2^n(l_1+l_2+1)l_1!l_2!j!(n-d)!(m-j-l_1)!(d-m-1-l_2)!},$$
$$p_{8,e} = -p_{7,e} e^{-\frac{(T-\mu)(l_1+l_2+2)}{\sigma}},$$
$$p_{8,o} = -p_{7,o} e^{-\frac{(T-\mu)(l_1+l_2+1)}{\sigma}}$$

$$p_9 = \frac{(-1)^{d-m-l-1} n! e^{-\frac{(T-\mu)(m-l-1)}{\sigma}}}{2^n m!(d-m-l-1)!(l+1)!(n-d)!(1-p_0)},$$
$$p_{10} = -p_9 e^{-\frac{(T-\mu)(l+1)}{\sigma}},$$
$$p_{11} = \frac{(-1)^{l_1+l_2} n! e^{-\frac{(T-\mu)(n-d+l_2)}{\sigma}}}{2^n m!(j-m-l_1-1)!l_1!(d-j-l_2)!l_2!(n-d)!(m+l_1+1)(1-p_0)},$$
$$p_{7\sigma} = \frac{(-1)^{l_1+d-m-1-l_2} n! e^{-\frac{(T-\mu)(m-1-l_2)}{\sigma}}}{(1-p_0)2^n(l_1+l_2+1)l_1!l_2!j!(n-d)!(m-j-l_1)!(d-m-1-l_2)!},$$
$$p_{8\sigma} = -p_{7\sigma} e^{-\frac{(T-\mu)(l_1+l_2+1)}{\sigma}},$$
$$p_{2\mu} = \frac{(-1)^l n! e^{-\frac{(T-\mu)m}{\sigma}}}{(m-l-1)!(l+1)!m!2^{m+l+1}(1-p_0)},$$
$$p_{3\mu} = -p_{2\mu} e^{-\frac{(T-\mu)(l+1)}{\sigma}},$$
$$p_{5\mu} = \frac{n!(-1)^{l_1+d-m-1-l_2} e^{-\frac{(T-\mu)(m-l_2-1)}{\sigma}}}{2^{m+l_1+1}(m-l_1-1)!(l_1+1)!(d-m-l_2-1)!(l_2+1)!(n-d)!(1-p_0)},$$
$$p_{6\mu} = -p_{5\mu} e^{-\frac{(T-\mu)(l_2+1)}{\sigma}},$$
$$p_{7\mu,e} = -\frac{l_2+1}{l_1+l_2+2} p_{5\mu},$$
$$p_{7\mu,o} = \frac{n!(-1)^{l_1+d-m-1-l_2} e^{-\frac{(T-\mu)(m-l_2)}{\sigma}}}{2^{m+l_1+1}(m-l_1)!l_1!(d-m-1-l_2)!l_2!(n-d)!(l_1+l_2+1)(1-p_0)},$$
$$p_{8\mu,e} = -p_{7\mu,e} e^{-\frac{(T-\mu)(l_1+l_2+2)}{\sigma}},$$
$$p_{8\mu,o} = -p_{7\mu,o} e^{-\frac{(T-\mu)(l_1+l_2+1)}{\sigma}},$$
$$p_{11\mu} = \frac{(-1)^{l_1} n! e^{-\frac{(T-\mu)(n-d)}{\sigma}} \left[1-\frac{1}{2}e^{-\frac{T-\mu}{\sigma}}\right]^{d-m-1-l_1}}{2^{m+l_1+1+n-d} m!(d-m-l_1-1)!l_1!(n-d)!(m+l_1+1)(1-p_0)},$$
$$q_1 = \frac{n!}{d!(n-d)!(1-q_0)} \left(\frac{1}{2}e^{-\frac{\mu-T}{\sigma}}\right)^d \left(1-\frac{1}{2}e^{-\frac{\mu-T}{\sigma}}\right)^{n-d},$$
$$q_2 = \frac{n!}{m!m!} \left(\frac{1}{2}e^{-\frac{\mu-T}{\sigma}}\right)^m \left[1-\frac{1}{2}e^{-\frac{\mu-T}{\sigma}}\right]^m,$$

$$q_3 = \frac{(-1)^l \left(1 - \frac{1}{2}e^{-\frac{\mu - T}{\sigma}}\right)^{n-d} \left(\frac{1}{2}e^{-\frac{(\mu - T)}{\sigma}}\right)^d n!}{(l + m + 1)m!l!(d - m - 1 - l)!(n - d)!(1 - q_0)},$$

$$Z_\sigma^{(7)} \stackrel{d}{=} \Gamma\left(j + d - m - 1, \frac{\sigma}{d}\right) + N\Gamma\left(m - j, \frac{\sigma}{d}\right) + E\left(\frac{(l_2 - l_1 + 1)\sigma}{(l_2 + l_1 + 1)d}\right) + \frac{(T - \mu)(m - 1 - l_2)}{d},$$

$$Z_\sigma^{(8)} \stackrel{d}{=} \Gamma\left(j + d - m - 1, \frac{\sigma}{d}\right) + N\Gamma\left(m - j, \frac{\sigma}{d}\right) + E\left(\frac{(l_2 - l_1 + 1)\sigma}{(l_2 + l_1 + 1)d}\right) + \frac{(T - \mu)(m - l_1)}{d},$$

$$Z_1^{(1)} \stackrel{d}{=} \Gamma\left(j, \frac{\sigma}{d}\right) + N\Gamma\left(d - j, \frac{\sigma}{d}\right) + \frac{(T - \mu)(d - l)}{d},$$

$$Z_2^{(1)} \stackrel{d}{=} \log\left(\frac{n}{2d}\right) Z_1^{(1)} + T,$$

$$Z_{1,e}^{(2)} \stackrel{d}{=} \Gamma\left(j, \frac{\sigma}{m}\right) + N\Gamma\left(m - 1 - j, \frac{\sigma}{m}\right) - \frac{\sigma}{m}E_2 + (T - \mu),$$

$$Z_{2,e}^{(2)} \stackrel{d}{=} \frac{\sigma}{2(l + 1)}E_2 + \frac{T + \mu}{2},$$

$$Z_1^{(3)} \stackrel{d}{=} \Gamma\left(j, \frac{\sigma}{m}\right) + N\Gamma\left(m - 1 - j, \frac{\sigma}{m}\right) - \frac{\sigma}{m}E_3 + \frac{(T - \mu)(m - l - 1)}{m},$$

$$Z_2^{(3)} \stackrel{d}{=} \frac{\sigma}{2(l + 1)}E_3 + T,$$

$$Z_1^{(4)} \stackrel{d}{=} \Gamma\left(m - 1, \frac{\sigma}{m}\right) + \frac{\sigma}{m}E_4 + (T - \mu),$$

$$Z_2^{(4)} \stackrel{d}{=} -\frac{\sigma}{n}E_4 + \frac{T + \mu}{2},$$

$$Z_{1,e}^{(5)} \stackrel{d}{=} \Gamma\left(d - m - 1 + j, \frac{\sigma}{d}\right) + N\Gamma\left(m - 1 - j, \frac{\sigma}{d}\right) + \frac{\sigma}{d}E_{5A} - \frac{\sigma}{d}E_{5B} + \frac{(T - \mu)(m - 1 - l_2)}{d},$$

$$Z_{2,e}^{(5)} \stackrel{d}{=} \frac{\sigma}{2(l_2 + 1)}E_{5A} + \frac{\sigma}{2(l_1 + 1)}E_{5B} + \mu,$$

$$Z_{1,e}^{(6)} \stackrel{d}{=} \Gamma\left(d - m - 1 + j, \frac{\sigma}{d}\right) + N\Gamma\left(m - 1 - j, \frac{\sigma}{d}\right) + \frac{\sigma}{d}E_{6A} - \frac{\sigma}{d}E_{6B} + \frac{(T - \mu)m}{d},$$

$$Z_{2,e}^{(6)} \stackrel{d}{=} \frac{\sigma}{2(l_2 + 1)}E_{6A} + \frac{\sigma}{2(l_1 + 1)}E_{6B} + \frac{T + \mu}{2},$$

$$Z_{1,e}^{(7)} \stackrel{d}{=} \Gamma\left(d - m - 1 + j, \frac{\sigma}{d}\right) + N\Gamma\left(m - 1 - j, \frac{\sigma}{d}\right) + \frac{(l_2 - l_1)\sigma}{(l_1 + l_2 + 2)d}E_{7A} - \frac{\sigma}{d}E_{7B} + \frac{(T - \mu)(m - l_2 - 1)}{d},$$

$$Z_{2,e}^{(7)} \overset{d}{=} \frac{\sigma}{l_1+l_2+2}E_{7A} + \frac{\sigma}{2(l_1+1)}E_{7B} + \mu,$$

$$Z_{1,o}^{(7)} \overset{d}{=} \Gamma\left(j+d-m-1, \frac{\sigma}{d}\right) + N\Gamma\left(m-j, \frac{\sigma}{d}\right) + \frac{(l_2-l_1+1)\sigma}{(l_2+l_1+1)d}E_7 + \frac{(T-\mu)(m-l_2)}{d},$$

$$Z_{2,o}^{(7)} \overset{d}{=} \frac{\sigma}{l_2+l_1+1}E_7 + \mu,$$

$$Z_{1,e}^{(8)} \overset{d}{=} \Gamma\left(d-m-1+j, \frac{\sigma}{d}\right) + N\Gamma\left(m-1-j, \frac{\sigma}{d}\right) + \frac{(l_2-l_1)\sigma}{(l_1+l_2+2)d}E_{8A} - \frac{\sigma}{d}E_{8B} + \frac{(T-\mu)(m-l_1-1)}{d},$$

$$Z_{2,e}^{(8)} \overset{d}{=} \frac{\sigma}{l_1+l_2+2}E_{8A} + \frac{\sigma}{2(l_1+1)}E_{8B} + T,$$

$$Z_{1,o}^{(8)} \overset{d}{=} \Gamma\left(j+d-m-1, \frac{\sigma}{d}\right) + N\Gamma\left(m-j, \frac{\sigma}{d}\right) + \frac{(l_2-l_1+1)\sigma}{(l_2+l_1+1)d}E_8 + \frac{(T-\mu)(m-l_1)}{d},$$

$$Z_{2,o}^{(8)} \overset{d}{=} \frac{\sigma}{l_2+l_1+1}E_8 + T,$$

$$Z_1^{(9)} \overset{d}{=} \Gamma\left(d-2, \frac{\sigma}{d}\right) + \frac{\sigma}{d}E_{9A} + \frac{\sigma}{d}E_{9B} + \frac{(T-\mu)(m-l-1)}{d},$$

$$Z_2^{(9)} \overset{d}{=} -\frac{\sigma}{n}E_{9A} + \frac{\sigma}{2(l+1)}E_{9B} + \mu,$$

$$Z_1^{(10)} \overset{d}{=} \Gamma\left(d-2, \frac{\sigma}{d}\right) + \frac{\sigma}{d}E_{10A} + \frac{\sigma}{d}E_{10B} + \frac{(T-\mu)m}{d},$$

$$Z_2^{(10)} \overset{d}{=} -\frac{\sigma}{n}E_{10A} + \frac{\sigma}{2(l+1)}E_{10B} + \frac{T+\mu}{2},$$

$$Z_{1,e}^{(11)} \overset{d}{=} \Gamma\left(d-j+m-1, \frac{\sigma}{d}\right) + N\Gamma\left(j-m-1, \frac{\sigma}{d}\right) + \frac{\sigma}{d}E_{11A} + \frac{(m-l_1-1)\sigma}{(m+l_1+1)d}E_{11B} + \frac{(T-\mu)(n-d+l_2)}{d},$$

$$Z_{2,e}^{(11)} \overset{d}{=} -\frac{\sigma}{n}E_{11A} - \frac{\sigma}{m+l_1+1}E_{11B} + \mu,$$

$$Z_{1,o}^{(11)} \overset{d}{=} \Gamma\left(d-j+m, \frac{\sigma}{d}\right) + N\Gamma\left(j-m-1, \frac{\sigma}{d}\right) + \frac{(m-l_1)\sigma}{(m+l_1+1)d}E_{11} + \frac{(T-\mu)(n-d+l_2)}{d},$$

$$Z_{2,o}^{(11)} \overset{d}{=} -\frac{\sigma}{m+l_1+1}E_{11} + \mu,$$

$$Z_1^{(12)} \overset{d}{=} \Gamma\left(d, \frac{\sigma}{d}\right),$$

$$
\begin{aligned}
Z_2^{(12)} &\stackrel{d}{=} \log\left(\frac{n}{2d}\right) Z_1^{(12)} + T,\\
Z_1^{(13)} &\stackrel{d}{=} \Gamma\left(m-1, \frac{\sigma}{m}\right) + \frac{\sigma}{m} E_{13},\\
Z_2^{(13)} &\stackrel{d}{=} -\frac{\sigma}{n} E_{13} + T,\\
Z_{1,e}^{(14)} &\stackrel{d}{=} \Gamma\left(m-1, \frac{\sigma}{d}\right) + N\Gamma\left(d-m-1, \frac{\sigma}{d}\right) + \frac{\sigma}{d} E_{14A} + \frac{(m-l-1)\sigma}{(m+l+1)d} E_{14B},\\
Z_{2,e}^{(14)} &\stackrel{d}{=} -\frac{\sigma}{n} E_{14A} - \frac{\sigma}{m+l+1} E_{14B} + T,\\
Z_{1,o}^{(14)} &\stackrel{d}{=} \Gamma\left(m, \frac{\sigma}{d}\right) + N\Gamma\left(d-m-1, \frac{\sigma}{d}\right) + \frac{(m-l)\sigma}{(m+l+1)d} E_{14},\\
Z_{2,o}^{(14)} &\stackrel{d}{=} -\frac{\sigma}{m+l+1} E_{14} + T,\\
E_{\cdot} &\stackrel{d}{=} E(1).
\end{aligned}
$$

$$
\begin{aligned}
ZQ_1 &\stackrel{d}{=} \frac{dT + (T-\mu)(d-l)\left(\log\left(\frac{n}{2d}\right) + q\right)}{d} + \Gamma^*\left(j, \frac{q + \log\left(\frac{n}{2d}\right)}{d}\sigma\right)\\
&\quad + \Gamma^*\left(d-j, -\frac{q + \log\left(\frac{n}{2d}\right)}{d}\sigma\right),\\
ZQ_2 &\stackrel{d}{=} \frac{(2q+1)T + (1-2q)\mu}{2} + \Gamma^*\left(j, \frac{q\sigma}{m}\right) + \Gamma^*\left(m-1-j, -\frac{q\sigma}{m}\right)\\
&\quad + E^*\left(\frac{m-2q(l+1)}{n(l+1)}\sigma\right),\\
ZQ_3 &\stackrel{d}{=} \frac{(n-2l-2)qT + nT + 2(l+1-m)q\mu}{n} + \Gamma^*\left(j, \frac{q\sigma}{m}\right)\\
&\quad + \Gamma^*\left(m-1-j, -\frac{q\sigma}{m}\right) + E^*\left(\frac{m-2q(l+1)}{n(l+1)}\sigma\right),\\
ZQ_4 &\stackrel{d}{=} \frac{(2q+1)T + (1-2q)\mu}{2} + \Gamma^*\left(m-1, \frac{q\sigma}{m}\right) + E^*\left(\frac{2q-1}{n}\sigma\right),\\
ZQ_5 &\stackrel{d}{=} \frac{(T-\mu)(m-1-l_2)q + d\mu}{d} + \Gamma^*\left(d-m-1+j, \frac{q\sigma}{d}\right)\\
&\quad + \Gamma^*\left(m-1-j, -\frac{q\sigma}{d}\right)\\
&\quad + E^*\left(\frac{2(l_2+1)q + d}{2d(l_2+1)}\sigma\right) + E^*\left(\frac{d-2(l_1+1)q}{2d(l_1+1)}\sigma\right),\\
ZQ_6 &\stackrel{d}{=} \frac{(T-\mu)nq + (T+\mu)d}{2d} + \Gamma^*\left(d-m-1+j, \frac{q\sigma}{d}\right)\\
&\quad + \Gamma^*\left(m-1-j, -\frac{q\sigma}{d}\right)\\
&\quad + E^*\left(\frac{2(l_2+1)q + d}{2d(l_2+1)}\sigma\right) + E^*\left(\frac{d-2(l_1+1)q}{2d(l_1+1)}\sigma\right),
\end{aligned}
$$

$$ZQ_{7,e} \overset{d}{=} \frac{(T-\mu)(m-1-l_2)q+d\mu}{d} + \Gamma^*\left(d-m-1+j, \frac{q\sigma}{d}\right) + \Gamma^*\left(m-1-j, -\frac{q\sigma}{d}\right) + E^*\left(\frac{(l_2-l_1)q+d}{d(l_1+l_2+2)}\sigma\right) + E^*\left(\frac{d-2(l_1+1)q}{2d(l_1+1)}\sigma\right),$$

$$ZQ_{7,o} \overset{d}{=} \frac{(T-\mu)(m-l_2)q+d\mu}{d} + \Gamma^*\left(d-m-1+j, \frac{q\sigma}{d}\right) + \Gamma^*\left(m-j, -\frac{q\sigma}{d}\right) + E^*\left(\frac{(l_2-l_1)q+d}{d(l_1+l_2+1)}\sigma\right),$$

$$ZQ_{8,e} \overset{d}{=} \frac{(T-\mu)(m-l_1-1)q+dT}{d} + \Gamma^*\left(d-m-1+j, \frac{q\sigma}{d}\right) + \Gamma^*\left(m-1-j, -\frac{q\sigma}{d}\right) + E^*\left(\frac{(l_2-l_1)q+d}{d(l_1+l_2+2)}\sigma\right) + E^*\left(\frac{d-2(l_1+1)q}{2d(l_1+1)}\sigma\right),$$

$$ZQ_{8,o} \overset{d}{=} \frac{(T-\mu)(m-l_1)q+dT}{d} + \Gamma^*\left(d-m-1+j, \frac{q\sigma}{d}\right) + \Gamma^*\left(m-j, -\frac{q\sigma}{d}\right) + E^*\left(\frac{(l_2-l_1)q+d}{d(l_1+l_2+1)}\sigma\right),$$

$$ZQ_9 \overset{d}{=} \frac{(T-\mu)(m-1-l)q+d\mu}{d} + \Gamma^*\left(d-2, \frac{q\sigma}{d}\right) + E^*\left(\frac{nq-d}{nd}\sigma\right) + E^*\left(\frac{2(l+1)q+d}{2d(l+1)}\sigma\right),$$

$$ZQ_{10} \overset{d}{=} \frac{(T-\mu)nq+d(T+\mu)}{2d} + \Gamma^*\left(d-2, \frac{q\sigma}{d}\right) + E^*\left(\frac{nq-d}{nd}\sigma\right) + E^*\left(\frac{2(l+1)q+d}{2d(l+1)}\sigma\right),$$

$$ZQ_{11,e} \overset{d}{=} \frac{(T-\mu)(n-d+l_2)q+\mu d}{d} + \Gamma^*\left(d-j+m-1, \frac{q\sigma}{d}\right) + \Gamma^*\left(j-m-1, -\frac{q\sigma}{d}\right) + E^*\left(\frac{nq-d}{nd}\sigma\right) + E^*\left(\frac{(m-l_1-1)q-d}{d(m+l_1+1)}\sigma\right),$$

$$ZQ_{11,o} \overset{d}{=} \frac{(T-\mu)(n-d+l_2)q+\mu d}{d} + \Gamma^*\left(d-j+m, \frac{q\sigma}{d}\right) + \Gamma^*\left(j-m-1, -\frac{q\sigma}{d}\right) + E^*\left(\frac{(m-l_1)q-d}{d(m+l_1+1)}\sigma\right),$$

$$ZQ_{12} \stackrel{d}{=} \Gamma^*\left(d, \frac{q+\log\left(\frac{n}{2d}\right)}{d}\sigma\right),$$

$$ZQ_{13} \stackrel{d}{=} \Gamma^*\left(m-1, \frac{q}{m}\sigma\right) + E^*\left(\frac{2q-1}{n}\sigma\right),$$

$$ZQ_{14,e} \stackrel{d}{=} \Gamma^*\left(m-1, \frac{q}{d}\sigma\right) + \Gamma^*\left(d-m-1, -\frac{q}{d}\sigma\right) + E^*\left(\frac{nq-d}{nd}\sigma\right) + E^*\left(\frac{(m-l-1)q-d}{d(m+l+1)}\sigma\right),$$

$$ZQ_{14,o} \stackrel{d}{=} \Gamma^*\left(m, \frac{q}{d}\sigma\right) + \Gamma^*\left(d-m-1, -\frac{q}{d}\sigma\right) + E^*\left(\frac{(m-l)q-d}{d(m+l+1)}\sigma\right).$$

Proof of Result 16.1

Here, we will present the detailed proof for the derivation of the MLEs for the case when $d < \frac{n}{2}$ and abstain from presenting the proofs for all other cases for the sake of brevity since their derivations are quite similar. Even though it will not be known whether T is greater than μ or not, it is clear that the density in (16.3) will take on two different forms and so we will first find the MLE of μ based on the two cases $T \geq \mu$ and $T \leq \mu$ separately. Then, finally the MLE of μ is determined by comparing the likelihood values under these two cases.

Case I: $T \geq \mu$

In this case, we readily obtain the MLE of μ as $\hat{\mu}_1 = T$, and the corresponding likelihood to be

$$L_1(T, \sigma) = \frac{C_d}{2^n \sigma^d} e^{-\frac{dT - \sum_{i=1}^{d} x_{i:n}}{\sigma}}. \tag{16.30}$$

Case II: $T \leq \mu$

In this case, from the likelihood function L_2, we obtain the MLE of μ as

$$\hat{\mu}_2 = T + \sigma \log\left(\frac{n}{2d}\right). \tag{16.31}$$

Since for any σ, $L_1(T, \sigma) = L_2(T, \sigma) < L_2(\hat{\mu}_2, \sigma)$, we now obtain

$$\hat{\mu} = T + \hat{\sigma} \log\left(\frac{n}{2d}\right), \tag{16.32}$$

as given in (16.4). Then, the MLE of σ can be obtained from the profile likelihood function to be

$$\hat{\sigma} = \frac{1}{d}\sum_{i=1}^{d}(T - X_{i:n}), \tag{16.33}$$

as given in (16.5).

Proof of Result 16.2.

We shall consider the two cases $\mu < T$ and $\mu \geq T$ separately.

Case I: $\mu < T$. In this case, we have

$$E[e^{t\hat{\sigma}}|D > 0] = \sum_{d=1}^{m}\sum_{j=0}^{d} E\left[e^{t\hat{\sigma}}|D = d, J = j\right] P(D = d, J = j|D > 0) + \sum_{d=m+1}^{n}\sum_{j=0}^{d} E\left[e^{t\hat{\sigma}}|D = d, J = j\right] P(D = d, J = j|D > 0). \tag{16.34}$$

The joint distribution of J and D, conditional on $D > 0$, is

$$\begin{aligned} P(D = d, J = j|D > 0) &= P(J = j|D = d)\frac{P(D = d, D > 0)}{P(D > 0)} \\ &= (1 - p_0)^{-1}2^{-n}\binom{d}{j}\binom{n}{d}\left(1 - e^{-\frac{T-\mu}{\sigma}}\right)^{d-j} e^{-\frac{(T-\mu)(n-d)}{\sigma}}. \end{aligned} \tag{16.35}$$

Now, the joint distribution of $X_{1:d}, \cdots, X_{d:d}$, conditional on $D = d$ and $J = j$, is given by

$$f(X_{1:d}, \cdots, X_{d:d}|D = d, J = j) = j!(d - j)!\prod_{i=1}^{j}\frac{1}{\sigma}e^{-\frac{\mu - x_{i:d}}{\sigma}}\prod_{i=j+1}^{d}\frac{\frac{1}{\sigma}e^{-\frac{x_{i:d}-\mu}{\sigma}}}{1 - e^{-\frac{T-\mu}{\sigma}}},$$
$$x_{1:d} < \cdots < x_{j:d} < \mu < x_{j+1:d} < \cdots < x_{d:d} < T. \tag{16.36}$$

For the case when $D \leq \frac{n}{2}$, and given $J = j$, we find

$$\hat{\sigma}|_{D=d,J=j} \stackrel{d}{=} \sum_{i=1}^{j} E\left(\frac{\sigma}{d}\right) + \sum_{i=j+1}^{d} E_R^*\left(\frac{\sigma}{d}, T - \mu\right) + T - \mu, \tag{16.37}$$

where $E^*(\theta)$ denotes the negative exponential distribution with scale parameter θ, that is, if X follows the exponential distribution, then $-X$ is negative exponentially distributed, i.e., $X \sim E(\theta)$, $-X \sim E^*(\theta)$, and $E_R^*(\sigma, T)$ denotes a negative exponential distribution right truncated at time T. Then, we have the conditional MGF of $\hat{\sigma}$ as

$$E[e^{t\hat{\sigma}}|D=d, J=j] = e^{t(T-\mu)}\left(1-\frac{t\sigma}{d}\right)^{-j}\left(1+\frac{t\sigma}{d}\right)^{-(d-j)}\left\{\frac{1-e^{-(T-\mu)(\frac{1}{\sigma}+\frac{t}{d})}}{1-e^{-\frac{T-\mu}{\sigma}}}\right\}^{d-j}$$
$$= \sum_{l=0}^{d-j}\binom{d-j}{l}(-1)^l\left(1-e^{-\frac{T-\mu}{\sigma}}\right)^{-(d-j)} e^{-\frac{(T-\mu)l}{\sigma}} e^{(T-\mu)\frac{(d-l)t}{d}}$$
$$\times\left(1-\frac{t\sigma}{d}\right)^{-j}\left(1+\frac{t\sigma}{d}\right)^{-(d-j)}. \quad (16.38)$$

For the case when $D > m$, we need to consider $J \le m$ and $J > m$ separately. When $J \le m$, similarly, we will have the first j failures as i.i.d. exponential random variables, denoted by $X_1, \cdots, X_j$. For the remaining $d-j$ failures, we may consider them as $m-j$ i.i.d. failures before $X_{m+1:d}$ and $d-m-1$ i.i.d. failures after $X_{m+1:d}$ with $\mu < X_{m+1:d} < T$, denoted by $X_{j+1}, \cdots, X_m$ and $X_{m+2}, \cdots, X_d$, respectively.

The joint pdf $\mathbf{X} = (X_1, \cdots, X_m, X_{m+1:d}, X_{m+2}, \cdots, X_d)$ is given by

$$f(\mathbf{X}|D=d, J=j) = \frac{(d-j)!}{(m-j)!(d-m-1)!}\left(\prod_{i=1}^{j}\frac{1}{\sigma}e^{-\frac{\mu-x_i}{\sigma}}\right)\left(\prod_{i=j}^{m}\frac{\frac{1}{\sigma}e^{-\frac{x_i-\mu}{\sigma}}}{1-e^{-\frac{T-\mu}{\sigma}}}\right)$$
$$\times\left(\frac{\frac{1}{\sigma}e^{-\frac{x_{m+1:d}-\mu}{\sigma}}}{1-e^{-\frac{T-\mu}{\sigma}}}\right)\left(\prod_{i=m+2}^{d}\frac{\frac{1}{\sigma}e^{-\frac{x_i-\mu}{\sigma}}}{1-e^{-\frac{T-\mu}{\sigma}}}\right),$$
$$x_1, \cdots, x_j < \mu < x_{j+1}, \cdots, x_m < x_{m+1:d} < x_{m+2}, \cdots, x_d < T. \quad (16.39)$$

Then, the conditional MGF can be derived as follows:

$$E[e^{t\hat{\sigma}}|J=j, D=d]$$
$$= \frac{(d-j)!}{(m-j)!(d-m-1)!}\left(1-e^{-\frac{T-\mu}{\sigma}}\right)^{-(d-j)} e^{\frac{(n-d)(T-\mu)t}{d}}\left[\int_{-\infty}^{\mu}\frac{1}{\sigma}e^{-(\mu-x)(\frac{1}{\sigma}-\frac{t}{d})}dx\right]^j$$
$$\times\int_{\mu}^{T}\left[\int_{\mu}^{x_{m+1:d}}\frac{1}{\sigma}e^{-(x-\mu)(\frac{1}{\sigma}+\frac{t}{d})}dx\right]^{m-j}\left[\int_{x_{m+1:d}}^{T}\frac{1}{\sigma}e^{-(x-\mu)(\frac{1}{\sigma}-\frac{t}{d})}dx\right]^{d-m-1}$$
$$\times\frac{1}{\sigma}e^{-(x_{m+1:d}-\mu)(\frac{1}{\sigma}-\frac{t}{d})}dx_{m+1:d}$$
$$= \sum_{l_1=0}^{m-j}\sum_{l_2=0}^{d-m-1}(-1)^{l_1+d-m-1-l_2}\binom{m-j}{l_1}\binom{d-m-1}{l_2}\frac{(d-j)!}{(m-j)!(d-m-1)!}$$
$$\times(l_1+l_2+1)^{-1}\left(1-e^{-\frac{T-\mu}{\sigma}}\right)^{-(d-j)} e^{(T-\mu)\left(\frac{(m-1-l_2)t}{d}-\frac{d-m-1-l_2}{\sigma}\right)}\left(1+\frac{t\sigma}{d}\right)^{-(m-j)}$$
$$\times\left(1-\frac{t\sigma}{d}\right)^{-(j+d-m-1)}\left\{1-\frac{t(l_2+1-l_1)\sigma}{d(l_1+l_2+1)}\right\}^{-1}\left\{1-e^{-(T-\mu)\left[\frac{l_1+l_2+1}{\sigma}-\frac{t(l_2+1-l_1)}{d}\right]}\right\}.$$

We can similarly derive the conditional MGF for the case when $J > m$.

Case II: $\mu > T$. In this case, we have

$$P(D = d|D > 0) = (1 - q_0)^{-1}\binom{n}{d}[F(T)]^d[1 - F(T)]^{n-d}$$
$$= (1 - q_0)^{-1}\binom{n}{d}\left(\frac{1}{2}e^{-\frac{\mu-T}{\sigma}}\right)^d\left(1 - \frac{1}{2}e^{-\frac{\mu-T}{\sigma}}\right)^{n-d} \quad (16.40)$$

Now, by adopting a similar procedure, we can obtain the corresponding conditional MGF. Finally, upon combining these expressions, we obtain the conditional MGF presented in Result 16.2.

Marginal and Joint CDF of W_1 and W_2

To derive the marginal and joint CDF of W_1 and W_2 as described in Lemma 16.1, we first need the following lemma.

Lemma 16.2 *Let $Y_1 \sim \Gamma(\alpha_1, \beta_1)$ and $Y_2 \sim \Gamma(\alpha_2, \beta_2)$ be independent variables with integer shape parameters α_1 and α_2 and $\beta_1, \beta_2 > 0$. Let $Y = Y_1 - Y_2$. Then, the CDF of Y, denoted by $\Gamma(y, \alpha_1, \alpha_2, \beta_1, \beta_2)$, is given by*

$$\begin{aligned}\Gamma(y, \alpha_1, \alpha_2, \beta_1, \beta_2) &= P(Y_1 \le y + y_2) = 1 - P(Y_1 > y + y_2)\\ &= 1 - \sum_{i=0}^{\alpha_1-1}\int_0^{\infty}\frac{1}{i!}\left(\frac{y+y_2}{\beta_1}\right)^i e^{-\frac{y+y_2}{\beta_1}}\frac{y_2^{\alpha_2-1}e^{-\frac{y_2}{\beta_2}}}{\Gamma(\alpha_2)\beta_2^{\alpha_2}}dy_2\\ &= 1 - \frac{\beta_1^{\alpha_2}}{\Gamma(\alpha_2)\,(\beta_1+\beta_2)^{\alpha_2}}\sum_{i=0}^{\alpha_1-1}\sum_{j=0}^{i}\frac{\Gamma(\alpha_2+j)\beta_1^{j-i}\beta_2^j y^{i-j}e^{-\frac{y}{\beta_1}}}{(i-j)!j!\,(\beta_1+\beta_2)^j}, \qquad y \ge 0;\end{aligned}$$

$$\begin{aligned}\Gamma(y, \alpha_1, \alpha_2, \beta_1, \beta_2) &= P(Y_2 \ge y_1 - y)\\ &= \frac{\beta_2^{\alpha_1}}{\Gamma(\alpha_1)\,(\beta_1+\beta_2)^{\alpha_1}}\sum_{i=0}^{\alpha_2-1}\sum_{j=0}^{i}\\ &\quad\times\frac{\Gamma(\alpha_1+j)\beta_2^{j-i}\beta_1^j(-y)^{i-j}e^{\frac{y}{\beta_2}}}{(i-j)!j!\,(\beta_1+\beta_2)^j}, \qquad y < 0.\end{aligned}$$

Now, the corresponding PDF is given by

$$f(y) = \begin{cases}\dfrac{\beta_1^{\alpha_2-\alpha_1}}{\Gamma(\alpha_2)(\beta_1+\beta_2)^{\alpha_2}}\displaystyle\sum_{j=0}^{\alpha_1-1}\frac{\Gamma(\alpha_2+j)\beta_1^j\beta_2^j y^{\alpha_1-j-1}e^{-\frac{y}{\beta_1}}}{(\alpha_1-j-1)!j!(\beta_1+\beta_2)^j}, & y \ge 0,\\[2ex] \dfrac{\beta_2^{\alpha_1-\alpha_2}}{\Gamma(\alpha_1)(\beta_1+\beta_2)^{\alpha_1}}\displaystyle\sum_{j=0}^{\alpha_2-1}\frac{\Gamma(\alpha_1+j)\beta_1^j\beta_2^j(-y)^{\alpha_2-j-1}e^{\frac{y}{\beta_2}}}{(\alpha_2-j-1)!j!(\beta_1+\beta_2)^j}, & y < 0.\end{cases}$$

The marginal distribution of W_2 is either exponential or is a linear combination of two exponential variables, and so its CDF is easy to obtain and is therefore omitted for brevity. By using Lemma 16.2, the marginal CDF of W_1 can be readily obtained as presented in the following lemma.

Lemma 16.3 *Let $Y_1 \sim \Gamma(\alpha_1, \beta_1)$, $Y_2 \sim N\Gamma(\alpha_2, \beta_2)$, with α_1 and α_2 being positive integer shape parameters and β_1 and $\beta_2 > 0$. Further, let $Z_1 \sim E(1)$ and $Z_2 \sim E(1)$, with $a_1 \neq a_2 \neq \beta_1$ (and β_2) > 0. If Y_1, Y_2, Z_1, and Z_2 are all independent, then the CDF of $W_1 = Y_1 + Y_2 + a_1 Z_1 - a_2 Z_2$ is as follows:*

$$P(W_1 \le w_1) = \frac{a_2 e^{\frac{w_1}{a_2}}}{a_1 + a_2} \sum_{j=0}^{\alpha_1 - 1} C_j F\left(w_1, \infty, \alpha_1 - j, \frac{1}{\beta_1} + \frac{1}{a_2}\right) + \Gamma(w_1, \alpha_1, \alpha_2, \beta_1, \beta_2)$$
$$- \frac{a_1 e^{-\frac{w_1}{a_1}}}{a_1 + a_2} \sum_{j=0}^{\alpha_2 - 1} C_j^* F\left(-\infty, 0, \alpha_2 - j, -\frac{1}{\beta_2} - \frac{1}{a_1}\right)$$
$$- \frac{a_1 e^{-\frac{w_1}{a_1}}}{a_1 + a_2} \sum_{j=0}^{\alpha_1 - 1} C_j F\left(0, w_1, \alpha_1 - j, \frac{1}{\beta_1} - \frac{1}{a_1}\right), \quad w_1 \ge 0; \tag{16.41}$$

$$P(W_1 \le w_1) = \frac{a_2 e^{\frac{w_1}{a_2}}}{a_1 + a_2} \sum_{j=0}^{\alpha_2 - 1} C_j^* F\left(w_1, 0, \alpha_2 - j, \frac{1}{a_2} - \frac{1}{\beta_2}\right)$$
$$+ \frac{a_2 e^{\frac{w_1}{a_2}}}{a_1 + a_2} \sum_{j=0}^{\alpha_1 - 1} C_j F\left(0, \infty, \alpha_1 - j, \frac{1}{\beta_1} + \frac{1}{a_2}\right) + \Gamma(w_1, \alpha_1, \alpha_2, \beta_1, \beta_2)$$
$$- \frac{a_1 e^{-\frac{w}{a_1}}}{a_1 + a_2} \sum_{j=0}^{\alpha_2 - 1} C_j^* F\left(-\infty, w_1, \alpha_2 - j, -\frac{1}{\beta_2} - \frac{1}{a_1}\right), \quad w_1 < 0. \tag{16.42}$$

The CDF of $W_1 = Y_1 + Y_2 + a_1 Z_1 + a_2 Z_2$ is as follows:

$$P(W_1 \le w_1) = \Gamma(w_1, \alpha_1, \alpha_2, \beta_1, \beta_2) - \frac{a_2}{a_2 - a_1} e^{-\frac{w_1}{a_2}} \sum_{j=0}^{\alpha_1 - 1} C_j F\left(0, w_1, \alpha_1 - j, \frac{1}{\beta_1} - \frac{1}{a_2}\right)$$
$$- \frac{a_2 e^{-\frac{w_1}{a_2}}}{a_2 - a_1} \sum_{j=0}^{\alpha_2 - 1} C_j^* F\left(-\infty, 0, \alpha_2 - j, -\frac{1}{\beta_2} - \frac{1}{a_2}\right)$$
$$+ \frac{a_1}{a_2 - a_1} e^{-\frac{w}{\theta_1}} \sum_{j=0}^{\alpha_1 - 1} C_j F\left(0, w_1, \alpha_1 - j, \frac{1}{\beta_1} - \frac{1}{a_1}\right)$$
$$+ \frac{a_1}{a_2 - a_1} e^{-\frac{w_1}{a_1}} \sum_{j=0}^{\alpha_2 - 1} C_j^* F\left(-\infty, 0, \alpha_2 - j, -\frac{1}{\beta_2} - \frac{1}{a_1}\right), \quad w_1 \ge 0; \tag{16.43}$$

$$P(W_1 \le w_1) = \Gamma(w_1, \alpha_1, \alpha_2, \beta_1, \beta_2) - \frac{a_2 e^{-\frac{w_1}{a_2}}}{a_2 - a_1} \sum_{j=0}^{\alpha_2 - 1} C_j^* F\left(-\infty, w_1, \alpha_2 - j, -\frac{1}{\beta_2} - \frac{1}{a_2}\right)$$
$$+ \frac{a_1 e^{-\frac{w_1}{a_1}}}{a_2 - a_1} \sum_{j=0}^{\alpha_2 - 1} C_j^* F\left(-\infty, w_1, \alpha_2 - j, -\frac{1}{\beta_2} - \frac{1}{a_1}\right), \quad w_1 < 0. \tag{16.44}$$

By using Lemmas 16.2 and 16.3, the joint CDF of W_1 and W_2 can be derived as presented in Tables 16.10, 16.11, 16.12, 16.13, 16.14, 16.15, 16.16, 16.17, 16.18,

16.19, 16.20, and 16.21. Note in these tables that all the coefficients a_1, a_2, b_1, and b_2 are positive, all the scale parameters β_1, β_2 are positive, and the shape parameters α_1 and α_2 are positive integers. Moreover, in these tables, we have used the notation

$$
\begin{aligned}
r_1 &= w_1 - \frac{a_1 w_2}{b_1},\\
r_2 &= w_1,\\
r_3 &= w_1 + \frac{a_2 w_2}{b_2},\\
r_4 &= w_1 + \frac{a_1 w_2}{b_1},\\
r_i^* &= \max(r_i, 0), \qquad i = 1, \cdots, 4,\\
S\Gamma\,(l, r, \alpha_1, \alpha_2, \beta_1, \beta_2) &= \Gamma\,(r, \alpha_1, \alpha_2, \beta_1, \beta_2) - \Gamma\,(l, \alpha_1, \alpha_2, \beta_1, \beta_2),\\
C_j &= \frac{\Gamma(\alpha_2 + j)\beta_1^{\alpha_2-\alpha_1+j}\beta_2^j}{\Gamma(\alpha_2)(\alpha_1 - j - 1)!j!\,(\beta_1 + \beta_2)^{\alpha_2+j}},\\
C_j^* &= \frac{\Gamma(\alpha_1 + j)\beta_1^j\beta_2^{\alpha_1-\alpha_2+j}}{\Gamma(\alpha_1)(\alpha_2 - j - 1)!j!\,(\beta_1 + \beta_2)^{\alpha_1+j}},\\
C_\Gamma &= \frac{1}{\Gamma(\alpha)\beta^\alpha},
\end{aligned}
$$

and

$$
\begin{aligned}
F\,(l, r, \theta_1, \theta_2) &= \int_l^r x^{\theta_1-1}e^{-x\theta_2}dx\\
&= \begin{cases}
\frac{\Gamma(\theta_1)}{\theta_2^{\theta_1}}\left(\Gamma(r, \theta_1, \theta_2^{-1}) - \Gamma(l, \theta_1, \theta_2^{-1})\right), & \theta_2 > 0, l > 0,\\
\frac{\Gamma(\theta_1)}{(-\theta_2)^{\theta_1}}\left(\Gamma(-l, \theta_1, \theta_2^{-1}) - \Gamma(-r, \theta_1, \theta_2^{-1})\right), & \theta_2 > 0, r < 0,\\
\frac{1}{\theta_1}\left(r^{\theta_1} - l^{\theta_1}\right), & \theta_2 = 0,\\
-\sum_{j=0}^{\theta_1-1}\frac{(\theta_1-1)!}{j!\theta_2^{\theta_1-j}}\left(r^j e^{-r\theta_2} - l^j e^{-l\theta_2}\right), & \theta_2 < 0.
\end{cases}
\end{aligned}
$$

By using these results, we can also obtain a more general result for the joint CDF of $W_1 = Y_1 + Y_2 + a_1 Z_1 + a_2 Z_2$ and $W_2 = b_1 Z_1 + b_2 Z_2$ by using the known results on the joint CDF of $-W_1$ and W_2 and the CDF of W_2 as

$$
\begin{aligned}
P(W_1 \le w_1, W_2 \le w_2) &= P(-W_1 \ge -w_1, W_2 \le w_2)\\
&= P(W_2 \le w_2) - P(-W_1 \le -w_1, W_2 \le w_2).
\end{aligned}
$$

Table 16.10 Joint CDF of $W_1 = Y_1 + Y_2 - a_1 Z_1 - a_2 Z_2$ and $W_2 = b_1 Z_1 + b_2 Z_2$

Case I: $a_1 \neq a_2, b_1 \neq b_2, w_1 \geq 0, a_1 b_2 > a_2 b_1$
$\Gamma(r_2, \alpha_1, \alpha_2, \beta_1, \beta_2) - \frac{b_2 e^{-\frac{w_2}{b_2}}}{b_2 - b_1} \Gamma(r_3, \alpha_1, \alpha_2, \beta_1, \beta_2) + \frac{b_1 e^{-\frac{w_2}{b_1}}}{b_2 - b_1} \Gamma(r_4, \alpha_1, \alpha_2, \beta_1, \beta_2)$
$+ \frac{a_1 e^{\frac{w_1}{a_1}}}{a_1 - a_2} \sum_{j=0}^{\alpha_1 - 1} C_j F\left(r_2, r_4, \alpha_1 - j, \frac{1}{a_1} + \frac{1}{\beta_1}\right)$
$+ \frac{e^{\frac{(b_2 - b_1) w_1 + (a_2 - a_1) w_2}{a_1 b_2 - a_2 b_1}}}{\left(\frac{a_1}{a_2 - a_1} - \frac{b_1}{b_2 - b_1}\right)^{-1}} \sum_{j=0}^{\alpha_1 - 1} C_j F\left(r_3, r_4, \alpha_1 - j, \frac{1}{\beta_1} + \frac{b_2 - b_1}{a_1 b_2 - a_2 b_1}\right)$
$+ \frac{a_2 e^{\frac{w_1}{a_2}}}{a_2 - a_1} \sum_{j=0}^{\alpha_1 - 1} C_j F\left(r_2, r_3, \alpha_1 - j, \frac{1}{a_2} + \frac{1}{\beta_1}\right)$
Case II: $a_1 \neq a_2, b_1 \neq b_2, w_1 < 0, r_3 \geq 0, a_1 b_2 > a_2 b_1$
$\Gamma(r_2, \alpha_1, \alpha_2, \beta_1, \beta_2) - \frac{b_2 e^{-\frac{w_2}{b_2}}}{b_2 - b_1} \Gamma(r_3, \alpha_1, \alpha_2, \beta_1, \beta_2) + \frac{b_1 e^{-\frac{w_2}{b_1}}}{b_2 - b_1} \Gamma(r_4, \alpha_1, \alpha_2, \beta_1, \beta_2)$
$+ \frac{a_1 e^{\frac{w_1}{a_1}}}{a_1 - a_2} \sum_{j=0}^{\alpha_2 - 1} C_j^* F\left(r_2, 0, \alpha_2 - j, \frac{1}{a_1} - \frac{1}{\beta_2}\right) + \frac{a_1 e^{\frac{w_1}{a_1}}}{a_1 - a_2} \sum_{j=0}^{\alpha_1 - 1} C_j F\left(0, r_4, \alpha_1 - j, \frac{1}{a_1} + \frac{1}{\beta_1}\right)$
$+ \frac{e^{\frac{(b_2 - b_1) w_1 + (a_2 - a_1) w_2}{a_1 b_2 - a_2 b_1}}}{\left(\frac{a_1}{a_2 - a_1} - \frac{b_1}{b_2 - b_1}\right)^{-1}} \sum_{j=0}^{\alpha_1 - 1} C_j F\left(r_3, r_4, \alpha_1 - j, \frac{1}{\beta_1} + \frac{b_2 - b_1}{a_1 b_2 - a_2 b_1}\right)$
$+ \frac{a_2 e^{\frac{w_1}{a_2}}}{a_2 - a_1} \sum_{j=0}^{\alpha_2 - 1} C_j^* F\left(r_2, 0, \alpha_2 - j, \frac{1}{a_2} - \frac{1}{\beta_2}\right)$
$+ \frac{a_2 e^{\frac{w_1}{a_2}}}{a_2 - a_1} \sum_{j=0}^{\alpha_1 - 1} C_j F\left(0, r_3, \alpha_1 - j, \frac{1}{a_2} + \frac{1}{\beta_1}\right)$
Case III: $a_1 \neq a_2, b_1 \neq b_2, w_1 < 0, r_3 < 0, r_4 \geq 0, a_1 b_2 > a_2 b_1$
$\Gamma(r_2, \alpha_1, \alpha_2, \beta_1, \beta_2) - \frac{b_2 e^{-\frac{w_2}{b_2}}}{b_2 - b_1} \Gamma(r_3, \alpha_1, \alpha_2, \beta_1, \beta_2) + \frac{b_1 e^{-\frac{w_2}{b_1}}}{b_2 - b_1} \Gamma(r_4, \alpha_1, \alpha_2, \beta_1, \beta_2)$
$+ \frac{a_1 e^{\frac{w_1}{a_1}}}{a_1 - a_2} \sum_{j=0}^{\alpha_2 - 1} C_j^* F\left(r_2, 0, \alpha_2 - j, \frac{1}{a_1} - \frac{1}{\beta_2}\right) + \frac{a_1 e^{\frac{w_1}{a_1}}}{a_1 - a_2} \sum_{j=0}^{\alpha_1 - 1} C_j F\left(0, r_4, \alpha_1 - j, \frac{1}{a_1} + \frac{1}{\beta_1}\right)$
$+ \frac{e^{\frac{(b_2 - b_1) w_1 + (a_2 - a_1) w_2}{a_1 b_2 - a_2 b_1}}}{\left(\frac{a_1}{a_2 - a_1} - \frac{b_1}{b_2 - b_1}\right)^{-1}} \left[\sum_{j=0}^{\alpha_2 - 1} C_j^* F\left(r_3, 0, \alpha_2 - j, \frac{b_2 - b_1}{a_1 b_2 - a_2 b_1} - \frac{1}{\beta_2}\right) + \sum_{j=0}^{\alpha_1 - 1} C_j F\left(0, r_4, \alpha_1 - j, \frac{1}{\beta_1} + \frac{b_2 - b_1}{a_1 b_2 - a_2 b_1}\right) \right]$
$+ \frac{a_2 e^{\frac{w_1}{a_2}}}{a_2 - a_1} \sum_{j=0}^{\alpha_2 - 1} C_j^* F\left(r_2, r_3, \alpha_2 - j, \frac{1}{a_2} - \frac{1}{\beta_2}\right)$

(continued)

Table 16.10 (continued)

Case IV: $a_1 \neq a_2, b_1 \neq b_2, w_1 < 0, b_1 w_1 + a_1 w_2 < 0, a_1 b_2 > a_2 b_1$
$\Gamma(r_2, \alpha_1, \alpha_2, \beta_1, \beta_2) - \frac{b_2 e^{-\frac{w_2}{b_2}}}{b_2-b_1} \Gamma(r_3, \alpha_1, \alpha_2, \beta_1, \beta_2) + \frac{b_1 e^{-\frac{w_2}{b_1}}}{b_2-b_1} \Gamma(r_4, \alpha_1, \alpha_2, \beta_1, \beta_2)$
$+\frac{a_1 e^{\frac{w_1}{a_1}}}{a_1-a_2} \sum_{j=0}^{\alpha_2-1} C_j^* F\left(r_2, r_4, \alpha_2 - j, \frac{1}{a_1} - \frac{1}{\beta_2}\right)$
$+\frac{e^{\frac{(b_2-b_1)w_1+(a_2-a_1)w_2}{a_1 b_2 - a_2 b_1}}}{\left(\frac{a_1}{a_2-a_1} - \frac{b_1}{b_2-b_1}\right)^{-1}} \sum_{j=0}^{\alpha_2-1} C_j^* F\left(r_3, r_4, \alpha_2 - j, \frac{b_2-b_1}{a_1 b_2 - a_2 b_1} - \frac{1}{\beta_2}\right)$
$+\frac{a_2 e^{\frac{w_1}{a_2}}}{a_2-a_1} \sum_{j=0}^{\alpha_2-1} C_j^* F\left(r_2, r_3, \alpha_2 - j, \frac{1}{a_2} - \frac{1}{\beta_2}\right)$
Case V: $a_1 \neq a_2, b_1 \neq b_2, w_1 \geq 0, a_1 b_2 = a_2 b_1$
$\Gamma(r_2, \alpha_1, \alpha_2, \beta_1, \beta_2) + \frac{b_1 e^{-\frac{w_2}{b_1}} - b_2 e^{-\frac{w_2}{b_2}}}{b_2-b_1} \Gamma(r_3, \alpha_1, \alpha_2, \beta_1, \beta_2)$
$+\frac{a_1 e^{\frac{w_1}{a_1}}}{a_1-a_2} \sum_{j=0}^{\alpha_1-1} C_j F\left(r_2, r_3, \alpha_1 - j, \frac{1}{a_1} + \frac{1}{\beta_1}\right)$
$+\frac{a_2 e^{\frac{w_1}{a_2}}}{a_2-a_1} \sum_{j=0}^{\alpha_1-1} C_j F\left(r_2, r_3, \alpha_1 - j, \frac{1}{a_2} + \frac{1}{\beta_1}\right)$
Case VI: $a_1 \neq a_2, b_1 \neq b_2, w_1 < 0, r_3 \geq 0, a_1 b_2 = a_2 b_1$
$\Gamma(r_2, \alpha_1, \alpha_2, \beta_1, \beta_2) + \frac{b_1 e^{-\frac{w_2}{b_1}} - b_2 e^{-\frac{w_2}{b_2}}}{b_2-b_1} \Gamma(r_3, \alpha_1, \alpha_2, \beta_1, \beta_2)$
$+\frac{a_1 e^{\frac{w_1}{a_1}}}{a_1-a_2} \sum_{j=0}^{\alpha_2-1} C_j^* F\left(r_2, 0, \alpha_2 - j, \frac{1}{a_1} - \frac{1}{\beta_2}\right)$
$+\frac{a_1 e^{\frac{w_1}{a_1}}}{a_1-a_2} \sum_{j=0}^{\alpha_1-1} C_j F\left(0, r_3, \alpha_1 - j, \frac{1}{a_1} + \frac{1}{\beta_1}\right) + \frac{a_2 e^{\frac{w_1}{a_2}}}{a_2-a_1} \sum_{j=0}^{\alpha_2-1} C_j^* F\left(r_2, 0, \alpha_2 - j, \frac{1}{a_2} - \frac{1}{\beta_2}\right)$
$+\frac{a_2 e^{\frac{w_1}{a_2}}}{a_2-a_1} \sum_{j=0}^{\alpha_1-1} C_j F\left(0, r_3, \alpha_1 - j, \frac{1}{a_2} + \frac{1}{\beta_1}\right)$
Case VII: $a_1 \neq a_2, b_1 \neq b_2, w_1 < 0, r_3 < 0, a_1 b_2 = a_2 b_1$
$\Gamma(r_2, \alpha_1, \alpha_2, \beta_1, \beta_2) + \frac{b_1 e^{-\frac{w_2}{b_1}} - b_2 e^{-\frac{w_2}{b_2}}}{b_2-b_1} \Gamma(r_3, \alpha_1, \alpha_2, \beta_1, \beta_2)$
$+\frac{a_1 e^{\frac{w_1}{a_1}}}{a_1-a_2} \sum_{j=0}^{\alpha_2-1} C_j^* F\left(r_2, r_3, \alpha_2 - j, \frac{1}{a_1} - \frac{1}{\beta_2}\right)$
$+\frac{a_2 e^{\frac{w_1}{a_2}}}{a_2-a_1} \sum_{j=0}^{\alpha_2-1} C_j^* F\left(r_2, r_3, \alpha_2 - j, \frac{1}{a_2} - \frac{1}{\beta_2}\right)$

(continued)

Table 16.10 (continued)

Case VIII: $a_1 = a_2 = a, b_2 > b_1, w_1 \geq 0$

$$\Gamma(r_2, \alpha_1, \alpha_2, \beta_1, \beta_2) - \frac{b_2 e^{-\frac{w_2}{b_2}}}{b_2 - b_1} \Gamma(r_3, \alpha_1, \alpha_2, \beta_1, \beta_2) + \frac{b_1 e^{-\frac{w_2}{b_1}}}{b_2 - b_1} \Gamma(r_4, \alpha_1, \alpha_2, \beta_1, \beta_2)$$

$$+ \frac{e^{\frac{w_1}{a}}}{a} \sum_{j=0}^{\alpha_1 - 1} C_j F\left(r_2, r_3, \alpha_1 + 1 - j, \tfrac{1}{a} + \tfrac{1}{\beta_1}\right) - \frac{(w_1 - a) e^{\frac{w_1}{a}}}{a} \sum_{j=0}^{\alpha_1 - 1} C_j F\left(r_2, r_3, \alpha_1 - j, \tfrac{1}{a} + \tfrac{1}{\beta_1}\right)$$

$$+ \frac{(b_1 w_1 + a w_2 - a b_1) e^{\frac{w_1}{a}}}{a(b_2 - b_1)} \sum_{j=0}^{\alpha_1 - 1} C_j F\left(r_3, r_4, \alpha_1 - j, \tfrac{1}{a} + \tfrac{1}{\beta_1}\right)$$

$$- \frac{b_1 e^{\frac{w_1}{a}}}{a(b_2 - b_1)} \sum_{j=0}^{\alpha_1 - 1} C_j F\left(r_3, r_4, \alpha_1 + 1 - j, \tfrac{1}{a} + \tfrac{1}{\beta_1}\right)$$

Case IX: $a_1 = a_2 = a, b_2 > b_1, w_1 < 0, r_3 \geq 0$

$$\Gamma(r_2, \alpha_1, \alpha_2, \beta_1, \beta_2) - \frac{b_2 e^{-\frac{w_2}{b_2}}}{b_2 - b_1} \Gamma(r_3, \alpha_1, \alpha_2, \beta_1, \beta_2) + \frac{b_1 e^{-\frac{w_2}{b_1}}}{b_2 - b_1} \Gamma(r_4, \alpha_1, \alpha_2, \beta_1, \beta_2)$$

$$+ \frac{e^{\frac{w_1}{a}}}{a} \sum_{j=0}^{\alpha_2 - 1} C_j^* F\left(r_2, 0, \alpha_2 + 1 - j, \tfrac{1}{a} - \tfrac{1}{\beta_2}\right) + \frac{e^{\frac{w_1}{a}}}{a} \sum_{j=0}^{\alpha_1 - 1} C_j F\left(0, r_3, \alpha_1 + 1 - j, \tfrac{1}{a} + \tfrac{1}{\beta_1}\right)$$

$$- \frac{(w_1 - a) e^{\frac{w_1}{a}}}{a} \sum_{j=0}^{\alpha_2 - 1} C_j^* F\left(r_2, 0, \alpha_2 - j, \tfrac{1}{a} - \tfrac{1}{\beta_2}\right) - \frac{(w_1 - a) e^{\frac{w_1}{a}}}{a} \sum_{j=0}^{\alpha_1 - 1} C_j F\left(0, r_3, \alpha_1 - j, \tfrac{1}{a} + \tfrac{1}{\beta_1}\right)$$

$$+ \frac{(b_1 w_1 + a w_2 - a b_1) e^{\frac{w_1}{a}}}{a(b_2 - b_1)} \sum_{j=0}^{\alpha_1 - 1} C_j F\left(r_3, r_4, \alpha_1 - j, \tfrac{1}{a} + \tfrac{1}{\beta_1}\right)$$

$$- \frac{b_1 e^{\frac{w_1}{a}}}{a(b_2 - b_1)} \sum_{j=0}^{\alpha_1 - 1} C_j F\left(r_3, r_4, \alpha_1 + 1 - j, \tfrac{1}{a} + \tfrac{1}{\beta_1}\right)$$

Case X: $a_1 = a_2 = a, b_2 > b_1, w_1 < 0, r_3 < 0, r_4 \geq 0$

$$\Gamma(r_2, \alpha_1, \alpha_2, \beta_1, \beta_2) - \frac{b_2 e^{-\frac{w_2}{b_2}}}{b_2 - b_1} \Gamma(r_3, \alpha_1, \alpha_2, \beta_1, \beta_2) + \frac{b_1 e^{-\frac{w_2}{b_1}}}{b_2 - b_1} \Gamma(r_4, \alpha_1, \alpha_2, \beta_1, \beta_2)$$

$$+ \frac{e^{\frac{w_1}{a}}}{a} \sum_{j=0}^{\alpha_2 - 1} C_j^* F\left(r_2, r_3, \alpha_2 + 1 - j, \tfrac{1}{a} - \tfrac{1}{\beta_2}\right) - \frac{(w_1 - a) e^{\frac{w_1}{a}}}{a} \sum_{j=0}^{\alpha_2 - 1} C_j^* F\left(r_2, r_3, \alpha_2 - j, \tfrac{1}{a} - \tfrac{1}{\beta_2}\right)$$

$$+ \frac{(b_1 w_1 + a w_2 - a b_1) e^{\frac{w_1}{a}}}{a(b_2 - b_1)} \sum_{j=0}^{\alpha_2 - 1} C_j^* F\left(r_3, 0, \alpha_2 - j, \tfrac{1}{a} - \tfrac{1}{\beta_2}\right)$$

$$+ \frac{(b_1 w_1 + a w_2 - a b_1) e^{\frac{w_1}{a}}}{a(b_2 - b_1)} \sum_{j=0}^{\alpha_1 - 1} C_j F\left(0, r_4, \alpha_1 - j, \tfrac{1}{a} + \tfrac{1}{\beta_1}\right)$$

$$- \frac{b_1 e^{\frac{w_1}{a}}}{a(b_2 - b_1)} \sum_{j=0}^{\alpha_2 - 1} C_j^* F\left(r_3, 0, \alpha_2 + 1 - j, \tfrac{1}{a} - \tfrac{1}{\beta_2}\right)$$

$$- \frac{b_1 e^{\frac{w_1}{a}}}{a(b_2 - b_1)} \sum_{j=0}^{\alpha_1 - 1} C_j F\left(0, r_4, \alpha_1 + 1 - j, \tfrac{1}{a} + \tfrac{1}{\beta_1}\right)$$

(continued)

Table 16.10 (continued)

Case XI: $a_1 = a_2 = a, b_2 > b_1, w_1 < 0, r_4 < 0$

$$\Gamma(r_2,\alpha_1,\alpha_2,\beta_1,\beta_2) - \frac{b_2 e^{-\frac{w_2}{b_2}}}{b_2-b_1}\Gamma(r_3,\alpha_1,\alpha_2,\beta_1,\beta_2) + \frac{b_1 e^{-\frac{w_2}{b_1}}}{b_2-b_1}\Gamma(r_4,\alpha_1,\alpha_2,\beta_1,\beta_2)$$

$$+\frac{e^{\frac{w_1}{a}}}{a}\sum_{j=0}^{\alpha_2-1} C_j^* F\left(r_2, r_3, \alpha_2+1-j, \tfrac{1}{a}-\tfrac{1}{\beta_2}\right) - \frac{(w_1-a)e^{\frac{w_1}{a}}}{a}\sum_{j=0}^{\alpha_2-1} C_j^* F\left(r_2, r_3, \alpha_2-j, \tfrac{1}{a}-\tfrac{1}{\beta_2}\right)$$

$$+\frac{(b_1w_1+aw_2-ab_1)e^{\frac{w_1}{a}}}{a(b_2-b_1)}\sum_{j=0}^{\alpha_2-1} C_j^* F\left(r_3, r_4, \alpha_2-j, \tfrac{1}{a}-\tfrac{1}{\beta_2}\right)$$

$$-\frac{b_1 e^{\frac{w_1}{a}}}{a(b_2-b_1)}\sum_{j=0}^{\alpha_2-1} C_j^* F\left(r_3, r_4, \alpha_2+1-j, \tfrac{1}{a}-\tfrac{1}{\beta_2}\right)$$

Case XII: $a_1 > a_2, b_1 = b_2 = b, w_1 \geq 0$

$$\Gamma(r_2,\alpha_1,\alpha_2,\beta_1,\beta_2) - \frac{b+w_2}{b}e^{-\frac{w_2}{b}}\Gamma(r_3,\alpha_1,\alpha_2,\beta_1,\beta_2)$$

$$+\frac{a_1 e^{\frac{w_1}{a_1}}}{a_1-a_2}\sum_{j=0}^{\alpha_1-1} C_j F\left(r_2, r_4, \alpha_1-j, \tfrac{1}{a_1}+\tfrac{1}{\beta_1}\right)$$

$$+\frac{a_2 e^{\frac{w_1}{a_2}}}{a_2-a_1}\sum_{j=0}^{\alpha_1-1} C_j F\left(r_2, r_3, \alpha_1-j, \tfrac{1}{a_2}+\tfrac{1}{\beta_1}\right) - \frac{(a_1b+a_1w_2+bw_1)e^{-\frac{w_2}{b}}}{b(a_1-a_2)} S\Gamma(r_3, r_4, \alpha_1, \alpha_2, \beta_1, \beta_2)$$

$$+\frac{e^{-\frac{w_2}{b}}}{a_1-a_2}\sum_{j=0}^{\alpha_1-1} C_j F\left(r_3, r_4, \alpha_1+1-j, \tfrac{1}{\beta_1}\right)$$

Case XIII: $a_1 > a_2, b_1 = b_2 = b, w_1 < 0, r_3 \geq 0$

$$\Gamma(r_2,\alpha_1,\alpha_2,\beta_1,\beta_2) - \frac{b+w_2}{b}e^{-\frac{w_2}{b}}\Gamma(r_3,\alpha_1,\alpha_2,\beta_1,\beta_2)$$

$$+\frac{a_1 e^{\frac{w_1}{a_1}}}{a_1-a_2}\sum_{j=0}^{\alpha_2-1} C_j^* F\left(r_2, 0, \alpha_2-j, \tfrac{1}{a_1}-\tfrac{1}{\beta_2}\right)$$

$$+\frac{a_1 e^{\frac{w_1}{a_1}}}{a_1-a_2}\sum_{j=0}^{\alpha_1-1} C_j F\left(0, r_4, \alpha_1-j, \tfrac{1}{a_1}+\tfrac{1}{\beta_1}\right) + \frac{a_2 e^{\frac{w_1}{a_2}}}{a_2-a_1}\sum_{j=0}^{\alpha_2-1} C_j^* F\left(r_2, 0, \alpha_2-j, \tfrac{1}{a_2}-\tfrac{1}{\beta_2}\right)$$

$$+\frac{a_2 e^{\frac{w_1}{a_2}}}{a_2-a_1}\sum_{j=0}^{\alpha_1-1} C_j F\left(0, r_3, \alpha_1-j, \tfrac{1}{a_2}+\tfrac{1}{\beta_1}\right) - \frac{(a_1b+a_1w_2+bw_1)e^{-\frac{w_2}{b}}}{b(a_1-a_2)} S\Gamma(r_3, r_4, \alpha_1, \alpha_2, \beta_1, \beta_2)$$

$$+\frac{e^{-\frac{w_2}{b}}}{a_1-a_2}\sum_{j=0}^{\alpha_1-1} C_j F\left(r_3, r_4, \alpha_1+1-j, \tfrac{1}{\beta_1}\right)$$

(continued)

Table 16.10 (continued)

Case XIV: $a_1 > a_2, b_1 = b_2 = b, w_1 < 0, r_3 < 0, r_4 \geq 0$
$\Gamma(r_2,\alpha_1,\alpha_2,\beta_1,\beta_2) - \frac{b+w_2}{b}e^{-\frac{w_2}{b}}\Gamma(r_3,\alpha_1,\alpha_2,\beta_1,\beta_2)$
$+\frac{a_1 e^{\frac{w_1}{a_1}}}{a_1-a_2}\sum_{j=0}^{\alpha_2-1} C_j^* F\left(r_2, 0, \alpha_2-j, \frac{1}{a_1}-\frac{1}{\beta_2}\right)$
$+\frac{a_1 e^{\frac{w_1}{a_1}}}{a_1-a_2}\sum_{j=0}^{\alpha_1-1} C_j F\left(0, r_4, \alpha_1-j, \frac{1}{a_1}+\frac{1}{\beta_1}\right) + \frac{a_2 e^{\frac{w_1}{a_2}}}{a_2-a_1}\sum_{j=0}^{\alpha_2-1} C_j^* F\left(r_2, r_3, \alpha_2-j, \frac{1}{a_2}-\frac{1}{\beta_2}\right)$
$-\frac{(a_1 b+a_1 w_2+b w_1)e^{-\frac{w_2}{b}}}{b(a_1-a_2)} S\Gamma(r_3,r_4,\alpha_1,\alpha_2,\beta_1,\beta_2) + \frac{e^{-\frac{w_2}{b}}}{a_1-a_2}\sum_{j=0}^{\alpha_2-1} C_j^* F\left(r_3, 0, \alpha_2+1-j, -\frac{1}{\beta_2}\right)$
$+\frac{e^{-\frac{w_2}{b}}}{a_1-a_2}\sum_{j=0}^{\alpha_1-1} C_j F\left(0, r_4, \alpha_1+1-j, \frac{1}{\beta_1}\right)$
Case XV: $a_1 > a_2, b_1 = b_2 = b, r_4 < 0$
$\Gamma(r_2,\alpha_1,\alpha_2,\beta_1,\beta_2) - \frac{b+w_2}{b}e^{-\frac{w_2}{b}}\Gamma(r_3,\alpha_1,\alpha_2,\beta_1,\beta_2)$
$+\frac{a_1 e^{\frac{w_1}{a_1}}}{a_1-a_2}\sum_{j=0}^{\alpha_2-1} C_j^* F\left(r_2, r_4, \alpha_2-j, \frac{1}{a_1}-\frac{1}{\beta_2}\right)$
$+\frac{a_2 e^{\frac{w_1}{a_2}}}{a_2-a_1}\sum_{j=0}^{\alpha_2-1} C_j^* F\left(r_2, r_3, \alpha_2-j, \frac{1}{a_2}-\frac{1}{\beta_2}\right) - \frac{(a_1 b+a_1 w_2+b w_1)e^{-\frac{w_2}{b}}}{b(a_1-a_2)} S\Gamma(r_3,r_4,\alpha_1,\alpha_2,\beta_1,\beta_2)$
$+\frac{e^{-\frac{w_2}{b}}}{a_1-a_2}\sum_{j=0}^{\alpha_2-1} C_j^* F\left(r_3, r_4, \alpha_2+1-j, -\frac{1}{\beta_2}\right)$
Case XVI: $a_1 = a_2 = a, b_1 = b_2 = b, w_1 \geq 0, r_2 \geq 0$
$\Gamma(r_2,\alpha_1,\alpha_2,\beta_1,\beta_2)\Gamma\left(\frac{w_2}{b_2}, 2, 1\right) - \frac{(b+w_2)e^{-\frac{w_2}{b}}}{b} S\Gamma(r_2,r_3,\alpha_1,\alpha_2,\beta_1,\beta_2)$
$\frac{(a-w_1)e^{\frac{w_1}{a}}}{a}\sum_{j=0}^{\alpha_1-1} C_j F\left(r_2, r_3, \alpha_1-j, \frac{1}{a}+\frac{1}{\beta_1}\right) + \frac{e^{\frac{w_1}{a}}}{a}\sum_{j=0}^{\alpha_1-1} C_j F\left(r_2, r_3, \alpha_1+1-j, \frac{1}{a}+\frac{1}{\beta_1}\right)$
Case XVII: $a_1 = a_2 = a, b_1 = b_2 = b, w_1 < 0, r_2 \geq 0$
$\Gamma(r_2,\alpha_1,\alpha_2,\beta_1,\beta_2)\Gamma\left(\frac{w_2}{b_2}, 2, 1\right) - \frac{(b+w_2)e^{-\frac{w_2}{b}}}{b} S\Gamma(r_2,r_3,\alpha_1,\alpha_2,\beta_1,\beta_2)$
$+\frac{(a-w_1)e^{\frac{w_1}{a}}}{a}\sum_{j=0}^{\alpha_2-1} C_j^* F\left(r_2, 0, \alpha_2-j, \frac{1}{a}-\frac{1}{\beta_2}\right) + \frac{(a-w_1)e^{\frac{w_1}{a}}}{a}\sum_{j=0}^{\alpha_1-1} C_j F\left(0, r_3, \alpha_1-j, \frac{1}{a}+\frac{1}{\beta_1}\right)$
$+\frac{e^{\frac{w_1}{a}}}{a}\sum_{j=0}^{\alpha_2-1} C_j^* F\left(r_2, 0, \alpha_2+1-j, \frac{1}{a}-\frac{1}{\beta_2}\right) + \frac{e^{\frac{w_1}{a}}}{a}\sum_{j=0}^{\alpha_1-1} C_j F\left(0, r_3, \alpha_1+1-j, \frac{1}{a}+\frac{1}{\beta_1}\right)$
Case XVIII: $a_1 = a_2 = a, b_1 = b_2 = b, w_1 < 0, r_3 < 0$
$\Gamma(r_2,\alpha_1,\alpha_2,\beta_1,\beta_2)\Gamma\left(\frac{w_2}{b_2}, 2, 1\right) - \frac{(b+w_2)e^{-\frac{w_2}{b}}}{b} S\Gamma(r_2,r_3,\alpha_1,\alpha_2,\beta_1,\beta_2)$
$+\frac{(a-w_1)e^{\frac{w_1}{a}}}{a}\sum_{j=0}^{\alpha_2-1} C_j^* F\left(r_2, r_3, \alpha_2-j, \frac{1}{a}-\frac{1}{\beta_2}\right) + \frac{e^{\frac{w_1}{a}}}{a}\sum_{j=0}^{\alpha_2-1} C_j^* F\left(r_2, r_3, \alpha_2+1-j, \frac{1}{a}-\frac{1}{\beta_2}\right)$

Table 16.11 Joint CDF of $W_1 = Y_1 + Y_2 + a_1 Z_1 + a_2 Z_2$ and $W_2 = b_1 Z_1 - b_2 Z_2$

Case I: $a_1 \neq a_2,\ w_1, w_2 \geq 0,\ r_1 \geq 0$
$\Gamma(r_2, \alpha_1, \alpha_2, \beta_1, \beta_2) - \frac{b_1 e^{-\frac{w_2}{b_1}}}{b_1+b_2} \Gamma(r_1, \alpha_1, \alpha_2, \beta_1, \beta_2)$
$-\frac{a_2 e^{-\frac{w_1}{a_2}}}{a_2-a_1} \sum_{j=0}^{\alpha_2-1} C_j^* F\left(-\infty, 0, \alpha_2 - j, -\frac{1}{a_2} - \frac{1}{\beta_2}\right)$
$-\frac{a_2 e^{-\frac{w_1}{a_2}}}{a_2-a_1} \sum_{j=0}^{\alpha_1-1} C_j F\left(0, r_2, \alpha_1 - j, \frac{1}{\beta_1} - \frac{1}{a_2}\right) + \frac{a_1 e^{-\frac{w_1}{a_1}}}{a_2-a_1} \sum_{j=0}^{\alpha_1-1} C_j F\left(r_1, r_2, \alpha_1 - j, \frac{1}{\beta_1} - \frac{1}{a_1}\right)$
$+\frac{e^{-\frac{(b_1+b_2)w_1+(a_2-a_1)w_2}{a_1 b_2+a_2 b_1}}}{\left(\frac{a_1}{a_2-a_1}+\frac{b_1}{b_1+b_2}\right)^{-1}} \left[\sum_{j=0}^{\alpha_2-1} C_j^* F\left(-\infty, 0, \alpha_2 - j, -\frac{b_1+b_2}{a_1 b_2+a_2 b_1} - \frac{1}{\beta_2}\right)\right.$
$\left.+\sum_{j=0}^{\alpha_1-1} C_j F\left(0, r_1, \alpha_1 - j, \frac{1}{\beta_1} - \frac{b_1+b_2}{a_1 b_2+a_2 b_1}\right)\right]$
Case II: $a_1 \neq a_2,\ w_1, w_2 \geq 0,\ r_1 < 0$
$\Gamma(r_2, \alpha_1, \alpha_2, \beta_1, \beta_2) - \frac{b_1 e^{-\frac{w_2}{b_1}}}{b_1+b_2} \Gamma(r_1, \alpha_1, \alpha_2, \beta_1, \beta_2)$
$-\frac{a_2 e^{-\frac{w_1}{a_2}}}{a_2-a_1} \sum_{j=0}^{\alpha_2-1} C_j^* F\left(-\infty, 0, \alpha_2 - j, -\frac{1}{a_2} - \frac{1}{\beta_2}\right)$
$-\frac{a_2 e^{-\frac{w_1}{a_2}}}{a_2-a_1} \sum_{j=0}^{\alpha_1-1} C_j F\left(0, r_2, \alpha_1 - j, \frac{1}{\beta_1} - \frac{1}{a_2}\right) + \frac{a_1 e^{-\frac{w_1}{a_1}}}{a_2-a_1} \sum_{j=0}^{\alpha_2-1} C_j^* F\left(r_1, 0, \alpha_2 - j, -\frac{1}{a_1} - \frac{1}{\beta_2}\right)$
$+\frac{a_1 e^{-\frac{w_1}{a_1}}}{a_2-a_1} \sum_{j=0}^{\alpha_1-1} C_j F\left(0, r_2, \alpha_1 - j, \frac{1}{\beta_1} - \frac{1}{a_1}\right)$
$+\frac{e^{\frac{(a_1-a_2)w_2-(b_1+b_2)w_1}{a_1 b_2+a_2 b_1}}}{\left(\frac{a_1}{a_2-a_1}+\frac{b_1}{b_1+b_2}\right)^{-1}} \sum_{j=0}^{\alpha_2-1} C_j^* F\left(-\infty, r_1, \alpha_2 - j, -\frac{b_1+b_2}{a_1 b_2+a_2 b_1} - \frac{1}{\beta_2}\right)$
Case III: $a_1 \neq a_2,\ w_1 < 0,\ w_2 > 0$
$\Gamma(r_2, \alpha_1, \alpha_2, \beta_1, \beta_2) - \frac{b_1 e^{-\frac{w_2}{b_1}}}{b_1+b_2} \Gamma(r_1, \alpha_1, \alpha_2, \beta_1, \beta_2)$
$-\frac{a_2 e^{-\frac{w_1}{a_2}}}{a_2-a_1} \sum_{j=0}^{\alpha_2-1} C_j^* F\left(-\infty, r_2, \alpha_2 - j, -\frac{1}{a_2} - \frac{1}{\beta_2}\right)$
$+\frac{a_1 e^{-\frac{w_1}{a_1}}}{a_2-a_1} \sum_{j=0}^{\alpha_2-1} C_j^* F\left(r_1, r_2, \alpha_2 - j, -\frac{1}{a_1} - \frac{1}{\beta_2}\right)$
$+\frac{e^{\frac{(a_1-a_2)w_2-(b_1+b_2)w_1}{a_1 b_2+a_2 b_1}}}{\left(\frac{a_1}{a_2-a_1}+\frac{b_1}{b_1+b_2}\right)^{-1}} \sum_{j=0}^{\alpha_2-1} C_j^* F\left(-\infty, r_1, \alpha_2 - j, -\frac{b_1+b_2}{a_1 b_2+a_2 b_1} - \frac{1}{\beta_2}\right)$

(continued)

Table 16.11 (continued)

Case IV: $a_1 = a_2 = a,\ w_1, w_2 \geq 0,\ r_1 \geq 0$
$-\frac{(ab_2+b_2w_1+aw_2)e^{-\frac{w_1}{a}}}{a(b_1+b_2)} \sum_{j=0}^{\alpha_2-1} C_j^* F\left(-\infty, 0, \alpha_2 - j, -\frac{1}{\beta_2} - \frac{1}{a}\right)$
$-\frac{(ab_2+b_2w_1+aw_2)e^{-\frac{w_1}{a}}}{a(b_1+b_2)} \sum_{j=0}^{\alpha_1-1} C_j F\left(0, r_1, \alpha_1 - j, \frac{1}{\beta_1} - \frac{1}{a}\right)$
$+\frac{b_2 e^{-\frac{w_1}{a}}}{a(b_1+b_2)} \sum_{j=0}^{\alpha_2-1} C_j^* F\left(-\infty, 0, \alpha_2 + 1 - j, -\frac{1}{\beta_2} - \frac{1}{a}\right)$
$+\frac{b_2 e^{-\frac{w_1}{a}}}{a(b_1+b_2)} \sum_{j=0}^{\alpha_1-1} C_j F\left(0, r_1, \alpha_1 + 1 - j, \frac{1}{\beta_1} - \frac{1}{a}\right)$
$+\Gamma(r_2, \alpha_1, \alpha_2, \beta_1, \beta_2) - \frac{b_1}{b_1+b_2} e^{-\frac{w_2}{b_1}} \Gamma(r_1, \alpha_1, \alpha_2, \beta_1, \beta_2)$
$-\frac{(a+w_1)e^{-\frac{w_1}{a}}}{a} \sum_{j=0}^{\alpha_1-1} C_j F\left(r_1, r_2, \alpha_1 - j, \frac{1}{\beta_1} - \frac{1}{a}\right)$
$+\frac{e^{-\frac{w_1}{a}}}{a} \sum_{j=0}^{\alpha_1-1} C_j F\left(r_1, r_2, \alpha_1 + 1 - j, \frac{1}{\beta_1} - \frac{1}{a}\right)$
Case V: $a_1 = a_2 = a,\ w_1, w_2 \geq 0,\ r_1 < 0$
$-\frac{(ab_2+b_2w_1+aw_2)e^{-\frac{w_1}{a}}}{a(b_1+b_2)} \sum_{j=0}^{\alpha_2-1} C_j^* F\left(-\infty, r_1, \alpha_2 - j, -\frac{1}{\beta_2} - \frac{1}{a}\right)$
$+\frac{b_2 e^{-\frac{w_1}{a}}}{a(b_1+b_2)} \sum_{j=0}^{\alpha_2-1} C_j^* F\left(-\infty, r_1, \alpha_2 + 1 - j, -\frac{1}{\beta_2} - \frac{1}{a}\right)$
$+\Gamma(r_2, \alpha_1, \alpha_2, \beta_1, \beta_2) - \frac{b_1}{b_1+b_2} e^{-\frac{w_2}{b_1}} \Gamma(r_1, \alpha_1, \alpha_2, \beta_1, \beta_2)$
$-\frac{(a+w_1)e^{-\frac{w_1}{a}}}{a} \sum_{j=0}^{\alpha_2-1} C_j^* F\left(r_1, 0, \alpha_2 - j, -\frac{1}{\beta_2} - \frac{1}{a}\right)$
$-\frac{(a+w_1)e^{-\frac{w_1}{a}}}{a} \sum_{j=0}^{\alpha_1-1} C_j F\left(0, r_2, \alpha_1 - j, \frac{1}{\beta_1} - \frac{1}{a}\right)$
$+\frac{e^{-\frac{w_1}{a}}}{a} \sum_{j=0}^{\alpha_2-1} C_j^* F\left(r_1, 0, \alpha_2 + 1 - j, -\frac{1}{\beta_2} - \frac{1}{a}\right)$
$+\frac{e^{-\frac{w_1}{a}}}{a} \sum_{j=0}^{\alpha_1-1} C_j F\left(0, r_2, \alpha_1 + 1 - j, \frac{1}{\beta_1} - \frac{1}{a}\right)$

(continued)

Table 16.11 (continued)

Case VI: $a_1 = a_2 = a,\ w_1 < 0,\ w_2 \geq 0$
$-\frac{(ab_2+b_2w_1+aw_2)e^{-\frac{w_1}{a}}}{a(b_1+b_2)} \sum_{j=0}^{\alpha_2-1} C_j^* F\left(-\infty, r_1, \alpha_2 - j, -\frac{1}{\beta_2} - \frac{1}{a}\right)$
$+\frac{b_2e^{-\frac{w_1}{a}}}{a(b_1+b_2)} \sum_{j=0}^{\alpha_2-1} C_j^* F\left(-\infty, r_1, \alpha_2 + 1 - j, -\frac{1}{\beta_2} - \frac{1}{a}\right)$
$+\Gamma(r_2, \alpha_1, \alpha_2, \beta_1, \beta_2) - \frac{b_1}{b_1+b_2} e^{-\frac{w_2}{b_1}} \Gamma(r_1, \alpha_1, \alpha_2, \beta_1, \beta_2)$
$-\frac{(a+w_1)e^{-\frac{w_1}{a}}}{a} \sum_{j=0}^{\alpha_2-1} C_j^* F\left(r_1, r_2, \alpha_2 - j, -\frac{1}{\beta_2} - \frac{1}{a}\right)$
$+\frac{e^{-\frac{w_1}{a}}}{a} \sum_{j=0}^{\alpha_2-1} C_j^* F\left(r_1, r_2, \alpha_2 + 1 - j, -\frac{1}{\beta_2} - \frac{1}{a}\right)$

Table 16.12 Joint CDF of $W_1 = Y_1 + Y_2 + a_1Z_1 - a_2Z_2$ and $W_2 = b_1Z_1 + b_2Z_2$

Case I: $w_1 \geq 0,\ b_1 \neq b_2,\ r_1 \geq 0$
$\frac{b_1e^{-\frac{w_2}{b_1}}}{b_2-b_1} \Gamma\left(r_1, \alpha_1, \beta_1, \alpha_2, \beta_2\right) + \Gamma\left(r_2, \alpha_1, \alpha_2, \beta_1, \beta_2\right) - \frac{b_2e^{-\frac{w_2}{b_2}}}{b_2-b_1} \Gamma\left(r_3, \alpha_1, \alpha_2, \beta_1, \beta_2\right)$
$+\frac{e^{\frac{(b_1-b_2)w_1-(a_1+a_2)w_2}{a_1b_2+a_2b_1}}}{\left(\frac{a_1}{a_1+a_2}+\frac{b_1}{b_2-b_1}\right)^{-1}} \sum_{j=0}^{\alpha_1-1} C_j F\left(r_1, r_3, \alpha_1 - j, \frac{1}{\beta_1} + \frac{b_1-b_2}{a_1b_2+a_2b_1}\right)$
$-\frac{a_1e^{-\frac{w_1}{a_1}}}{a_1+a_2} \sum_{j=0}^{\alpha_1-1} C_j F\left(r_1, r_2, \alpha_1 - j, \frac{1}{\beta_1} - \frac{1}{a_1}\right)$
$+\frac{a_2}{a_1+a_2} e^{\frac{w_1}{a_2}} \sum_{j=0}^{\alpha_1-1} C_j F\left(r_2, r_3, \alpha_1 - j, \frac{1}{\beta_1} + \frac{1}{a_2}\right)$

(continued)

Table 16.12 (continued)

Case II: $w_1 \geq 0, b_1 \neq b_2, r_1 < 0$

$$\frac{b_1 e^{-\frac{w_2}{b_1}}}{b_2-b_1}\Gamma\left(r_1,\alpha_1,\beta_1,\alpha_2,\beta_2\right)+\Gamma\left(r_2,\alpha_1,\alpha_2,\beta_1,\beta_2\right)-\frac{b_2 e^{-\frac{w_2}{b_2}}}{b_2-b_1}\Gamma\left(r_3,\alpha_1,\alpha_2,\beta_1,\beta_2\right)$$

$$+\frac{e^{\frac{(b_1-b_2)w_1-(a_1+a_2)w_2}{a_1b_2+a_2b_1}}}{\left(\frac{a_1}{a_1+a_2}+\frac{b_1}{b_2-b_1}\right)^{-1}}\left[\sum_{j=0}^{\alpha_2-1}C_j^*F\left(r_1,0,\alpha_2-j,-\frac{1}{\beta_2}+\frac{b_1-b_2}{a_1b_2+a_2b_1}\right)\right.$$

$$\left.+\sum_{j=0}^{\alpha_1-1}C_jF\left(0,r_3,\alpha_1-j,\frac{1}{\beta_1}+\frac{b_1-b_2}{a_1b_2+a_2b_1}\right)\right]$$

$$-\frac{a_1e^{-\frac{w_1}{a_1}}}{a_1+a_2}\sum_{j=0}^{\alpha_2-1}C_j^*F\left(r_1,0,\alpha_2-j,-\frac{1}{\beta_2}-\frac{1}{a_1}\right)-\frac{a_1e^{-\frac{w_1}{a_1}}}{a_1+a_2}\sum_{j=0}^{\alpha_1-1}C_jF\left(0,r_2,\alpha_1-j,\frac{1}{\beta_1}-\frac{1}{a_1}\right)$$

$$+\frac{a_2e^{\frac{w_1}{a_2}}}{a_1+a_2}\sum_{j=0}^{\alpha_1-1}C_jF\left(r_2,r_3,\alpha_1-j,\frac{1}{\beta_1}+\frac{1}{a_2}\right)$$

Case III: $w_1 < 0, b_1 \neq b_2, r_3 \geq 0$

$$\frac{b_1 e^{-\frac{w_2}{b_1}}}{b_2-b_1}\Gamma\left(r_1,\alpha_1,\beta_1,\alpha_2,\beta_2\right)+\Gamma\left(r_2,\alpha_1,\alpha_2,\beta_1,\beta_2\right)-\frac{b_2 e^{-\frac{w_2}{b_2}}}{b_2-b_1}\Gamma\left(r_3,\alpha_1,\alpha_2,\beta_1,\beta_2\right)$$

$$+\frac{e^{\frac{(b_1-b_2)w_1-(a_1+a_2)w_2}{a_1b_2+a_2b_1}}}{\left(\frac{a_1}{a_1+a_2}+\frac{b_1}{b_2-b_1}\right)^{-1}}\left[\sum_{j=0}^{\alpha_2-1}C_j^*F\left(r_1,0,\alpha_2-j,-\frac{1}{\beta_2}+\frac{b_1-b_2}{a_1b_2+a_2b_1}\right)\right.$$

$$\left.+\sum_{j=0}^{\alpha_1-1}C_jF\left(0,r_3,\alpha_1-j,\frac{1}{\beta_1}+\frac{b_1-b_2}{a_1b_2+a_2b_1}\right)\right]$$

$$-\frac{a_1e^{-\frac{w_1}{a_1}}}{a_1+a_2}\sum_{j=0}^{\alpha_2-1}C_j^*F\left(r_1,r_2,\alpha_2-j,-\frac{1}{\beta_2}-\frac{1}{a_1}\right)+\frac{a_2e^{\frac{w_1}{a_2}}}{a_1+a_2}\sum_{j=0}^{\alpha_2-1}C_j^*F\left(r_2,0,\alpha_2-j,-\frac{1}{\beta_2}+\frac{1}{a_2}\right)$$

$$+\frac{a_2e^{\frac{w_1}{a_2}}}{a_1+a_2}\sum_{j=0}^{\alpha_1-1}C_jF\left(0,r_3,\alpha_1-j,\frac{1}{\beta_1}+\frac{1}{a_2}\right)$$

Case IV: $w_1 < 0, b_1 \neq b_2, r_3 < 0$

$$\frac{b_1 e^{-\frac{w_2}{b_1}}}{b_2-b_1}\Gamma\left(r_1,\alpha_1,\beta_1,\alpha_2,\beta_2\right)+\Gamma\left(r_2,\alpha_1,\alpha_2,\beta_1,\beta_2\right)-\frac{b_2 e^{-\frac{w_2}{b_2}}}{b_2-b_1}\Gamma\left(r_3,\alpha_1,\alpha_2,\beta_1,\beta_2\right)$$

$$+\frac{e^{\frac{(b_1-b_2)w_1-(a_1+a_2)w_2}{a_1b_2+a_2b_1}}}{\left(\frac{a_1}{a_1+a_2}+\frac{b_1}{b_2-b_1}\right)^{-1}}\sum_{j=0}^{\alpha_2-1}C_j^*F\left(r_1,r_3,\alpha_2-j,-\frac{1}{\beta_2}+\frac{b_1-b_2}{a_1b_2+a_2b_1}\right)$$

$$-\frac{a_1e^{-\frac{w_1}{a_1}}}{a_1+a_2}\sum_{j=0}^{\alpha_2-1}C_j^*F\left(r_1,r_2,\alpha_2-j,-\frac{1}{\beta_2}-\frac{1}{a_1}\right)$$

$$+\frac{a_2e^{\frac{w_1}{a_2}}}{a_1+a_2}\sum_{j=0}^{\alpha_2-1}C_j^*F\left(r_2,r_3,\alpha_2-j,-\frac{1}{\beta_2}+\frac{1}{a_2}\right)$$

(continued)

Table 16.12 (continued)

Case V: $w_1 \ge 0, b_1 = b_2 = b, r_1 \ge 0$
$\Gamma(r_1,\alpha_1,\beta_1,\alpha_2,\beta_2)\left(1-e^{-\frac{w_2}{b}}-\frac{w_2}{b}e^{-\frac{w_2}{b}}\right)-\left(1+\frac{a_2w_2+bw_1}{b(a_1+a_2)}\right)e^{-\frac{w_2}{b}}S\Gamma(r_1,r_3,\alpha_1,\alpha_2,\beta_1,\beta_2)$ $+\frac{e^{-\frac{w_2}{b}}}{a_1+a_2}\sum_{j=0}^{\alpha_1-1}C_jF\left(r_1,r_3,\alpha_1+1-j,\frac{1}{\beta_1}\right)+S\Gamma(r_1,r_2,\alpha_1,\alpha_2,\beta_1,\beta_2)$ $+\frac{a_1e^{\frac{-w_2}{b}}}{a_1+a_2}S\Gamma(r_1,r_3,\alpha_1,\alpha_2,\beta_1,\beta_2)-\frac{a_1e^{-\frac{w_1}{a_1}}}{a_1+a_2}\sum_{j=0}^{\alpha_1-1}C_jF\left(r_1,r_2,\alpha_1-j,\frac{1}{\beta_1}-\frac{1}{a_1}\right)$ $+\frac{a_2e^{\frac{w_1}{a_2}}}{a_1+a_2}\sum_{j=0}^{\alpha_1-1}C_j\left(r_2,r_3,\alpha_1-j,\frac{1}{\beta_1}+\frac{1}{a_2}\right)$
Case VI: $w_1 \ge 0, b_1 = b_2 = b, r_1 < 0$
$\Gamma(r_1,\alpha_1,\beta_1,\alpha_2,\beta_2)\left(1-e^{-\frac{w_2}{b}}-\frac{w_2}{b}e^{-\frac{w_2}{b}}\right)-\left(1+\frac{a_2w_2+bw_1}{b(a_1+a_2)}\right)e^{-\frac{w_2}{b}}S\Gamma(r_1,r_3,\alpha_1,\alpha_2,\beta_1,\beta_2)$ $+\frac{e^{-\frac{w_2}{b}}}{a_1+a_2}\sum_{j=0}^{\alpha_2-1}C_j^*F\left(r_1,0,\alpha_2+1-j,-\frac{1}{\beta_2}\right)+\frac{e^{-\frac{w_2}{b}}}{a_1+a_2}\sum_{j=0}^{\alpha_1-1}C_jF\left(0,r_3,\alpha_1+1-j,\frac{1}{\beta_1}\right)$ $+S\Gamma(r_1,r_2,\alpha_1,\alpha_2,\beta_1,\beta_2)+\frac{a_1e^{\frac{-w_2}{b}}}{a_1+a_2}S\Gamma(r_1,r_3,\alpha_1,\alpha_2,\beta_1,\beta_2)$ $-\frac{a_1e^{-\frac{w_1}{a_1}}}{a_1+a_2}\sum_{j=0}^{\alpha_2-1}C_j^*F\left(r_1,0,\alpha_2-j,-\frac{1}{\beta_2}-\frac{1}{a_1}\right)$ $-\frac{a_1e^{-\frac{w_1}{a_1}}}{a_1+a_2}\sum_{j=0}^{\alpha_1-1}C_jF\left(0,r_2,\alpha_1-j,\frac{1}{\beta_1}-\frac{1}{a_1}\right)+\frac{a_2e^{\frac{w_1}{a_2}}}{a_1+a_2}\sum_{j=0}^{\alpha_1-1}C_j\left(r_2,r_3,\alpha_1-j,\frac{1}{\beta_1}+\frac{1}{a_2}\right)$
Case VII: $w_1 < 0, b_1 = b_2 = b, bw_1 + a_2w_2 \ge 0$
$\Gamma(r_1,\alpha_1,\beta_1,\alpha_2,\beta_2)\left(1-e^{-\frac{w_2}{b}}-\frac{w_2}{b}e^{-\frac{w_2}{b}}\right)-\left(1+\frac{a_2w_2+bw_1}{b(a_1+a_2)}\right)e^{-\frac{w_2}{b}}S\Gamma(r_1,r_3,\alpha_1,\alpha_2,\beta_1,\beta_2)$ $+\frac{e^{-\frac{w_2}{b}}}{a_1+a_2}\sum_{j=0}^{\alpha_2-1}C_j^*F\left(r_1,0,\alpha_2+1-j,-\frac{1}{\beta_2}\right)+\frac{e^{-\frac{w_2}{b}}}{a_1+a_2}\sum_{j=0}^{\alpha_1-1}C_jF\left(0,r_3,\alpha_1+1-j,\frac{1}{\beta_1}\right)$ $+S\Gamma(r_1,r_2,\alpha_1,\alpha_2,\beta_1,\beta_2)+\frac{a_1e^{\frac{-w_2}{b}}}{a_1+a_2}S\Gamma(r_1,r_3,\alpha_1,\alpha_2,\beta_1,\beta_2)$ $-\frac{a_1e^{-\frac{w_1}{a_1}}}{a_1+a_2}\sum_{j=0}^{\alpha_2-1}C_j^*F\left(r_1,r_2,\alpha_2-j,-\frac{1}{\beta_2}-\frac{1}{a_1}\right)+\frac{a_2e^{\frac{w_1}{a_2}}}{a_1+a_2}\sum_{j=0}^{\alpha_2-1}C_j^*\left(r_2,0,\alpha_2-j,-\frac{1}{\beta_2}+\frac{1}{a_2}\right)$ $+\frac{a_2e^{\frac{w_1}{a_2}}}{a_1+a_2}\sum_{j=0}^{\alpha_1-1}C_j\left(0,r_3,\alpha_1-j,\frac{1}{\beta_1}+\frac{1}{a_2}\right)$

(continued)

Table 16.12 (continued)

Case VIII: $w_1 < 0, b_1 = b_2 = b, bw_1 + a_2w_2 < 0$
$\Gamma(r_1, \alpha_1, \beta_1, \alpha_2, \beta_2)\left(1 - e^{-\frac{w_2}{b}} - \frac{w_2}{b}e^{-\frac{w_2}{b}}\right) - \left(1 + \frac{a_2w_2+bw_1}{b(a_1+a_2)}\right)e^{-\frac{w_2}{b}}S\Gamma(r_1, r_3, \alpha_1, \alpha_2, \beta_1, \beta_2)$
$+\frac{e^{-\frac{w_2}{b}}}{a_1+a_2}\sum_{j=0}^{\alpha_2-1} C_j^* F\left(r_1, r_3, \alpha_2 + 1 - j, -\frac{1}{\beta_2}\right) + S\Gamma(r_1, r_2, \alpha_1, \alpha_2, \beta_1, \beta_2)$
$+\frac{a_1e^{\frac{-w_2}{b}}}{a_1+a_2}S\Gamma(r_1, r_3, \alpha_1, \alpha_2, \beta_1, \beta_2) - \frac{a_1e^{-\frac{w_1}{a_1}}}{a_1+a_2}\sum_{j=0}^{\alpha_2-1} C_j^* F\left(r_1, r_2, \alpha_2 - j, -\frac{1}{\beta_2} - \frac{1}{a_1}\right)$
$+\frac{a_2e^{\frac{w_1}{a_2}}}{a_1+a_2}\sum_{j=0}^{\alpha_2-1} C_j^* F\left(r_2, 0, \alpha_2 - j, -\frac{1}{\beta_2} + \frac{1}{a_2}\right)$

Table 16.13 Joint CDF of $W_1 = Y_1 - a_1Z_1 - a_2Z_2$ and $W_2 = b_1Z_1 + b_2Z_2$

Case I: $a_1 \neq a_2, b_1 \neq b_2, a_1b_2 > a_2b_1$
$\Gamma(r_2^*, \alpha, \beta) - \frac{b_2e^{-\frac{w_2}{b_2}}}{b_2-b_1}\Gamma(r_3^*, \alpha_1, \beta_1) + \frac{b_1e^{-\frac{w_2}{b_1}}}{b_2-b_1}\Gamma(r_4^*, \alpha_1, \beta_1) + \frac{a_1e^{\frac{w_1}{a_1}}}{a_1-a_2}C_\Gamma F\left(r_2^*, r_4^*, \alpha_1, \frac{1}{a_1} + \frac{1}{\beta_1}\right)$
$+\frac{e^{\frac{(b_2-b_1)w_1+(a_2-a_1)w_2}{a_1b_2-a_2b_1}}}{\left(\frac{a_1}{a_2-a_1} - \frac{b_1}{b_2-b_1}\right)^{-1}}C_\Gamma F\left(r_3^*, r_4^*, \alpha_1, \frac{1}{\beta_1} + \frac{b_2-b_1}{a_1b_2-a_2b_1}\right) + \frac{a_2e^{\frac{w_1}{a_2}}}{a_2-a_1}C_\Gamma F\left(r_2^*, r_3^*, \alpha_1, \frac{1}{a_2} + \frac{1}{\beta_1}\right)$
Case II: $a_1 \neq a_2, b_1 \neq b_2, a_1b_2 = a_2b_1$
$\Gamma(r_2^*, \alpha_1, \beta_1) + \frac{b_1e^{-\frac{w_2}{b_1}} - b_2e^{-\frac{w_2}{b_2}}}{b_2-b_1}\Gamma(r_3^*, \alpha_1, \beta_1) + \frac{a_1e^{\frac{w_1}{a_1}}}{a_1-a_2}C_\Gamma F\left(r_2^*, r_3^*, \alpha_1, \frac{1}{a_1} + \frac{1}{\beta_1}\right)$
$+\frac{a_2e^{\frac{w_1}{a_2}}}{a_2-a_1}C_\Gamma F\left(r_2^*, r_3^*, \alpha_1, \frac{1}{a_2} + \frac{1}{\beta_1}\right)$
Case III: $a_1 = a_2 = a, b_2 > b_1$
$\Gamma(r_2^*, \alpha_1, \beta_1) - \frac{b_2e^{-\frac{w_2}{b_2}}}{b_2-b_1}\Gamma(r_3^*, \alpha_1, \beta_1)$
$+\frac{b_1e^{-\frac{w_2}{b_1}}}{b_2-b_1}\Gamma(r_4^*, \alpha_1, \beta_1)$
$+\frac{e^{\frac{w_1}{a}}}{a}C_\Gamma F\left(r_2^*, r_3^*, \alpha_1 + 1, \frac{1}{a} + \frac{1}{\beta_1}\right)$
$-\frac{(w_1-a)e^{\frac{w_1}{a}}}{a}C_\Gamma F\left(r_2^*, r_3^*, \alpha_1, \frac{1}{a} + \frac{1}{\beta_1}\right) + \frac{(b_1w_1+aw_2-ab_1)e^{\frac{w_1}{a}}}{a(b_2-b_1)}C_\Gamma F\left(r_3^*, r_4^*, \alpha_1, \frac{1}{a} + \frac{1}{\beta_1}\right)$
$-\frac{b_1e^{\frac{w_1}{a}}}{a(b_2-b_1)}C_\Gamma F\left(r_3^*, r_4^*, \alpha_1 + 1, \frac{1}{a} + \frac{1}{\beta_1}\right)$

(continued)

Table 16.13 (continued)

Case IV: $a_1 > a_2, b_1 = b_2 = b$
$\Gamma(r_2^*, \alpha_1, \beta_1) - \frac{b+w_2}{b} e^{-\frac{w_2}{b}} \Gamma(r_3, \alpha_1, \beta_1) + \frac{a_1 e^{\frac{w_1}{a_1}}}{a_1 - a_2} C_\Gamma F\left(r_2^*, r_4^*, \alpha_1, \frac{1}{a_1} + \frac{1}{\beta_1}\right)$
$+\frac{a_2 e^{\frac{w_1}{a_2}}}{a_2 - a_1} C_\Gamma F\left(r_2^*, r_3^*, \alpha_1, \frac{1}{a_2} + \frac{1}{\beta_1}\right)$
$+\frac{e^{-\frac{w_2}{b}}}{a_1 - a_2} C_\Gamma F\left(r_3^*, r_4^*, \alpha_1 + 1, \frac{1}{\beta_1}\right) - \frac{(a_1 b + a_1 w_2 + b w_1) e^{-\frac{w_2}{b}}}{b(a_1 - a_2)} S\Gamma(r_3^*, r_4^*, \alpha, \beta)$
Case V: $a_1 = a_2 = a, b_1 = b_2 = b$
$\Gamma(r_2^*, \alpha_1, \beta_1) \Gamma\left(\frac{w_2}{b_2}, 2, 1\right) - \frac{(b+w_2) e^{-\frac{w_2}{b}}}{b} S\Gamma(r_2^*, r_3^*, \alpha_1, \beta_1)$
$+\frac{(a-w_1) e^{\frac{w_1}{a}}}{a} C_\Gamma F\left(r_2^*, r_3^*, \alpha_1, \frac{1}{a} + \frac{1}{\beta_1}\right)$
$+\frac{e^{\frac{w_1}{a}}}{a} C_\Gamma F\left(r_2^*, r_3^*, \alpha_1 + 1, \frac{1}{a} + \frac{1}{\beta_1}\right)$

Table 16.14 Joint CDF of $W_1 = Y_1 + a_1 Z_1 + a_2 Z_2$ and $W_2 = b_1 Z_1 - b_2 Z_2$

Case I: $a_1 \neq a_2$
$\Gamma(r_2^*, \alpha_1, \beta_1) - \frac{b_1 e^{-\frac{w_2}{b_1}}}{b_1 + b_2} \Gamma\left(r_1^*, \alpha_1, \beta_1\right) - \frac{a_2 e^{-\frac{w_1}{a_2}}}{a_2 - a_1} C_\Gamma F\left(0, r_2^*, \alpha_1, \frac{1}{\beta_1} - \frac{1}{a_2}\right)$
$+\frac{a_1 e^{-\frac{w_1}{a_1}}}{a_2 - a_1} C_\Gamma F\left(r_1^*, r_2^*, \alpha_1, \frac{1}{\beta_1} - \frac{1}{a_1}\right)$
$+\frac{e^{-\frac{(b_1+b_2) w_1 + (a_2 - a_1) w_2}{a_1 b_2 + a_2 b_1}}}{\left(\frac{a_1}{a_2 - a_1} + \frac{b_1}{b_1 + b_2}\right)^{-1}} C_\Gamma F\left(0, r_1^*, \alpha_1, \frac{1}{\beta_1} - \frac{b_1 + b_2}{a_1 b_2 + a_2 b_1}\right)$
Case II: $a_1 = a_2 = a$
$-\frac{(a b_2 + b_2 w_1 + a w_2) e^{-\frac{w_1}{a}}}{a(b_1 + b_2)} C_\Gamma F\left(0, r_1^*, \alpha_1, \frac{1}{\beta_1} - \frac{1}{a}\right) + \frac{b_2 e^{-\frac{w_1}{a}}}{a(b_1 + b_2)} C_\Gamma F\left(0, r_1^*, \alpha_1 + 1, \frac{1}{\beta_1} - \frac{1}{a}\right)$
$-\frac{b_1 e^{-\frac{w_2}{b_1}}}{b_1 + b_2} \Gamma(r_1^*, \alpha_1, \beta_1)$
$+\Gamma(r_2^*, \alpha, \beta) - \frac{(a+w_1) e^{-\frac{w_1}{a}}}{a} C_\Gamma F\left(r_1^*, r_2^*, \alpha_1, \frac{1}{\beta_1} - \frac{1}{a}\right) + \frac{e^{-\frac{w_1}{a}}}{a} C_\Gamma F\left(r_1^*, r_2^*, \alpha_1 + 1, \frac{1}{\beta_1} - \frac{1}{a}\right)$

Table 16.15 Joint CDF of $W_1 = Y_1 + a_1 Z_1 - a_2 Z_2$ and $W_2 = b_1 Z_1 + b_2 Z_2$

Case I: $b_1 \neq b_2$
$\Gamma\left(r_2^*, \alpha_1, \beta_1\right) - \frac{b_2 e^{-\frac{w_2}{b_2}}}{b_2 - b_1} \Gamma\left(r_3^*, \alpha_1, \beta_1\right) + \frac{b_1 e^{-\frac{w_2}{b_1}}}{b_2 - b_1} \Gamma\left(r_1^*, \alpha_1, \beta_1\right)$
$+ \frac{e^{-\frac{(a_1+a_2)w_2+(b_2-b_1)w_1}{a_1 b_2 + b_1 a_2}}}{\left(\frac{a_1+a_2}{a_1} + \frac{b_1}{b_2-b_1}\right)^{-1}} C_\Gamma F\left(r_1^*, r_3^*, \alpha_1, \frac{1}{\beta_1} + \frac{b_1 - b_2}{a_1 b_2 + b_1 a_2}\right)$
$-\frac{a_1 e^{-\frac{w_1}{a_1}}}{a_1 + a_2} C_\Gamma F\left(r_1^*, r_2^*, \alpha_1, \frac{1}{\beta_1} - \frac{1}{a_1}\right) + \frac{a_1 e^{\frac{w_1}{a_2}}}{a_1 + a_2} C_\Gamma F\left(r_2^*, r_3^*, \alpha_1, \frac{1}{\beta_1} + \frac{1}{a_2}\right)$
Case II: $b_1 = b_2 = b$
$\Gamma\left(r_2^*, \alpha_1, \beta_1\right) - e^{-\frac{w_2}{b}} \Gamma\left(r_3^*, \alpha_1, \beta_1\right) - \frac{w_2}{b} e^{-\frac{w_2}{b}} \Gamma\left(r_1^*, \alpha_1, \beta_1\right)$
$-\frac{a_2 w_2 + b w_1 - a_1 b}{b(a_1 + a_2)} e^{-\frac{w_2}{b}} S\Gamma\left(r_1^*, r_3^*, \alpha_1, \beta_1\right)$
$+\frac{e^{-\frac{w_2}{b}}}{a_1 + a_2} C_\Gamma F\left(r_1^*, r_3^*, \alpha_1 + 1, \frac{1}{\beta_1}\right) - \frac{a_1 e^{-\frac{w_1}{a_1}}}{a_1 + a_2} C_\Gamma F\left(r_1^*, r_2^*, \alpha_1, \frac{1}{\beta_1} - \frac{1}{a_1}\right)$
$+\frac{a_2 e^{\frac{w_1}{a_2}}}{a_1 + a_2} C_\Gamma F\left(r_2^*, r_3^*, \alpha_1, \frac{1}{\beta_1} + \frac{1}{a_2}\right)$

Table 16.16 Joint CDF of $W_1 = Y_1 + Y_2 + a_1 Z_1$ and $W_2 = b_1 Z_1 + b_2 Z_2$

Case I: $b_1 \neq b_2, r_1 \geq 0$
$\Gamma\left(r_2, \alpha_1, \beta_1, \alpha_2, \beta_2\right)\left(1 - \frac{b_2 e^{-\frac{w_2}{b_2}}}{b_2 - b_1}\right) + \frac{b_1 e^{-\frac{w_2}{b_1}}}{b_2 - b_1} \Gamma\left(r_1, \alpha_1, \beta_1, \alpha_2, \beta_2\right)$
$-e^{-\frac{w_1}{a_1}} \sum_{j=0}^{\alpha_1 - 1} C_j F\left(r_1, r_2, \alpha_1 - j, \frac{1}{\beta_1} - \frac{1}{a_1}\right)$
$+\frac{b_2 e^{-\frac{a_1 w_2 + (b_2 - b_1) w_1}{a_1 b_2}}}{b_2 - b_1} \sum_{j=0}^{\alpha_1 - 1} C_j F\left(r_1, r_2, \alpha_1 - j, \frac{1}{\beta_1} + \frac{b_1 - b_2}{a_1 b_2}\right)$
Case II: $b_1 \neq b_2, w_1 > 0, r_1 < 0$
$\Gamma\left(r_2, \alpha_1, \beta_1, \alpha_2, \beta_2\right)\left(1 - \frac{b_2 e^{-\frac{w_2}{b_2}}}{b_2 - b_1}\right) + \frac{b_1 e^{-\frac{w_2}{b_1}}}{b_2 - b_1} \Gamma\left(r_1, \alpha_1, \beta_1, \alpha_2, \beta_2\right)$
$-e^{-\frac{w_1}{a_1}} \sum_{j=0}^{\alpha_1 - 1} C_j F\left(0, r_2, \alpha_1 - j, \frac{1}{\beta_1} - \frac{1}{a_1}\right) - e^{-\frac{w_1}{a_1}} \sum_{j=0}^{\alpha_2 - 1} C_j^* F\left(r_1, 0, \alpha_2 - j, -\frac{1}{\beta_2} - \frac{1}{a_1}\right)$
$-\frac{b_2 e^{-\frac{a_1 w_2 + (b_2 - b_1) w_1}{a b_2}}}{b_1 - b_2} \sum_{j=0}^{\alpha_2 - 1} C_j^* F\left(r_1, 0, \alpha_2 - j, \frac{b_1 - b_2}{a_1 b_2} - \frac{1}{\beta_2}\right)$
$-\frac{b_2}{b_1 - b_2} e^{-\frac{a_1 w_2 + (b_2 - b_1) w_1}{a b_2}} \sum_{j=0}^{\alpha_1 - 1} C_j F\left(0, r_2, \alpha_1 - j, \frac{1}{\beta_1} + \frac{b_1 - b_2}{a_1 b_2}\right)$

(continued)

Table 16.16 (continued)

Case III: $b_1 = b_2 = b, r_1 \geq 0$
$\Gamma(r_1, \alpha_1, \beta_1, \alpha_2, \beta_2)\left(1 - e^{-\frac{w_2}{b}} - \frac{w_2}{b}e^{-\frac{w_2}{b}}\right) + S\Gamma(r_1, r_2, \alpha_1, \alpha_2, \beta_1, \beta_2)\left(1 - \frac{w_1}{a_1}e^{-\frac{w_2}{b}}\right)$ $-e^{-\frac{w_1}{a_1}}\sum_{j=0}^{\alpha_1-1} C_j F\left(r_1, r_2, \alpha_1 - j, \frac{1}{\beta_1} - \frac{1}{a_1}\right) + e^{-\frac{w_2}{b}}\sum_{j=0}^{\alpha_1-1} C_j F\left(r_1, r_2, \alpha_1 + 1 - j, \frac{1}{\beta_1}\right)$
Case IV: $b_1 = b_2 = b, r_1 < 0$
$\Gamma(r_1, \alpha_1, \beta_1, \alpha_2, \beta_2)\left(1 - e^{-\frac{w_2}{b}} - \frac{w_2}{b}e^{-\frac{w_2}{b}}\right) + S\Gamma(r_1, r_2, \alpha_1, \alpha_2, \beta_1, \beta_2)\left(1 - \frac{w_1}{a_1}e^{-\frac{w_2}{b}}\right)$ $-e^{-\frac{w_1}{a_1}}\sum_{j=0}^{\alpha_1-1} C_j F\left(0, r_2, \alpha_1 - j, \frac{1}{\beta_1} - \frac{1}{a}\right) + e^{-\frac{w_2}{b}}\sum_{j=0}^{\alpha_1-1} C_j F\left(0, r_2, \alpha_1 + 1 - j, \frac{1}{\beta_1}\right)$ $-e^{-\frac{w_1}{a_1}}\sum_{j=0}^{\alpha_2-1} C_j^* F\left(r_1, 0, \alpha_2 - j, -\frac{1}{\beta_2} - \frac{1}{a}\right) + e^{-\frac{w_2}{b}}\sum_{j=0}^{\alpha_2-1} C_j F\left(r_1, 0, \alpha_2 + 1 - j, -\frac{1}{\beta_2}\right)$

Table 16.17 Joint CDF of $W_1 = Y_1 + Y_2 + a_1 Z_1$ and $W_2 = b_1 Z_1$

Case I: $r_1 \geq 0$
$\Gamma(r_2, \alpha_1, \alpha_2, \beta_1, \beta_2) - e^{-\frac{w_2}{b_1}}\Gamma(r_1, \alpha_1, \alpha_2, \beta_1, \beta_2) - e^{-\frac{w_1}{a_1}}\sum_{j=0}^{\alpha_1-1} C_j F\left(r_1, r_2, \alpha_1 - j, \frac{1}{\beta_1} - \frac{1}{a_1}\right)$
Case II: $r_1 < 0, w_1 \geq 0$
$\Gamma(r_2, \alpha_1, \alpha_2, \beta_1, \beta_2) - e^{-\frac{w_2}{b_1}}\Gamma(r_1, \alpha_1, \alpha_2, \beta_1, \beta_2) - e^{-\frac{w_1}{a_1}}\sum_{j=0}^{\alpha_2-1} C_j^* F\left(r_1, 0, \alpha_2 - j, -\frac{1}{\beta_2} - \frac{1}{a_1}\right)$ $-e^{-\frac{w_1}{a_1}}\sum_{j=0}^{\alpha_1-1} C_j F\left(0, r_2, \alpha_1 - j, \frac{1}{\beta_1} - \frac{1}{a_1}\right)$
Case III: $w_1 < 0$
$\Gamma(r_2, \alpha_1, \alpha_2, \beta_1, \beta_2) - e^{-\frac{w_2}{b_1}}\Gamma(r_1, \alpha_1, \alpha_2, \beta_1, \beta_2) - e^{-\frac{w_1}{a_1}}\sum_{j=0}^{\alpha_2-1} C_j^* F\left(r_1, r_2, \alpha_2 - j, -\frac{1}{\beta_2} - \frac{1}{a_1}\right)$

Table 16.18 Joint CDF of $W_1 = Y_1 + a_1 Z_1$ and $W_2 = b_1 Z_1 + b_2 Z_2$

Case I: $b_1 \neq b_2$
$\Gamma\left(r_2^*, \alpha_1, \beta_1, \alpha_2, \beta_2\right)\left(1 - \frac{b_2 e^{-\frac{w_2}{b_2}}}{b_2 - b_1}\right) + \frac{b_1 e^{-\frac{w_2}{b_1}}}{b_2 - b_1}\Gamma\left(r_1^*, \alpha_1, \beta_1, \alpha_2, \beta_2\right)$
$-e^{-\frac{w_1}{a_1}} \sum_{j=0}^{\alpha_1 - 1} C_j F\left(r_1^*, r_2^*, \alpha_1 - j, \frac{1}{\beta_1} - \frac{1}{a_1}\right)$
$+\frac{b_2 e^{-\frac{a_1 w_2 + (b_2 - b_1) w_1}{a b_2}}}{b_2 - b_1} \sum_{j=0}^{\alpha_1 - 1} C_j F\left(r_1^*, r_2^*, \alpha_1 - j, \frac{1}{\beta_1} + \frac{b_1 - b_2}{a_1 b_2}\right)$
Case II: $b_1 = b_2 = b$
$\Gamma\left(r_1^*, \alpha_1, \beta_1, \alpha_2, \beta_2\right)\left(1 - e^{-\frac{w_2}{b}} - \frac{w_2}{b} e^{-\frac{w_2}{b}}\right) + S\Gamma\left(r_1^*, r_2^*, \alpha_1, \alpha_2, \beta_1, \beta_2\right)\left(1 - \frac{w_1}{a_1} e^{-\frac{w_2}{b}}\right)$
$-e^{-\frac{w_1}{a_1}} \sum_{j=0}^{\alpha_1 - 1} C_j F\left(r_1^*, r_2^*, \alpha_1 - j, \frac{1}{\beta_1} - \frac{1}{a_1}\right) + e^{-\frac{w_2}{b}} \sum_{j=0}^{\alpha_1 - 1} C_j F\left(r_1^*, r_2^*, \alpha_1 + 1 - j, \frac{1}{\beta_1}\right)$

Table 16.19 Joint CDF of $W_1 = Y_1 - a_1 Z_1$ and $W_2 = b_1 Z_1 + b_2 Z_2$

Case I: $b_1 \neq b_2$
$\Gamma(r_2^*, \alpha_1, \beta_1) - \frac{b_1 e^{-\frac{w_2}{b_1}}}{b_1 - b_2}\Gamma(r_4^*, \alpha_1, \beta_1) + \frac{b_2 e^{-\frac{w_2}{b_2}}}{b_1 - b_2}\Gamma(r_4^*, \alpha_1, \beta_1)$
$+e^{\frac{w_1}{a_1}} \sum_{j=0}^{\alpha_1 - 1} C_j F\left(r_2^*, r_4^*, \alpha_1 - j, \frac{1}{\beta_1} + \frac{1}{a_1}\right)$
$+\frac{b_2}{b_1 - b_2} e^{-\frac{a_1 w_2 + (b_1 - b_2) w_1}{a_1 b_2}} \sum_{j=0}^{\alpha_1 - 1} C_j F\left(r_2^*, r_4^*, \alpha_1 - j, \frac{1}{\beta_1} + \frac{b_2 - b_1}{a_1 b_2}\right)$
Case II: $b_1 = b_2 = b$
$\Gamma(r_2^*, \alpha_1, \beta_1) - \frac{(b + w_2) e^{-\frac{w_2}{b}}}{b}\Gamma(r_4^*, \alpha_1, \beta_1) - \frac{w_1 e^{-\frac{w_2}{b}}}{a_1} S\Gamma(r_2^*, r_4^*, \alpha_1, \beta_1)$
$+e^{\frac{w_1}{a_1}} \sum_{j=0}^{\alpha_1 - 1} C_j F\left(r_2^*, r_4^*, \alpha_1 - j, \frac{1}{\beta_1} + \frac{1}{a_1}\right)$
$+e^{-\frac{w_2}{b}} \sum_{j=0}^{\alpha_1 - 1} C_j F\left(r_2^*, r_4^*, \alpha_1 + 1 - j, \frac{1}{\beta_1}\right)$

Table 16.20 Joint CDF of $W_1 = Y_1 + a_1 Z_1$ and $W_2 = b_1 Z_1$

$\Gamma(r_2^*, \alpha_1, \beta_1) - e^{-\frac{w_2}{b_1}} \Gamma(r_1^*, \alpha_1, \beta_1) - e^{-\frac{w_1}{a_1}} \sum_{j=0}^{\alpha_1 - 1} C_j F\left(r_1^*, r_2^*, \alpha_1 - j, \frac{1}{\beta_1} - \frac{1}{a_1}\right)$

Table 16.21 Joint CDF of $W_1 = Y_1 - a_1 Z_1$ and $W_2 = b_1 Z_1$

$\Gamma(r_2^*, \alpha_1, \beta_1) - e^{-\frac{w_2}{b_1}} \Gamma(r_4^*, \alpha_1, \beta_1) + e^{\frac{w_1}{a_1}} \sum_{j=0}^{\alpha_1 - 1} C_j F\left(r_2^*, r_4^*, \alpha_1 - j, \frac{1}{\beta_1} + \frac{1}{a_1}\right)$

References

1. Arnold, B.C., N. Balakrishnan, and N.H. Nagaraja. 1992. *A first course in order statistics*. New York: Wiley.
2. Bain, L.J., J.A. Eastman, M. Engelhardt, N. Balakrishnan, and C.E. Antle. 1992. Reliability estimation based on MLEs for complete and censored samples. In *Handbook of logistic distribution*, ed. N. Balakrishnan. New York: Marcel Dekker.
3. Bain, L.J., and M. Engelhardt. 1973. Interval estimation for the two-parameter double exponential distribution. *Technometrics* 15: 875–887.
4. Balakrishnan, N., and M.P. Chandramouleeswaran. 1996. Reliability estimation and tolerance limits for Laplace distribution based on censored samples. *Mircoelectronics Reliability* 36: 375–378.
5. Balakrishnan, N., and A.C. Cohen. 1991. *Order statistics and inference: Estimation methods*. Boston: Academic Press.
6. Balakrishnan, N., and C.D. Cutler. 1995. Maximum likelihood estimation of Laplace parameters based on Type-II censored samples. In *Statistical theory and applications: Papers in honor of herbert A. David*, eds.: Nagaraja, H.N.,P.K. Sen, and D.F. Morrison, 45–151. New York: Springer.
7. Balakrishnan, N., and D. Kundu. 2013. Hybrid censoring: Models, inferential results and applications (with discussions). *Computational Statistics & Data Analysis* 57: 166–209.
8. Balakrishnan, N., and X. Zhu. 2016. Exact likelihood-based point and interval estimation for Laplace distribution based on Type-II right censored samples. *Journal of Statistical Computation and Simulation* 86: 29–54.
9. Childs, A., and N. Balakrishnan. 1996. Conditional inference procedures for the Laplace distribution based on Type-II right censored samples. *Statistics & Probability Letters* 31: 31–39.
10. Childs, A., and N. Balakrishnan. 1997. Maximum likelihood estimation of Laplace parameters based on general Type-II censored samples. *Statistical Papers* 38: 343–349.
11. Childs, A., and N. Balakrishnan. 2000. Conditional inference procedures for the Laplace distribution when the observed samples are progressively censored. *Metrika* 52: 253–265.
12. Davis, D. 1952. An analysis of some failure data. *Journal of the American Statistical Association* 47: 113–150.
13. Iliopoulos, G., and N. Balakrishnan. 2011. Exact likelihood inference for Laplace distribution based on Type-II censored samples. *Journal of Statistical Planning and Inference* 141: 1224–1239.
14. Iliopoulos, G., and S.M.T.K. MirMostafaee. 2014. Exact prediction intervals for order statistics from the Laplace distribution based on the maximum-likelihood estimators. *Statistics* 48: 575–592.
15. Johnson, N.L., S. Kotz, and N. Balakrishnan. 1994. *Continuous Univariate distributions*, vol. 1, 2nd ed. New York: Wiley.

16. Johnson, N.L., S. Kotz, and N. Balakrishnan. 1995. *Continuous Univariate Distributions*, vol. 2, 2nd ed. New York: Wiley.
17. Kappenman, R.F. 1975. Conditional confidence intervals for double exponential distribution parameters. *Technometrics* 17: 233–235.
18. Kappenman, R.F. 1977. Tolerance intervals for the double exponential distribution. *Journal of the American Statistical Association* 72: 908–909.
19. Kotz, S., T.J. Kozubowski, and K. Podgorski. 2001. *The laplace distribution and generalizations: A revisit with applications to communications, economics, engineering, and finance*. New York: Wiley.
20. Mann, N.R., and K.W. Fertig. 1973. Tables for obtaining Weibull confidence bounds and tolerance bounds based on best linear invariant estimates of parameters of the extreme-value distribution. *Technometrics* 15: 87–101.
21. Puig, P., and M.A. Stephens. 2000. Tests of fit for the Laplace distribution, with applications. *Technometrics* 42: 417–424.
22. Zhu, X., and N. Balakrishnan. 2016. Exact inference for Laplace quantile, reliability and cumulative hazard functions based on Type-II censored data. *IEEE Transactions on Reliability* 65: 164–178.

Erratum to: Environmental Applications Based on Birnbaum–Saunders Models

Víctor Leiva and Helton Saulo

Erratum to:
Chapter 14 in: A. Adhikari et al. (eds.), *Mathematical and Statistical Applications in Life Sciences and Engineering* https://doi.org/10.1007/978-981-10-5370-2_14

The original version of the book was inadvertently published with incorrect affiliations in Chapter 14

V. Leiva
Avenida Brasil 2241, Valparaíso 2362807, Chile
e-mail: victorleivasanchez@gmail.com

which have been corrected as

V. Leiva
School of Industrial Engineering, Pontificia Universidad católica de Valparaíso, Avenida Brasil 2241, Valparaíso 2362807, Chile
e-mail: victorleivasanchez@gmail.com

The udpated online version of this chapter can be found at
https://doi.org/10.1007/978-981-10-5370-2_14

A. Adhikari et al. (eds.), *Mathematical and Statistical Applications in Life Sciences and Engineering*, https://doi.org/10.1007/978-981-10-5370-2_17

Printed in the United States
By Bookmasters